FUNDAMENTALS OF ORTHOGNATHIC SURGERY AND NON SURGICAL FACIAL AESTHETICS

Third Edition

FUNDAMENTALS OF ORTHOGNATHIC SURGERY AND NON SURGICAL FACIAL AESTHETICS

Third Edition

Editors

Malcolm Harris

Nigel Hunt

University College London, UK

World Scientific

NEW JERSEY • LONDON • SINGAPORE • BEIJING • SHANGHAI • HONG KONG • TAIPEI • CHENNAI • TOKYO

Published by

World Scientific Publishing Co. Pte. Ltd.
5 Toh Tuck Link, Singapore 596224
USA office: 27 Warren Street, Suite 401-402, Hackensack, NJ 07601
UK office: 57 Shelton Street, Covent Garden, London WC2H 9HE

Library of Congress Cataloging-in-Publication Data
Names: Harris, Malcolm, 1934– editor. | Hunt, Nigel, Ph. D., editor.
Title: Fundamentals of orthognathic surgery and non surgical facial aesthetics / edited by Malcolm Harris & Nigel Hunt.
Other titles: Fundamentals of orthognathic surgery
Description: 3rd edition. | New Jersey : World Scientific, 2018. | Preceded by Fundamentals of orthognathic surgery / editors, Malcolm Harris, Nigel Hunt. 2nd ed. c2008. | Includes bibliographical references and index.
Identifiers: LCCN 2018025846 | ISBN 9789813221833 (hardcover : alk. paper)
Subjects: | MESH: Maxillofacial Abnormalities--surgery | Oral Surgical Procedures--methods | Orthodontics--methods
Classification: LCC RK529 | NLM WU 600 | DDC 617.6/43--dc23
LC record available at https://lccn.loc.gov/2018025846

British Library Cataloguing-in-Publication Data
A catalogue record for this book is available from the British Library.

For any available supplementary material, please visit
https://www.worldscientific.com/worldscibooks/10.1142/10485#t=suppl

Typeset by Stallion Press
Email: enquiries@stallionpress.com

Contributors

Peter Ayliffe

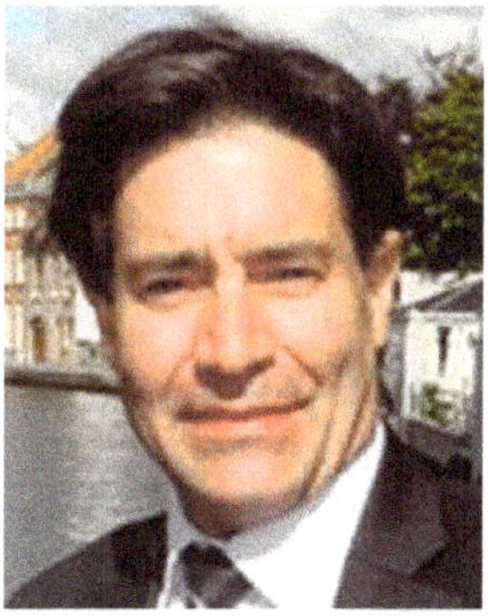

FDRCS, FRCS (OMFS)
Consultant Oral and Maxillofacial Surgeon
Great Ormond Street Hospital for Children and University College London Hospital
Honorary Senior Lecturer
Eastman Dental Institute and Institute of Child Health, University College London, UK
peter.ayliffe@ucl.ac.uk (p.ayliffe@live.co.uk)

Mohammad Anwar Bamber

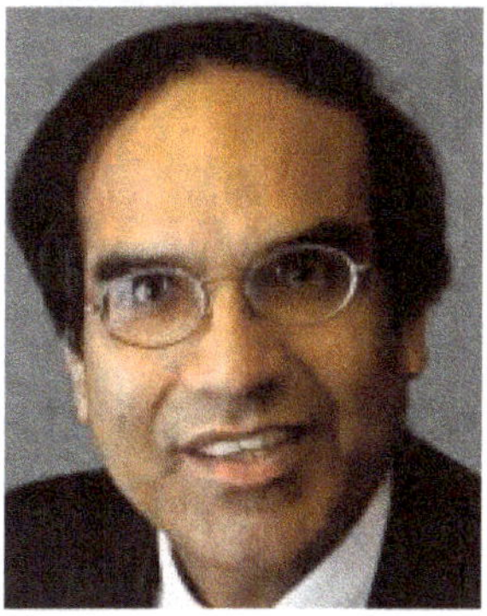

PhD, BA, MSSCh, FIMPT, MBRCP, LFHom, ILTM
Retired Senior Maxillofacial Instructor
Department of Oral and Maxillofacial Surgery,
Eastman Dental Institute,
University College London, UK
bambermn@gmail.com
(ma161@hotmail.co.uk)

Tara Brantley

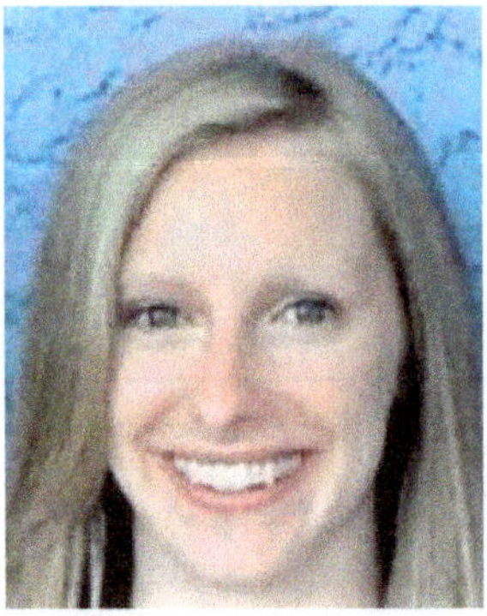

DMD. BSc
Oral and Maxillofacial Surgery Resident
University of California,
San Francisco, USA
tara.brantley@ucsf.edu

Kieran Coghlan

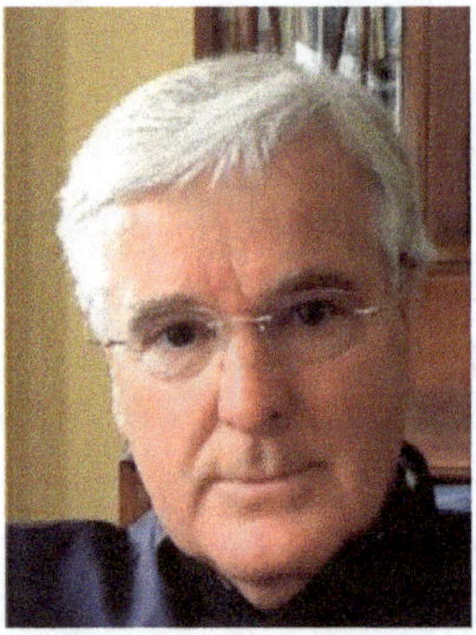

MB, BCh, BDS, FRCS (Edin), FFD, RCSI
Consultant Oral and Maxillofacial Surgeon
Princess Alexandra Hospital NHS Trust, Harlow
Honorary Consultant, Barts & the London, NHS Trust London, UK
kierancoghlan@doctors.org.uk

Susan J. Cunningham

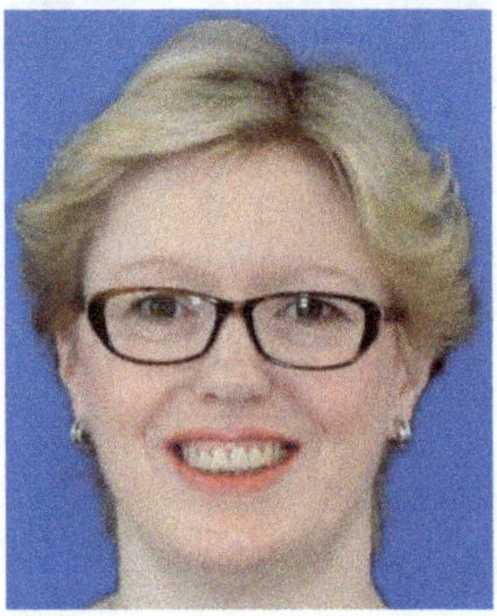

PhD, MSc, BChD, FDS RCS (Eng), MOrth RCS, FDS (Orth) RCS
Professor and Honorary Consultant
Unit of Orthodontics: Eastman Dental Institute, University College London and UCLH NHS Foundation Trust, UK
s.cunningham.ucl.ac.uk

Dan Harris

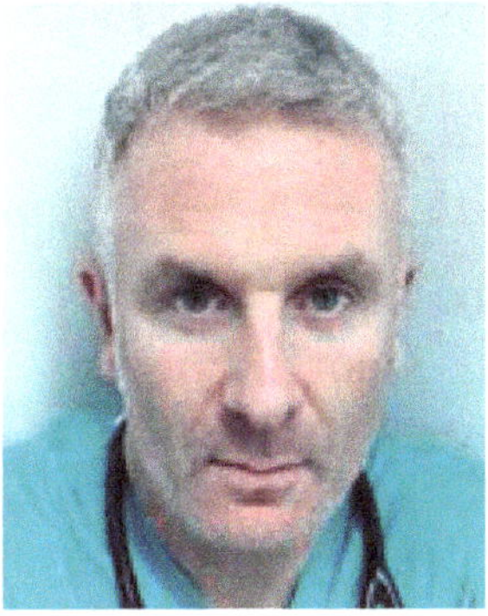

FCEM, MBBS, BSc, MRCS
Consultant Accident and Emergency Physician
Clinical Associate: Emergency Care Improvement Programme, UK
dndanharris71@gmail.com

Malcolm Harris

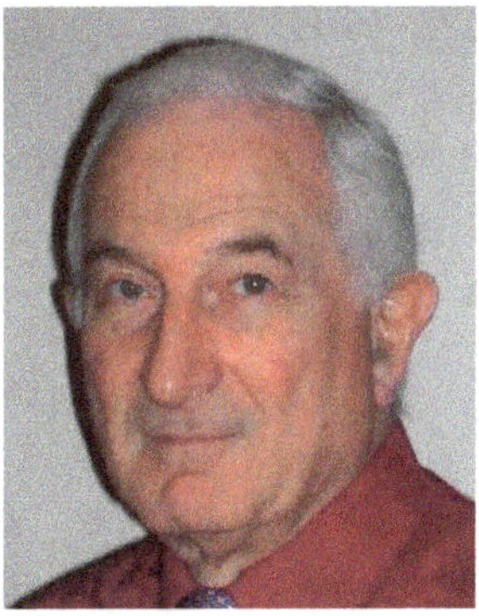

DSc, MD, FRCS (Edin), FDSRCS
Emeritus Professor: Oral and Maxillofacial Surgery
University College London, UK
malcolm.harrise@ucl.ac.uk

Rui Ming Ho

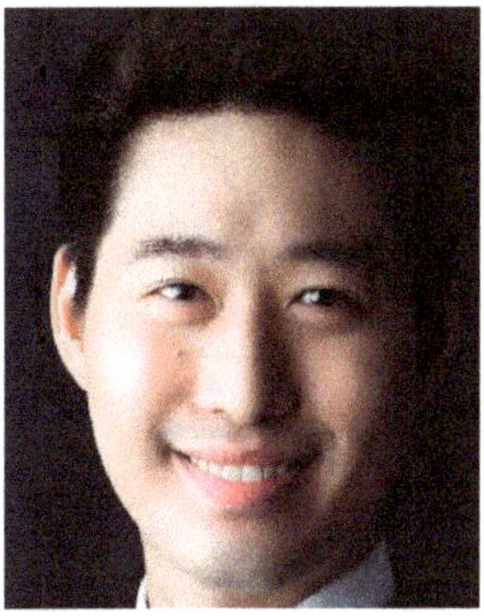

MBBS (Monash University, Australia)
MSc Clinical Dermatology (King's College London, UK)
Dip. Aesthetic Medicine (American Academy of Aesthetic Medicine)
Physician Non Surgical Facial Aesthetics
Director of Chrysalis Medical Aesthetics Clinic Singapore
ruimingho@hotmail.com/gmail.com

Nigel Hunt

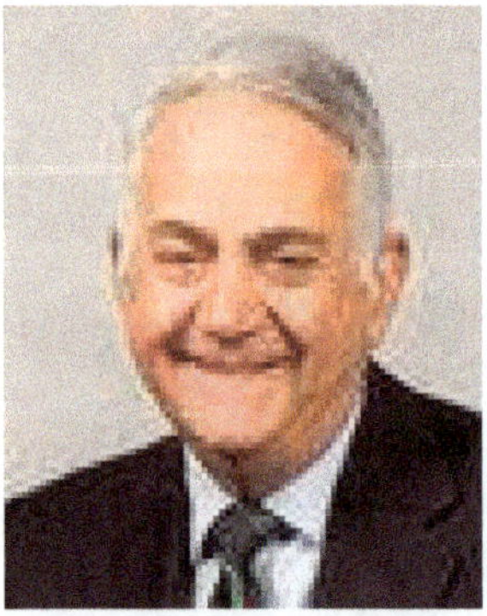

OBE, PhD, MSc, BDS, FDS RCS (Eng), FDS RCS (Ed), FDS RCPS, DOrth, MOrth RCS
Chairman of Division of Craniofacial and Developmental Sciences
Head of Unit of Orthodontics. Eastman Dental Institute, University College London, UK
n.hunt@ucl.ac.uk

Sabah Kalamchi

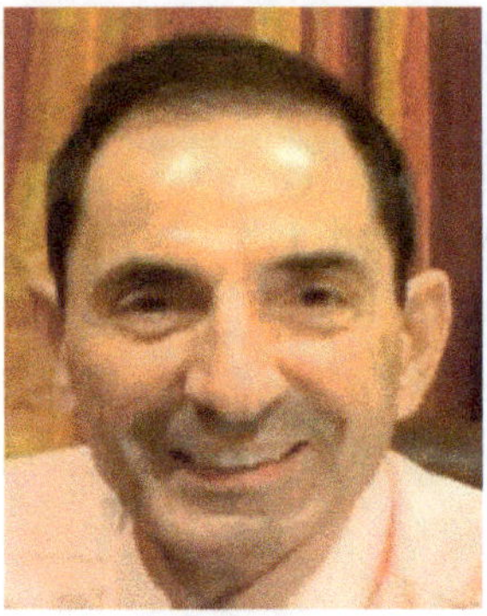

BDS., LDSRCS., DDS. FFD. RCS
Professor and Director
Oral & Maxillofacial Surgery Department, Arizona School of Dentistry & Oral Health
Mesa, Arizona, USA
skalamchi@atsu.edu

Fooi Chin NG

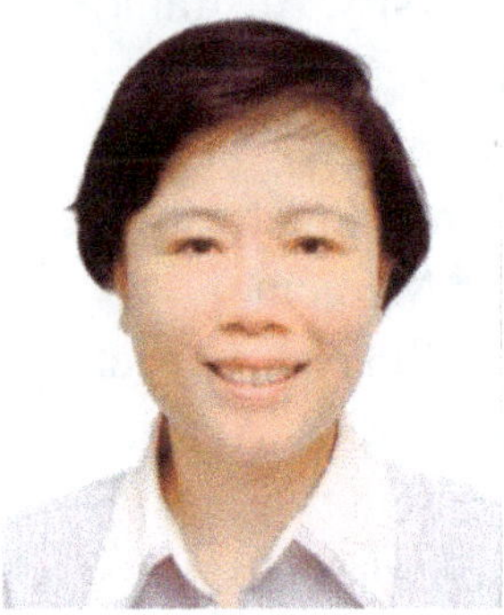

BDS (Singapore), MDS (Oral Maxillofacial Surgery), FDSRCS (England)
Oral & Maxillofacial Surgeon
Coden Specialists, Paragon Medical Centre,
Singapore
nfc@codenspecialists.com

Santdeep H. Paun

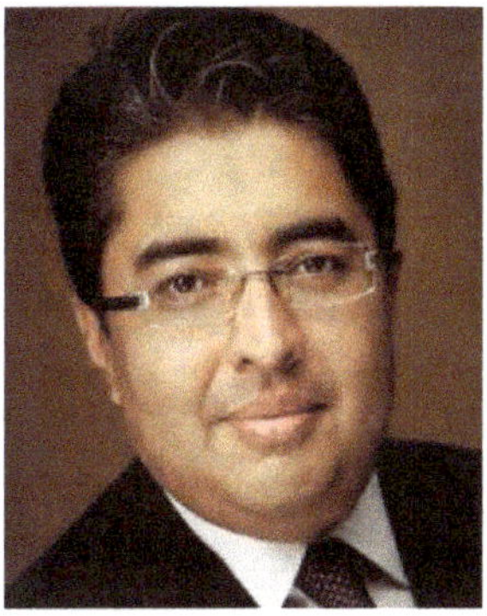

FRCS (ORL-HNS)
Consultant Rhinologist and Facial Plastic Surgeon
Barts and the London Hospital Trust, London, UK
mail@spaun.co.uk [spaun@me.com]

Edwin Payne

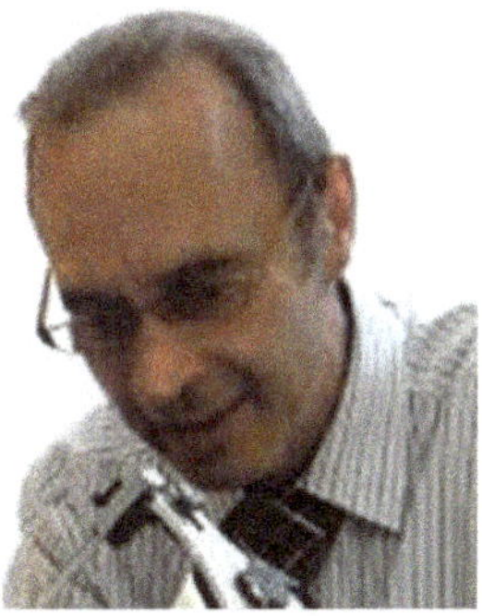

Chief Technical Instructor
Division of Craniofacial Developmental Sciences
Eastman Dental Institute, University College London, UK

Paul M. Thomas

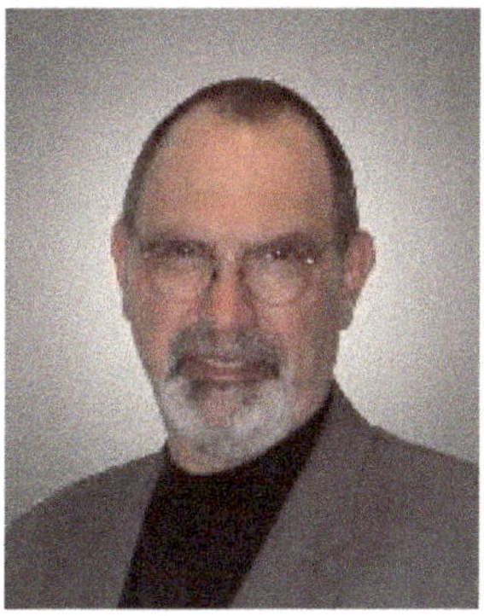

DMD, MS, FDS [RCS Ed]
Adjunct Professor, Department of Orthodontics,
UNC School of Dentistry, Chapel Hill, North Carolina, USA
Former Senior Research Fellow:
Eastman Dental Institute, University College London, UK
p.thomas@earthlink.net
(p.thomas@dolphinimaging.com)

Mr Tom W M Walker

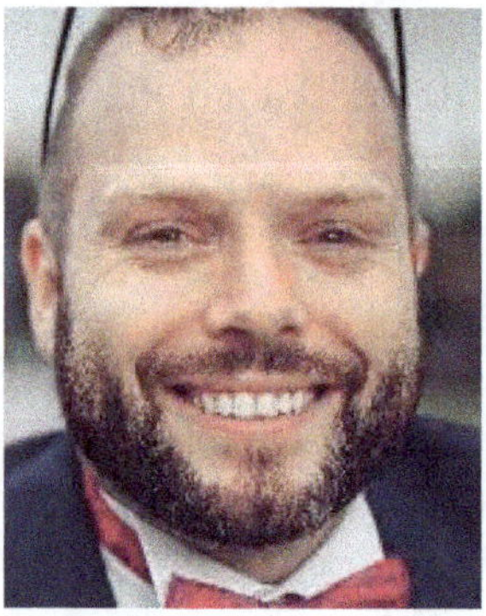

MBChB BDS DOHNS(RCSEd) MRCSI MFDRCSI AKC
Specialist Registrar & Honorary Clinical Lecturer
Department of Oral & Maxillofacial Surgery
Bristol Royal Infirmary
Children's Hospital & Dental School
University Hospitals Bristol NHS Foundation Trust
Bristol, UK
tom.walker@bristol.ac.uk

Preface and Acknowledgements

The first edition of the "Fundamentals" was published in 1991 by Malcolm Harris and Ian Reynolds shortly after Ian's untimely death and is now coedited for the second time by Nigel Hunt. This 3rd Edition of the "Fundamentals of Orthognathic Surgery has been substantially extended with completely new chapters covering Non Surgical Facial Aesthetics by Rui Ming Ho and Fooi Chin Ng and the application of Cone Beam Computer Scanning for Surgical Planning which was created by Paul Thomas and Sabah Kalamchi with the advice of Tarik Kramcha, a Biomedical Engineer of Healthcare 3D Systems. Although Computer Assisted Surgical Simulation (CASS) may supersede the traditional multi-stage manual orthognathic planning process, this means of record transfer by Mohammad Anwar Bamber and Ed Payne has been retained as an essential clinical skill.

Both fresh disciplines have made the "Fundamentals" an up-to-date operative manual for surgical and orthodontic consultants, their trainees as well as theatre and ward staff.

The important major deformity sections are still the Secondary Management of Clefts by Peter Ayliffe and Tom Walker, the Role of Distraction Osteogenesis by Kieran Coghlan, Rhinoplasty by Santdeep Paun and Temporomandibular Joint Ankylosis*. The invaluable knowledge of nutrition for the Maxillofacial Surgery patient is by Tara Brantley and Sabah Kalamchi. Susan Cunningham has refined her essential chapter "The Psychosocial Aspects of Facial Deformity" to reconfirm the crucial borderland between the psyche and cosmesis, and warn how the unstable patient can create unexpected problems for the clinician.

The chapter on Emergencies and Complications has been modernised by Dan Harris, and Gemma Harris provided the digital rescue service. The illustration for the cover was produced by Paul Thomas. Many of the drawings from the original text have been retained and were by Mohamed Nour Awang, David Banks, Helen McParland, Daljit S. Gill and Cristina Nacher. There are no references as very few clinicians consult an ever changing scene which is readily available through Google Chrome or Pubmed etc.

Nigel and I must express our gratitude for the continued patience and inspiration of our wives Susan and Naomi and are also grateful to Joy Quek of World Scientific Press for her generous support.

With our best regards to all readers, Malcolm Harris* and Nigel Hunt.

Contents

Chapter 1

General Assessment

Malcolm Harris and Nigel Hunt

Introduction

The overall management of a patient with facial deformity requiring orthognathic surgery is both an art and a science. The management must be based on a team approach. Whilst the team may vary according to local circumstances, the optimum would consist of an orthodontist, an oral and maxillofacial surgeon, a liaison psychiatrist or clinical psychologist, a specialist in restorative dentistry, supported by a maxillofacial technician. A speech therapist is essential for cleft cases and plastic surgery expertise should also be available on an individual patient basis. Whilst a patient may be referred to any of the above specialists, it is important that all patients follow an agreed care pathway to ensure patient satisfaction with the outcome. It is imperative that as part of the initial consultation, patients are encouraged to state precisely what aspects of their facial features or dentition they would like corrected, for what reason and the length of time that they have sought treatment. Whilst the patient can be guided to what constitutes an ideal facial appearance, it is vital that the clinician does not lose sight of the patient's underlying concerns.

The motivation behind the request for treatment is very important and special consideration is required when psychological factors appear to influence both the diagnosis and the treatment.

The combined orthodontic and surgical treatment goals are:

- Improve facial aesthetics
- Improve dental aesthetics
- A functional, balanced and stable occlusion
- A satisfied patient.

The management protocol for facial deformity should comprise the:

- History
- Clinical examination
- Investigations
- Initial diagnosis
- Treatment plan
- Presurgical orthodontics
- Final treatment plan
- Surgery
- Postsurgical orthodontics
- When appropriate, restorative dentistry, psychological intervention or support and speech therapy will be required.

History

The purpose of the history is to identify the patient's orofacial problems and their cause. This may be a family trait, congenital deformity, or the result of trauma in infancy or adolescence. It is useful to ask the patient to draw up a problem list in order of priority of the specific features they wish to have corrected and for the clinician to note where the drive for treatment has arisen. For example, a patient may complain of having a prominent chin, which they have noticed ever since adolescence and for which they have frequently requested treatment through the general dental practitioner. This differs from the sudden desire to change minimal deformity as a response to a personal crisis. The long term success in terms of patient satisfaction is far better when driven by the patient than that of a patient seeking surgery driven by a parent, partner or close relative. Many orthognathic procedures have a secondary effect on other aspects of facial appearance. For example, correction of a "gummy smile" with a maxillary impaction will also increase the fullness of the cheeks over the malar region and widen the alar width of the nose It is important to inform the patient of these changes. The overall treatment goals must be to improve facial and dental aesthetics, and to provide a functional and stable occlusion but with the underlying premise that these satisfy the patient's reasonable wishes.

The Medical History

Most orthognathic patients are young and fit to undergo a general anaesthetic and prolonged surgery. Occasional disorders, which require specific attention include:

i) haemophilia or similar clotting disorders which require pre- and intraoperative correction
ii) acromegaly patients may be a cardiomyopathy risk
iii) antibiotic or analgesic idiosyncrasy or allergy
iv) rheumatic or congenital heart valve lesions
v) obstructive sleep apnoea should warrant a sleep study and specific assessment.

Body Dysmorphic Disorder (Formerly Dysmorphophobia)

A small but significant proportion of patients may present with varying degrees of concern about one or more aspects of their facial appearance without appropriate clinical signs. This may be a manifestation of the psychiatric disturbance now called the Body Dysmorphic Disorder (formerly dysmorphophobia). This condition will create problems in surgical management as the patient is often dissatisfied with the final result. The condition invariably raises the conflict as to whether one does,

i) what the patient wants
ii) what the patient needs
iii) or nothing.

It is therefore worth consideration in some detail. See Chapter 16.

Evaluation of the Patient

Patient Evaluation

- Clinical examination
- Radiographic examination and if necessary a Cone Beam Computer Tomographic (CBCT) scan
- Analysis of study models
- Psychological examination where appropriate.

Introduction

The full examination must include the basic scrutiny of the patient, radiographs, cephalometry and study casts. The evaluation should begin with a systematic examination of the patient's facial features from the frontal perspective (vertical proportions) and the lateral profile (horizontal relations). It is important to consider the vertical facial proportions and their balance in relation to the patient's general build, and personality. Examples of patients who may not need surgery are: (i) a young female patient who possesses a vivacious and extrovert personality suited to a mild Class II malocclusion accompanied by a broad smile and marked incisor exposure and (ii) similarly, a well-built male may be suited to a mild Class III malocclusion with a minor degree of mandibular prognathism. It is also important to take into consideration the overall facial shape, as there is extreme variation from a square shaped facial appearance to one of a long ovoid appearance. In the former case this may fit in well with a shorter stature whereas a longer face may be more suited to a tall individual. At the moment these decisions are based on experience and intuition.

Clinical Examination

The clinical examination should be undertaken with the patient comfortably seated with the Frankfort plane horizontal. Not only is it easy to visualise a line running from the inferior orbital margin to the upper end of the tragal cartilage, but this can be readily compared with the same horizontal plane on the lateral skull radiograph (cephalogram) and photographs.

Frontal Assessment

There are several important facial features to note. These include:

a) *The facial proportions*
The useful classic guide is to consider the face as having three equal vertical components (Figure 1.1): The distance from the hairline to the soft tissue bridge of the nose; from the soft tissue bridge of the nose to the alar base and from the alar base to the lower border of the chin. It is also important to determine whether or not there is a relative excess or deficiency in the vertical height of either the maxillary or mandibular thirds.

b) *The alar base width*
Traditionally in a westernised population it is accepted that the alar base width, as measured from the lateral aspects of the alar cartilages of the nose, should be approximately equal to the distance between the inner canthi of the eyes (Figure 1.2). This measurement has importance when planning a maxillary impaction.

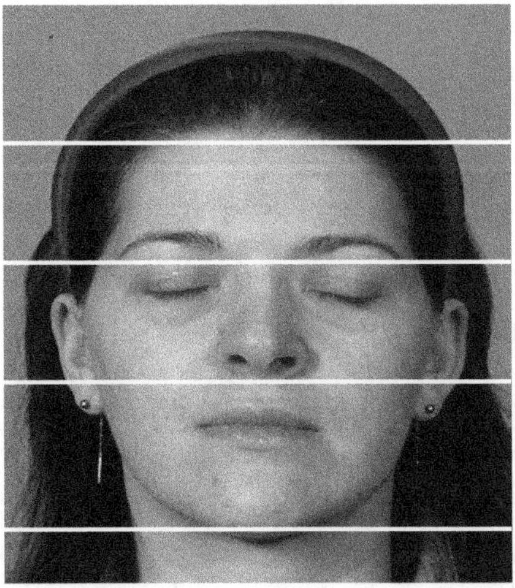

Figure 1.1 The superficial aesthetic proportions of the face can be divided into equal thirds. However the underlying cephalometric proportions of the upper to the lower facial height are 45:55 (see Figure 2.3).

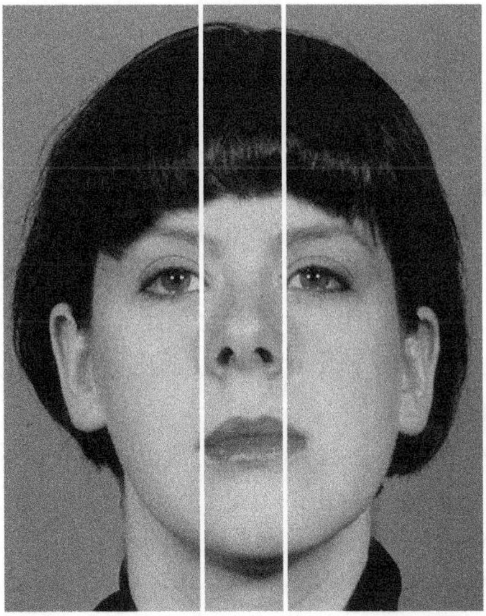

Figure 1.2 The alar base width should approximate the inner intercanthal distance.

c) *Incisor exposure* (*the lip — incisor relationship*)
For a patient with an average upper lip length of 20–25 mm, the standard exposure for orthognathic planning of the upper labial segment with the lips parted at rest should be 2–4 mm of the incisor crown. On smiling, the exposure should increase to the level of the gingival margin of the upper labial segment. This assessment is crucial when planning the vertical height of the mid face where the amount of incisor exposure should be inversely proportional to the length of the upper lip (Figure 1.3). Where the upper lip length is very short then the patient would expect to show more of the upper incisors. Any attempt to reduce the incisor exposure in relation to a short upper lip will lead to an unaesthetic reduced middle face height. Similarly, with a long upper lip, the patient would be expected to show less or no upper incisor, both at rest and during facial animation. The lip incisor measurement should be undertaken with the face at rest. Animation especially smiling will enhance the face and make planning difficult.

The harmony between the components of the lower third of the face is also important, in that the subnasale to the upper lip vermillion border should be a third of the total (i.e. half of the lower lip vermillion border to the soft tissue menton). In those cases where the lower third of the face appears overclosed, it is wise to re-evaluate both the upper lip length and the incisor exposure with the mouth open so that the lips are taken just out of contact.

d) *Facial asymmetry and centre line relationships*
It is important to note any asymmetry of the middle or lower third of the face, including the position and levels of the eyes. This may be facilitated by marking the midlines on the patient's face and also by analysing a clinical photograph or surface laser scan.

The patient's maxillary and mandibular dental midlines may not be coincident nor match their skeletal midlines (Figure 1.4).

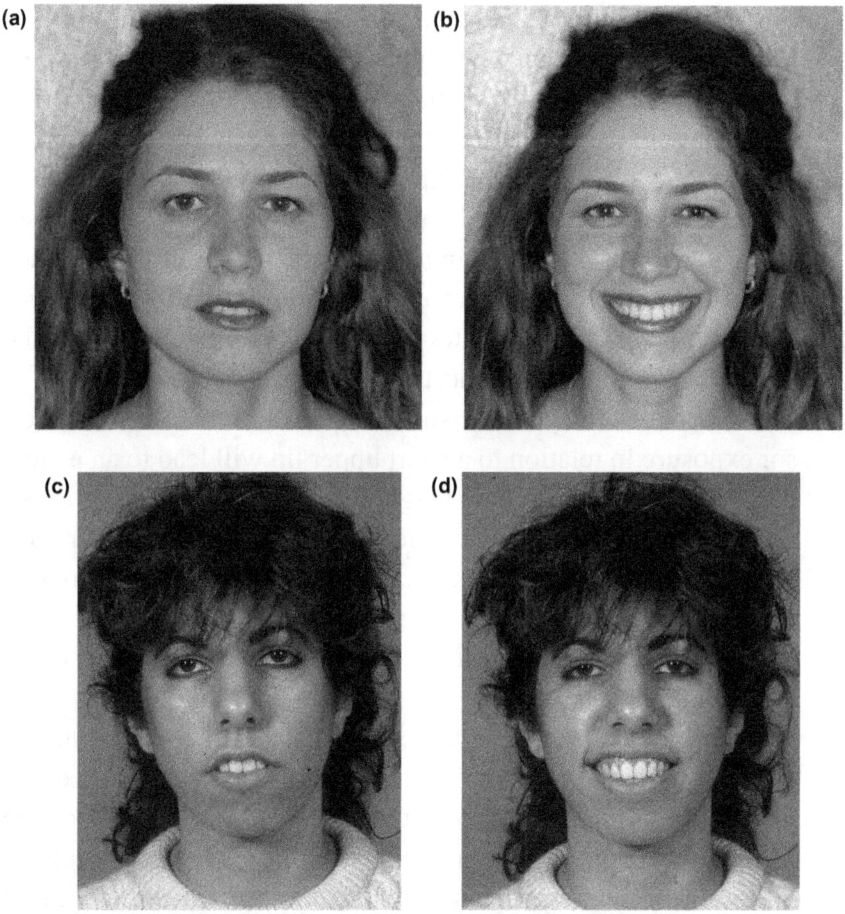

Figure 1.3 With an average upper lip length, a useful aesthetic proportion is (**a**) 2–4 mms of maxillary incisor crown visible with the lips apart at rest. (**b**) This increases to the level of the gingival margin on smiling. (**c**) Here the excess incisor exposure of vertical maxillary excess at rest is important for the estimation of the required vertical impaction. (**d**) The aesthetic animated face makes this estimation difficult.

Generally where the maxillary dental midline is displaced to one side of the skeletal midline, there is an indication for orthodontic correction rather than attempting to rotate the maxilla in order to produce a dental midline coincident with the midface. Where a mandibular dental midline discrepancy is noted in

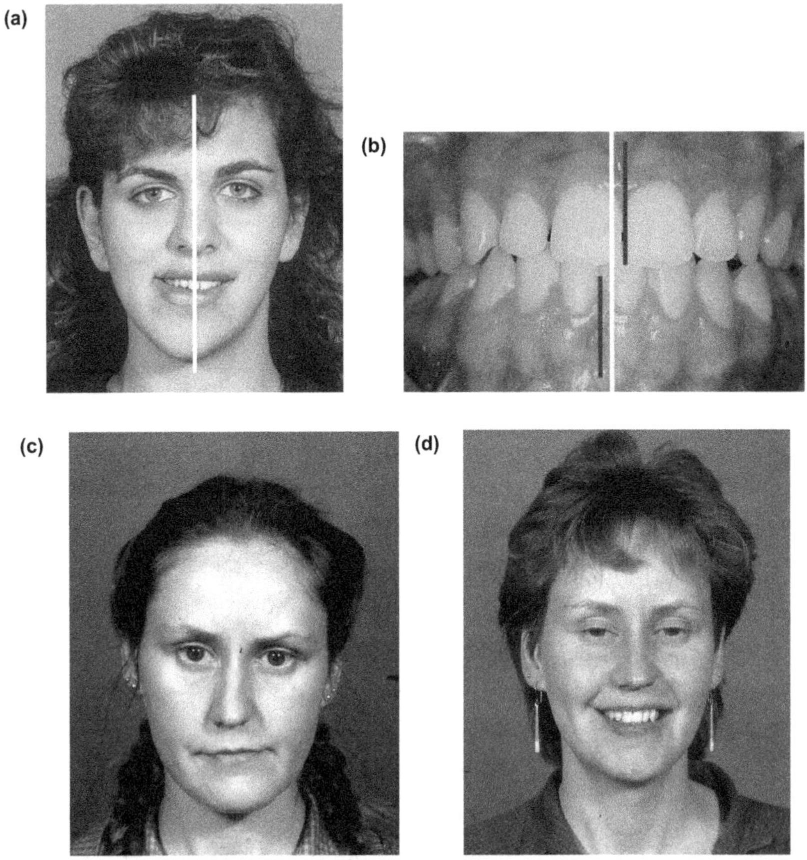

Figure 1.4 (**a**) The facial asymmetry of a left-sided hemimandibular elongation with the chin point displaced to the right. The lower dental midline mirrors the mandibular skeletal asymmetry and will be corrected as part of the surgery. (**b**) The maxillary dental midline is displaced to the left of a symmetrical maxilla and therefore should be corrected as part of the orthodontic preparation of the case. (**c**) Postural camouflage showing tilting of the head to level the lip line, in an asymmetrical face can give a false impression of orbital dystopia. (**d**) Levelling the occlusal plane with bimaxillary osteotomies also "levels" the eyes!

relation to the upper midline, it is important to determine whether it is coincident with a mandibular skeletal asymmetry or of purely dental origin. Where the skeletal asymmetry and dental midlines coincide the centre lines will be corrected as part of the surgical procedure.

Postural camouflage can be a problem with the asymmetrical face as shown in Figures 1.4c and 1.4d. This patient with a marked occlusal cant habitually tilted her head to level the lip line which gave the impression of orbital dystopia. This was corrected by bimaxillary levelling of the occlusal plane.

Profile Assessment

As with frontal evaluation it is important to work down the profile from above to observe key features.

a) *Relative protrusion of the maxilla and mandible*
The relations of the maxilla and mandible to each other and to the skull base will be discussed in greater detail in Chapter 2. It is common for patients to complain of a protruding chin, whereas it is the relationship of the maxilla to the skull base which is at fault, i.e. a hypoplastic maxilla related to a normal mandible. This can be clinically demonstrated by simply padding out the upper lip with soft wax or cotton wool (Figure 1.5) until the lip relationship and facial profile appear normal. Similarly, the surgical correction of a retrognathic mandible may be visualised by asking the patient to slide the mandible forwards (Figure 1.6). Most orthognathic cases require a combination of both maxillary and mandibular surgery and an assessment of the protrusion of the mid third and mandible can be made by assessing their position relative to the coronal facial plane which divides the head into dorsal and ventral (posterior and anterior) portions and passes downwards through the nasion (Figure 1.8). With normal facial proportions the soft tissue profile of the maxilla should be approximately 2–3 mm in front, and the soft tissue pogonion should lie 2 mm behind this facial plane (Figure 1.7). However the face will vary with ethnic norms, giving anterognathic, mesognathic or posterognathic profiles (Figure 1.8b).

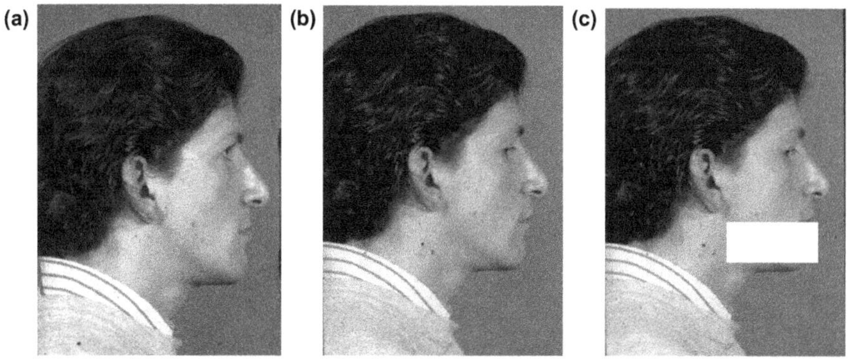

Figure 1.5 (**a**) Apparent mandibular prognathism. (**b**) Padding the upper lip suggests a maxillary advancement will harmonise the profile and maintain a "strong chin". (**c**) Masking the mandible facilitates judging the mid face.

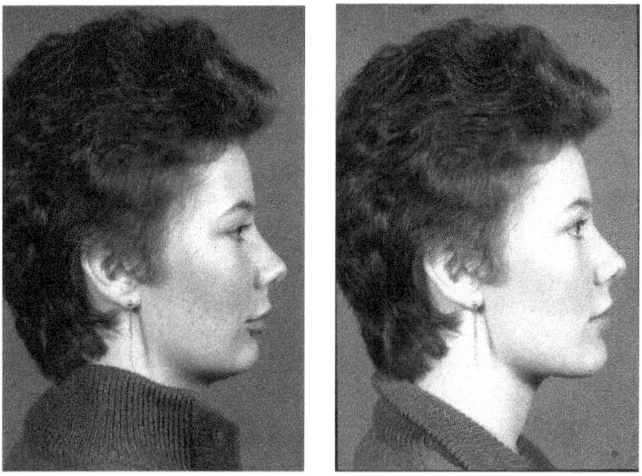

Figure 1.6 Forward posturing of the mandible will help to visualize the horizontal and vertical effects of a mandibular advancement to correct a marked Class II deformity.

b) *Position of the infra-orbital margin*

A good indicator of middle third hypoplasia arises from the relative protrusion of the maximum convexity of the globe of

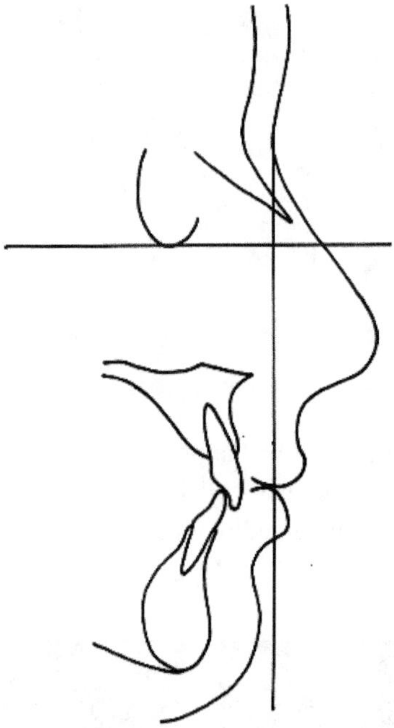

Figure 1.7 The relative projection of the maxilla and mandible can be assessed by the coronal facial plane which is perpendicular to the Frankfort plane passing downwards from the soft tissue nasion. With "normal facial proportions" the soft tissue profile of the maxilla should be 2–3 mm in front of the line and that of the mandible 2–3 mm behind.

the eye in relation to the infra-orbital margin. Ideally the globe should be just 2–3 mm in advance of the infra-orbital margin (Figure 1.9).

c) *Nasal morphology*
The appearance of the nose will often change both relatively and anatomically with many osteotomies. For instance, an apparent large nose may appear more acceptable following a bimaxillary correction (Figure 1.10) due to the change in the adjacent soft tissue drape. Alternatively, a Le Fort I maxillary advancement and/or impaction will tend to raise the nasal tip and straighten a nasal hump unless modifications to the surgical procedure are

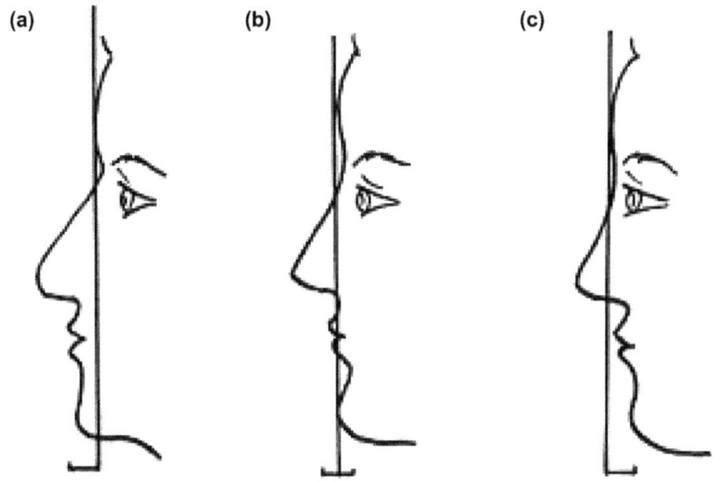

Figure 1.8 The "normal profile" can vary with concepts of beauty and ethnic variation as is seen above showing: (**a**) the anterognathic, (**b**) mesognathic, and (**c**) posterognathic norms.

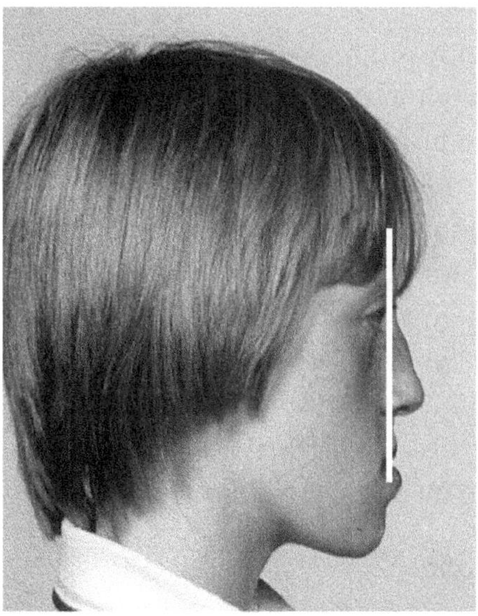

Figure 1.9 A patient with midface hypoplasia. Note the retruded infra-orbital margin relative to the globe of the eye. The globe should only be 2–3 mm in front of the orbital margin.

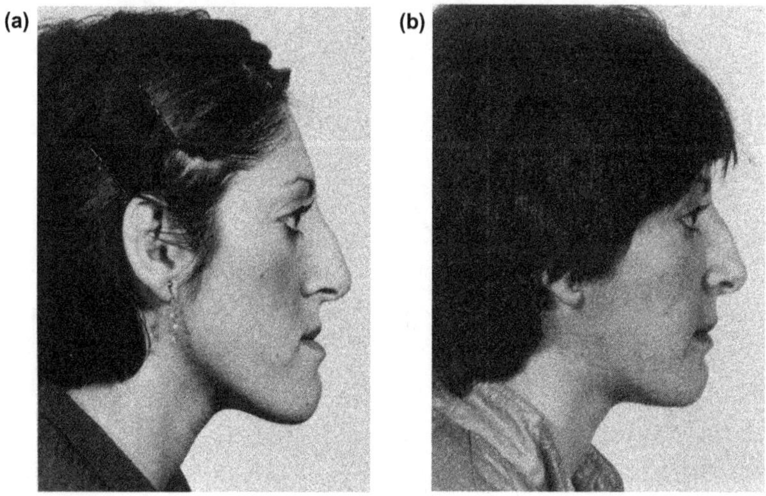

Figure 1.10 (**a**) The relative prominence of the nose seen preoperatively is diminished with a bimaxillary correction, (**b**) which has radically changed the facial soft tissue drape.

included (Figure 1.11). Where a formal rhinoplasty is considered essential, it should always be undertaken as a separate surgical procedure once the changes produced by the jaw surgery have stabilised. See Chapter 14.

The importance of the nasolabial angle in the surgical planning process will be discussed in greater detail in Chapter 5. However it is important to record the nasolabial angle, which is the angle formed by the intersection of tangents to the lower border of the nose and upper lip. Ideally, in Caucasians this angle should be slightly greater than 90 degrees indicating optimum lip support by the maxillary alveolus (Figure 1.12).

d) *Morphology of the ears*

The ears, being first arch derivatives, may concurrently suffer with a gross facial deformity. The ear deformity associated with hemifacial hypoplasia (microsomia) will require reconstruction at a later stage (Figure 1.13). It is not uncommon for the external auditory meati to lie at unequal levels. This creates difficulties

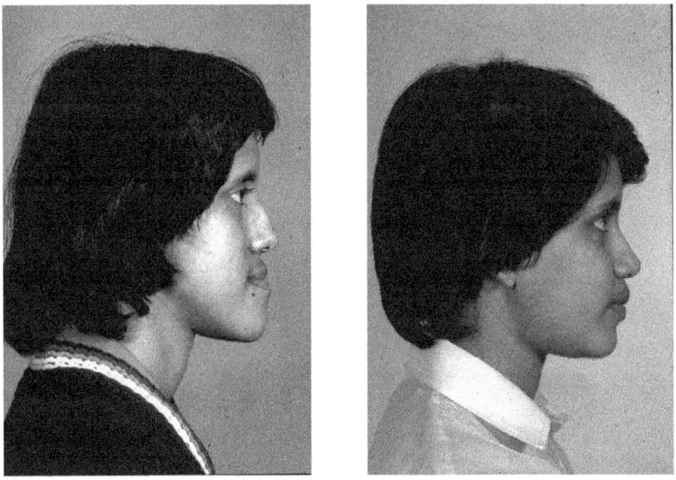

Figure 1.11 This bimaxillary correction consisted of a maxillary impaction with advancement and a mandibular setback. The maxilla has elevated the nasal tip and the combination enhanced the facial tissue drape.

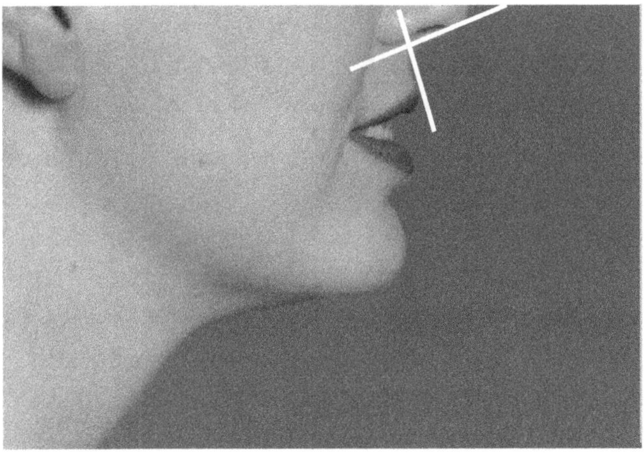

Figure 1.12 The nasolabial angle is assessed at the intersection of tangents to the columella (the lower border of the nasal septum) and the upper lip.

when taking a facebow recording for transfer to the articulator. See Chapter 6. Bat ears appear to be an independent abnormality and do not seem to concern most adults.

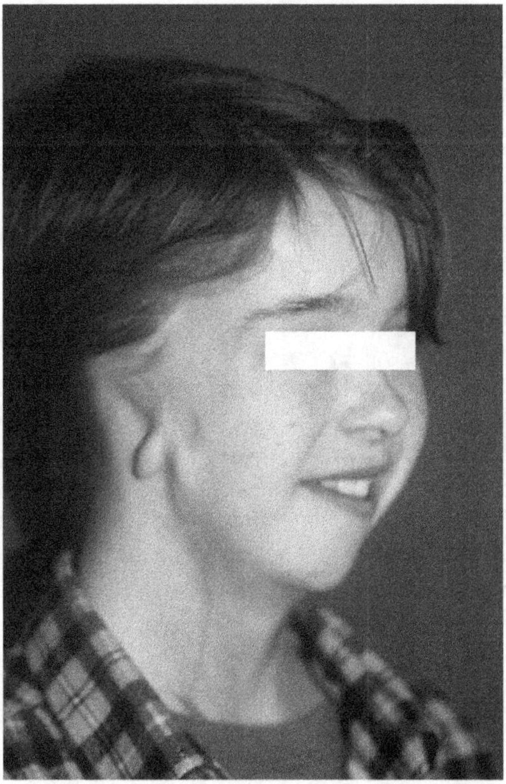

Figure 1.13 Severe ear deformity in a patient with hemifacial microsomia.

e) *Chin depth*

When assessing the facial height in the frontal (coronal) and sagittal planes, the lower facial third can be further subdivided into the upper lip which forms one-third, whilst the distance from the lower lip margin (stomion) to the chin margin (soft tissue menton) should comprise two-thirds of the lower facial height. Taken together with the chin profile this is an important component for correcting jaw disproportion (Figure 1.14).

f) *Chin-Throat angle*

Some patients request cosmetic surgery for an excess fat deposit in the throat region. This should be distinguished from

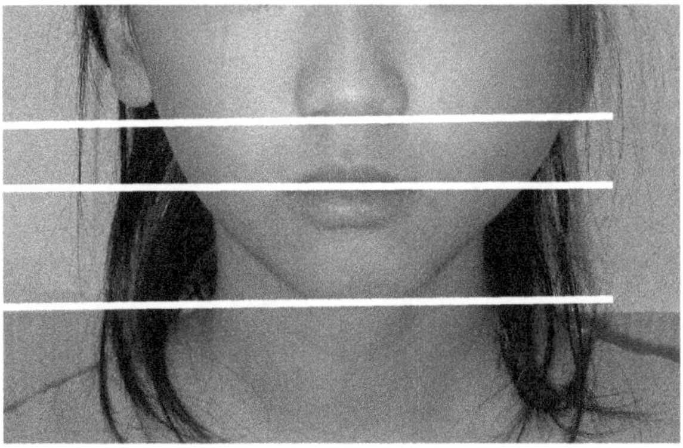

Figure 1.14 The upper lip length should be a third of the lower facial height.

a dewlap which is a fold of loose skin. As a consequence the fat gives a bulky contour below the chin. Surgery to setback the mandible may occasionally accentuate this build up of submental soft tissue, in which case liposuction or plastic surgery procedures may need to be incorporated into the postoperative surgical plan. However in the young patient the submental neck area usually remodels spontaneously following a mandibular setback.

Temporomandibular Joint Examination

Although there is no evidence of malocclusion or jaw deformity causing temporomandibular joint symptoms, it is important to record any abnormalities present in patients considering surgery. The examination of the joint should include observation of the path of opening and closure of the mandible, noting any clicking sounds whilst palpating the joints. If a click is present, it should be noted how this relates to the opening or closing cycle. Also, the extent of maximum opening should be recorded.

Intraoral Examination

The intraoral dental examination must be carried out with the study models and radiographs.

1. Record the teeth that are present or unerupted and any that are impacted, carious, overerupted or periodontally involved. This is often overlooked.
2. The following orthodontic base line notes should include:
   a) A definition of the dental occlusion and dental base relationships.
   b) Any dental centre line discrepancies relative to each other and the facial midline and chin point.
   c) Any crossbite indicating a discrepancy in the transverse relations. This includes both anteroposterior and buccal crossbites. It is important to check and record whether there is any associated displacement or deviation of the mandible on closing. In the buccal segments, it is also important to note whether the segments have attempted to compensate for the discrepancy by tipping of the dentition.
   d) The upper and lower incisor inclinations and in particular, compensatory changes due to the jaw disproportion, e.g. retroclined lower incisors and proclined upper incisors in a prognathous mandible.
   e) The biotype (thickness) of the periodontal attachment and soft tissues overlying the roots of the lower incisors. This is important when considering incisor decompensation. Where there is a thin biotype or signs of gingival recession consideration should be given to a periodontal graft.
   f) The presence of crowding or spacing together with any tooth size discrepancies. Note also any tilting and rotation of teeth.
   g) The levels and shape of the occlusal planes, both the anteroposterior curves of Spee, and the transverse occlusal plane.

A wooden spatula placed across the transverse occlusal plane can help identify any cant in relation to extraoral structures, for example, the interpupillary line.

h) The depth of the overbite and whether it is complete or incomplete. The size of the overjet from the most prominent incisor should also be recorded.
i) Whether the maxillary intercanine width can accommodate the lower arch.
j) The arch form and the coordination of upper and lower arches.

3. Examine and record the tongue size and mobility, and the speech pattern.
4. Enlarged tonsils may jeopardise the patency of the airway. Adenoids are rarely a problem as they have usually regressed in size during early adolescence. However, remember that the micrognathic mandible will create an intubation problem for the anaesthetist.
5. Cleft cases require careful analysis of the cleft site and bony defects that will require grafting. Velopharyngeal competence should be examined by endoscopy and speech recorded by a speech therapist.

Investigations

Radiographic Imaging

Digital radiographic imaging has largely replaced plain film processing. Nevertheless the recorded information should include the following:

1. A panoramic film, e.g. orthopantomograph shows at a glance:
   a) Any unerupted and impacted teeth.
   b) The shape and relative size of each half of the mandible, including the condyles, in two dimensions.

c) The presence of any pathological condition such as impacted unerupted teeth, caries, periodontal disease, any apical root resorption that may have arisen as a consequence of earlier orthodontic treatment, apical granulomas or cysts.
d) The trabeculation pattern of the bone, especially at the lingula, which when visible is an indication of adequate thickness of the ascending ramus and ease with which the ramus can be split.

2. The true lateral skull radiograph is taken with the head in a reproducible position with the aid of a cephalostat. The tube is set 1.5 m from the film so that the central parallel rays are used, producing a life-sized image with minimal distortion. Ideally the teeth should be in centric relation (retruded contact position), i.e. the mandible should be gently closed to the natural retruded cuspal contact position to approximate to the supine anaesthetised centric relation during surgery. However, the influence of centric occlusion and centric relation on planning will be discussed in Chapter 6.
3. A cephalostat posteroanterior view of the skull helps to reveal facial bone asymmetry. However, remember that the head may be tilted in the craniostat if the external auditory meati are asymmetrically placed, giving a misleading image.
4. Long cone periapical films are essential for assessing the space between teeth when segmental surgery is required.
5. A maxillary occlusal radiograph defines the bone defect in cleft cases.
6. Unusual anatomy or pathology will require additional investigation using a Cone Beam Computerised Tomograph scan (CBCT).

If the patient elects to have surgery, a preoperative chest radiograph is required by some surgeons but is only justified where a costochondral graft is to be harvested.

Study Models (Casts)

The use of intra-oral scanners to record the condition, and relationships of the teeth, and facilitate virtual planning will be covered in Chapter 7. However, traditional methods are still relevant. Impressions are taken for study models, together with a careful interocclusal record ("squash bite") so that the models can be trimmed in centric relation. This is done with the patient in a relaxed supine position. The models must show all the teeth present as well as the sulci. The patient's name, hospital number and the date of taking the impressions must be marked on them after trimming in a standardised manner (e.g. Angle or Tweed).

Initially two replicas are made of the originals and one set is mounted on an anatomical articulator using a facebow recording, although a simple plasterless articulator is suitable for those cases involving mandibular surgery alone. Model surgery is discussed in detail in Chapter 6.

Photographs

The basic orthognathic series of colour images consists of (Figure 1.15):

i) Full face at rest and smiling.
ii) Right profile but both profiles with any asymmetry.
iii) Anterior teeth and right and left buccal segments in occlusion.
iv) Some also include occlusal views of the upper and lower dentition.
v) Cleft cases require a palatal view.
vi) Cleft and rhinoplasty patients also need an inferior view of the alar margins to capture problems of asymmetry.

In addition, some use black and white prints of the patient's profile for treatment planning but the 1:1 object-image profile photograph is not exactly comparable to the lateral skull tracing. These

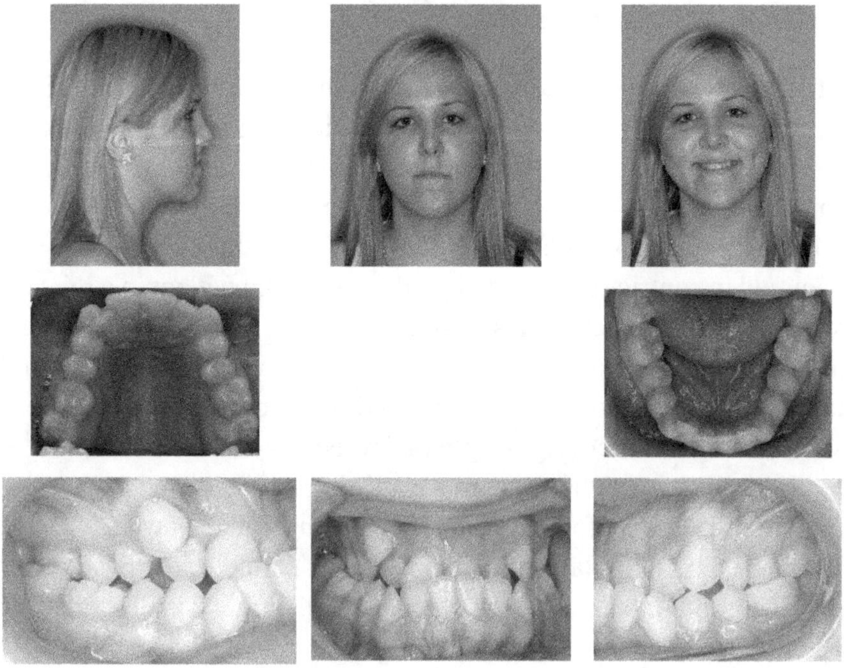

Figure 1.15 A basic orthognathic series of photographic records.

techniques have been largely superseded by computer imaging and morphing software programmes which are used to simulate surgical changes (Chapter 3).

Photographs should be taken pre- and postoperatively as a surgical audit, for teaching and rarely for medico-legal reasons. If photographs are to be of value, hair must be retracted from the face and moustaches and beards removed.

Lateral Skull Tracing

The "true lateral skull" radiograph is traced manually or digitised by computer for cephalometric analysis.

These will be discussed in detail in Chapters 2 and 3 and in the sections on deformities.

The Diagnosis

With many patients this can be readily stated, for example, "mandibular prognathism requiring a sagittal split osteotomy pushback". However, without more formal scrutiny, bimaxillary, orthodontic, restorative and periodontal problems will be overlooked.

Complex deformities require a detailed appraisal by the surgeon and orthodontist jointly, even then a surgical solution may not suggest itself immediately. Hence it is useful to describe the case under the following headings, in the form of a "problem list".

1. The jaw relationship and facial proportions, including the nose and ears
2. Orthodontic diagnosis
3. Restorative, including periodontal problems
4. Speech
5. Psychological assessment.

Chapter 2

Radiographic Analysis and Imaging

Nigel Hunt

The standard radiographic views which are fundamental to orthognathic surgery planning consist of a panoramic screening radiograph, for example, an orthopantomogram, and a lateral skull radiograph taken in a cephalostat. In addition the posteroanterior skull radiograph may be used in cases where there is clinical evidence of asymmetry. More detailed radiographs, for example, long cone periapical views or an upper standard occlusal radiograph may be taken for clarification of specific areas of pathology. It is not uncommon for surgical patients to have previously undergone some form of orthodontic treatment and therefore it is important to ensure that the roots of the teeth are perfectly sound.

The Need

Cephalometric analysis will establish the relations of:

1. The maxilla and the mandible to the base of the skull.
2. The maxilla to the mandible.

3. The maxillary teeth to the maxilla.
4. The mandibular teeth to the mandible.
5. The upper incisors to the lower incisors.

In order for these measurements and relationships to be meaningful it is important that the radiograph is taken in the standardised centric relation position (retruded contact position) with the patient's Frankfort Plane (the line from the lower border of the orbital rim to the upper border of the cephalostat ear post) horizontal. It is also important to ensure that the soft tissues are at rest when the radiograph is recorded.

Modern radiological guidelines require that intensifying screens should be used and that the radiographic beam has undergone appropriate collimation so as to avoid excessive exposure of structures considered unnecessary in the planning process.

Ethical approval is also required for repeated radiographs used for research purposes.

The Tracing

A sheet of clear, matt acetate paper is fixed securely with adhesive tape to the lateral skull radiograph placed on a horizontal viewing box. The radiographic image is enhanced by tracing in a darkened room with any peripheral light from the viewing box masked off. Many operators will have their preferred landmarks and analyses but the following outlines and points are commonly registered (Figure 2.1).

Outlines:

1. The soft tissue profile including glabella, nasion, nasal tip, upper lip, lower lip and the soft tissue chin.
2. The inner outline of the sella turcica, the anterior aspect of the nasal bones together with the frontonasal suture and the outline of the lower bony margin of the orbit.

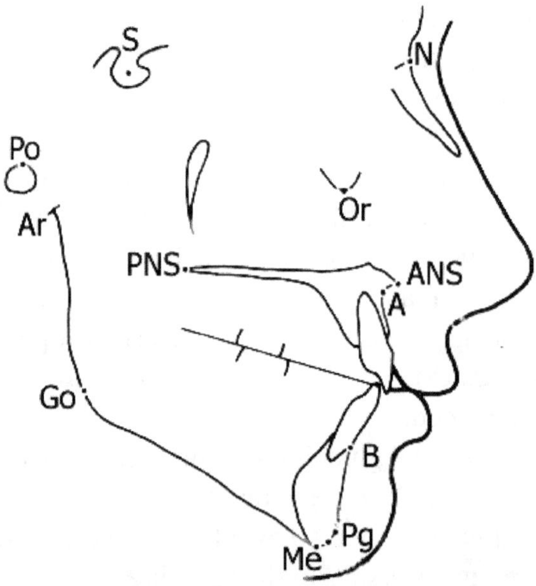

Figure 2.1 Cephalometric outlines and landmarks: A, point A; ANS, anterior nasal spine; Ar, articulare; B, point B; Go, gonion; Me, menton; N, nasion; Or, orbitale; PNS, posterior nasal spine; Pg, pogonion; Po, porion; S, sella.

3. The maxillary outline, upper incisors and upper first molar.
4. The mandibular outline with the mandibular incisors and first molar and articulare. As a result of superimposition it is often difficult to identify the head of the condyle but it is easy to register the articulare where the posterior margin of the ramus crosses the cranial base. In general, where bilateral landmarks present two images, the average of the two should be drawn. The exceptions to this are those cases where there is an obvious asymmetry of the mandible, which has resulted in two distinct lower borders to the mandible. From the point of view of measurement, it is normal practice to take the lower border which conforms to the normal side of the face, as assessed clinically.

Points:

- S Sella: The centre of the sella turcica determined by visual inspection.

- N Nasion: The anterior point of the frontonasal suture.
- ANS. Anterior nasal spine: Where the tip of the anterior nasal spine deviates markedly upwards or downwards, it is taken as the mid-point of the upper and lower spine outlines where it is 2 mm wide.
- PNS. Posterior nasal spine.
- Point A. The deepest midline point on the maxillary alveolus outlined between the anterior nasal spine and the maxillary alveolar crest.
- Point B. The deepest midline point between the mandibular alveolar crest and pogonion.
- Me Menton: The most inferior point on the lower border of the bony symphysis.
- Pg Pogonion: The most anterior point on the bony symphysis.
- Go Gonion: Is determined by bisecting the angle formed by tangents to the lower and posterior borders of the mandible. It is the point where the bisector cuts the angle of the mandible.
- Ar Articulare: The intersection of the posterior border of the ramus and the temporal bone.
- Co Condylion: The superior point on the condylar head.
- Or Orbitale: The most inferior point on the orbital margin.
- Po Porion: The upper margin of the bony external auditory meatus. The upper margin of the condylar head (Co) may also be used as it is often more easily determined.
- UMC. The tip of the mesio-buccal cusp of the upper first permanent molar.
- LMC. The tip of the mesio-buccal cusp of the lower first permanent molar.
- UIA. The tip of the most prominent maxillary incisor root apex.
- UIE. The most prominent maxillary incisor crown edge.
- LIE. The most prominent mandibular incisor crown edge.
- LIA. The tip of the most prominent mandibular incisor root apex.

The following lines are then drawn (Figure 2.2):

- S-N (the anterior cranial base).
- S-Ar.

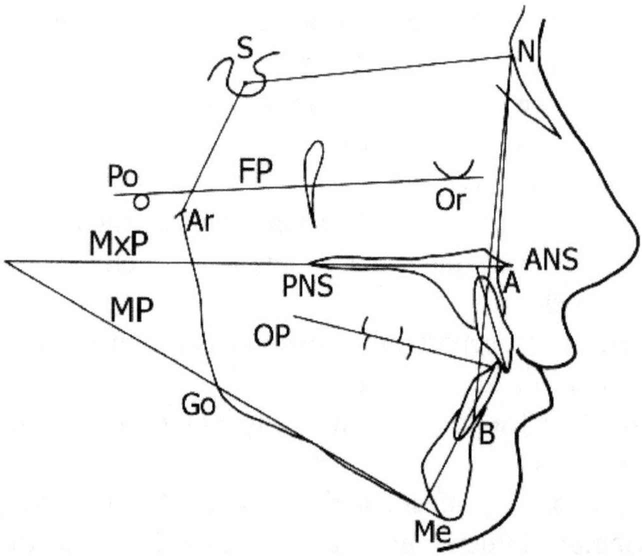

Figure 2.2 The planes and angles. Using the cephalometric points the following planes are constructed; SN plane (SN), mandibular plane (MP), maxillary plane (MxP) and Frankfort plane (FP). The long axes of the maxillary and mandibular incisors are considered relative to the maxillary and mandibular planes respectively. The important cephalometric angles can be readily derived from these points and planes. For key, see Table 2.1.

- N-A.
- N-B.
- Or-Po (the Frankfort plane-FP).
- ANS-PNS (the maxillary plane-MxP).
- Me-Go (mandibular plane-MP).
- Long axes of the upper (UI) and lower (LI) incisors.
- The occlusal plane (OP) is drawn through the occlusal outline of the buccal segment teeth, including the premolars. However, it may be difficult to determine the outline of the molars due to superimposition. Therefore for simplicity, the tips of the upper and lower mesial cusps (UMC and LMC) and the upper and lower distal cusps only are drawn.

The Analysis

The accuracy when undertaking a cephalometric tracing of a radiograph by hand and its analysis only permits linear and angular measurements to be expressed to the nearest whole millimetre or degree. The values obtained can then be compared with the population normal values to determine the patient's problems (Tables 2.1–2.3). It is important to appreciate that they will vary with age, sex and ethnic origin. Table 2.1 presents the mean angular cephalometric values based on a Caucasian population. As can be seen from these tables, there is considerable variation for all values.

Although cephalometric analysis is helpful in providing information for diagnosis and treatment planning, it has to be borne in mind that the ultimate goal is not necessarily to achieve ideal values near to the mean but to produce a proportional and harmonious

Table 2.1 Mean angular cephalometric values (Caucasians)

Measurement	Mean ^{0}± SD
SNA	81 ± 3
SNB	78 ± 3
ANB	3 ± 2
SN/MxP	8 ± 3
SN/MP	35 ± 4
FP/OP	8 ± 4
NSAr (saddle angle)	125 ± 5
SArGo (articular angle)	140 ± 6
ArGoMe (gonial angle)	128 ± 7
MxP/MP	27 ± 4
UI/MxP	109 ± 6
UI/LI	130 ± 6
LI/MP	93 ± 6

For explanations of abbreviations, see text.

Table 2.2 Mean linear cephalometric values (Caucasians)

Measurement		Mean mm ± SD
Facial Heights		
Total anterior	TAFH (N-Me)	124 ± 8
Lower anterior	LAFH	68 ± 8
Total posterior	TPFH (S-Go)	79 ± 6
Lower posterior	LPFH	34 ± 5
	Ar – Go	54 ± 4
Lower anterior face height ratio	LAFH/TAFH%	55 ± 2
Lower posterior face height ratio	LPFH/TPFH%	44 ± 1
Dentoalveolar Heights		
Lower posterior	LPDH (LMC-MP)	38 ± 3
Lower anterior	LADH (LIE-MP)	40 ± 2 (females) 44 ± 2 (males)
Upper anterior	UADH (UIE- MxP)	33 ± 3
Upper posterior	UPDH (UMC-MxP)	28 ± 3

For explanations of abbreviations, see text.

Table 2.3 Angular cephalometric values (Negroes and Chinese)

	Value^0	
Measurement	Negroes	Chinese
SNA	85	83
SNB	80	80
ANB	5	3
MxP/MP	28	28
UI/MxP	118	113
LI/MP	98	96

For explanation of abbreviations, see text.
These figures may be used for Negro and Oriental patients instead of those in Table 2.1 but should be regarded as a broad guide, rather than an exact ideal, bearing in mind that numbers in some surveys are small and may be the average of a wide range. Because of natural incisor proclination, the aesthetic nasolabial angles are invariably acute, i.e. significantly less than the Caucasian range.

facial structure. To that end, where there are discrepancies between clinical observation and cephalometric values, the analysis of the clinical presentation is always more important.

Vertical Values

Vertical cephalometric analysis is of great value in orthognathic planning.

Linear

The total anterior face height (TAFH) is the sum of the upper anterior face height (UAFH), measured from nasion to the maxillary plane, and the lower anterior face height (LAFH), maxillary plane to menton. The lower anterior face height is usually 55 ± 2% of the total anterior face height.

Posterior face height is similarly measured from sella to gonion using the maxillary plane to divide the upper posterior face height (UPFH) from the lower posterior face height (LPFH). The lower posterior face height being approximately 44 ± 1% of the total posterior face height (Figure 2.3).

The anterior dentoalveolar heights are measured from the incisal edges of the upper and lower incisors (UIE and LIE) to the maxillary plane and mandibular plane respectively. It should be noted that these measurements reflect the components of the lower face height. In other words, if the lower anterior face height value is high, then the upper and lower anterior dentoalveolar heights (UADH and LADH) will also be increased, except in some cases of anterior open bite.

The upper and lower posterior dentoalveolar heights (UPDH and LPDH) can be recorded from the tips of the mesial cusps of the upper and lower molars (UMC and LMC) to the maxillary and mandibular planes respectively.

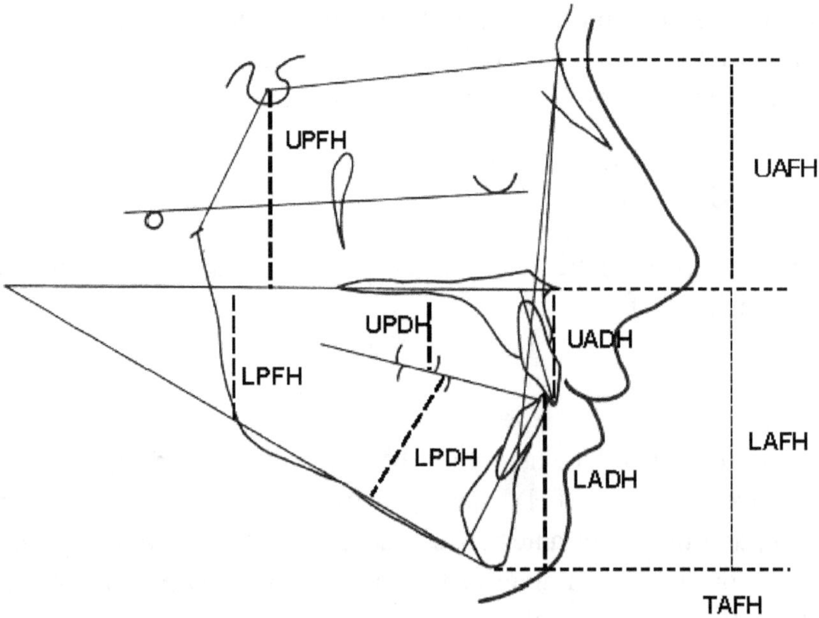

Figure 2.3 Linear measurements for the vertical dimensions. See Table 2.2 for details.

Angular

The relationship of the anterior and posterior face heights is reflected by the angles between the skull base and the maxillary and mandibular planes.

The angle of the maxillary to the mandibular plane (MxP/MP) is normally 27 ± 4°. This angle is important because as with the posterior face height measurement, it reflects the surgically important pterygomasseteric sling length (muscle, fascia and ligaments). For instance, a patient with a high angle, i.e. greater than 35°, tends to have a relatively short posterior face height and therefore posterior musculo-ligamentous height. Any attempt to stretch this posterior connective tissue by rotating the anterior body of the mandible upwards, in an anticlockwise direction, around a fulcrum produced by the posterior molar occlusion, is doomed to failure and will lead to early surgical relapse.

Anteroposterior Relationships

In clinical practice anteroposterior lengths are rarely measured or used to relate the jaws to each other. It has become conventional to study the angular relationship of the jaws to the cranial base (SN). Orientation to the Frankfort plane is also used to compare these structures. However, in extremes of skeletal variation some angular measurements may be misleading. A typical example is the problem of SNA and SNB to analyse the anteroposterior relationship of the maxilla to the mandible (Figure 2.4). In the normal Class I patient, SNA is 81° with a standard deviation of 3°, and the normal maxillary-mandibular relationship (ANB) is 3°. An increased ANB angle suggests a Class II relationship, whereas a negative ANB angle suggests a Class III case. However, variations in the positions of N will influence both the SNA and SNB. For example, with a shorter anterior cranial base length (SN) increasing SNA by 10° alters the ANB angle to 7° giving the impression of a skeletal Class II jaw relationship (Figure 2.4). These variations, due to an "abnormal" SNA, may be corrected by subtracting 0.5° from the ANB angle for every degree by which SNA exceeds the normal value of 81°. In the above example, applying the conversion would reduce the apparent ANB angle from 7° to 2°. Conversely, where the SNA is below the normal value of 81°, 0.5° should be added to the ANB angle for every degree that SNA is below the normal figure. This conversion is only possible providing the SN/MxP values are within the normal range of $8^0 \pm 3^0$. If the SN/MxP value is outside this range then alternate analyses of the anteroposterior skeletal pattern should be employed as detailed in cephalometric specific texts.

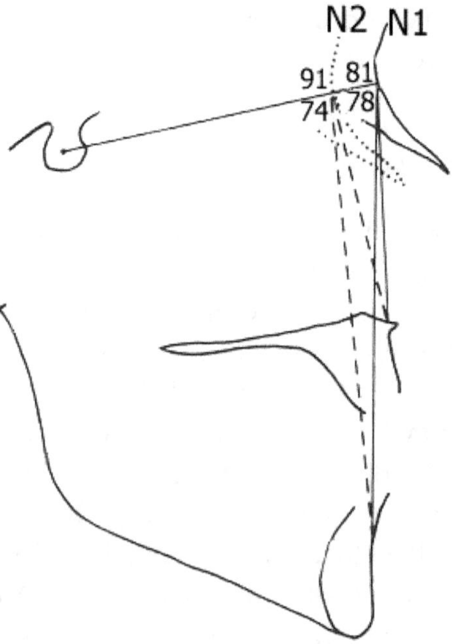

Figure 2.4 Cephalometric idiosyncrasies. The tracing shows how variations in skull base length (SN) can influence the angular values relating to A point and B point. With SNA 81° and SNB 78°, ANB is 3° indicating a Class I skeletal pattern (continuous line). With an unchanged jaw relationship, a shorter skull base SN (from N1 to N2) changes the SNA and SNB angles, i.e. SNA 91°, SNB 74° and ANB becomes 7°, suggesting a Class II skeletal pattern (broken line).

Analysis of the Incisor Angulations to the Maxillary and Mandibular Bases

Skeletal deformity with its disturbed muscular skeletal pattern will lead to changes in the angles of the upper incisor to the maxillary plane (UI/MxP) and the lower incisor to the mandibular plane (LI/MP) adding a degree of secondary deformity (dental compensation) to any underlying skeletal discrepancy (Figure 2.5). Thus with a mandibular prognathism the lower incisors tend to be retroclined and the maxillary incisors proclined. In some severe Class II deformities the lower lip may become trapped behind the maxillary

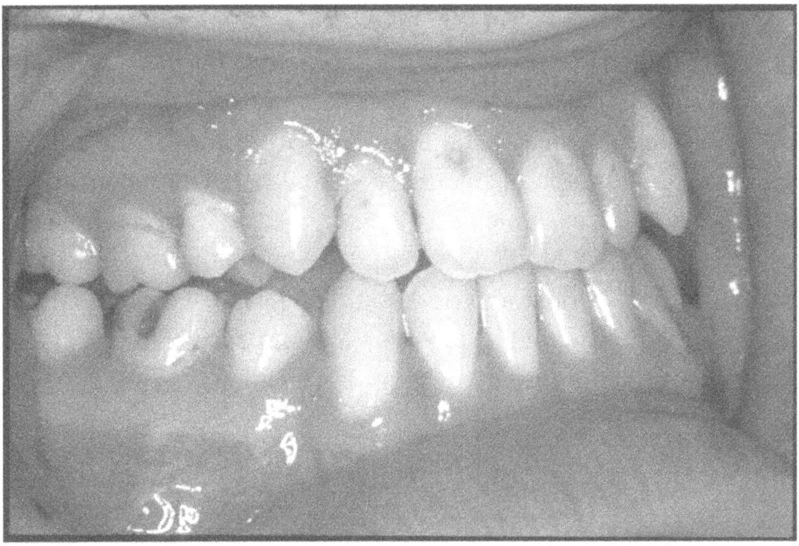

Figure 2.5 Dental compensation in a Class III case with proclination of the maxillary incisors and retroclination of the mandibular incisor teeth. See also Figures 4.8 and 4.9.

incisors with the effect that the upper incisors may actually procline, whilst the lower incisors may be retroclined. This "compensation" requires correction, i.e decompensation, as part of the overall treatment plan.

The Surgical Application of Cephalometry

Caution must be used in the interpretation of precise linear measurements such as the anterior face height. Measurements from different samples can vary by as much as 10 mm. This problem is diminished when the components are expressed as a percentage. In addition, too many measurements may cause confusion, defeating the purpose of the analysis. However, the exercise is an important means of studying the clinical problem. The geometry can also be checked by the use of diagnostic templates.

Various templates to be matched to the patient for age and sex have been developed from population studies. The Bolton ("unisex") template, provides a simple means of diagnosis when superimposed over the cranial base and calvarium of the patient's lateral skull radiograph or tracing (Figure 2.6a). The Jacobson templates are alternatives, which provide racial separation (Figure 2.6b). This direct method of diagnosis may be particularly attractive to those who find cephalometrics confusing. However, a template should not be considered in any way a treatment goal but rather an aid in establishing the exact areas of discrepancy.

Computerised Cephalometrics

Many computer software packages are now available which with direct digitisation of radiographs, store the data as co-ordinates. Computerised cephalometrics have the advantage that any number of identical copies of the computerised tracing can be produced, and superimpositions can be achieved readily by incorporating normal template tracings into the data bank. But they also have the disadvantage of removing the "personal touch". Many operators still prefer undertaking a hand tracing as it gives a greater appreciation of any difficulties of a particular case, identified during the planning process. Computerised cephalometrics are discussed in detail in Chapter 3.

Posteroanterior Radiograph Tracings

The major use of posteroanterior skull radiograph tracings is for the identification of facial asymmetries. By constructing a series of horizontal and vertical reference planes the exact extent of the asymmetry can be readily demonstrated (Figure 2.7).

In the vertical plane it is normal to draw a median reference line passing through the centre of the nasal bones, through the majority of the nasal septum (unless there is gross deviation) and this line

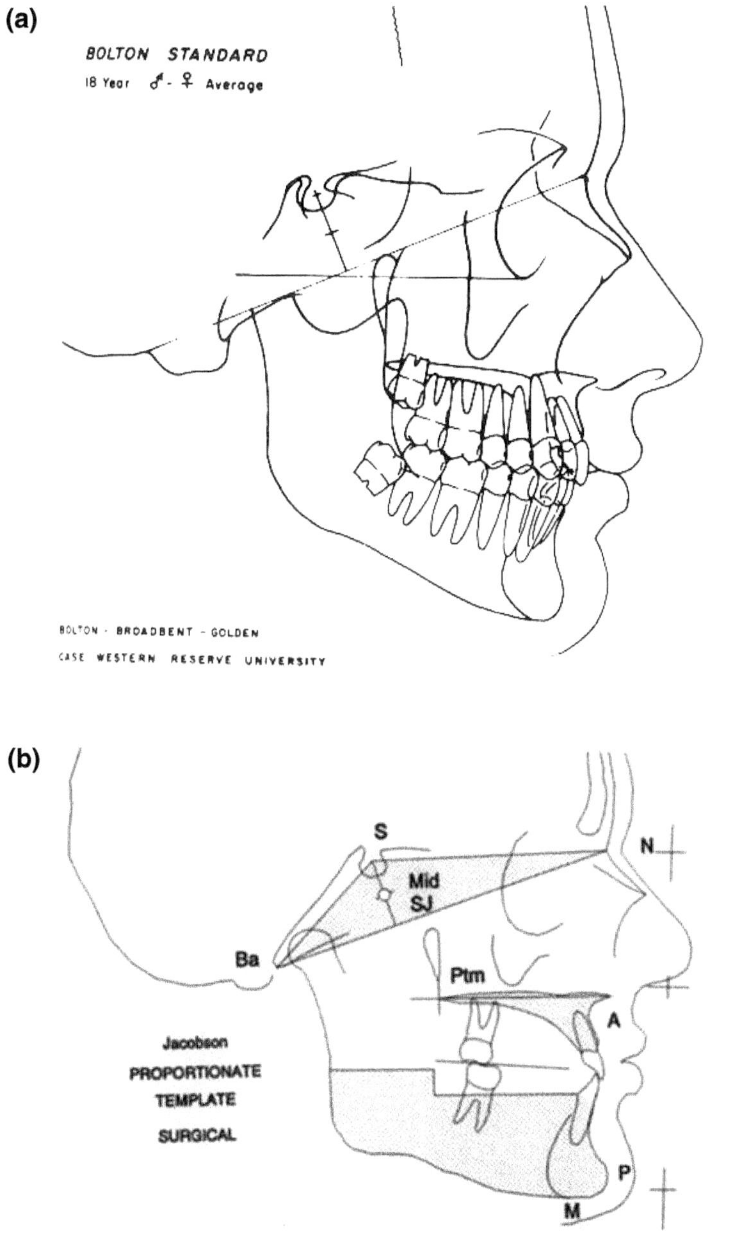

Figure 2.6 (**a**) Bolton standard template. (**b**) Jacobson proportional template.

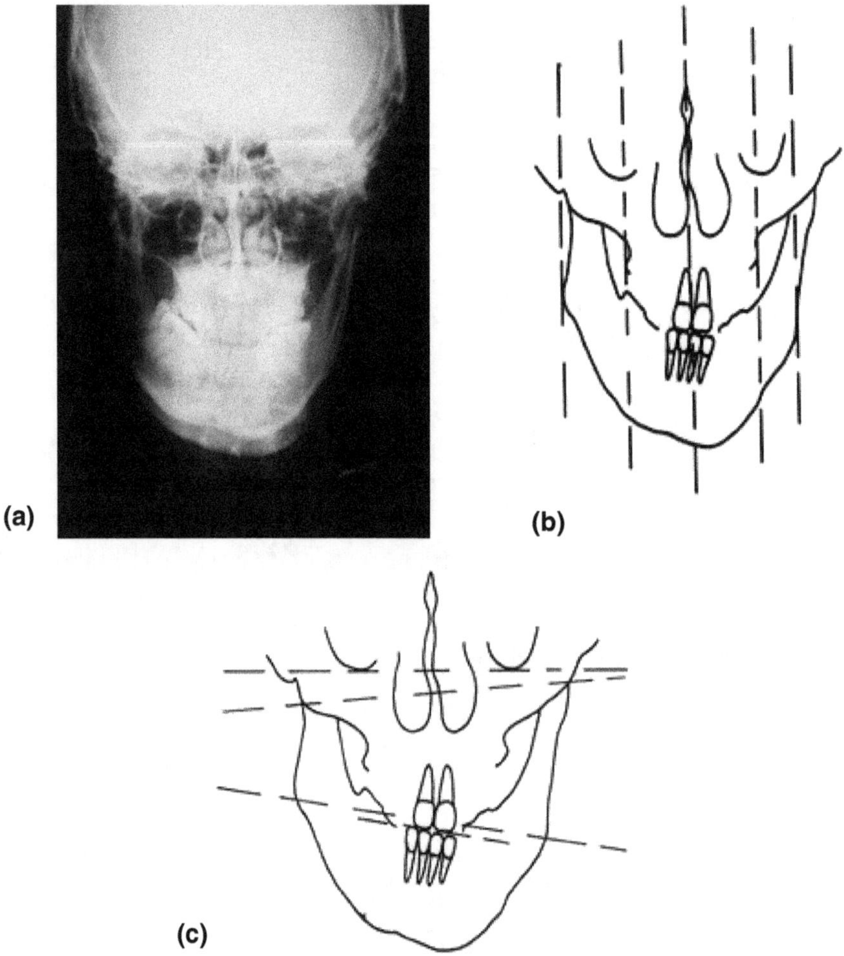

Figure 2.7 (**a**) Posteroanterior cephalogram used in the assessment of facial asymmetry. Vertical (**b**) and horizontal (**c**) reference lines give an indication of the site of the asymmetry. See text for details.

when extended inferiorly should coincide with the midline of the upper central incisors, midline of the lower central incisors and the midpoint of the chin. Two more vertical reference planes should then be drawn, parallel to the median reference line, and forming a tangent to the most lateral point of the contour of the maxillary tuberosity region. Moving further laterally, additional vertical lines should be drawn, again parallel to the median reference line, and passing as a tangent to the most lateral point of the gonial angle region on both sides of the face. As such the face has been divided up into four vertical segments which should be of equal transverse width.

A second series of lines is then drawn in the horizontal plane. The horizontal reference plane should be taken as a line which passes as a tangent to the lower border of the infra-orbital margins, and ideally this should intersect the median vertical plane at a right angle. The second and third lines, should link both inferior borders of the right and left tuberosities and the gonial angles respectively, revealing any horizontal discrepancies. Finally, lines drawn across the incisal edges of the upper and lower incisors represent the upper and lower occlusal planes as seen in the PA view.

Through a combination of these vertical and horizontal reference lines the exact source of bony and dental asymmetries can be identified. This form of analysis is particularly useful in identifying the presence and extent of any cants to the occlusal plane but is dependent on an accurately positioned cephalogram.

Orthopantomogram Tracing

Tracing of the orthopantomogram is not undertaken as part of routine assessment. However, when considering asymmetries in the lower border of the mandible a full tracing of the radiograph may prove useful. An example of a tracing is seen in Figure 2.8 where a tracing of the normal side of the radiograph has been superimposed on the abnormal side using the occlusal plane as a guide. The discrepancy of the mandibular borders can be seen readily (Figure 2.8b). In marked cases of mandibular asymmetry, a procedure to reduce the lower border of the mandible may be

(a)

(b)

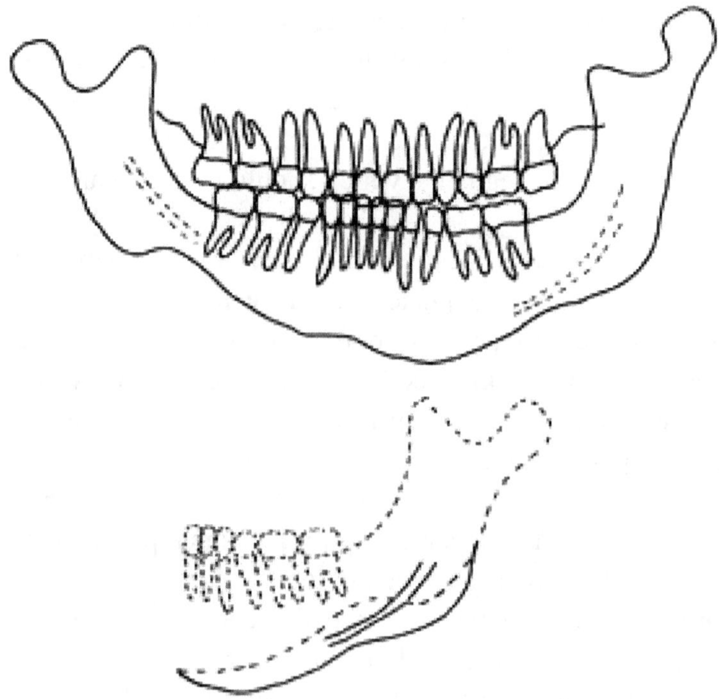

Figure 2.8 (**a**) Orthopantomogram tracing of a patient with hemimandibular hyperplasia. (**b**) The "normal" side tracing has been superimposed over the "abnormal" side, using the occlusal plane as a reference, indicating the extent of bone removal necessary to achieve a symmetrical lower border to the mandible and that repositioning of the dentoalveolar nerve would be required.

considered. This tracing can give information as to the extent of the bone to be removed and whether or not the inferior dental nerve is likely to need repositioning. The advent of Computer Assisted Surgical Simulation (CASS) provides a 3 dimensional image for surgical guidance. However, tracing the orthopantomogram provides a simple approach when such techniques are unavailable.

Chapter 3

Computerised Cephalometrics for Orthodontic and Orthognathic Planning

Paul Thomas

Although basic cephalometric methodology has remained unchanged for many years the application of information technology, to store, display and manipulate cephalometric images has evolved so that;

i) Analysis is significantly faster and more reliable when compared to manual measurement.
ii) Reformation of digital data enables the simulation of several treatment alternatives almost simultaneously.

These benefits are seen with direct digital imaging in which the X-ray beam is recorded by photoelectric sensors or a plate with phosphor emulsion. These images require a reduced radiation exposure and can be read as a soft copy on a monitor or a hard copy printed out on transparency film or paper. Indirect digital imaging methods include copying the radiograph film from a view box with a digital camera or by converting the radiograph to a digital image with a flatbed scanner. Both systems provide multiple advantages such as ease of storage, manipulation and enhancement, duplication and the possibility of automated landmark identification.

Regardless of the method used to produce the digital image, the data storage and display are very different from conventional film.

Images on a monitor display are composed of small dots called picture elements or pixels. The resolution or clarity of the image is directly proportional to the number of pixels which make up the image. More pixels mean a sharper image but also involves the manipulation and storage of more information. The contrast of a digital radiograph is also determined by the number of shades of grey which can be displayed. Depending on the complexity of the software the number of shades can vary from 64 to 1024. Most dental radiology applications display 256 shades of grey.

A limiting factor when viewing digital images is the monitor itself. Typical monitors can display 72–96 pixels per inch (ppi). However the full potential of any image with higher resolution can only be displayed with clarity after being printed as a hard copy.

Digital images are further limited by the monitor's ability to display contrast. Analogue films have an almost infinite or continuous greyscale. As stated, most dental digital images are viewed with only 256 shades of grey. The problem is compounded by the fact that digital images are often displayed more brightly than analogue film images which tends to reduce the limited greyscale resolution. It is important to bear in mind that the optimum number of shades of grey is dependent on what is being diagnosed from the image. A medical radiologist would require the maximum shades of grey possible to discern subtleties in diagnosing pathology.

Once the spatial resolution and contrast have been optimized, the capacity of the human eye becomes the limiting factor. The smallest detail the human eye can resolve is approximately 0.1 mm by 0.1 mm. Therefore, we are unable to appreciate more detail in any image with a smaller pixel size. Conversely, images with pixels

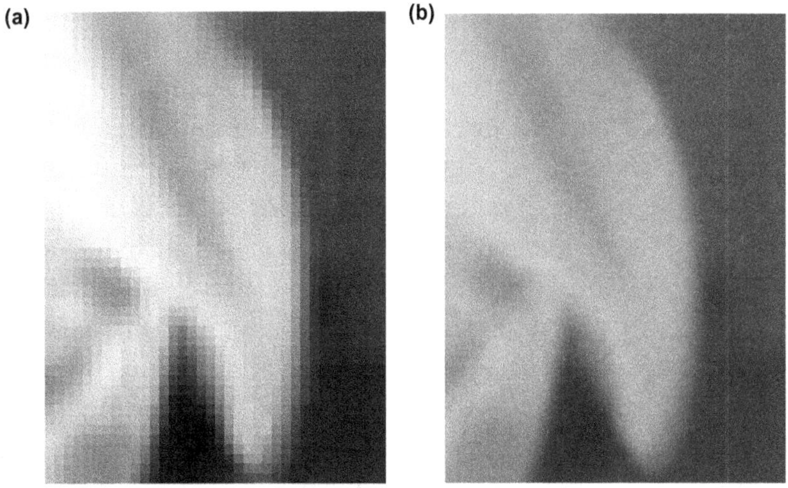

Figure 3.1 These digital images are identical except for spatial resolution, that is pixel size. (**a**) The left image has a pixel dimension of 0.084 mm. × 0.084 mm. which is at the limit the human eye can resolve. (**b**) The pixel dimension of the image on the right is 0.35 mm × 0.35 mm. Note the fuzzy appearance with loss of definition.

of a much larger size, for example 0.7 mm by 0.7 mm, may seem blurred (Figure 3.1). A pixel size of 0.1 mm should be equal to X-ray film when identifying landmarks on cephalometric radiographs.

Digital imaging technology is becoming the standard of care. It has the advantages of storage, accessibility, portability, ease of duplication, manipulation and communication which outweigh the disadvantages. However, with these advantages come responsibilities. The ease of duplication create problems of confidentiality. The DICOM (Digital Imaging and Communication in Medicine) Standards have been developed to attain compatibility between imaging systems and other information systems. The standards also include security in record transmission and storage as well as record "locking" or digital signatures. The contemporary clinician must be vigilant of changes in hardware, software and the responsibilities for their use.

Treatment Planning with Digital Images

Orthognathic treatment planning requires a method of predicting the anticipated outcome. In clinical practice this has been based on experience and intuition. Digital simulation is based on the tracing of the landmarks identified on a standardised lateral cephalometric radiograph. The dental and skeletal structures are moved to correct the malocclusion and the predicted soft tissue response is based on data collected from the analysis of previous treatments tempered with clinical experience (Figure 3.2). Such simulation gives the patient and family a glimpse of the aesthetic change. Various terms have been given to this process including the Visualised Treatment Objective (VTO) and Surgical Treatment Objective (STO). These simulations are usually limited to a profile view due to the lack of data provided by PA cephalometry. Surface laser scans and photogrammetry provide alternative techniques to overcome this limitation.

Although acetate tracings are adequate for most clinicians, patients may view them as arcane. To improve patient understanding a photographic likeness can be incorporate into the process. Initially, this was limited to a photographic montage created by rearranging cut-outs of profile photographs. The computer has streamlined this process so that cephalometric data can be digitally stored and recalled for manipulation. These graphic reproductions of tracings can be viewed on screen or printed on paper. Other advances in software engineering have produced programmes which have replaced manual digitizing with auto-recognition of landmarks which will not be covered here. Regardless of the digitizing method, the clinician will always need to verify landmark accuracy prior to proceeding to diagnosis and treatment planning. However despite technological advances, the result is no better than the data used to predict the soft tissue response.

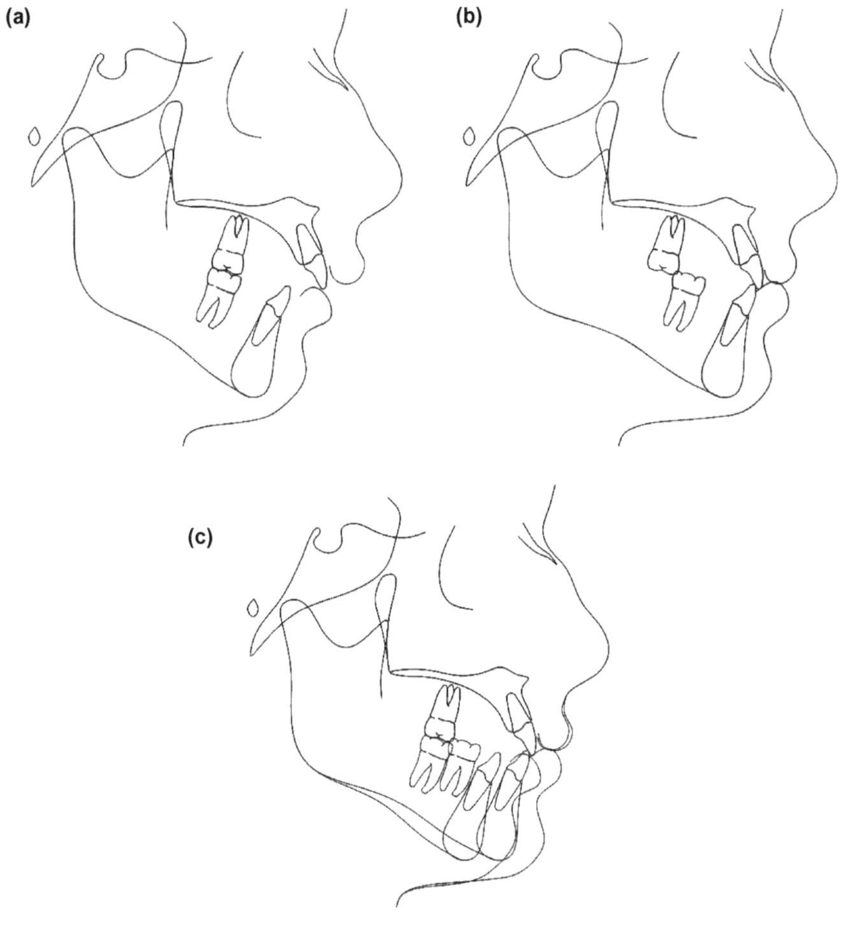

Figure 3.2 Simulation tracings can be done by hand on acetate or are computer generated. The preoperative cephalometric tracing (**a**) is altered to simulate the mandibular advancement (**b**). The superimposition (**c**) graphically demonstrates the amount of movement needed for correction.

Patient Education is Important

The breakthrough in treatment simulation for patient education came with the ability to manipulate patient's photographs, or video images or slides which were converted from analogue to digital form prior to being linked to the cephalometric tracing. Although the result was still limited to a profile view, both patient and clinician had a representation which was much closer to a credible likeness.

Patients need to have the nature of their problem presented in a language they can understand. For both educational and a medico-legal reasons, those involved must understand the risk versus benefit of any treatment involving a change in appearance. Although facial appearance is invariably the primary motivator for those seeking surgical correction it may not be the principal underlying reason (See Chapter 16).

There is concern that the use of digital imaging for patient communication creates the possibility of legal action if the treatment outcome does not approximate to the simulation. For this reason a disclaimer may be printed on a copy of the image. Although there is no history of litigation related to such disappointment good communication is essential especially when patients have a mild or moderate rather than severe aesthetic problems. Such patients are in a borderline area where the alternatives could range from no treatment to correction by extractions and orthodontic compensation. It is generally easier for the patient and family to accept a surgical treatment plan when there is a severe dentofacial deformity.

The decision is crucial as the objectives for orthodontic compensation are the opposite to those for orthodontic decompensation prior to orthognathic surgery. For example, the anterior teeth are compensated for the orthodontic solution but decompensated prior to surgery. The extraction patterns differ between compensation and surgical preparation. The approach to levelling mechanics and space closure is also different with each option. Since it is difficult if not impossible to cope with a "change of heart" patient, all the information required to choose between the treatment options must be presented prior to the start of treatment. Digital treatment simulation is a valuable tool in making this decision. Treatment simulation may also be used immediately prior to surgery.

Interactive and Simulation Programmes

Digital imaging technology can offer several options for treatment planning and patient education. Interactive programmes are useful during the preliminary consultations. This type of software employs a mixture of still photographs, graphic art and multimedia which can demonstrate specific problems and their potential solutions. For instance the clinician can demonstrate the difference between orthodontic compensation and surgical correction (Figure 3.3).

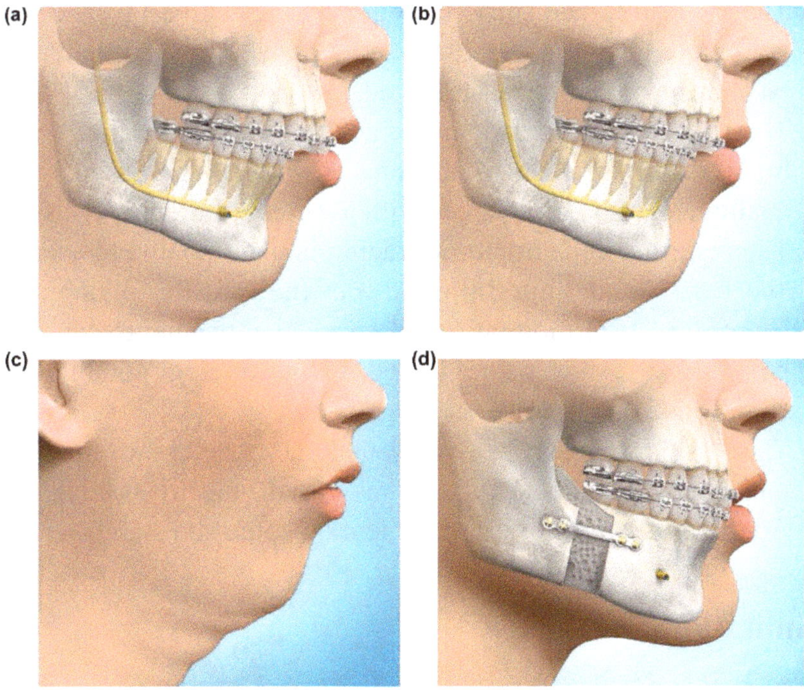

Figures 3.3 This multimedia programme demonstrates the contrast between correcting mandibular deficiency with orthodontic camouflage versus orthognathic surgery. Images **(a)** and **(b)** show extraction of the upper first premolars with retraction of the incisors and upper lip. Images **(c)** and **(d)** demonstrate the changes seen with surgical lengthening of the mandible. (Courtesy of Dolphin Imaging & Management Solutions, 9200 Oakdale Ave. Suite 500, Chatsworth, CA 91311 U.S.A.

The artist's representations of treatment outcome can be stylized to demonstrate the facial change seen with each option. If there is continued interest on the part of the patient and or family, full diagnostic records should be taken and the patient's data is used for the treatment simulation.

Although the data entry approach varies among programmes, the following steps are common to each:

- The patient's photographic series is directly entered with a digital camera or scanned into the computer from photographs or slides.
- The lateral cephalometric radiograph is imported into the programme using direct digital radiography or by scanning the radiograph with a transparency adapter.
- The conventional cephalometric analysis can be done on-screen by digitising the requisite landmarks. Radiographs of marginal quality can also be enhanced with a variety of graphic tools.
- The resulting cephalometric tracing is manipulated to achieve "best fit" and superimposed on the profile photograph (Figure 3.4). Orthodontic and surgical movements can now be simulated using the linked image-tracing combination (Figure 3.5).
- The soft tissue response from dental and skeletal movements is modelled by computer algorithms based on retrospective data from long-term studies of treatment outcome and stability.

Limitations

- Simulation is no better than the data on which it is based and which may be flawed by small sample size and patient heterogeneity, treatment instability, and errors in surgical management.
- Mean values are used to develop ratios which determine soft tissue movements relative to a skeletal landmark. The assumption is that the soft tissue response is a fixed percentage of skeletal

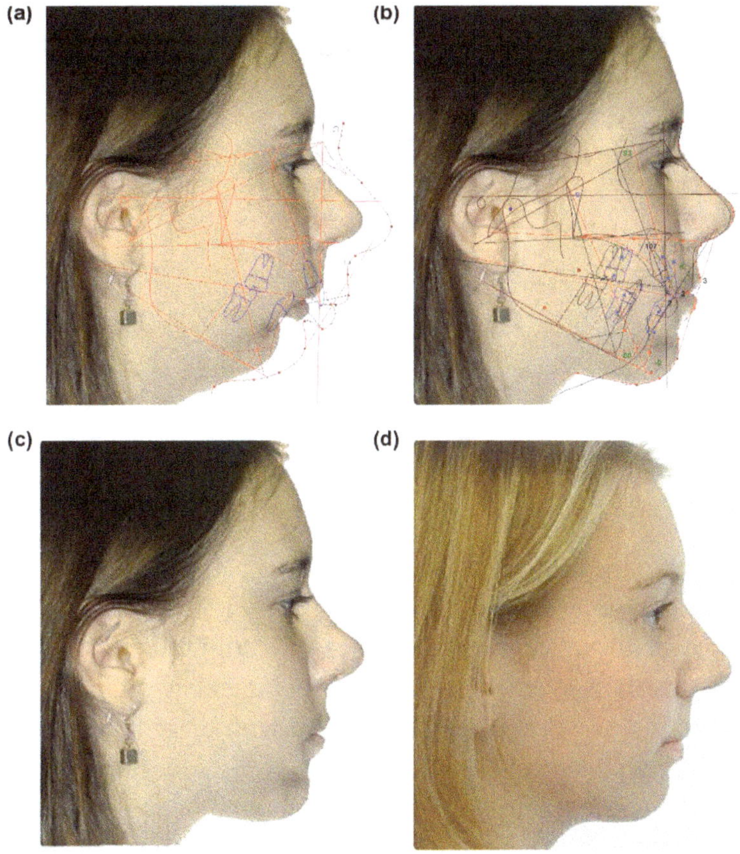

Figure 3.4 (**a**) Digital treatment simulation requires linking of the profile image with the tracing digitised from the lateral cephalometric film. The process is facilitated by having the head and soft tissue posture as identical as possible. (**b**) The image-tracing pair is manipulated with the software to simulate the surgical advancement of the mandible. The final simulation (**c**) is a close approximation of the actual outcome (**d**). All software programmes have difficulty creating the natural contours of the lips and mentolabial fold.

movement, regardless of the extent of skeletal change. This approach fails to account for local variations due to muscle tone, soft tissue compression and tissue redundancy.

- Studies have shown that most programmes now produce reasonable simulations when the surgical movements are moderate,

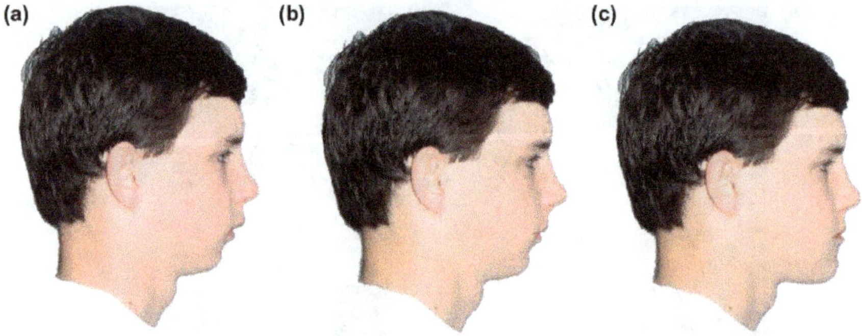

Figure 3.5 Treatment simulation software has been used to alter this patient's pretreatment image **(a)** to portray the outcome of orthodontic camouflage **(b)** versus surgical mandibular advancement **(c)**. Compared to cephalometric tracings, these images are more easily understood by patients and their family.

limited to the sagittal plane, and involve patients with competent lips and little eversion.

- However these same programmes have difficulty with simulations involving vertical movements in patients with increased lip separation or a deep labiomental fold with lip redundancy.
- A second source of variability is the technique for linking the cephalometric tracing and profile photograph. Factors influencing this variability include the number and location of the landmarks on the soft tissue profile; and the ability to adjust for differences in the radiographic and photographic scales.
- These recognised differences in orientation between the radiograph and profile photograph invariably need some adjustment in linking.
- Finally, most programmes have image refinement tools which allow the clinician to adjust the simulation's soft tissue response according to personal experience with certain surgical movements. These adjustments introduce potential sources of inaccuracy but are often needed to correct the predicted lip posture.

Chapter 4

Orthodontic Preparation

Nigel Hunt

Timing and Duration

The objectives of presurgical orthodontic treatment are to enable maximal surgical correction of the deformity, to facilitate any segmental surgical procedures and to enable the production of an ideal stable occlusion. An essential feature of the treatment plan is to decompensate the dento-alveolar results of the jaw deformity which is very different from the "compensatory" approach of the pure orthodontic management of the case. Hence the need for careful consideration by the patient and clinicians as to the desired choice of treatment. The majority of orthodontic treatment is undertaken prior to surgery, although some prefer to undertake minimal orthodontic treatment prior to surgery leaving the major proportion to the post-operative phase. Both of these approaches have advantages and disadvantages. Extensive presurgical preparation is usually better accepted by the patient giving maximum compliance. However, the dental movements may be hindered by the underlying skeletal and soft tissue discrepancy. Conversely, although the orthodontic changes may be easier once a normal skeletal and soft tissue relationship has become established, prolonged postoperative orthodontics may not be tolerated by the patient and leads to poor patient satisfaction.

Presurgical Orthodontics

Presurgical preparation usually takes 18–24 months, whilst postsurgical refinement should be completed within 6 months of the operation.

The goals of presurgical orthodontics are to facilitate the surgery by:

- Alignment of the dentition.
- Levelling of the occlusal plane, either as a continuous arch or segmentally prior to surgical levelling.
- Incisor decompensation.
- Buccal segment decompensation.
- Coordination of the upper and lower arches.
- Providing a means of fixation.

Alignment of the Dentition — The Technology

Dental arch alignment requires 3-dimensional control of tooth position. Most use a pre-adjusted Edgewise appliance system with a slot dimension of 0.022" × 0.028" or variants upon this. The term pre-adjusted appliance refers to the bracket design such that adjustments are incorporated into the brackets to create a final position of the teeth with the correct mesiodistal angulation (tip), buccopalatal or buccolingual inclination (torque) and horizontal positions (in/out) relative to each other. Individual teeth within the dental arch therefore have specific adjustments built into their appropriate bracket (Figure 4.1). A variety of pre-adjusted systems are available each with minor variations in the tip and torque values. This is referred to as the bracket prescription. Segmental surgery requires the added facility of a double tube on the mandibular molars and/or a triple tube on the maxillary molars. The Tip-Edge™ appliance system is equally applicable to presurgical alignment although individual operators will have their preferred bracket prescription.

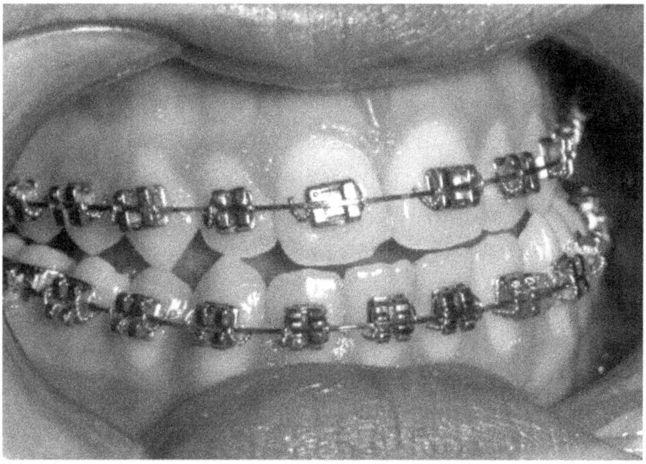

Figure 4.1 Pre-adjusted Edgewise appliances with individual brackets designed for specific teeth.

It is worthwhile considering the variations in bracket tip and torque required in specific cases. In an ideal occlusion, the crown of the lower incisor lies labial to the apex for ideal tooth inclination. In Class II cases where proclined lower incisor require decompensation, the use of MBT™ brackets with the 6^0 of additional lingual crown torque can aid the mechanics. Conversely, Super-torque™ brackets, with additional palatal root torque to the upper incisors, can be useful in correcting severely retroclined incisors in Class II division 2 cases. Mesiodistal tooth angulation (tip) becomes important when considering the preparation of a case for segmental surgery as it is important to facilitate the surgery (see below) by ensuring the roots adjacent to the osteotomy site are either parallel or slightly divergent. Again in an ideal functioning occlusion, the crown of the canine should lie mesial to the apex. Where the osteotomy cuts are to be made distal to the canines, the use of the canine bracket of the opposite side ensures that the tip incorporated into the bracket keeps the apices forward and out of the way of the surgical cuts.

The choice of archwire material and sequence is to a large extent, driven by operator preference. The use of modern "superelastic" shape-memory, nickel titanium wires is frequently beneficial for initial alignment. However, where the interbracket span is minimal, for example with mutually rotated lower incisors or premolars, the efficiency of these wires is reduced. In this situation, archwires with loops for flexibility may be preferable, for example 0.014" or 0.016" stainless steel or Titanium/Molybdenum (TMA) wires. Ultimately, heavy rectangular stainless steel archwires should be placed at the time of surgery (0.019" × 0.028" or 0.022" × 0.028") for maximal tooth control and with the addition of hooks to facilitate fixation.

Arch Levelling

The decision as to whether to fully level the arches is very much dependent on the patient's facial height and the upper lip/incisor relationship. In Class II corrections, where the facial height is reduced, it is preferable to preserve a Curve of Spee in the lower arch so that when the mandible is advanced, the lower incisors slide down the cingulum plateau of the upper incisors thereby increasing the lower facial height (Figure 4.2). Although this may occur in some Class II division 1 cases, it is especially common in patients with Class II division 2 incisor relationships where the presurgical orthodontic preparation converts the incisors into a Class II division 1 pattern.

Following surgery this results in buccal segment lateral open bites with occlusal contact in only the incisor and terminal molar regions. This tripod of contacts is referred to as a "3-point landing". The lateral open bites (Figure 4.3) require closure as part of the postsurgical orthodontic phase of treatment (see Chapter 11).

In Class II cases where the intention is to avoid increasing the facial height, the lower arch should be levelled as part of the presurgical orthodontic preparation, or by segmental surgical procedures. With a shallow curve of Spee (approximately 2 mm), it may be possible to level the arches orthodontically through a combination of buccal segment extrusion, incisor intrusion and/or incisor proclination (Figure 4.4). Levelling the Curve of Spee without space will procline the lower incisors, and reduce the potential for

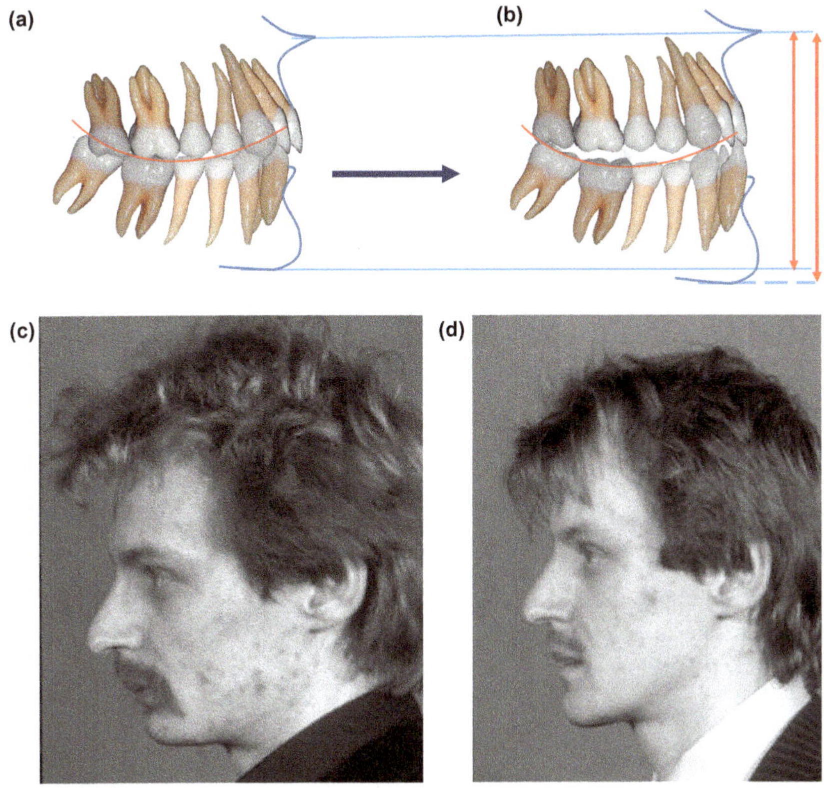

Figure 4.2 (**a**) and (**c**) Class II deep overbite cases, with an increased curve of Spee, facilitates an increase in anterior face height as the mandible is advanced (**b**) and (**d**). The resulting contact between the upper and lower incisors and the terminal molars of each side of the arch is referred to as a "3-point landing". Note the significant increase in lower facial height accompanying the advancement.

mandibular advancement. If the intention is to maintain antero-posterior arch length, then premolar extractions will be required, especially if there is any crowding present (Figure 4.5).

Segmental Levelling

a) *In cases of reduced vertical dimension*

In cases with a severe overbite the so-called "3-point landing" may produce lateral open bites which are too large to close by orthodontic

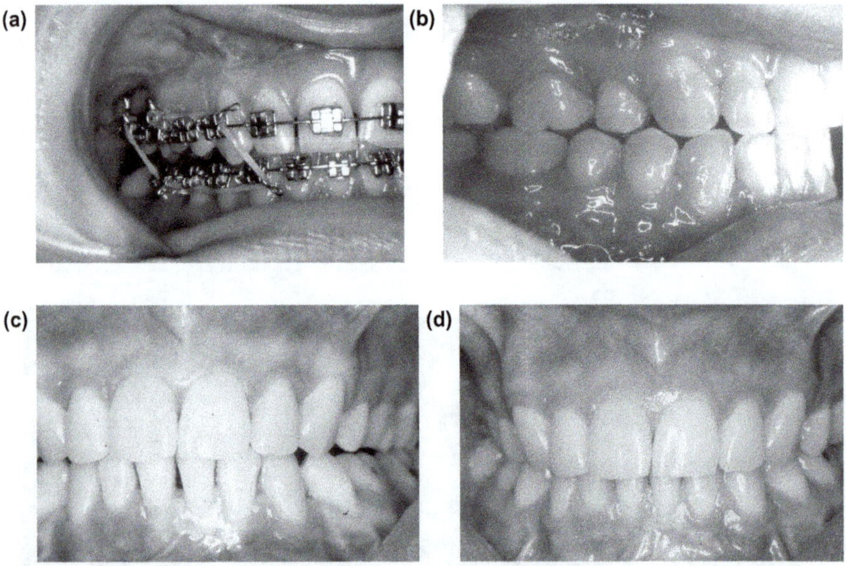

Figure 4.3 Following mandibular advancement the resulting lateral open bites can (**a**) be closed in the postoperative orthodontic phase (**b**) or may even close spontaneously (**c**) and (**d**). See also Figure 4.16.

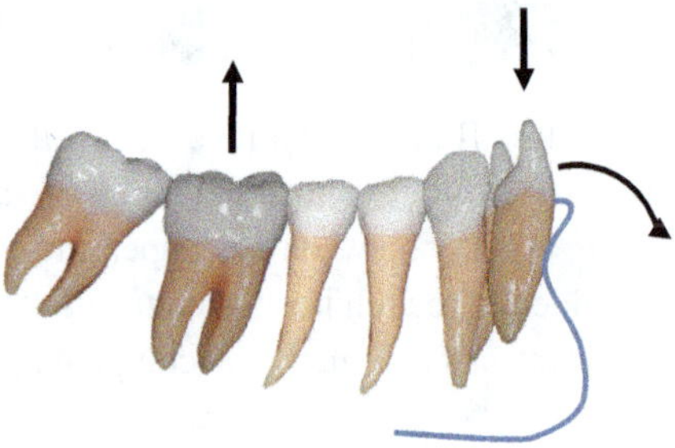

Figure 4.4 Orthodontic levelling of an increased curve of Spee can be achieved as a combination of premolar/molar extrusion, incisor intrusion or incisor proclination.

extrusion of the premolars and canines. Many operators consider 2 mm of extrusion from each arch as the absolute maximum that can be achieved and remain stable without rebound. Beyond this, levelling should be achieved through surgery, usually through a set-down

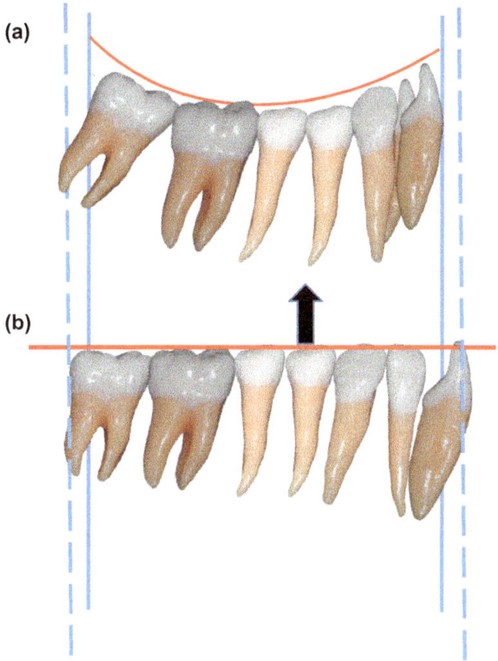

Figure 4.5 (**a**) Levelling the curve of Spee orthodontically will lead to (**b**) incisor proclination and an increase in arch length unless space is created through extractions.

of the lower labial segment with a mandibulotomy (see Chapter 11). Where there is a reverse Curve of Spee in the upper arch, as in some Class II division 2 cases, it may be necessary to undertake intrusive segmental surgery to both the upper and lower labial segments.

With all segmental surgery cases, the presurgical orthodontics should facilitate the alveolar section by diverging the canine and premolar roots. The mesiodistal tip incorporated into the canine brackets is such that the root apex will align distal to the crown encroaching into the site of the surgical cuts. When planning cases for segmental surgery it may be desirable to use the right canine bracket on the left canine and *vice versa* in order to keep the roots away from the osteotomy site. The brackets can then be replaced with those of the correct side in the postsurgical period.

Segmental orthodontic levelling is designed to place the buccal segments at one level and the incisor segments at a different level. This can be achieved by three segmental archwires, two running in the buccal segments from premolar to molar on each side together with a third segment for the canine and incisors. This approach tends to produce a lack of control of the tooth positions and therefore a continuous arch is preferred, from molar to molar but with an anterior step for the canines and incisors.

In the latter case, the surgeon will cut the archwire across the osteotomy site at the time of surgery. Although the segments are immobilised using rigid internal fixation, it is essential to provide additional fixation at the occlusal level. This can be done with a prefabricated continuous archwire bent to the planned postoperative segments. However, insertion of this wire intraoperatively can be extremely time-consuming. It is preferable to use a rigid prefabricated horseshoe shaped 1.0 mm steel supplemental arch wire, engaged passively into double or triple tubes on the molars and secured by ligatures to the three archwire segments (Figure 4.6). Ultimately, the sectional arches can be replaced with a continuous archwire once the patient has recovered.

b) *In cases of increased vertical dimension*

In anterior open bite cases, the presurgical orthodontics must not be allowed to extrude the incisors as this is potentially unstable and will jeopardise the surgical correction. Unfortunately incisor extrusion can occur all too readily, even with the initial flexible aligning archwire, and can take several visits to retrieve. Therefore, even initial alignment should be undertaken with steps incorporated into the archwire. This will dictate the choice of archwire material used. The presurgical orthodontics should then accentuate the open bite through intrusion of the labial segments and extrusion of the buccal segments. In this way maximal surgical correction can be achieved and any postsurgical incisor change will ensure closure of the anterior open bite (Figures 4.7a and 4.7b).

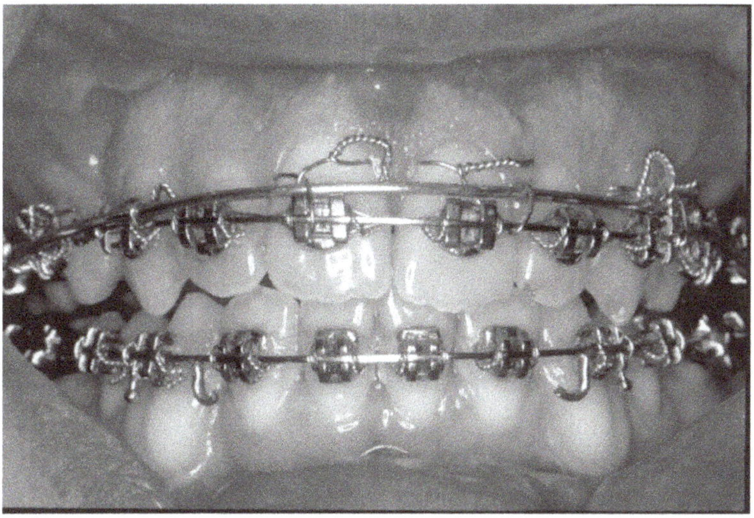

Figure 4.6 To control the occlusal relationship after segmental surgery the segmented arch (upper) is fixed at the occlusal level using a heavy 1mm stainless steel archwire. This is engaged passively into a headgear tube on the molar bands. Auxillary steel ligatures lash the segmented orthodontic archwire in the anterior and buccal segments to the heavy buccal arch.

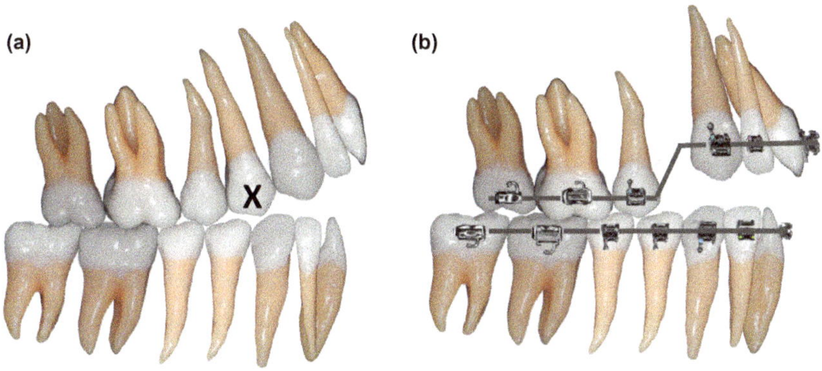

Figure 4.7 (**a**) and (**b**) Segmental orthodontic levelling of the Curve of Spee with a continuous archwire. The step in the archwire is designed to accentuate the anterior open bite by incisor intrusion and buccal segment extrusion. Any post-surgical rebound of the teeth will help maintain closure of the open bite.

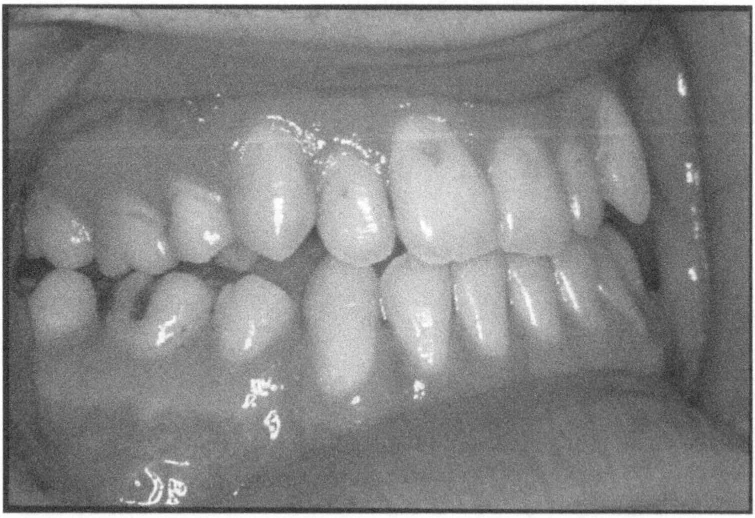

Figure 4.8 The secondary dental deformity of a prognathous mandible is the so called "compensation" with proclination of the maxillary incisors and retroclination of the mandibular incisor teeth.

Incisor Decompensation

In the majority of cases of severe antero-posterior disproportion, the soft tissues of the lips and tongue produce a secondary deformity of incisor inclination. In skeletal Class III cases, so-called compensation presents with proclined upper incisors and retroclined lower incisors (Figure 4.8). Presurgical preparation (decompensation) corrects the axial inclinations to maximise the mandibular setback (Figure 4.9). Although dictated by the amount of crowding, it is common for the lower arch to be treated non-extraction, aligning the labial segment by proclination. Care should be taken not to breach the labial alveolar plate, destroying the periodontal attachment, producing a dehiscence of the gingival margin. Periodontal grafting should be considered.

Severely crowded cases may need extractions to provide the space for arch alignment. With simultaneous decompensation of the lower incisors, the extractions of choice are the lower second

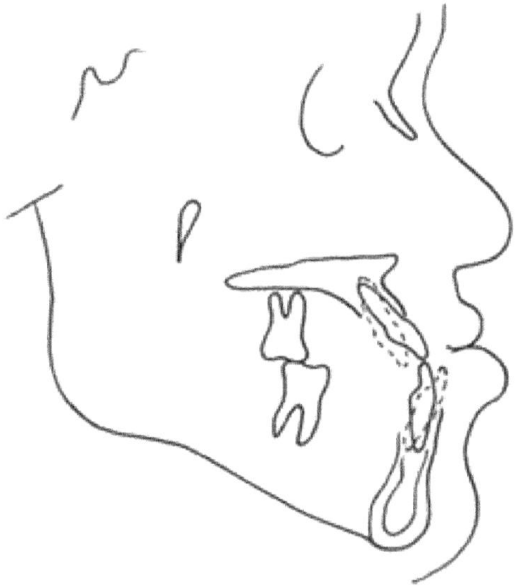

Figure 4.9 Dental "compensation" in a Class III case with proclination of the maxillary incisors and retroclination of the mandibular incisor teeth (continuous outline), compared with the ideal incisor inclination (broken outline) as seen on a lateral skull radiograph. The correction of the incisor angulation is termed decompensation.

premolars, assuming all teeth to be of good prognosis. This also adds to the anchorage balance in the lower arch through the incorporation of eight teeth in the anterior segment.

When using the pre-adjusted Edgewise brackets the orthodontist can take advantage of the mesiodistal tip incorporated into the canine bracket slot to aid lower incisor decompensation. During the alignment phase, the tip in the bracket would tend to throw the canine crown anteriorly, which in turn leads to proclination of the incisors (Figure 4.10a). Therefore the technique of "laceback" ligatures to the lower canine crown should be avoided (Figure 4.10b).

The upper incisors generally need to be retracted, a procedure, which may necessitate premolar extractions. In moderately crowded cases these will be the upper first premolars to aid the anchorage balance. In very mildly crowded cases, some would opt to move the upper arch distally using anchorage-reinforcing devices. In order to

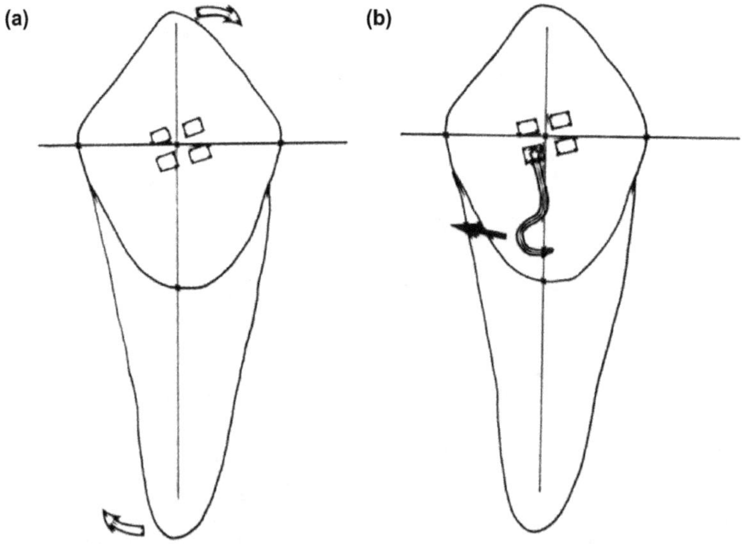

Figure 4.10 Once engaged with an initial aligning archwire, the mesiodistal tip incorporated into the mandibular canine bracket tends to throw the crown anteriorly (**a**) so aiding lower incisor decompensation in Class III cases. The technique of tying the crown back to the molar through the use of a "laceback" ligature (**b**) should be avoided in these cases.

avoid the undesirable effects of the tip incorporated into the brackets, laceback ligatures should be employed during the aligning phase. The clinician may also use Class II directed interarch elastics to aid mutual decompensation of upper and lower arches.

Most cases with an anterior open bite, require a differential posterior impaction of the maxilla. The posterior maxilla is impacted by a greater amount than the anterior segment. The effect of this surgery is to retrocline the incisors (Figure 4.11). Hence when undertaking orthodontics in this situation, the presurgical preparation may intentionally leave the upper incisors slightly proclined.

Decompensation in Class II Cases

The soft tissue influence in Class II cases is variable nevertheless the goal is to place the incisor segments at the correct inclination to

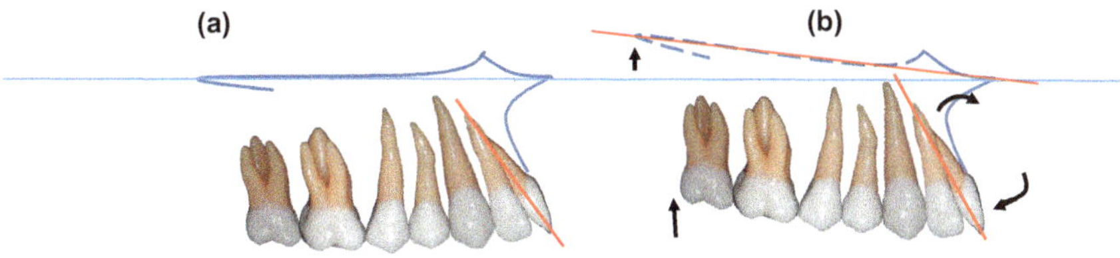

Figure 4.11 Impacting the maxilla posteriorly (dotted outline) has the effect of retroclining the maxillary incisors, and so presurgical orthodontics may intentionally leave the incisors proclined.

the dental bases. In the lower arch, the incisors may be proclined ("compensated"), in which case decompensation by retraction is indicated and usually involves premolar extractions (Figure 4.12). As in the upper arch in Class III cases, laceback ligatures will aid decompensation.

In the maxillary arch, especially in patients with a low vertical dimension, the lower lip may become trapped palatal to the upper incisors which become proclined. Presurgical preparation will involve retraction of the upper incisors back to a normal inclination. If the proclined maxillary incisors are naturally spaced, retraction may be undertaken without the need to resort to extractions. However in many cases, especially where there is crowding, the loss of premolars is indicated.

Arch Coordination

Anteroposterior changes in skeletal relationships frequently require an alteration in the transverse widths of the arches for coordination, especially expansion of the upper arch. Whether this can be achieved by orthodontics alone, or through a combination of orthodontics and surgery depends upon:

- the amount of expansion required;
- the initial inclination of the buccal segment dentition;
- the relative degree of expansion required throughout the buccal segments.

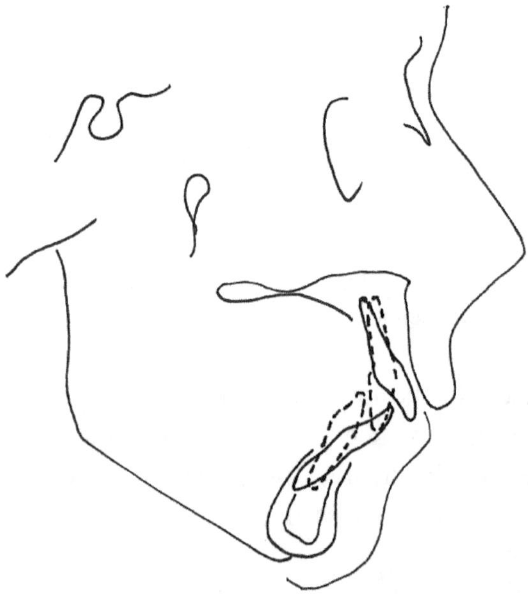

Figure 4.12 Decompensation in Class II cases will depend on the position of the incisors, which in most cases require retroclining in both upper and lower arches. Here shown as moving from the continuous to the broken outlines.

Orthodontic expansion is achieved by tipping movement. Where the teeth are initially tipped palatally, uprighting will allow a good dental interdigitation, which is important for stability. Where the buccal teeth are either upright or even already flared buccally, further expansion will not produce a satisfactory stable occlusion. In such cases surgical expansion is required (see Chapter 11).

Methods of Orthodontic Arch Expansion

Quadhelix

The quadhelix appliance is the most frequently used appliance for expanding the maxillary dentition (Figure 4.13a). Although producing an overall tipping movement, it has the advantage of enabling differential expansion within the buccal segments.

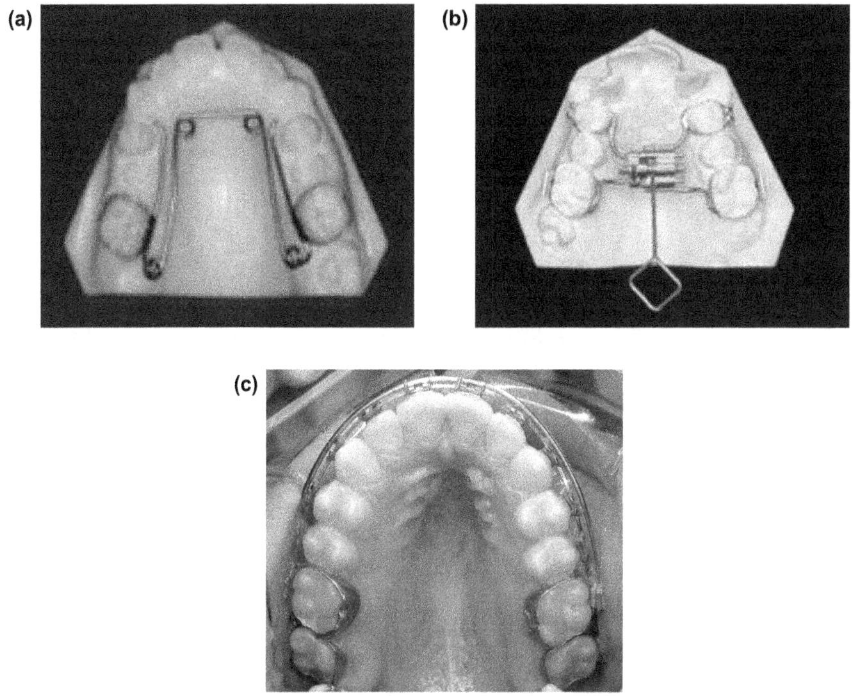

Figure 4.13 Examples of arch expansion methods: (**a**) quadhelix, (**b**) hyrax screw, and (**c**) auxillary expansion arch engaged in headgear tubes on molar bands.

Hyrax Screw

The hyrax screw (Figure 4.13b) is principally used for expansion prior to the fusion of the mid-palatal suture. The age at which this occurs may vary but it is usually complete by 21 years. Some suggest that the mechanism of expansion is more bodily movement rather than tipping in nature although this has been questioned.

Expansion Arch

Minor degrees of tooth movement can be achieved through expansion with a rectangular orthodontic archwire (usually of 0.018×0.025 minimum size). Use of a rectangular wire enables active buccal root torque to be placed in the buccal segments of the wire in order to achieve a positive overbite of the buccal cusps. Occasionally, the rectangular archwire can be used in conjunction with a 1 mm rigid and expanded stainless steel arch fitted into the headgear tubes of the upper molars (Figure 4.13c).

Alternative Arch Expanders

The development of Nickel/Titanium materials has led to an array of expansion devices which incorporate the shape/memory and superelasticity properties of these materials.

Monitoring Arch Coordination During Treatment

When preparing the arches for correction of Class II problems, testing of arch co-ordination in the transverse dimension can be achieved by simple forward posturing of the mandible. In Class III corrections the use of an acrylic template of the occlusal surfaces of the lower arch is invaluable. The template can be prepared by taking an alginate impression of the aligned lower arch and pouring cold cure acrylic resin into the occlusal portion of the impression. At successive visits, the template of the lower arch can then be occluded with the upper arch to check compatibility and avoid the need for repeated study models (Figure 4.14).

Facilitating Surgical Correction

Towards the end of the presurgical phase, upper and lower rectangular archwires should be in position and surgical hooks or soldered brass wires are added in the midline and throughout the buccal segments (Figure 4.15). These provide a means of attaching temporary intermaxillary fixation during surgery. They can also be used to attach seating elastics or intermaxillary elastics during the immediate postoperative period.

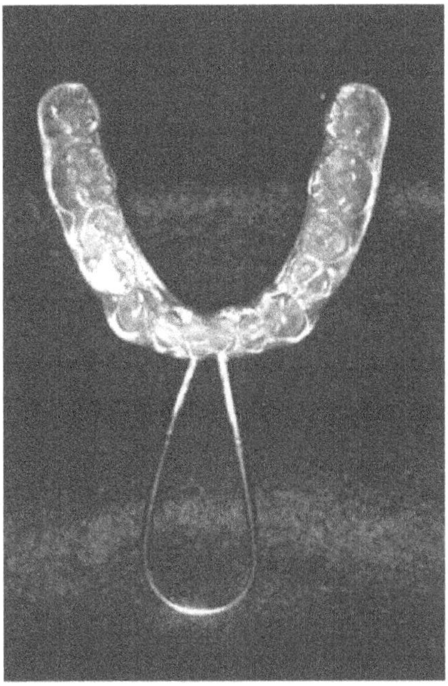

Figure 4.14 An acrylic template of the aligned lower arch can be used to check coordination with the upper arch expansion at successive visits.

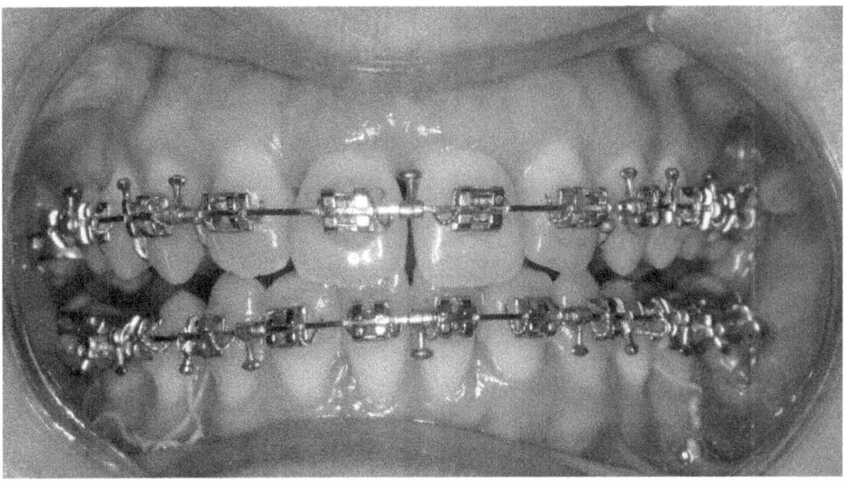

Figure 4.15 Rectangular archwires with surgical hooks. Note the archwires are engaged in the brackets using stainless steel ligatures.

Postsurgical Orthodontics

The goals of postsurgical orthodontics are to refine the occlusion, ensure a balanced occlusion and to plan the retention regime.

In cases of segmental surgery, where canine brackets have been reversed preoperatively, it is necessary to re-bond the canine brackets, placing brackets of the correct side in order to produce a normal canine angulation.

Postsurgical settling of a "3-point landing" usually involves a combination of flexible archwires together with vertical intra-oral seating elastics between the upper and lower arches (Figures 4.16a and 4.16b). Where the maxillary arch is level, a rigid upper rectangular archwire is maintained whereas a flexible wire, for example a braided steel wire, can be placed in the lower arch. When both arches need extrusion, the rectangular wires can be sectioned and seating elastics applied between the segments.

Retention

As in routine orthodontics, the tooth movements undertaken as part of orthognathic surgery require a period of retention following removal of the fixed appliances. This is to allow the alveolar bone and periodontal tissues to consolidate. Where there has been correction of incisor rotations or closure of large spaces, a permanent fixed bonded lingual or palatal retainer is employed. In other cases, a removable retainer of varying designs may be used. In general, it is good practice to avoid any retainer wirework passing through embrasures where extraction spaces have been closed (Figure 4.17).

(a)

(b)

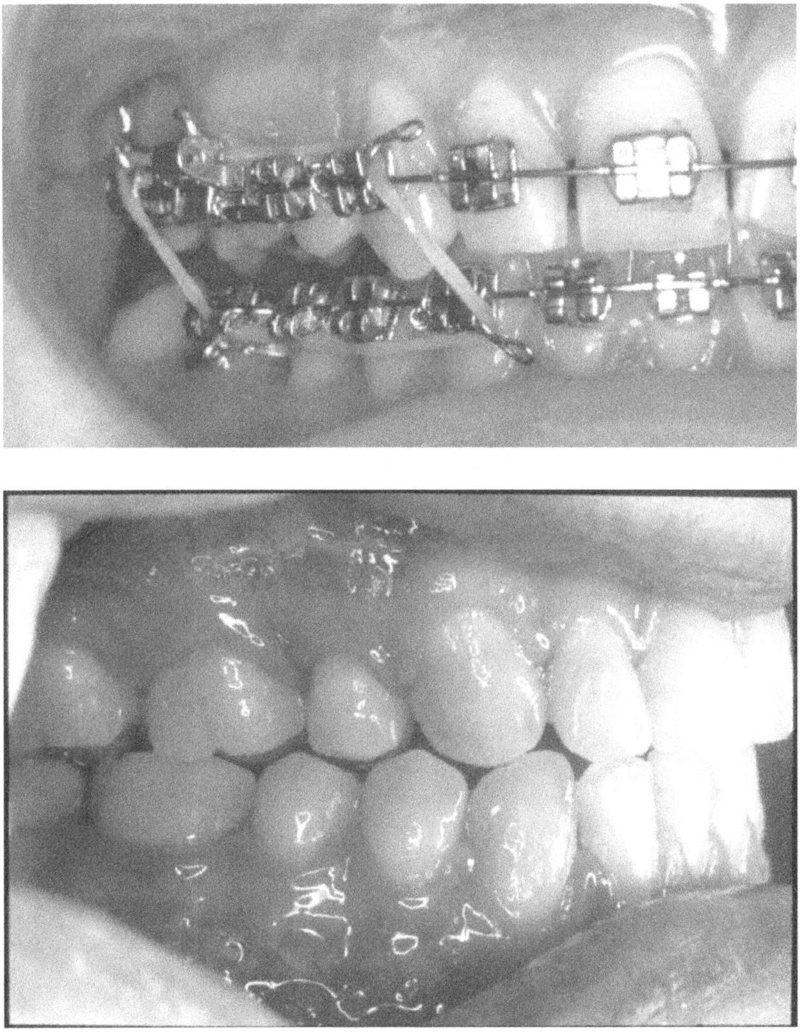

Figure 4.16 Closure of a lateral open-bite using postoperative intraoral elastics.

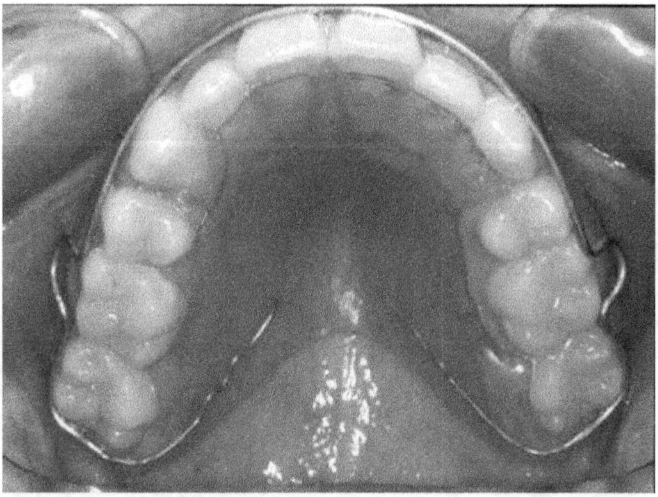

Figure 4.17 A removable retainer designed to avoid wirework passing through previously closed extraction sites.

Chapter 5

The Definitive Treatment Plan

Malcolm Harris and Nigel Hunt

Treatment planning can only be undertaken after a thorough history and clinical examination of the patient, together with an analysis of the radiographs and study casts.

Manual Planning of the Maxillary Move

The key to successful surgery is to place the maxilla and the decompensated maxillary incisors in the optimum anteroposterior and vertical position in relation to the upper lip and face. The orthodontically corrected mandible is then placed in a Class I incisor relationship to the maxilla.

The profile of the seated patient is assessed with the Frankfort plane horizontal to decide the horizontal anteroposterior movement of the maxilla.

Changes of the naso-labial angle can be predicted with a moist cotton roll or soft pink wax. **The frontal view** is assessed by:

i) The ratio of the cephalometric upper to lower facial height — 45:55%.

ii) The incisor exposure with the lips parted at rest — will decide the vertical movement of the maxilla. Aesthetic exposure may vary from 1 to 4 mm. This is inversely proportional to the upper lip length which ranges from 20–25 mm.

iii) Excessive or unaesthetic incisor exposure is corrected with the estimated maxillary impaction.

iv) Where the upper lip is unduly short, the patient can show a greater amount of incisor. If not, the resulting midfacial appearance will be disproportionately small in the vertical dimension.

v) Rarely the patient has marked dento-alveolar hypoplasia and shows little or no incisor with a normal lip length. This is corrected with an inferior movement of the anterior maxilla.

vi) Horizontal maxillary movements will also affect the incisor exposure. The advanced maxilla will lead to greater incisor exposure which will need to be adjusted for when considering the vertical move.

vii) Coronal occlusal cants and minor midline rotations must also be corrected at this stage.

viii) Moving the maxilla will affect the nose. Vertical impaction widens the alar base and forward movements will elevate the nasal tip. Depending upon the initial appearance these changes may or may not be desirable. If not, then a record should be made to provide a "cinch suture" across the lateral alar cartilages or to reduce the anterior nasal spine at the time of surgery.

ix) The inherent inaccuracy of the planning and surgical techniques and the eye's inability to perceive small anatomical changes, determine the most reliable units of horizontal advancement should be no less than 3 mm. This also facilitates planning as a 3 mm minor advancement; a 6 mm intermediate; and a 9 mm major move. Cleft cases usually require 9 mm or more.

x) Similarly vertical moves of 2 mm for minor; 4 mm intermediate and 6 mm for major impactions are appropriate for all cases. These three categories simplify the decision making process.

Planning the Mandibular Move

- Having planned where the maxilla is to be placed, the next step is to place the mandible in a Class I incisor relationship. This is built into the final wafer.
- If the definitive occlusion is not immediately possible and requires further orthodontics or restorative treatment, the wafer maintains the jaw relationship until orthodontics or restorative treatment can be commenced.
- The repositioned mandible may result from autorotation, antero-posterior, vertical, axial rotational or rarely transverse movements.

Autorotation

Any changes in the vertical and horizontal position of the maxilla will necessitate a change in the vertical position of the mandible. This is mediated naturally through neuromuscular feedback mechanisms and the mandibular elevator muscles. Impacting the maxilla will lead to a shortening of the elevator muscles and will re-establish the freeway space. This closing autorotation of the mandible will also lead to a greater anterior prominence of the lower jaw.

Anterior Movements

The downward and forward movement of the mandible to establish a Class I incisor relationship in Class II cases, will also increase lower face height. This is particularly the case with a deep overbite, when advancing the mandible without levelling the curve of Spee. The vertical facial height will increase and the everted lip will unroll and upright. The consequent lateral open bites needs to be closed with postsurgical orthodontics to a stable position. If too severe for orthodontic closure, then surgery must incorporate a levelling of the occlusal plane with an anterior mandibulotomy setdown procedure.

Posterior Movements

Mandibular setbacks will reduce the anterior facial height and evert the lip. Occasionally this may correct the occlusion but reduce the chin prominence which will require a genioplasty advancement.

Horizontal Rotation

A horizontal rotation is required in asymmetry cases, for example hemimandibular elongation where this needs arch coordination especially with an adequate maxillary intercanine width.

Chin Position

Both anteroposterior and vertical movements of the mandible will affect the position of the chin. It is important that the final chin profile be carefully predicted to avoid further surgery.

A common example is the need to correct a Class II division 1 malocclusion by a mandubular advancement which invariably leaves the patient with a deficient chin requiring a simultaneous advancement genioplasty.

With rare excess chin depth a combination of a vertical reduction and anterior sliding genioplasty helps provide a harmonious and balanced appearance.

Planning based on cephalometric assessment and the study model analysis.

Cephalometric Tracing Planning

The movements of the maxilla based on the clinical prediction of the incisor position, can then be repeated on a digital image or tracing of the patient's lateral cephalometric radiograph. Many still prefer to undertake this tracing procedure by hand although cephalometric software packages are available (see Chapter 3). When planning using hand tracing it is important to trace all the teeth in order to avoid missing potential premature contacts which may interfere with the planned movements.

Having traced the revised maxillary position, the next step is to autorotate the mandibular tracing into the initial contact position. In reality, mandibular autorotation is not a simple hinge but a 3-dimensional movement with an envelope of adjustment within the temporomandibular joint. Despite this, it is useful to use as a 2-dimensional tracing despite its uncertainty as to the true centre of rotation. Some use the centre of the condyle, others use the point "condylion" whilst geometric constructions suggest that the point of rotation lies in the region of the mastoid air cells. Despite these differences the mandible in life appears to have an adequate envelope of condylar movement to adapt to crude planning geometry.

Assessment of the incisor position of the autorotated mandible is also important to determine if further adjustment of the maxillary position is required in order to establish a positive overbite.

1. With an anterior open bite autorotation leads to initial buccal segment contact. Closure of the residual anterior open bite by (anticlockwise) rotation of the mandible around this posterior pivot will lead to an elongation of the pterygo-masseteric sling and relapse. In such cases it is essential to impact the posterior part of the maxilla differentially to that of the anterior maxilla. The extent of the differential impaction can be ascertained from the tracing.
2. With impactions for vertical maxillary excess, any minor incisor discrepancy on simple autorotation can be overcome by forward or backward adjusted movement of the maxilla. A significant discrepancy will require a bimaxillary procedure to achieve the incisor Class I relationship without compromising the upper lip incisor relationship.

3. Finally, the predicted profile can then be drawn on the composite planning tracing although this requires an estimate of the facial soft to hard tissue movements.

Imaging Simulations

The use of computerised software packages and the morphing of facial images as a means of planning the dental and surgical moves, together with the display of the predicted surgical outcome have been covered in Chapters 3 and 7.

Chapter 6

The Recording and Transfer of Orthognathic Planning Data

Mohammad Anwar Bamber and Edwin Payne

Introduction

Orthognathic surgery involves three-dimensional movements based on non-surgical and surgical procedures. This is particularly evident in osteotomies which change the occlusal level.

The main planning concerns are:

- prediction of the tooth, bone and soft tissue changes,
- the operative reproduction of the treatment plan,
- postoperative dentoskeletal stability.

Confounding factors are:

a) planning data transfer inadequacies,
b) the adaptation of the temporomandibular joints,
c) diversity of surgical skills, and
d) relapse forces.

The conventional preoperative planning process has the following 10 stages, which are gradually being replaced by computerised virtual planning. This follows in **Chapter 7**.

- clinical estimated measurements,
- impressions,
- occlusal record (squash bite),
- face bow registration,
- face bow transfer to the articulator and mounting of the maxillary model,
- mounting of the mandibular model,
- maxillary model surgery,
- intermediate occlusal wafer fabrication,
- mandibular model surgery, and
- final occlusal wafer fabrication.

These ten processes despite care are subject to inaccuracies. With a single jaw mandibular osteotomy, precise model surgery planning using a facebow and anatomical articulator may not be required. However, all maxillary and bimaxillary procedures require an accurate transfer of the jaw relationship to the articulator, for surgical control.

The Planning Process

1. *Clinical Measurements*

There are inherent difficulties in accurately recording the clinical data. For instance patients may camouflage an occlusal cant by tilting the head and many Class II division 1 patients posture their mandible forwards. There are also important occlusal changes due to the effects of gravity in the conscious patient compared to the loss of muscle tone in the anaesthetised patient.

2. *Impression Procedure*

a) The impression procedure is more demanding than for standard impressions for dental appliances. Apart from the jaw deformity, malocclusion and postural camouflage, the presence of orthodontic brackets create a challenge for the inexperienced. It is important that the orthdodontic archwire is passive in the brackets at the time of taking the impressions.
b) The impressions must be taken as near to the surgery as possible. Soft red wax is applied on the gingival side of the orthodontic brackets to avoid splitting adherent alginate. Avoid the application or flow of wax onto the occlusal side of the bracket which can obliterate the occlusion. Two full upper and lower impressions which detail all the teeth are taken using irreversible hydrocolloid impression material (Claudius Ash. UK). It is essential to include the terminal cusps of the most posterior molars as failure to record these could lead to unplanned prematurities in occlusal contact at the time of surgery. The impressions are cast in Crystacal R Class III stone plaster (Newark Works, Bowbridge Lane, Newark, Nottinghamshire) and based in plaster (British Gypsum). One set of models is anatomically trimmed for model surgery (Figure 6.1a) and the second angle trimmed as study models (Figure 6.1b).

3. *Recording the Occlusal Relationship*

The dental occlusion is dynamic with a three-dimensional envelope of movement which will change with altered patterns of neuromuscular function such as, postural habits, gravity, the level of consciousness and even psychiatric factors. It is crucial to recognise that preoperative planning is conventionally done on a conscious upright patient using centric occlusal records (CO), i.e maximal intercuspation in the X axis, despite the osteotomy taking place with the mandible in an anaesthetised supine centric relation position

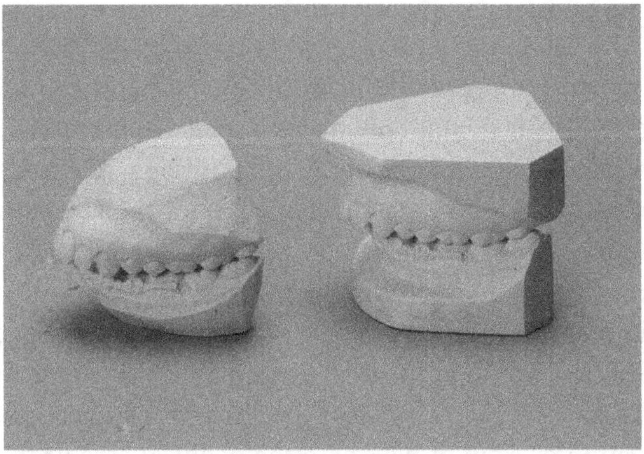

Figure 6.1 (**a**) Upper and lower models after removing non-anatomical parts, ready to articulate. (**b**) Standard angle trimmed study models.

(CR), i.e the occlusal retruded position in the Y-axis (Figures 6.2a and 6.2b).

A significant difference between the conscious upright CO and supine anaesthetised CR will produce unexpected discrepancies between the planned and postoperative occlusion, for instance when the osteotomised maxilla is temporarily fixed to the unoperated mandible and rotated upwards and forwards into its planned position for plate fixation. The anaesthetised mandibular CR will give rise to a loss of maxillary advancement which is seen when the patient wakes and sits up with the mandible recoiling forwards.

This may not be apparent in the bimaxillary procedure as the osteotomised mandible is then related to the previously fixed maxilla.

Conversely with a Class III mandibular setback there will be a loss of push back with the conscious upright recoil (Figures 6.3a and 6.3b). This is beneficial in a Class II division 1 mandibular advancement and helps to compensate for any distal relapse.

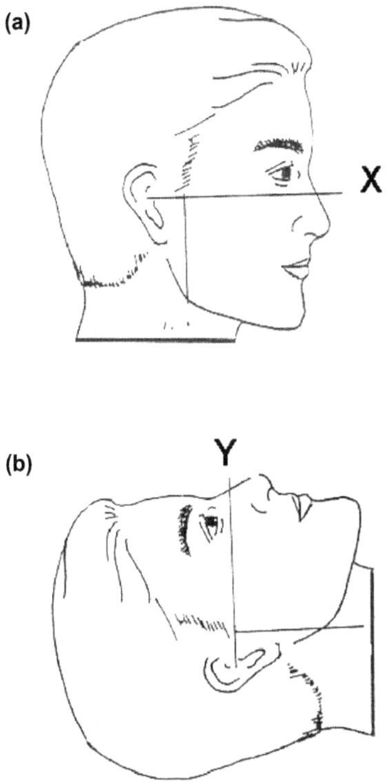

Figure 6.2 (**a**) and (**b**) Osteotomies are planned in the upright X-axis but carried out in a supine anaesthetised Y-axis.

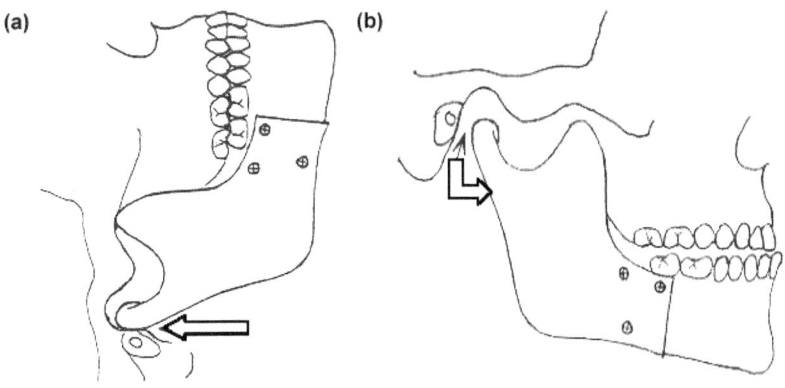

Figure 6.3 (**a**) Fixation in supine and (**b**) occlusion when upright.

To avoid these potential problems the osteotomy should be planned from the CR occlusal registration, taken in a relaxed supine patient. Any minor residual CO-CR discrepancies are usually compensated for by proprioceptive adaptation within the envelope of movement of the condyle-disc-fossa relationship.

The Registration of Supine Centric Relation

Centric relation is recorded using the bilateral manipulation technique, with the patient in a relaxed supine position and the operator seated behind and with the patient's head between the two arms. The operator supports the patient's mandible bilaterally by placing the fingers of each hand below the lower border of the mandible on each side and the thumbs in the depression of the labiomental fold (Figure 6.4). This technique emphasises the "posterior" placement of the condyles in the fossae. With the softened wax occlusal wafer in place the mandible is then guided into the centric relation position.

Appreciation of this plasticity of the condyle-disc-fossa relationship is essential in orthognathic surgery planning.

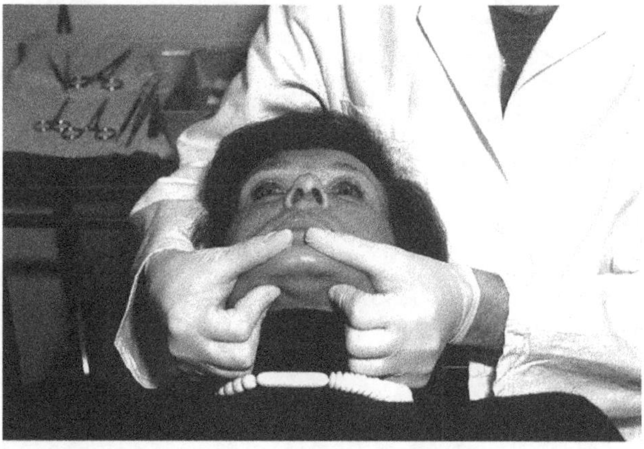

Figure 6.4 The centric jaw relation recording in supine conscious posture using bilateral manipulation technique.

4. *Facebow Recording*

a) The facebow is designed to record the relationship of the maxilla to the terminal hinge axis of the patient's mandibular condyles and a Frankfort-like plane. When transferred to the articulator this becomes the relationship of the maxillary cast to the condylar assemblies of an articulator. Although this axis can vary with posture, when carefully standardised, the facebow/articulator transfer method has proved to be reproducible for orthognathic planning.

  a) The Denar and similar systems are clinically reliable except where there is gross facial asymmetry. It has a facial reference point of 43 mm above the lateral incisor edge which defines the anterior point on an arbitrary plane within the maxilla (Figure 6.5). The posterior reference point of this plane is the

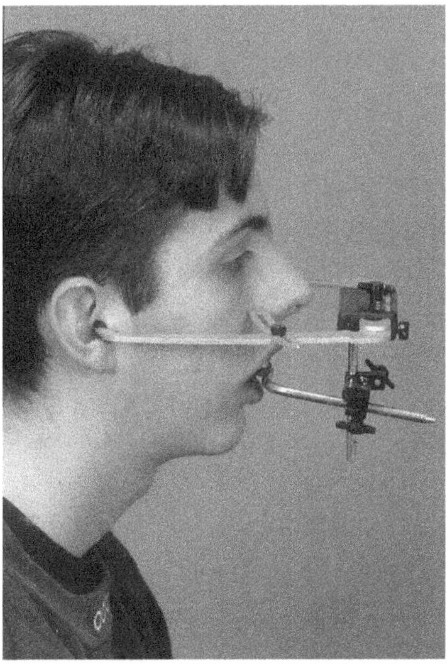

Figure 6.5 Clinical picture of Denar Slidematic facebow with ear plugs for hinge axis point and an anterior reference point 43 mm above central incisor.

bony margin of the external auditory meatus, conveniently located by the facebow earplugs.

Although careful facebow registration shows a high degree of accuracy in the vertical plane there is variation in the horizontal plane which together with the eight other variables in the transfer process, may invalidate small planning movements. Similarly small variations cannot be controlled surgically or perceived by the eye. For this reason forward and backward movements of the maxilla are most reliably planned in 3 mm units which also simplifies clinical decision making when translated into minor 3 mm, moderate 6 mm and major 9 mm moves. Similarly vertical movements are more accurately estimated as 2, 4 or 6 mm. impactions again representing the correction of minor, intermediate and major defects. The exception to this "3-unit rule" is the cleft palate case with a major iatrogenic disturbance to facial growth.

b) The facebow registration procedure: Facebow ear pieces are placed into the external auditory meati and manipulated until the subject feels equal pressure in both ears. The anterior reference pointer is adjusted to the pre-determined reference mark 43 mm above the incisal edge of the right maxillary lateral incisor and the transfer jig screws are tightened (Figure 6.5).

The facebow bite fork occlussal registration can be taken using a silicon based material which gives precise definition of the occlusal surfaces (Figure 6.6a) and can be easily trimmed with a scalpel should the material inadvertently encapsulate the orthodontic brackets.

Prior to mounting the upper and lower models, silicon moulds of the master casts/models can be prepared (Figure 6.6b). This enables copies of the models to be prepared should damage occur during the construction of the splints and for one set to be kept in the patient's study model box for record purposes.

(a)

(b)

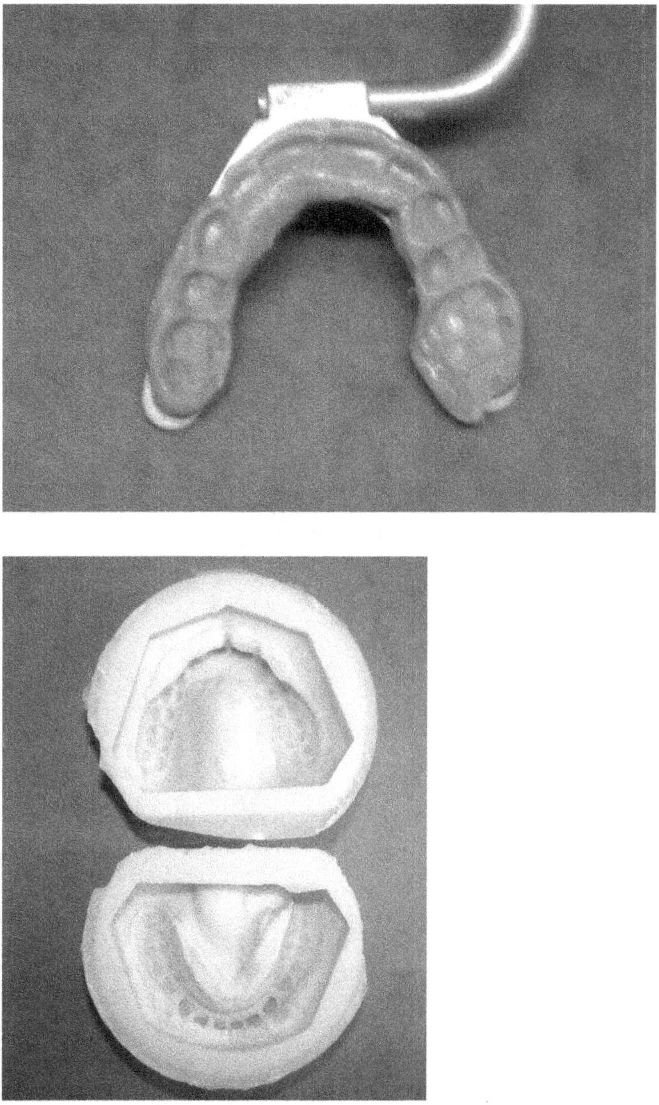

Figure 6.6 (**a**) Silicon bite fork registration. (**b**) Silicon mould of master models for duplication and record keeping.

5. Facebow Transfer to the Articulator and the Mounting of the Casts

Only the Denar transfer jig and bite fork need to be sent to the laboratory, the facebow does not have to leave the clinic. Unless the procedure is carried out very carefully, errors can be introduced when seating the cast into the bite fork indentation and during the subsequent mounting

Using a small amount of dental plaster mixed with an anti-expansion solution (Alan Pharmaceuticals Ltd., London) the maxillary model is mounted on the articulator (Figure 6.7a).

(a)

(b)

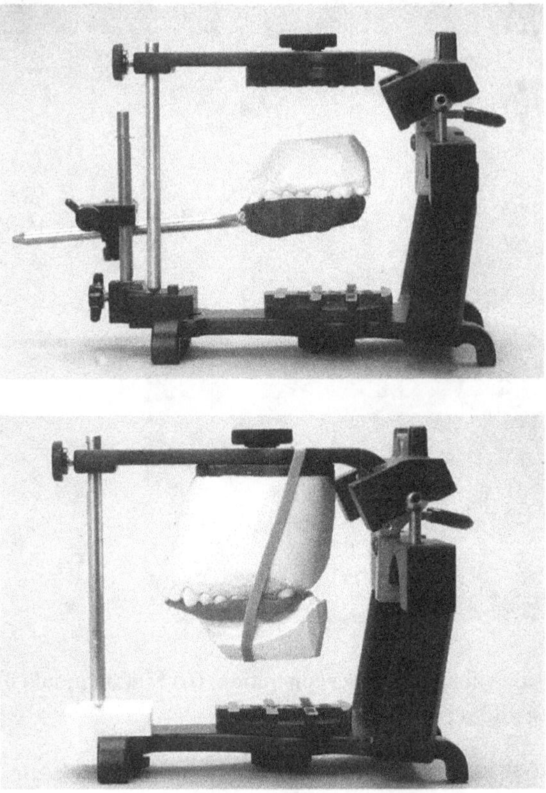

Figure 6.7 (**a**) The Denar facebow transfer jig assembled in an articulator with upper cast ready to be mounted. (**b**) Lower cast ready to be mounted in the Denar articulator.

This is followed by mounting the mandibular cast using the supine centric relation record (Figure 6.7b). The models are mounted in two stages; firstly using plaster mixed with anti-expansion solution as described, to eliminate any potential distortion. When set, the models together with their respective assembly plates are removed from the articulator and "anatomically" shaped with vacuum mixed white plaster in plain water.

The upright centric occlusal record is used for articulation of the study models.

Facial Asymmetry

The planning and correction of transverse occlusal plane asymmetry can be a challenge. Unfortunately articulators, facebows and cephalostats are designed for symmetrical faces.

With a facebow record, the patient's anatomical hinge axis (the external auditory meati) determine the orientation of the maxillary cast within the articulator. If this anatomic hinge axis is at right angles to the mid-sagittal plane, the resulting articulator model assembly will accurately represent the facial midline of the patient in an upright position (Figure 6.8).

With an asymmetrical face or external auditory meati, the patient's eccentric anatomical hinge axis will be transferred by the facebow to the articulator but made to coincide with its horizontal mechanical hinge axis (Figure 6.9a). This will rotate the maxilla in the articulator space and so the facial and the dental midlines will not coincide with the articulator incisal pin. When due to asymmetrical external auditory meati, a pseudocant will suggest the need to correct a facial midline discrepancy, which does not exist (Figures 6.9b and 6.9c). For this reason it is very important that the patient's facial midline is recorded clinically and independently of the facebow with a facial midline jig, and transferred to the articulated models for the preoperative work-up. Figure 6.9c shows how the inferiorly placed left ear has been recorded as a pseudocant with the true midline traced obliquely to the left.

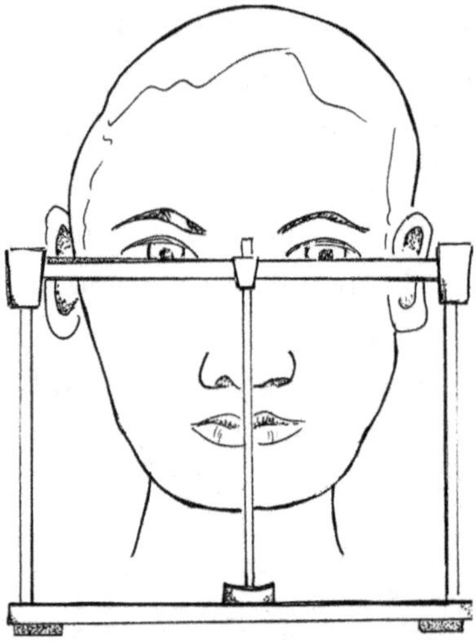

Figure 6.8 Symmetrical ears give symmetrical alignment with facebow recording.

Planning is done supporting the articulator in space to render the midline vertical.

The anatomical structures used to record the vertical facial midline are:

(i) from the centre of the glabella to the centre of the chin, unless the chin is deviated to one side with adhesive discs or a water soluble pen;
(ii) the centre of the philtrum unless it is deformed; and
(iii) a right angle to the interpupillary line at a point midway between the pupils when the patient is looking directly forward (Figures 6.10a and 6.10b).

The Transfer of the Facebow Record of a Maxillary Asymmetry

The facebow record is taken with the midline mark on the facebow bite fork matching the patient's facial midline, not the dental midline. With asymmetry a facial midline indicator (FMI) jig is

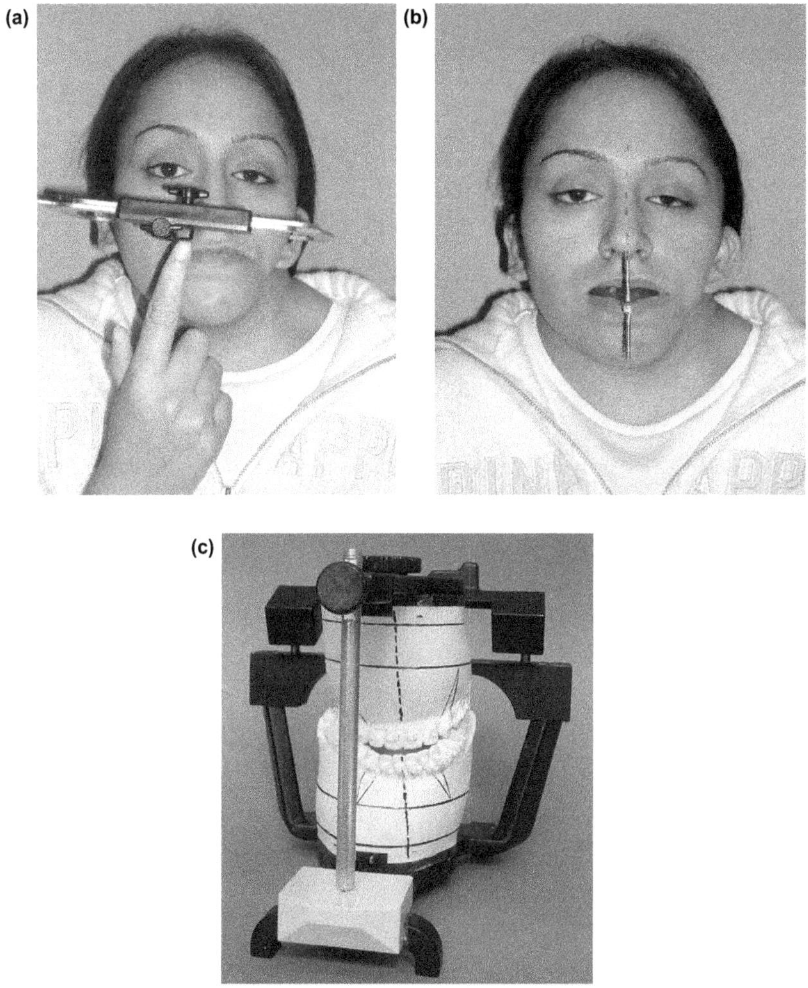

Figure 6.9 (**a**) Asymmetrical ears would give asymmetrical recording when using a standard facebow transfer. (**b**) The midline jig records the true facial midline. (**c**) The ear asymmetry is reflected in the mounted models as a pseudo cant when using the facebow record.

used which has a U shaped nickel silver wire tray, to take composition, silicon or wax, similar to a facebow bite fork. Its extraoral extension has two parallel vertical bars to register the long axis of the face. Each bar has notches on the upper and lower ends to help

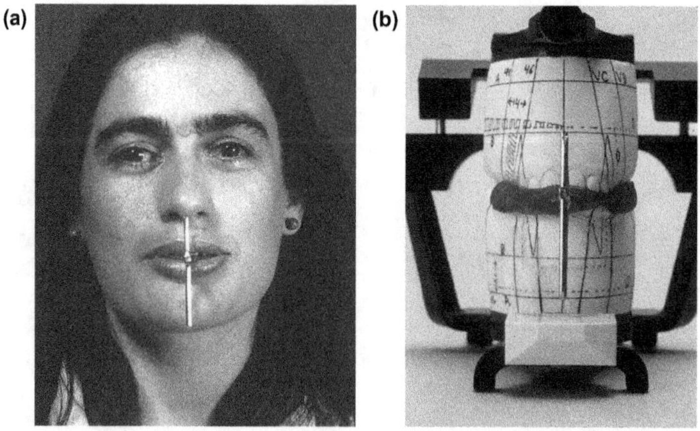

Figure 6.10 (**a**) Clinical picture of a midline jig in use with facial midline marker. (**b**) Jig transfer of midline to articulated models.

to align them to the facial midline (Figures 6.11a to 6.11d). Wax or composition is softened and applied to the U shaped part of the jig. While soft, the jig is placed in the mouth and the patient asked to close slowly into centric occlusion while the operator adjusts the vertical bars so that they match exactly the patients facial midline (Figure 6.10a). Heavy body silicon can also be used. When the material has set the jig is removed from the mouth and chilled.

The dental casts are mounted in the articulator using the face-bow record. The jig is then located by the impression of the cast teeth. Using the notches on the parallel vertical bars two reference points are marked on the surfaces of upper and lower mounting assembly plaster work. A third reference point is then taken from the facebow bite fork midline mark and the facial midline is drawn, using these three reference points, from the upper mounting plate A line to the lower mounting plate A line (Figures 6.10 and 6.12). This line represents the patient's true facial midline and the long axis of the face. This jig is an invaluable device, which

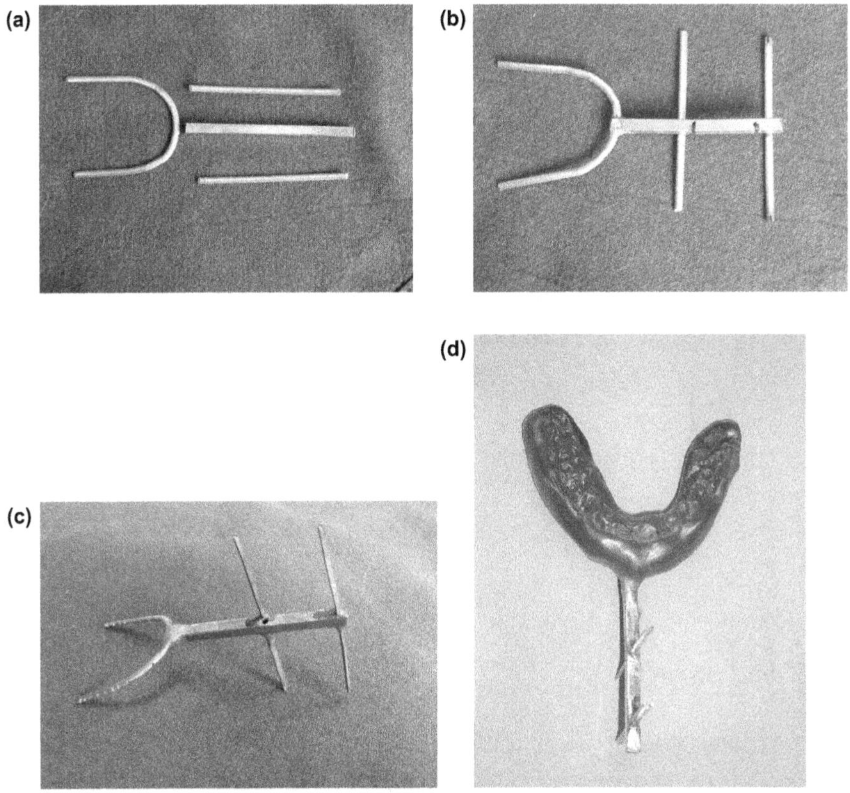

Figure 6.11 Midline jig: (**a**) Components: 4 mm nickel silver (NS) tube and 3 mm oval wire. (**b**) 3 mm oval NS wire is bent into a U shape and soldered on the end of the 4 mm NS tube, and two 3 mm NS wires with V cut are ready to be soldered on the tube at right angle to the U shape bite fork. (**c**) Midline jig with all components soldered together (**d**) with wax squash bite.

facilitates the correction of the maxillary midline and occlusal cant with accuracy. Figure 6.10 shows a true occlusal cant with a symmetrical face. The maxillary model shows the planned bone removal to level the occlusion. Figures 6.9 and 6.12 are both pseudocants where the occlusal plane is at right angles to the midline jig alignment.

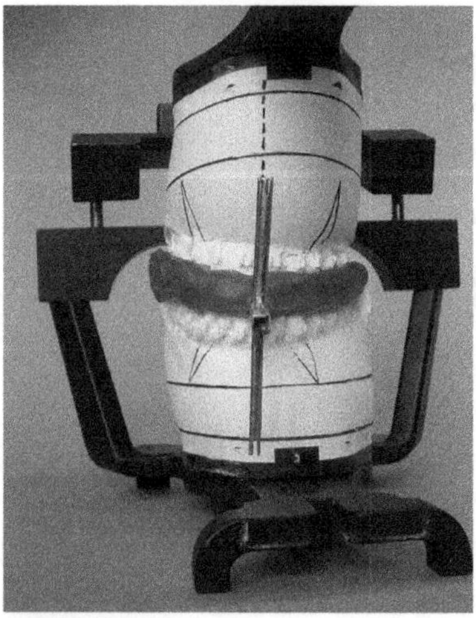

Figure 6.12 The midline jig is transferred to the articulator for midline cast marking.

6. *Model Surgery*

Bimaxillary surgery is usually sequenced with the maxilla mobilised and repositioned first although some surgeons correct the mandible at the outset. Regardless of which jaw, it is imperative that it is planned accurately because once fixed, it becomes the basis for repositioning the other jaw. For example a false asymmetrical maxilla will show itself by asymmetry of the mandible.

The following are important.

a) Midline dental discrepancies or an occlusal cant are corrected to the facial midline as drawn on the articulated models from the midline jig and not the articulator pin (Figure 6.9c).
b) The angular relationship of the occlusal to the Frankfort horizontal plane;

   ($8° \pm 4°$) is also important in treatment planning.
   Changes in the occlusal plane angle are used to

i) close an anterior open bite and
ii) retrocline maxillary incisal inclination.

In both cases the amount of occlusal plane alteration be carefully estimated clinically and radiolographically and then carried out on the articulated models.

c) Model Surgery Technique (Figures 6.13a to 6.13e)

- The preoperative relationships of the maxillary and mandibular models are recorded by horizontal lines (A, B and O) and vertical lines.
- The A lines are within half a centimetre of their mounting plates and the B line is at the estimated apices of the canines (Figure 6.13a).
- The O line (Figure 6.13b) is drawn to represent the site of the estimated osteotomy cut. The vertical lines are drawn through the following reference points: VM, molar buccal cusp tip; VB, buccal cusp tip of the second bicuspid; VC, canine cusp tip; and VF, interincisal edge or marker of the facial midline. The distance from each cusp reference point to its A line and the transpalatal intercanine and intermolar distances are measured with a Vernier calliper and metal ruler or Ericsson model platform and recorded on the models (Figures 6.13c to 6.13e).
- The model is cut at the O osteotomy line with a hand or electric saw, and where a vertical impaction is to be carried out, the required amount of plaster is removed with the saw or electric sander to achieve the planned jaw movements. The segments are assembled in the postoperative position using red ribbon wax, which allows easy manipulation into the required position. When the final position is achieved the red soft wax is replaced with sticky wax. If any adjustments are necessary the wax can be softened and the maxillary or mandibular segments repositioned.

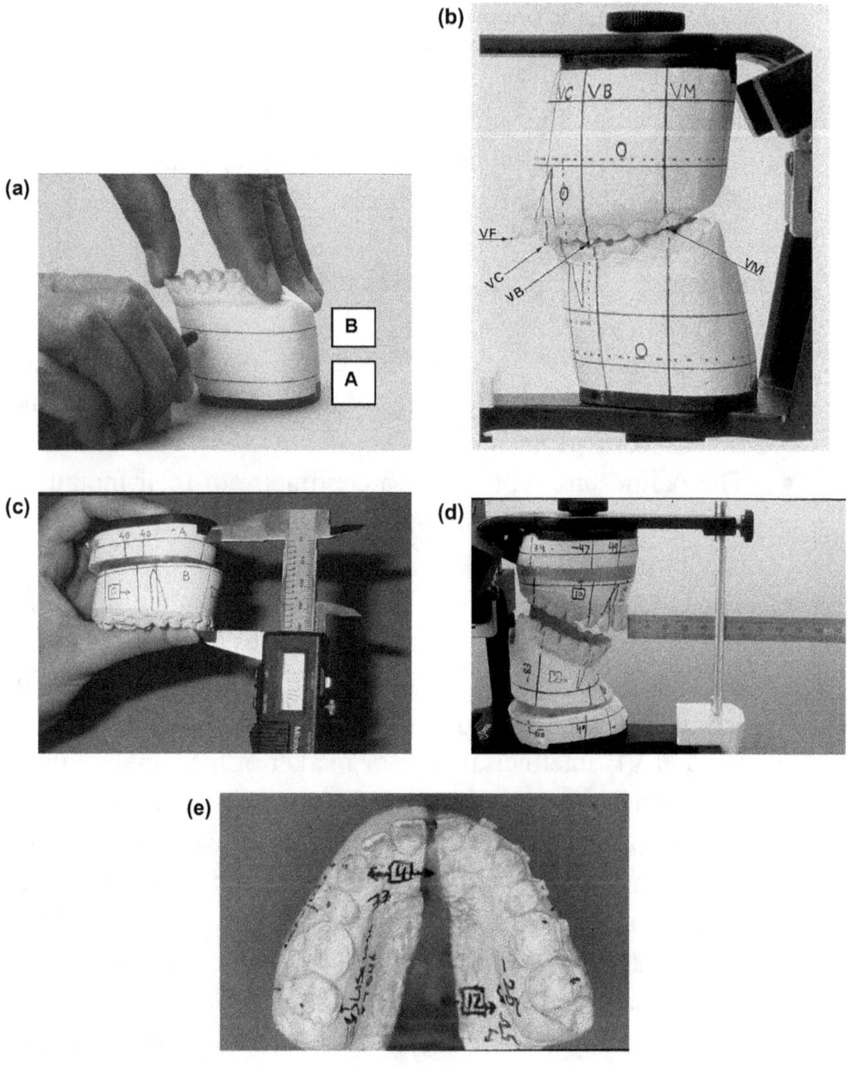

Figure 6.13 (**a**) Horizontal reference lines A and B are drawn with a fine tipped felt pen. (**b**) Models mounted in the preoperative position on the Denar articulator, using the Slidematic facebow and centric relation records, The anatomically-orientated models in preoperative positions showing the cusp reference points (as pointed out with arrows) used for pre- and postoperative measurements. VM = Mesial buccal cusp of a molar tooth; VB = buccal cusp of a premolar; VC = canine cusp; and VF = interincisor midline at the crown tip, unless the teeth or the maxilla are asymmetrically rotated in which case the most anterior

- The relative postoperative positions of the jaw segments are measured as the distances between the references points and the actual movements are indicated in boxes with direction arrows.
- It is advisable to complete the whole model surgery procedure, check the final occlusion and see if any adjustment is required in the maxillary position before making any occlusal wafer.
- For the intermediate wafer fabrication the postoperative mandibular model can be replaced with the preoperative mandibular model mounted with the supine CR wax occlusal record (Figures 6.14a and 6.14b).

The Ericsson Table for Model Surgery (Great Lakes Orthodontics)

This is a precise tool for carrying out the model surgery. The registration bite and transfer jig are used for the articulation of the upper then lower models as described previously. Once the plaster has set both mountings are allowed to dry completely overnight in a drying oven.

- The Ericsson system consists of a highly polished smooth granite platform (Figure 6.15a) with an electronic calliper mount inserted into the base at 90 degrees to the surface platform and a model block (Figure 6.15b). The models mounted on the model block can be measured in three planes. The calliper's tip

---

point at the incisor edge is used, where it coincides with the facial midline. Note: A and B base lines, O = simulated osteotomy line and the vertical reference lines. **(c)** The vertical maxillary movements measured with a digital Vernier calliper from the A line to the cusp tips of maxillary teeth. **(d)** The modified articulator anterior pin with a slot for the steel rule is used to confirm anteroposterior jaw movements. **(e)** Occlusal view of a patient cast showing 4 mm intercanine and 12 mm intermolar maxillary expansion.

(a) (b)

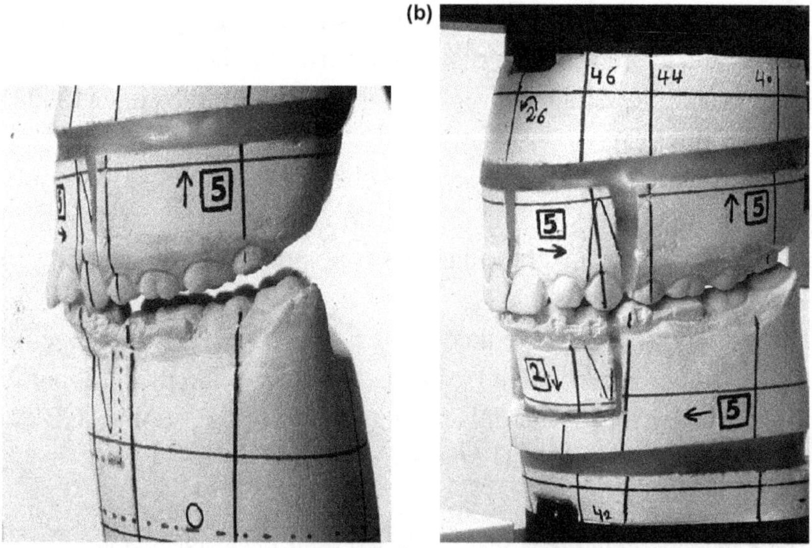

Figure 6.14 Models in **(a)** intermediate and **(b)** final position after the model surgery and before making intermediate and final occlusal wafers.

in addition to measuring can also be used to scribe lines onto the plaster models.

- The plaster model with its articulator ring is mounted on the rectangular model block in an identical manner to that on the anatomical articulator. The surface of the model block is therefore equivalent to the mounting surface of the articulator arm and is the reference plane for measuring vertical impaction changes (Y) (Figure 6.15b).
- With the model block on its posterior side on the granite table measurements are recorded from the platform surface to the dental midline and cusp reference points to simulate "horizontal — anteroposterior (X) movements.
- Transverse measurements (Z). are recorded with the block on its lateral side (Figures 6.15c and 6.15d).
- The measurements are taken as described in the previous technique, from the tip of the mesio-buccal cusps of the maxillary

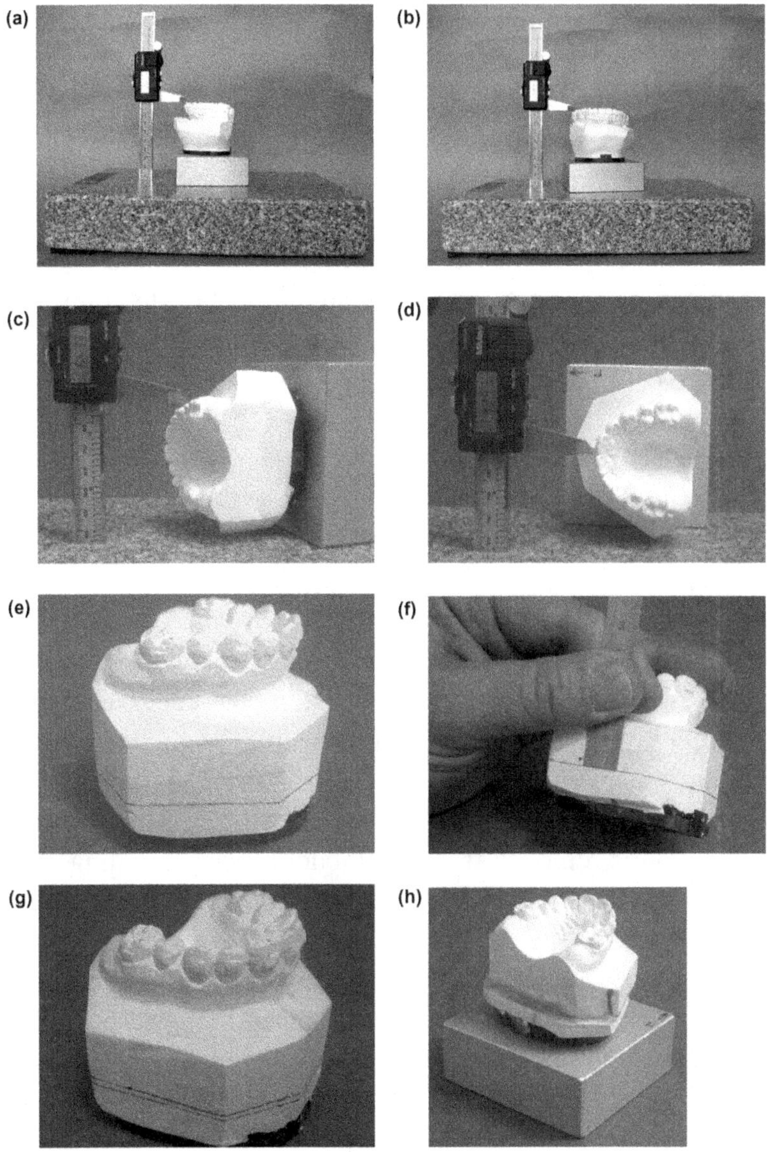

Figure 6.15 (**a**) Ericsson model platform with caliper and mounted casts. (**b**) Model with mounting ring on block. (**c**) and (**d**) Electronic caliper assembly showing identification of incisor and bicuspid reference points. To be measured against platform plane. (**e**) O osteotomy line for sectioning the model. (**f**) and (**g**) Measuring planned impaction to be removed from plaster base. (**h**) Assembled model after "surgery".

right and left first molars, the tips of the maxillary right and left canines, and the incisal edges of the maxillary central incisors to the mounting block surface.

- All measurements are recorded on a model surgery planning grid, drawn on a blank paper or lab-card and are repeated to ensure accuracy.
- The facial midline has already been drawn on the model when mounted on the articulator. The simulated O osteotomy line is drawn parallel to the granite base on the plaster mounting (Figure 6.15e).

When undertaking model surgery it is important to ensure that the clinically planned movements are in agreement with the reference points and measurements applied during the model surgery procedure.

- Planned vertical impaction movements can be first measured from the O line opposite the first molar cusps and incisor reference points and scribed on the plaster model mounting. (Figures 6.15f and 6.15g). Using a band saw, the mounting is cut along the O line. Plaster corresponding to the amount of maxillary impaction is removed from the model plaster mounting using a model trimmer. The total amount of plaster removed will be slightly greater that that required. This is taken up by flowing a thin layer of warmed carding wax between the cut model and the mounting base to relocate the two elements (Figure 6.15h).
- Planned anteroposterior or rotational movements of the maxilla are checked against the marked centre line and cusp reference points.
- Transverse or segmental surgery requires additional cuts to the plaster model but the same principal is applied.
- The recombined cut maxilla is then replaced on the model block and Ericcson table and the measurements are confirmed using the electronic calliper.

- Warming the interpositional wax by flaming, allows fine adjustments to be made to to ensure the new planned postsurgical measurements to correspond to those recorded on the planning grid. The model is then sealed to the mount using either sticky wax or a glue gun, and rechecked.
- Fabrication of the intermediate and final wafers is as described below.

7. *Occlusal Wafers*

Osteotomy wafers locate the dental arches in any preplanned relationship and eliminate unreliable intraoperative guesswork.

Wafers are used for the following purposes.

a) To reposition the mobilised maxilla relative to the intact mandible or the mobilised sectioned mandible to the intact maxilla. The intermediate wafer has a horizontal inaccuracy of about 2 mm of the planned position due to the discrepancy between the distalised centre of mandibular rotation in the supine anaesthetised patient and the mandibular rotation in the conscious upright patient. Overcorrection of the maxilla is therefore essential in a single jaw maxillary osteotomy to achieve the planned advancement. This maxillary discrepancy is masked in a bimaxillary procedure when the mandible is placed in a Class I incisor relationship to the maxilla regardless of its position.
b) To achieve the planned intermediate and final occlusion. After rigid fixation of the mandible the wafer may be wired to the maxilla or mandible to provide postoperative proprioceptive guidance for up to two weeks, with or without the help of elastics. However this causes discomfort to the patient and appears to have no proven value except to reassure the surgeon.
c) To stabilise the segments in the planned position when the dental arch is segmented and mobilised an orthodontic

supplemental arch wire or arch bar is secured into place. Without an occlusal wafer, this can be difficult and will give poor results. And without the supplemental arch wire the planned occlusal relationship will be unstable.

d) The wafer is most invaluable when the postoperative occlusion is not sufficiently stable after the release of intraoperative IMF in cases requiring substantial postoperative orthodontics or with poorly contoured crowns or bridges which need to be replaced.

Wafer Fabrication (Figures 6.16a to 6.16d)

Wafers may be fabricated from cold cured (autopolymerising) or quick cure methylmethacrylate. A poorly designed inaccurate wafer

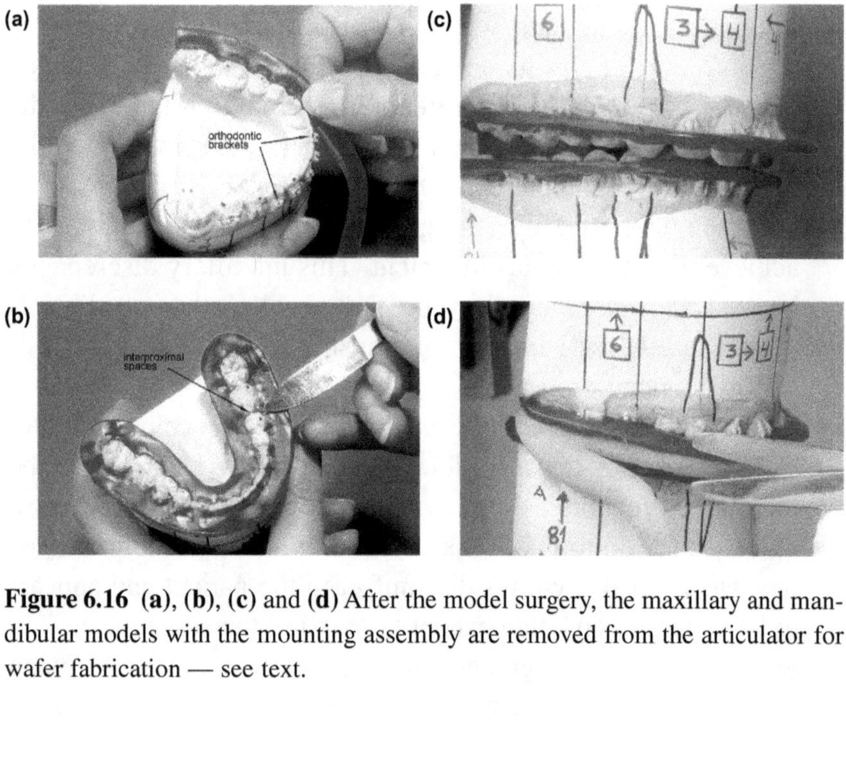

Figure 6.16 **(a)**, **(b)**, **(c)** and **(d)** After the model surgery, the maxillary and mandibular models with the mounting assembly are removed from the articulator for wafer fabrication — see text.

will spoil the most skilful surgical technique. It is common practice to construct both the intermediate and the final wafers as thin as possible. The justification has been that thick wafers introduce discrepancies in the final occlusion.

As stated the condylar recoil from the distalised anaesthetised centric relation to functional conscious centric occlusion can reduce the setback in Class III corrections. This is anticipated by overcorrection of the planned posterior position of the mandible by at least 2 mm.

Similarly, the inevitable degree of postoperative distal relapse in the Class II mandibular advancement justifies a forward overcorrection to an incisor edge to edge final occlusion.

The Construction Technique Using Quick Cure Acrylic

After the model surgery, the maxillary and mandibular models with the mounting assembly are removed from the articulator. All the undercuts along the palatal, lingual and buccal aspects of the dental arches are relieved by applying a strip of soft red beading wax (Utility Wax, Kem-Dent, Associated Dental Products Ltd, UK).

The occlusal margins of the orthodontic brackets are the limit of the coronal extension of the wafer. It is advisable to have about 1 mm space between the acrylic wafer and the orthodontics brackets or arch bar to avoid any interference at the time of insertion. The Interproximal spaces are blocked out with the wax to ensure that the wafer does not extend into these unwanted areas and impair fit during the surgery.

The tips of the plaster teeth are soaked in the water for 10 minutes and the dental arches are coated with sodium alginate separating medium for easy separation of the acrylic from the casts. The upper postoperative and the lower preoperative models are placed back onto the articulator to fabricate the intermediate occlusal wafer.

A quick cure high impact acrylic is mixed using 70% high impact polymer (Austenal Dental Products Ltd., The Crystal Centre, Harrow, UK), and 30% rapid repair polymer with its monomer. When the mix is at the dough stage, a U-shaped role is placed over the occlusal surface of the mandibular arch. The acrylic dough is moulded and directed towards the buccal and lingual surfaces of the teeth with a spatula, ensuring full coverage of the occlusal surfaces.

The upper arm of the articulator is closed down firmly until its incisal pin touches the incisal table. The acrylic material is thus sandwiched between the maxillary and mandibular dental arches indexing the occlusal surfaces of the teeth. While still soft, the excess acrylic is trimmed with a pair of scissors. At the initial polymerisation stage, the articulator is carefully opened and closed, to ensure that the wafer could be removed from both the upper and lower models when processed. This will also eliminate acrylic contraction around the incisal tips and minimise any damage to the teeth at wafer removal, when fully polymerised and hard.

After removal of the excess acrylic ensure that the dental arches are fully covered. The articulator with the models and wafer are then secured with a rubber band and placed in the hydro-flask or a Palamate (Hereous Kulzer), England for 20 minutes at 45°C for curing. Once processed, the upper arm of the articulator is unlocked and removed gently before removing the wafer. It is then trimmed and polished, avoiding frictional heat, which may warp the acrylic. The process is repeated with both postsurgical models for the final wafer.

The completed wafers are seated on each model for a final check. The buccal, labial and lingual aspects should blend into the tooth morphology. On the buccal sides, small holes are drilled using a round No. 5 bur for suspensory wires to orthodontic brackets or arch bar (Figures 6.17a to 6.17d).

It is essential for intraoperative identification to engrave I (intermediate) or F (final) with a No. 5 round bur. A groove representing the facial midline should also be marked with a No. 2 flat fissure bur. These are reinforced with a Lumocolor permanent pen

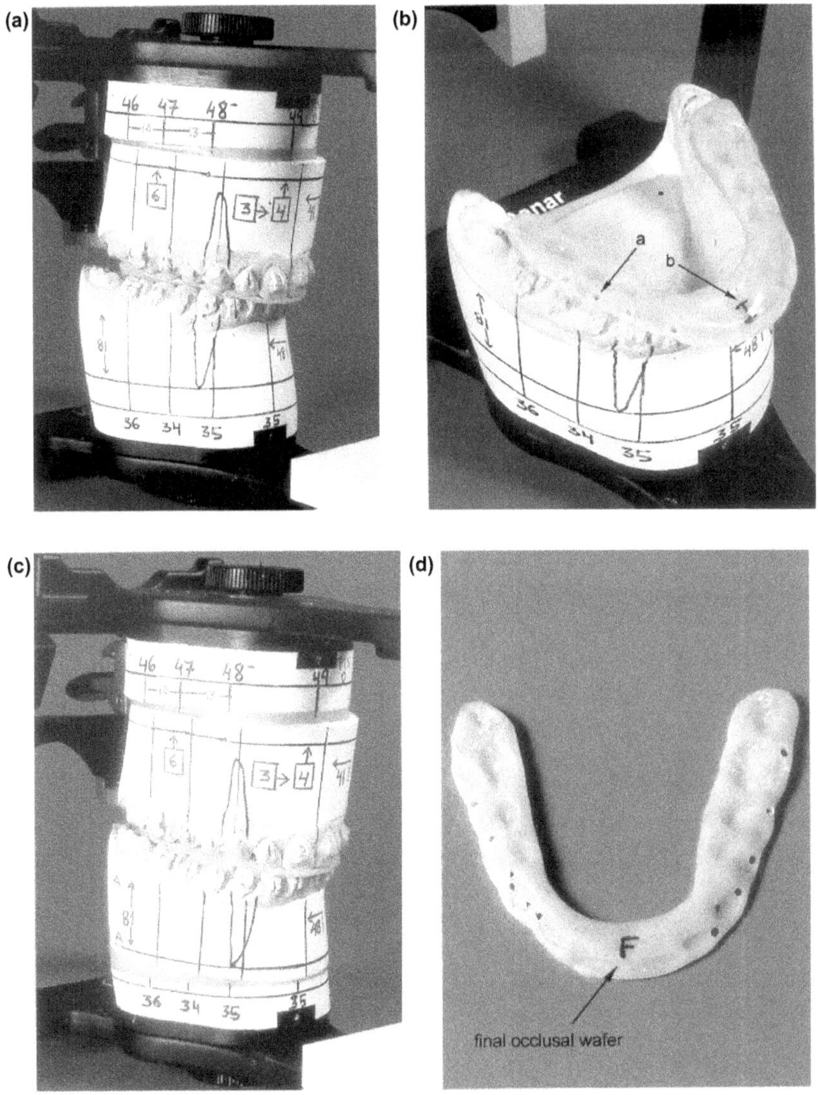

Figure 6.17 (**a**) The buccal and lingual aspect of the wafers should blend into the tooth morphology. (**b**) On buccal aspects of the wafer small holes are drilled using a round bur No. 5 to pass wires through to suspend the wafer to orthodontic brackets or arch bars. (**c**) Final occlusal wafer is tried in on the models. (**d**) For identification letter (I) for intermediate and (F) for final is engraved and a groove representing the midline can also be marked with No. 2 bur. These letters can be reinforced with lumocolor permanent pen (Staedtler, Germany).

(Staedtler, Germany) and can be embedded with self-curing clear resin, thus ensuring ready identification.

Although it is convenient to drill small holes for wire loop maxillary suspension, embedded ball end clasps are occasionally a useful alternative.

Chapter 7

Computer-Aided Surgical Simulation (CASS) for Orthognathic Surgery

Paul Thomas and Sabah Kalamchi

Introduction

Digital imaging technology has revolutionized the diagnosis and surgical management of dentofacial anomalies with its combined use of the patients' 3D computed tomographic data, virtual dental models and 3D digital photographic images. These are integrated by computer planning software in the process known as Computer-Aided Surgical Simulation (CASS). Alternative titles are Virtual Surgical Planning, (VSP®[1]) or Computer Aided Design/Computer Aided Manufacture (CAD/CAM). This methodology when applied to orthognathic surgery provides a surgical planning process and also the fabrication of surgical splints and occlusal wafers which transform the virtual plan into clinical reality. A major challenge is the use of computer terminology such as "virtual", which is a subject or

[1]VSP® is a registered trademark of 3D Systems (formerly Medical Modeling). Their primary planning software is the Dolphin Imaging and Management Solutions which was used to produce the virtual image illustrations in this chapter.

process which does not exist except as software data. It is electronically simulated. Such esoteric terms will require searching for online sources. The orthognathic technique uses cone beam computerized tomography (CBCT) where the X-rays form a divergent cone and the scanner rotates around the patient's head to obtain up to 600 distinct images of the orofacial volume, hence the term volumetric data (Figures 7.1 and 7.2). The patient is stabilised by a head positioning device ideally with a wax bite in centric occlusion. A fiducial marker (a reference marker) may also be placed in the wax to appear in the computer image as a point of reference. The bite registration and fiducial marker enables an accurate fusion of the patients digital dento alveolar models with the CBCT volume image of the facial skeleton.

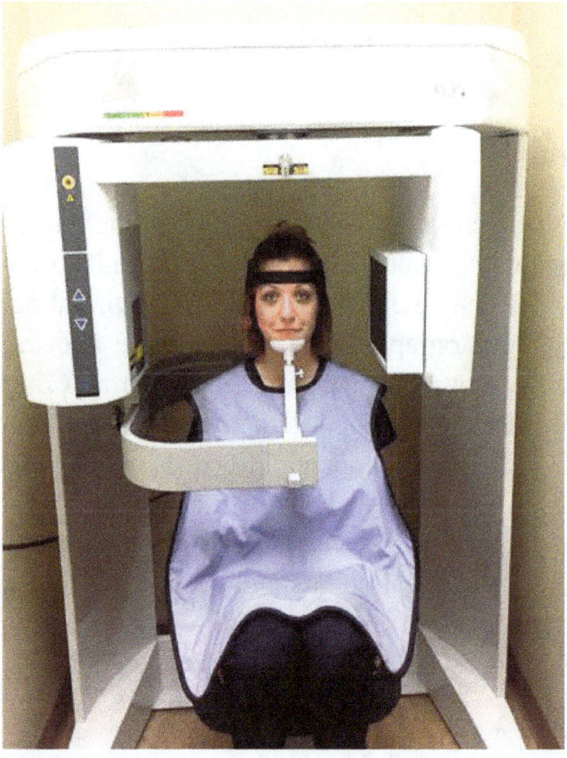

Figure 7.1 This technique uses cone beam computerized tomographic scan (CBCT).

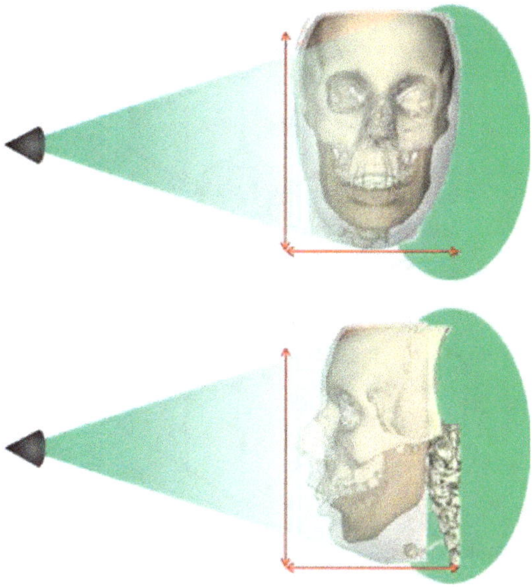

Figure 7.2 The scanned volume of the CBCT scanner.

Source: Swennen GR, Mollemans W, Schutyser F, Three-dimensional treatment planning of orthognathic surgery in the era of virtual imaging. *J Oral Maxillofac Surg* 67(10): 2080–2092 (2009).

A 200 degree rotation over the region of surgical importance records the anatomical data by the scanning software and reconstructs it to produce a digital volume made up of three-dimensional voxels which can be manipulated and visualized with specialized software (Figure 7.3).

These data can be derived either from a medical grade computed tomography (CT) scan or a Cone Beam Computed Tomography (CBCT) scan. The medical grade CT has the disadvantages of higher radiation exposure and an increase in artifact "noise" from dental restorations and orthodontic appliances. All CT studies are composed of voxels (volume elements) which are three dimensional rectangular cuboids (Figure 7.3). The medical grade CT "cuboids" are not isometric which reduces the image clarity when imported into the planning software, whereas the CBCT scan involves significantly less radiation exposure, lower scan times and

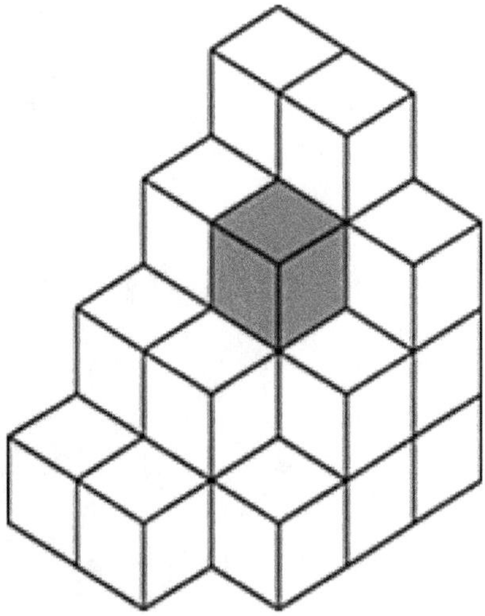

Figure 7.3 Computerised tomography (CT) studies are composed of three dimensional voxels.

isometric cuboids as low as 0.2 mm per side which are less prone to create noise artifact. The latest CBCT technology has reduced the radiation exposure below that seen with digital panoramic and cephalometric images.

The scan is often prescribed to be carried out with the head in the neutral head position which is defined as the relaxed head and neck posture with the gaze at infinity. Unfortunately many patients with jaw disproportion adopt a subjective aesthetic posture which may tilt the head and produce a false orbital dystopia. This can be avoided at the time of the scan by positioning the head with the Frankfort and orbital planes horizontal, unless the patient has a true orbital dystopia. The CBCT system has the option to incorporate a 3D camera which captures the image at the same time as the volumetric skeletal study. Although desirable, the 3D camera is an expensive option. An alternative is "photo-wrapping" which superimposes a frontal 2D digital image on to the soft tissues of the volumetric scan. This creates a virtual 3D face from the 2D data and is a feature of the VSP® software and has no cost implications.

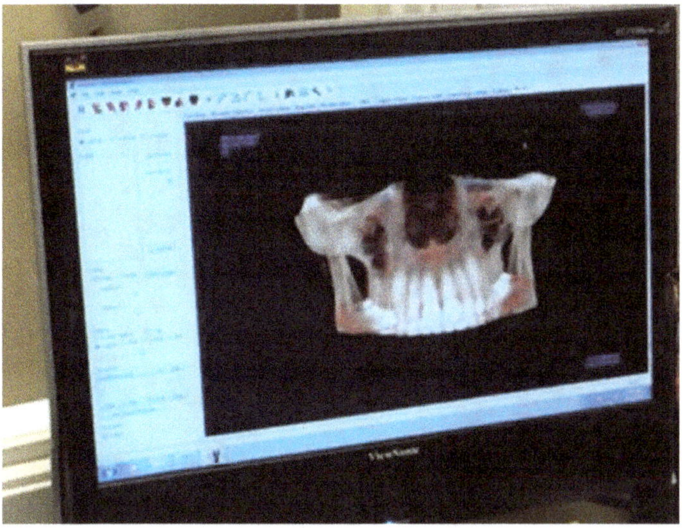

Figure 7.4 Processing the CBCT data to create a 3D virtual image of the patient's jaws and teeth.

The axial CBCT slices and their coronal and sagittal reconstructions, create a detailed 3D study of the facial anatomy by a process called volume rendering. This can produce a virtual 3D image from a sample of 2D millimetre slices. Here the term rendering means image synthesis and is invaluable for the roots of the teeth and the temporomandibular joints (Figure 7.4).

Similarly surface rendering can provide a virtual surface presentation of the face or even a partially transparent 3D image revealing the underlying bone and teeth (Figure 7.5).

The varied but realistic opacity and colour of the facial image can also be created by a computer graphics programme where every voxel is capable of an appropriate colour using the so called RGBA values for red, green, blue, and alpha where alpha stands for opacity. If alpha is 0% the voxel is transparent. In this way the facial soft-tissue mask can have a natural looking skin texture or a transparent window.

Both "volume rendering" and "surface rendering" produce 3D images which are derived from the axial CBCT slices and their

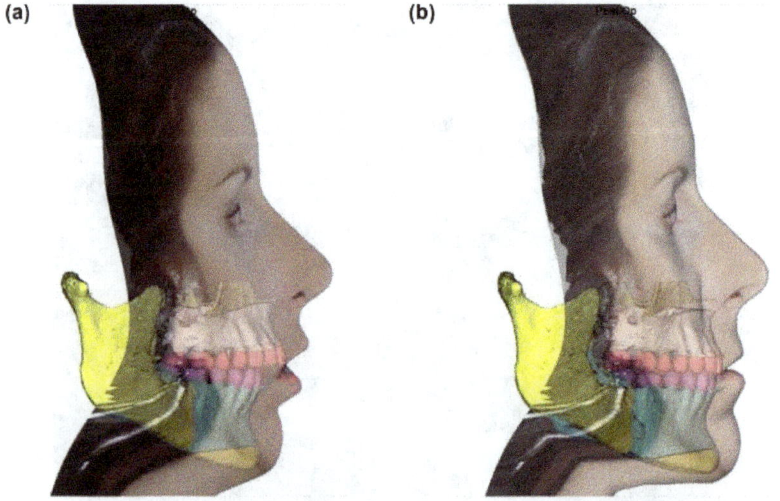

Figure 7.5 (**a**) Virtual preoperative. (**b**) Virtual postoperative correction.

coronal and sagittal reconstructions. In this way orthognathic virtual treatment planning has the advantage of a 3D facial image rather than being restricted to the mid sagittal facial profile and cephalometry, which rely on the clinicians experience and intuition.

Figure 7.5 is an in depth surface rendering of a 3D profile showing (a) the virtual preoperative and (b) the predicted post-operative mandible and dentition, in the context of the virtual face. This 3D simulation can be viewed from all dimensions using a multilayered slice format. The profile shows the sagittal split has advanced the pogonion with opening of the labiomental fold but the lip closure has not been programmed to be completely competent. Any soft tissue response to osteotomy movements is a prediction by the software based on the estimated percentage of the soft tissue movement in response to the underlying hard tissue landmarks. Here the amount of virtual lip closure can be controlled by the software operator.

The clinical potential of the CASS process is illustrated in the following case where 3D digital images show the deformity as left and right profiles and a full face (**Figure 7.6a**).

The case can be managed by several surgical solutions, which can be tried and compared within an hour. A simple Lefort 1

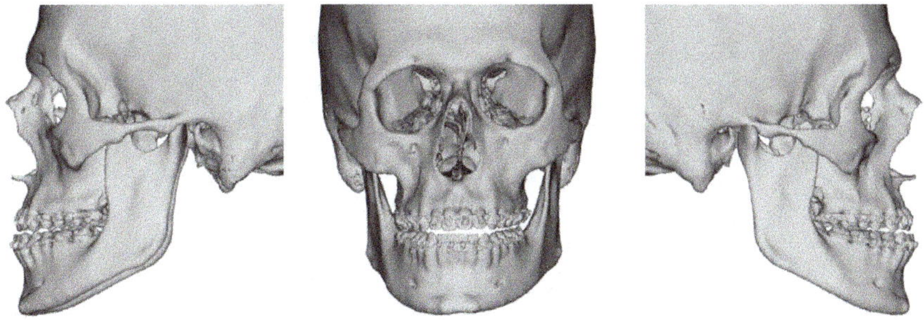

Figure 7.6a A preoperative CBCT scan illustrating a case diagnosed as a maxillary retrusion with an increased posterior vertical height and anterior open bite.

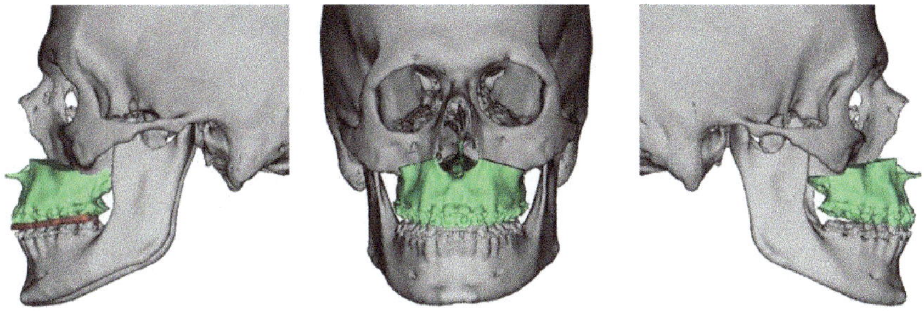

Figure 7.6b These virtual postoperative images show a Le Fort 1 osteotomy with anterior movement of the maxilla which has closed the anterior open bite at the expense of the molar occlusion.

advancement is virtually carried out to correct the diagnosis of a retruded maxilla and anterior open bite. Figure 7.6b shows the precise bone sections and their movements, which can also reveal sites which require bone removal or graft insertion.

However the 3D images of this solution which has corrected the anterior open bite has created a posterior open bite.

Figure 7.6c illustrates the outcome of a complex treatment plan of this case consisting of:

(i) extraction of the upper first premolars with integration of the 3 osteotomised maxillary segments,
(ii) surgical coordination of the modified maxilla with the intact mandibular dental arch by:

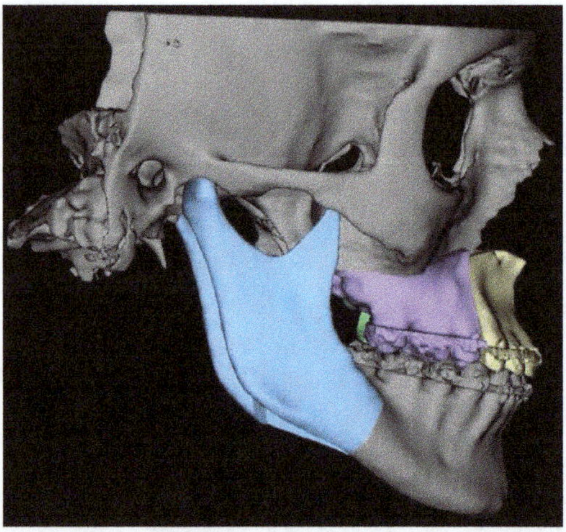

Figure 7.6c This complex bimaxillary approach included 4/4 extractions, enabling segmental coordination of the osteotomised maxilla with the mandibular dental arch, then advancement of the segmentalised Le Fort 1 maxilla and a mandibular sagittal split set back. The colour coding represents the different osteotomy segments.

(iii) advancement of the segmentalised maxilla and
(iv) a mandibular sagittal split set back.

The colour code identifies the osteotomy sections and if acceptable, prototype surgical splints and occlusal wafers will be manufactured for the intermediate and final stages of the actual operation.

The Virtual (Stereolithic) Dental Cast (STL)

A crucial part of the virtual treatment plan is to integrate high resolution dental occlusal surfaces into the patient's relatively low resolution volumetric CBCT jaws. This replaces the traditional mounting of plaster dental models onto an articulator with a face bow prior to model surgery. The virtual CBCT jaws are the articulator. For CASS the plaster models can be rendered digital with a bench top optical scanner so that impressions and plaster are completely avoided by using an intraoral wand scanner (Figure 7.7).

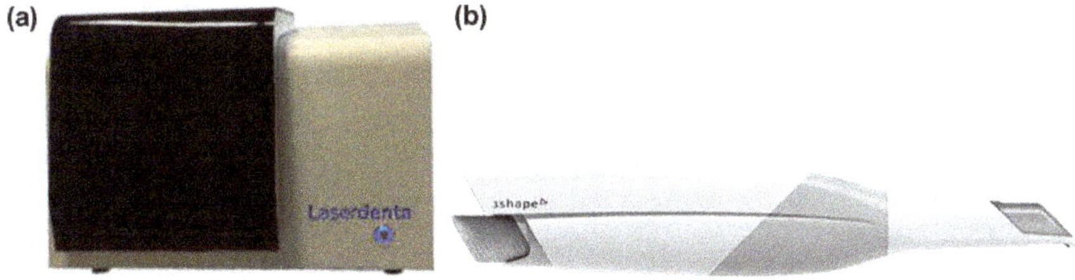

Figure 7.7 (**a**) Dental benchtop optical scanner and (**b**) a hand held wand laser scanner. Recent advances have resulted in a wireless intraoral scanner capable of producing a full-mouth scan in 3 minutes.

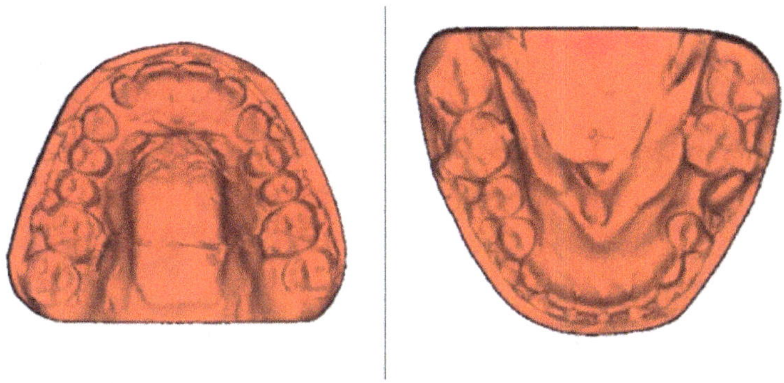

Figure 7.8 (**a**) and (**b**) Virtual models produced from plaster models by an optical benchtop scanner.

Plaster casts can also be scanned with CBCT but this requires increased radiation and a small field of view to produce acceptable resolution. The resulting volume is converted to surface data with the VSP® software. Optical scans are generally of better quality than the CBCT (Figures 7.8a and 7.8b).

These methods enable high resolution digital data to be grafted onto the CBCT volumetric data to create an accurate 3-dimensional composite model of the patient's maxillary and mandibular jaws and teeth (**Figure 7.9**). Once obtained this integrated CBCT data can be used for in-house osteotomy planning or sent to a specialist centre for processing and simulated surgery.

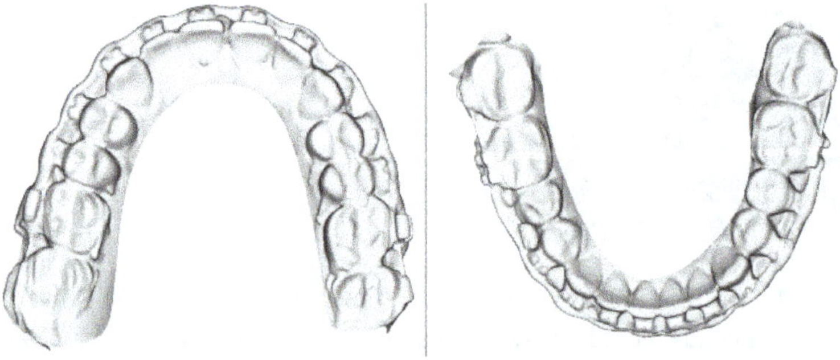

Figure 7.8b Virtual models from an intraoral wand scanner with no base added. This format is fused with the volumetric data (Figure 7.9).

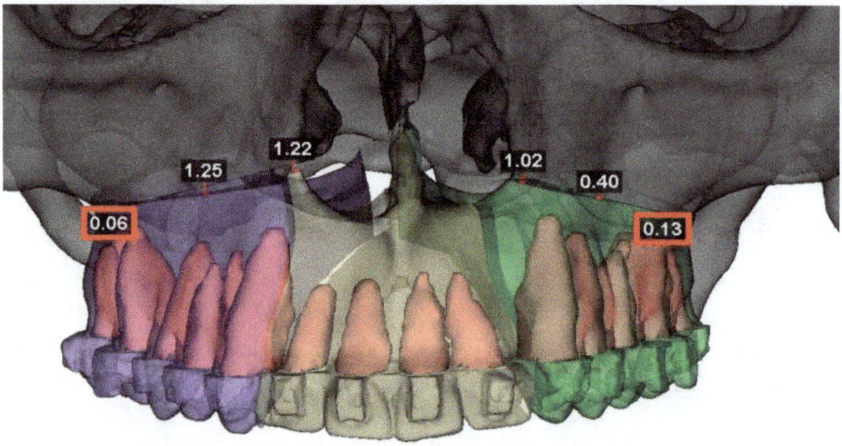

Figure 7.9 This is a virtual 3D post-operative image of a Le Fort 1 osteotomy with an incisor segmental modification. It shows the clarity of the high definition virtual dental models fused onto the volumetric CBCT data of the whole maxilla. The red boxes are the measured overlap of the osteotomy margins which may need to be trimmed whereas the black boxes are gaps, in millimetres. The colour coded alveolus represents the alveolar segments of the osteotomy.

In House CASS Processing

A complete in-house planning process is usually confined to a hospital department with specialized biomedical engineers. Traditionally the maxillofacial technician undertakes the orthognathic planning process from impressions, bite registration, face-bow transfer, pouring of plaster casts, articulator mounting, model surgery to the mid and final occlusal wafer fabrication (see Chapter 6). The time involved with this process is estimated to be 7–8 hours per case depending on its complexity. By contrast, the planning process using CASS requires 45–60 minutes once the data has been integrated into the planning software. Currently the primary obstacle to the in-house process is the cost of the hardware. Optical or wand scanners are expensive as is a 3D printer. However in-house laboratories in the future may justify the hardware expenditure by significant savings in dental technician time.

The Remote CASS Service Centre

Patient data collected by the clinician can be conveyed to a remote specialist service centre by a File Transfer Protocol (FTP), which is a computer network enabling the transmission of computer files to be assessed for surgical planning.

The CASS Programme

Traditionally, the patient requires the following when referred for correction of a dentofacial deformity by a dental practitioner or orthodontist;

i. Initial imaging which is minimally an orthopantomograph, a lateral skull radiograph with cephalometric tracing and a postero-anterior radiograph of the facial bones.
ii. Clinical photographs
iii. Alginate impressions for upper and lower study models with a centric occlusion wax bite registration

All may be provided by or for the orthodontist.

Discussion with the orthodontist is essential to establish if one or two jaw surgery, or a segmental osteotomy will be required. Also to be discussed is whether spaces are needed to be made available or closed and whether any anticipated postsurgical space will be closed orthodontically?

The patient then undergoes decompensation orthodontics in preparation for surgery, and on completion returns for the definitive surgical treatment plan.

The Alternative CASS Treatment Plan

CASS is alien to traditional maxillofacial surgeons because it is computer based, however the process consists of a preoperative CBCT scan following orthodontic preparation and upper and lower study models with a centric occlusion wax bite. Some operators insert a fiducial marker in the wax bite which is worn by the patient during the CBCT scan and is used in the digital model production. This facilitates the process of fusion of the digital models or the intraoral scanned dentition with the volumetric data. Plaster models are obsolete if an intraoral scanner is available.

When the planning is done by an external service centre, the recorded CBCT scan, and models can be sent by registered post, or the total digital data is transmitted to the centre by FTP protocol to be processed. A clean-up of the volumetric data is a manual process which involves the review of the CBCT data, slice by slice to remove the noise.

This is not necessary if the production of the wafers and splints is limited to the dentition but is required for accuracy if skeletal structures or drilling and cutting guides are generated by rapid prototyping. Stereolithographic splints, generated by the CAD/CAM technique, have a high degree of accuracy equal to conventional surgical splints.

The "clean-up" process includes the removal of "noise" (Figure 7.10), which includes cutting away the CBCT volumetric

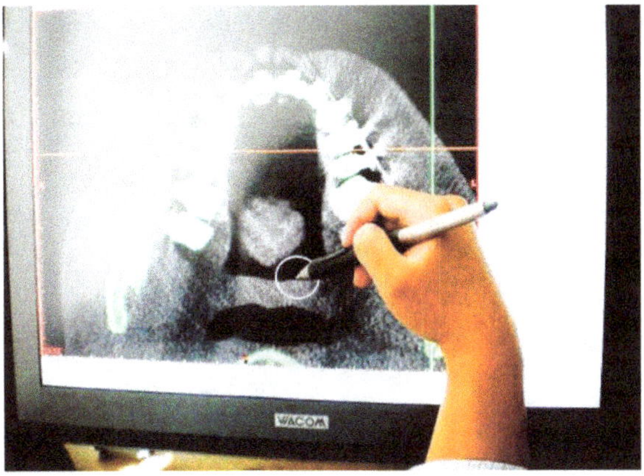

Figure 7.10 Initial preparation involves a manual clean-up on a slice by slice basis by the biomedical engineer, this process can take 45–60 minutes.

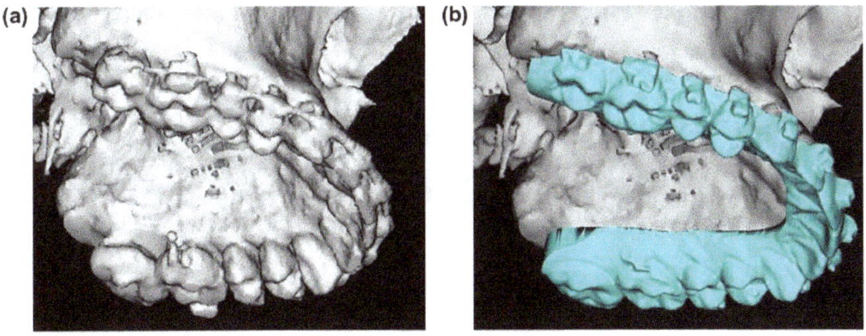

Figure 7.11 (**a**) and (**b**) This stereolithic file is created from the combined CBCT scan and the blue high resolution optically scanned plaster casts. The view shows the integration of the virtual dental models onto the CT volumetric data. If there is limited noise in the study, an automated superimposition programme can be used.

teeth and associated artifacts such as orthodontic bands, to be replaced by the virtual dental models. Figure 7.11 show the blue-green digitized occlusal anatomy from the high resolution scans of the teeth have replaced the anatomy of the CBCT teeth to create a composite model of the volumetric data maxilla and teeth from the dental cast or intraoral surface scan. This combination of virtual 3D

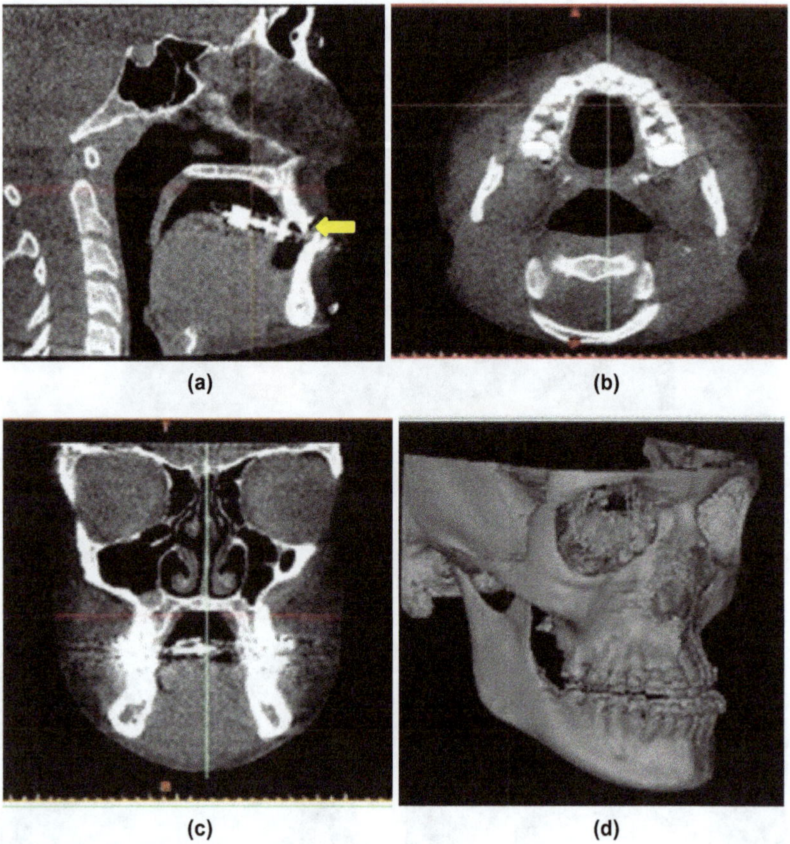

Figures 7.12 (**a**) to (**d**) These CBCT 3D slices; (**a**) sagittal; (**b**) axial, and (**c**) coronal illustrate the detailed skeletal anatomy (**d**) which can be examined by the CBCT surgical planning process. The fiducial marker, if used, is embedded in a centric occlusion wax bite (see a).

model of the patient's dental and skeletal anatomy is used for the rest of the planning process.

The CASS Remote Service Centre

A teleconference is scheduled when the service centre has performed the initial workup with the submitted clinical examination details, the proposed diagnosis and the CBCT data. This conference can take between 30 minutes to 2 hours depending on the complexity of the case. The centre creates a 3D simulation of the dentofacial deformity which is used for the virtual operation options. See example case (Figures 7.6a to 7.6c). This is carried out by the combined expertise of the recipient biomedical engineer, the referring surgeon, and orthodontist.

The following are reviewed online by all the participants:

i. The differential diagnosis.
ii. The verification of the CBCT head position orientation.
iii. The laser scanned dental image integration into the CBCT volumetric file of the jaws.
iv. The possible surgical alternatives to be considered.

Exploring the Possible Operations

The biomedical engineer performs on the screen so that all can observe the:

i. Bone cuts and bone removal.
ii. Segment movements.
iii. Areas that necessitate trimming or a bone graft.
iv. Confirmation of the occlusal outcome.
v. Verification of the occlusal symmetry.
vi. Prediction of soft tissue changes.

Example — The Le Fort 1 osteotomy

Once the osteotomy design is agreed the amount of maxillary antral wall and septum to be removed can be identified and measured to:

i. Close an anterior open bite by vertical impaction.
ii. Trim overlapping antral wall margins to eliminate interference on reduction.
iii. Identify voids which may need to be grafted (see Figure 7.9).

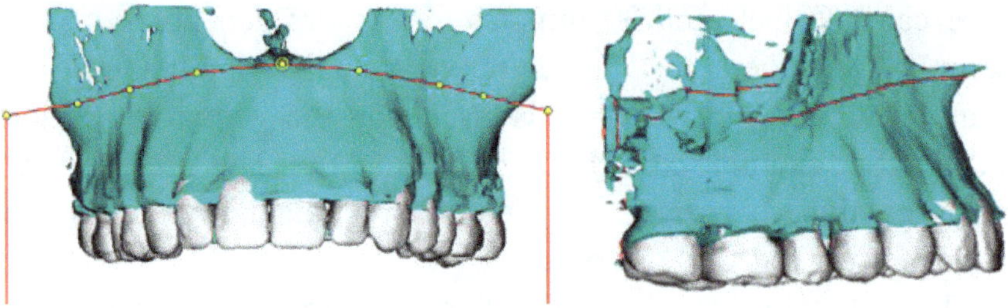

Figure 7.13a Le Fort 1 planning software has pre-existing red osteotomy cutting lines. The engineer can modify these lines by clicking and dragging the intervening dots to define the appropriate osteotomy bone sections.

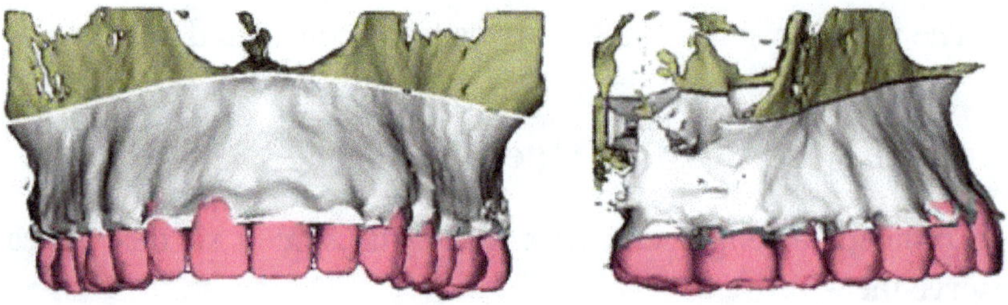

Figure 7.13b Once the osteotomy cuts are agreed they are applied to the maxilla so the sections are incorporated into the treatment plan. The images can also be rendered translucent to visualise the roots and prevent inadvertent damage during surgery (see Figure 7.13b).

The Bilateral Sagittal Split (BSSO). The mouse and cursor are used to create a closed figure around the ramus image. Each dot is a mouse click and the process of virtual cutting is done by on screen digitizing (see Figure 7.14). If a two jaw procedure, in reality most surgeons mobilize the maxilla first as the primary means of establishing the altered occlusion. Others first carry out the mandibular operation to avoid displacing the maxillary bone fixation with the jaw gag when carrying out the BSSO. This can be avoided by creating all the BSSO cortical cuts first but leaving the "sagittal

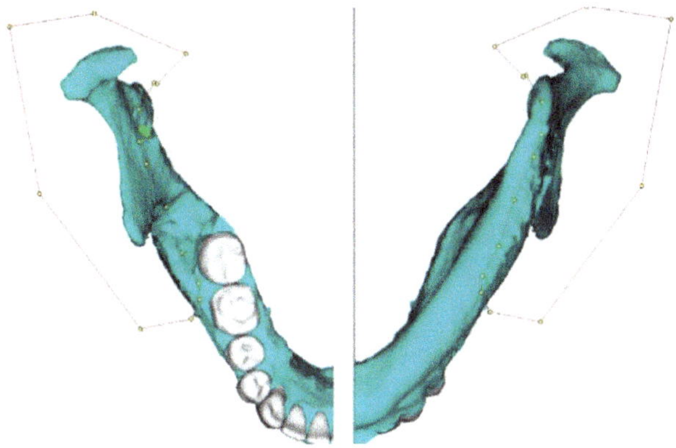

Figure 7.14 The superior and submento-vertex views of the BSSO cuts which were designed on-screen.

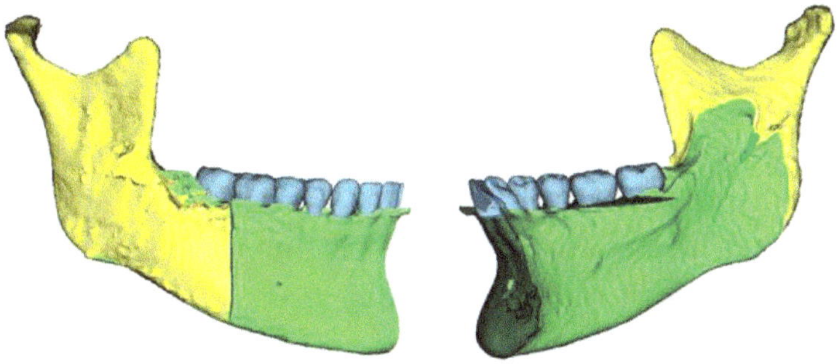

Figure 7.15 The lateral and medial view of the sagittal split bone sections: body (green) and ramus (yellow).

splits" until the maxillary osteotomy mobilization and fixation are complete.

Surgical Cutting Guides

It is possible to make cutting guides which will ensure the surgeon follows the operative design to place the cuts and fixation hardware. But these are cumbersome and unnecessary for most cases (Figure 7.16).

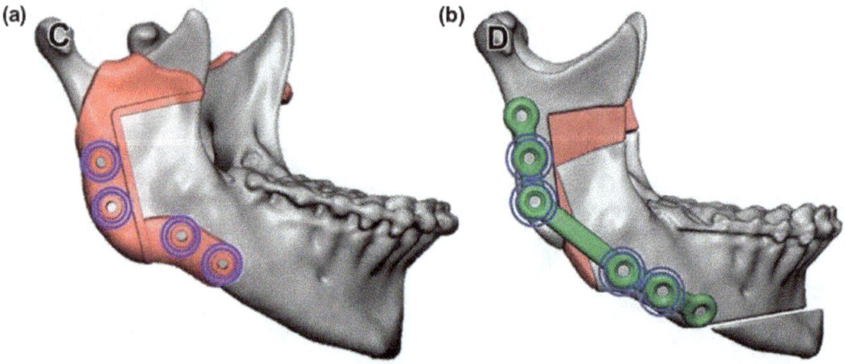

Figure 7.16 (a) An inverted "L" cutting and drilling guide with (b) the custom fixation plate on the right mandible.

These guides are rapid-prototyped in the same manner as the occlusal wafers and are placed over the bone and secured with fixation screws prior to making the osteotomy cuts. Custom made fixation plates have been designed by the same software which uses the same holes as the cutting/drilling guide. Similar processes are available for designing the Intraoral Vertical Ramus Osteotomy (IVRO).

Establishing Facial Dimensions for an Anterior Open Bite (Figures 7.17a and 7.17b)

The achievement of aesthetics is usually the most important aim of orthognathic surgery. CASS can contribute a precise aid for this purpose. The two frontal images (a) and (b) show red horizontal reference lines with orthogonal measurements in millimetres to the canine tips and the mesial- buccal cusps of the first molar.

(a) Although described as an arbitrary reference line, its bilateral orthogonal measurements are used to correct or prevent an occlusal cant. It also has the advantage of being movable to cover the most appropriate location for the CBCT scan. Note that the default computer settings shown here result in

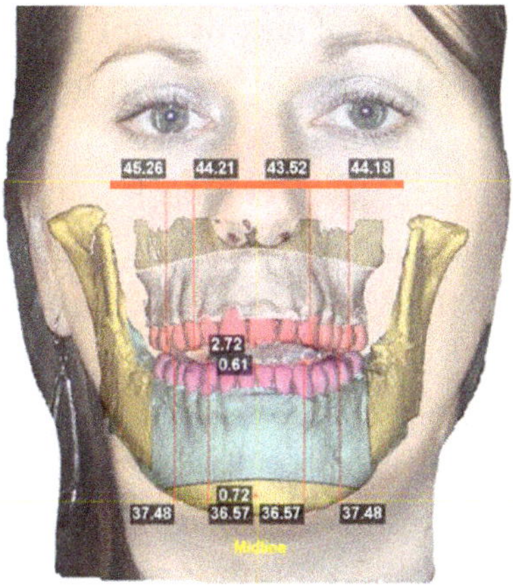

Figure 7.17a A frontal image of the untreated anterior open bite with the arbitrary horizontal reference line and the orthogonal measurements to the first molar mesial buccal cusps and the canine cusp tips. The measurements of 2.72 and 0.61 represent the deviation of the maxillary and mandibular dental midline from the mid-sagittal plane.

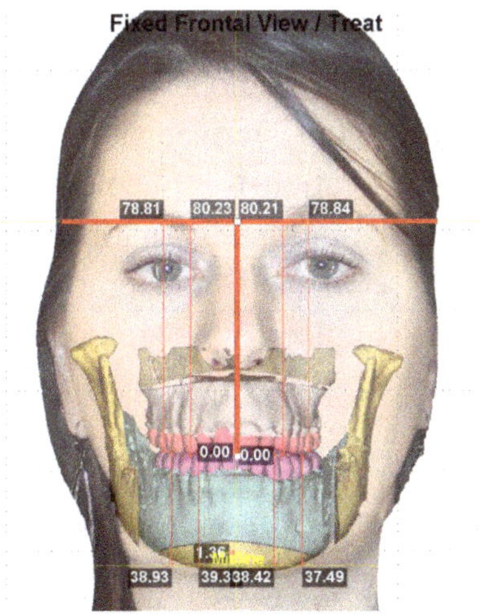

Figure 7.17b The horizontal glabella and mid-sagittal reference lines are highlighted in red. The planned postoperative measurements are from the glabellar reference line to the mid incisal edge (or mid arch wire), the canine cusp tips, and the first molar mesial buccal cusps. The midline orthogonal distance to the incisal edge is 82 mm, but is not shown on this diagram. The measurements over the incisors indicate the midline dental asymmetry has been corrected.

measures to 2 decimal places of a millimetre, which is surgically impractical and can be rounded off to the nearest whole millimetre.

(b) This horizontal glabella reference line (Figure 7.17b) and its virtual midline measurement extends to the central incisor margin or mid arch wire, which here is 82 mm and has the dual role of localising the virtual mobilised maxilla preoperatively and literally at operation. Hence the glabella is an invaluable skeletal marker both for virtual planning and the actual surgery.

(c) The vertical glabella midline measure of the maxilla height is readily confirmed at operation by a caliper and its anterio- posterior position by the intermediate wafer.

(d) The interincisal gap of the anterior open bite corresponds to the required amount of distal maxillary wall and nasal septum to be excised in order to raise the posterior occlusal plane. This measurement subtracted from the glabella to molar reference point is a useful guide for placement of the maxillary segment when repositioned. However the final decision which determines bone and septum resection is made intraoperatively on rotating the mobilised maxilla ligated to the intermediate splint and mandible.

(e) An important consideration is to achieve an aesthetic incisor exposure with the lips minimally apart at rest. This lip-incisor refinement may be estimated preoperatively on the screen by the surgeon and engineer with reference to the patient's photographs.

3D Printing Technology for Surgical Guides and Wafers

The terms surgical guides, splints, or wafers are unfortunately used interchangeably but have in common their design by rapid prototyping software and are created by 3D printing which if done overnight saves an estimated 7–8 hours in the preoperative workup process.

Once the surgical plan is approved the intermediate splint which relates the virtual corrected maxilla to the unchanged mandible and a final wafer relating the maxillary occlusion to that of the corrected mandible, are designed with the CASS software as 3D prototypes and printed in acrylic or epoxy-photopolymer.

Occlusal wafer surface contours and holes for ligation to the arch-wires are part of this process and largely eliminate the need for any post-printing refinement. The software reproduces the wafer surface contours and so the surgical splint thickness is accurately produced. The final design is exported as an STL file which is used by the rapid prototyping 3D printer to enable multiple cases to be printed in one session (Figures 7.18 and 7.19). Subtraction techniques by milling are possible but inefficient and result in much wasted material.

If fabricated by an external specialist centre they are sent non-sterilized to the surgeon with instructions for their preparation for use in the operating theatre. Also included are colour coded copies of the pre and post-operative CASS images which define the osteotomy sections and movements. This precise planning process must not be used if there has been any change in the preoperative anatomy.

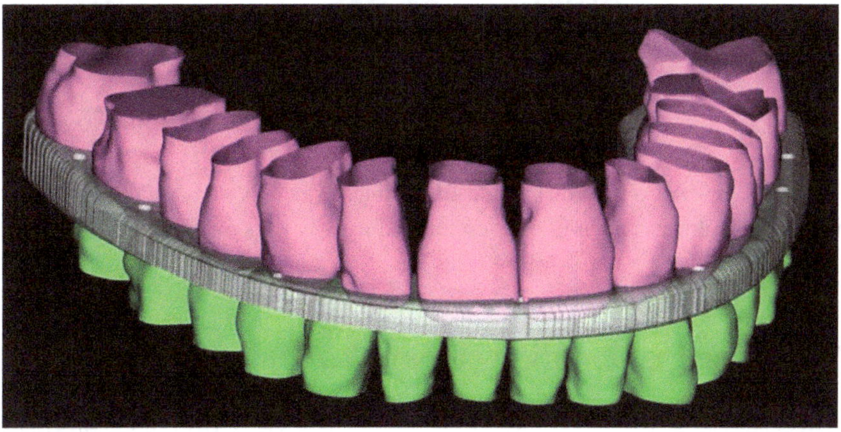

Figure 7.18a Virtual image of the final wafer with "drill" holes for the retaining wire ligatures.

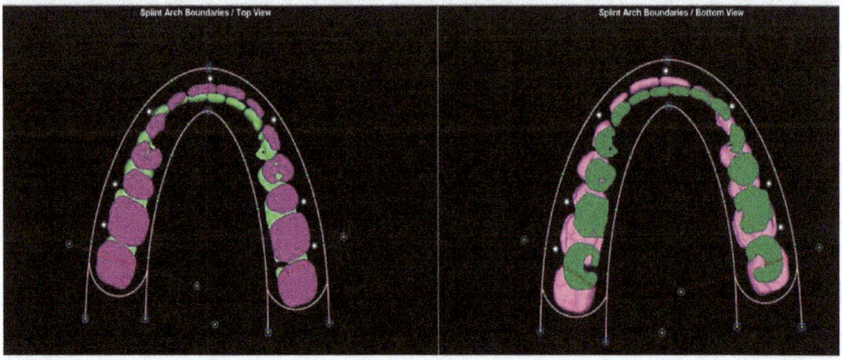

Figure 7.18b Virtual images of the upper and lower surfaces of the final wafer during the design process. The surfaces of the final wafer confirm the planned occlusion. Note the holes for wire ligation to the arch wires and the wafer outline which is scribed on the screen by the cursor.

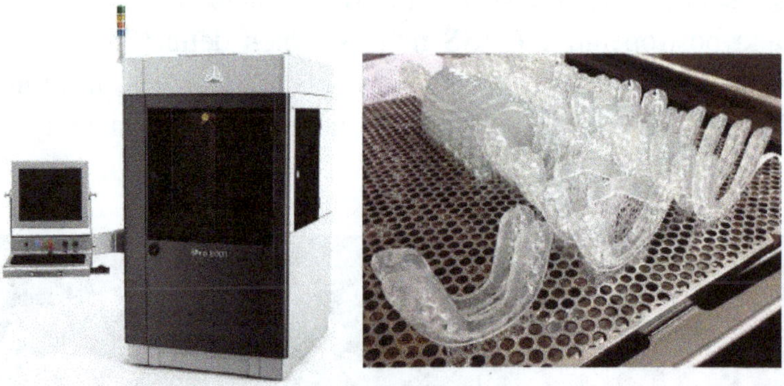

Figure 7.19 A commercial grade 3D printer which is capable of producing multiple wafers as shown in one session and usually runs overnight.

The Case Presentation (Figure 7.20)

This patient's clinical and cephalometric evaluation indicated an asymmetric skeletal open bite, increased facial height due to excess posterior maxillary growth and mandibular hypoplasia.

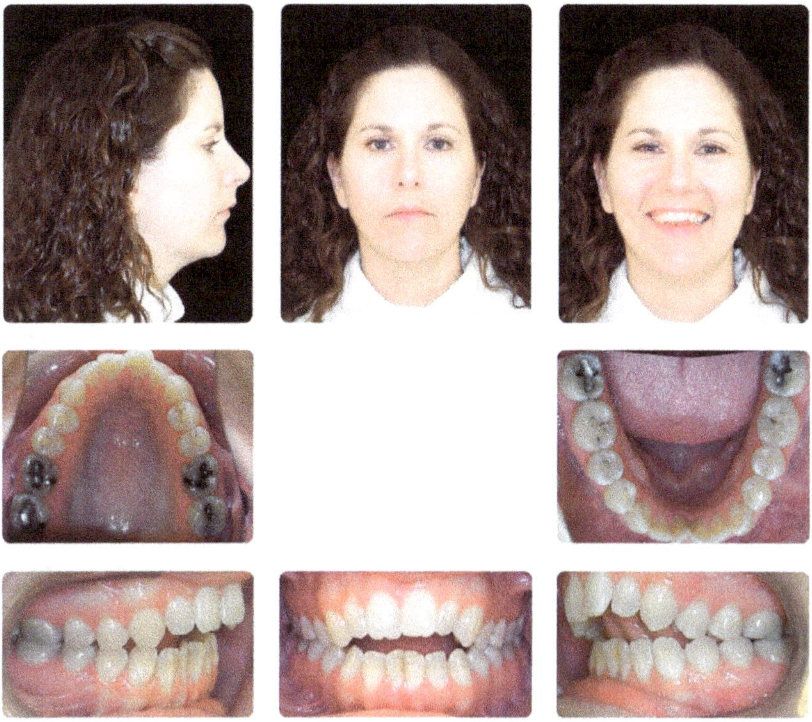

Figure 7.20 This 34 year old female presented to the orthodontic clinic with a principal complaint of difficulty in chewing and a secondary concern for her dental and facial appearance.

Cephalometric Data

The treatment plan included full orthodontic appliances to create inter-arch compatibility, followed by a Le Fort 1 osteotomy with differential posterior impaction of the maxilla and a sagittal split mandibular advancement. The orthodontic levelling of the occlusal planes was completed prior to the CBCT scan.

The Virtual Surgical Planning (CASS) is initiated at a conference call with the biomedical engineer who has prepared the case with the fusion of the scanned dental models to the CBCT dentoalveolar data using Dolphin Imaging Software.

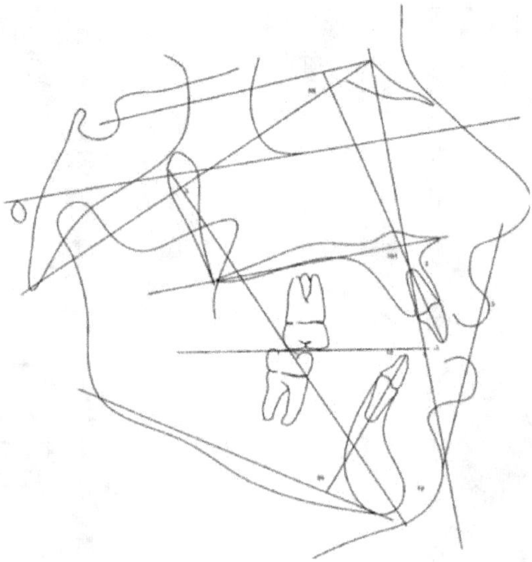

Figure 7.21 Cephalometric tracing resulting from on-screen digitizing of the lateral image which has been created from the CBCT data.

	Value	Norm	Std Dev	Dev Nor
-=Sagittal=-				
Maxillary Skeletal (A-Na Perp) (mm)	3.1	0.0	3.1	1.0 *
Mand. Skeletal (Pg-Na Perp) (mm)	-11.8	-1.5	5.3	-1.9 *
Mx Unit Length (Co-ANS)	92.7	90.0	5.0	0.5
Md Unit Length (Co-Pog)	114.2	113.0	8.0	0.1
Wits Appraisal (mm)	10.3	-1.0	1.0	11.3 *******
Harvold (CoPog)-(CoANS)	21.4	20.0	3.0	0.5
-=Vertical=-				
Facial Axis Angle (Ba-Na^Pt-Gn) (°)	-3.2	0.0	4.0	-0.8
FMA (MP-FH) (°)	33.9	23.9	4.5	2.2 **
MP - SN (°)	37.8	33.0	6.0	0.8
Occ Plane to SN (°)	13.0	14.4	2.5	-0.6
UFH (Na-ANS) (%)	41.5	46.0	5.0	-0.9
LFH (ANS-Me || FH) (%)	58.5	54.0	5.0	0.9
UFH:LFH, Upper (N-ANS/N-Gn) (%)	39.4	45.0	1.0	-5.6 *****
-=Dental=-				
Overbite (mm)	-3.4	2.5	2.0	-2.9 **
Overjet (mm)	9.4	2.5	2.5	2.8 **
U1 exposure, lips at rest (mm)	3.0	4.0	2.5	-0.4
U1 Angulation (U1 - SN) (°)	98.7	102.8	5.5	-0.7
U1 - Palatal Plane (°)	101.1	110.0	5.0	-1.8 *
IMPA (L1-MP) (°)	94.8	95.0	7.0	0.0
Interincisal Angle (U1-L1) (°)	128.6	135.0	6.0	-1.1 *
-=Soft Tissue=-				
st UFH RATIO (G'-Sn/G'-Me')(%)	48.1	50.0	5.0	-0.4
Upper Lip - S Line (mm)	1.0	0.0	2.0	0.5
Lower Lip - S Line (mm)	2.6	0.0	2.0	1.3 *

Figure 7.22 Cephalometric data quantifying the tracing findings. Linear data is used to describe skeletal structures and angular data indicates dental orientation.

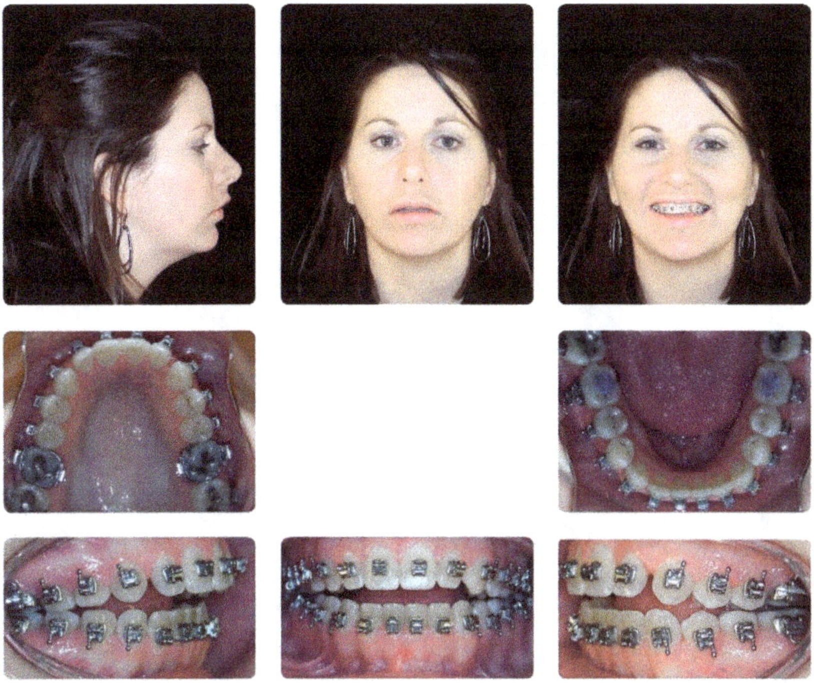

Figure 7.23 Preoperative clinical photos of the orthodontic preparation. The archwires have been removed to decrease noise artifact in the CBCT.

The treatment plan was to mobilize and realign the jaws with a LeFort 1 posterior superior maxillary impaction and a mandibular sagittal split advancement. The aims establish:-

i. Elimination of the anterior open bite.
ii. An optimum occlusion.
iii. Harmonious vertical facial proportions.
iv. An aesthetic lip-incisor relationship at rest and when animated.

The agreed treatment plan was superimposed over the preoperative volumetric data (the 3D CBCT facial image) to confirm the planned changes (Figure 7.24). The proposed surgical changes of

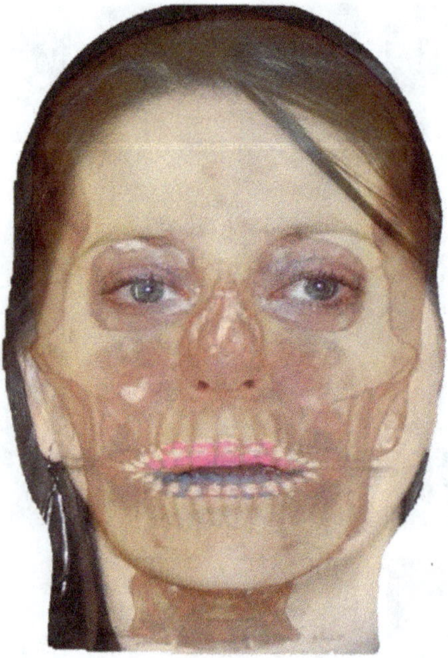

Figure 7.24 This illustration shows the fusion of the high definition scanned dental models to the CBCT dentoalveolar data, overlayed by a frontal photograph mapped (matched) to the cone beam soft tissue contours.

the maxilla and mandible can be seen as a blue "wire mesh" overlying the original skeletal volume (Figure 7.25). The closure of the anterior open bite was primarily achieved by the posterior maxillary impaction (PMS) leaving a degree of anterior downward rotation (ADR) which required a bone graft. The sagittal split image shows the planned amount of mandibular advancement. This solution also provided an aesthetic lip-incisor relationship at rest (see photographs Figure 7.28).

CASS and the Operative Methodology

The key intraoperative means of controlling a LeFort 1 osteotomy is the measurement from the glabella to the upper central incisal edge or midpoint of the upper arch wire. A Kirschner wire or a fine screw is inserted in the mid glabella and the real time measurement to the central incisor edge is recorded from which the measured amount anterior change is calculated. Once the osteotomy has mobilized the maxilla it is wired to the intact mandible with the intermediate wafer interposed to determine the final transverse and antero-posterior relationships. This maxillomandibular complex is carefully rotated about the condyles to the planned glabella — incisor measurement. This measure is confirmed with a caliper (Figure 7.27). Care must be taken on closure to remove any interfering bone or nasal septum contacts which can be anticipated on the virtual planning image (see Figure 7.9).

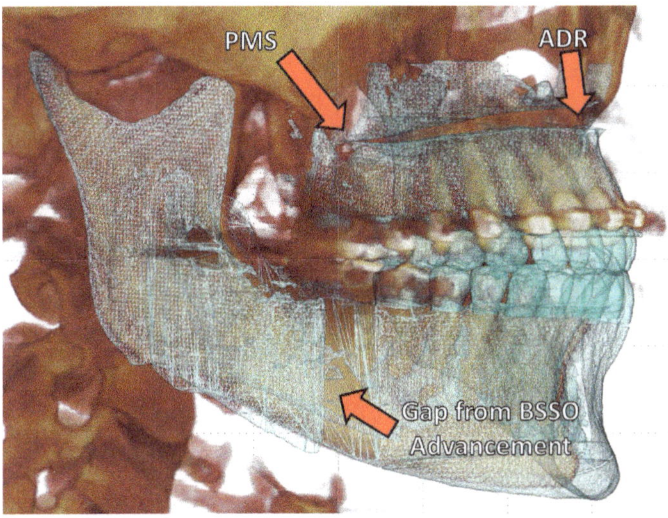

Figure 7.25 Superimposition of the surgical plan on the preoperative CBCT. The plan is represented as a wire mesh to allow visualization of the underlying volumetric anatomy.

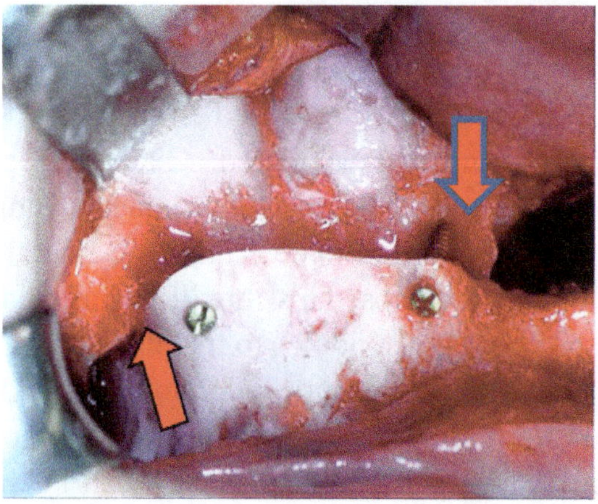

(a)

Figure 7.26 (**a**) The arrows show superior repositioning of the mobilized maxilla has resulted in medial displacement of the maxillary sinus wall. The only resection necessary was from the inferior nasal septum and the creation of notches at points of interference to allow the superior movement.

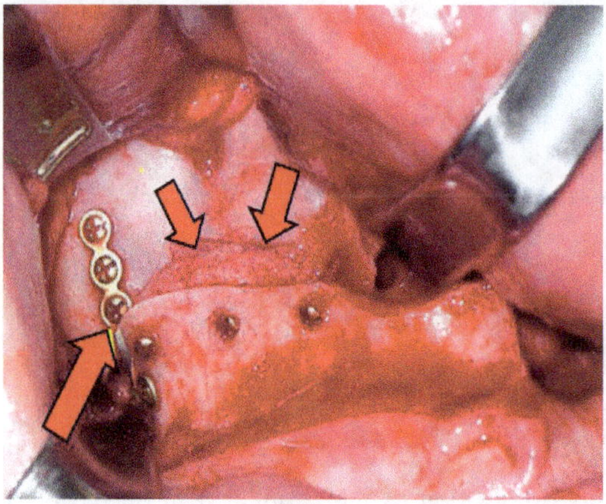

(b)

Figure 7.26 (**b**) An "L" plate is adapted for fixation at this point and bicortical screws used to secure the sinus walls. A cancellous graft has been fashioned to fill the void and is stabilized by a third bicortical screw.

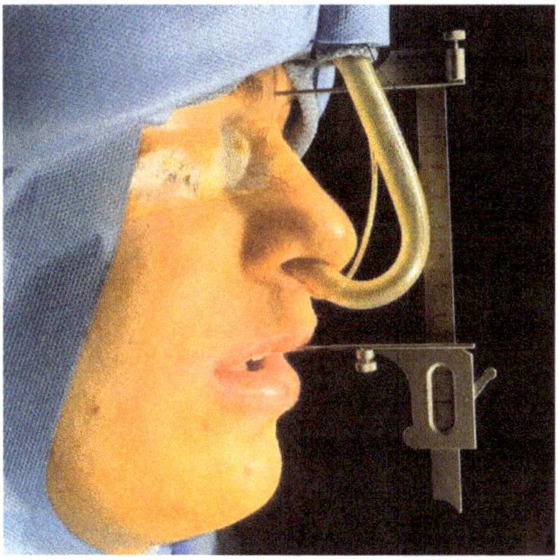

Figure 7.27 Caliper checking the vertical position of the postoperative maxilla. The transverse and antero-posterior positions are controlled by the CBCT/CADCAM intermediate and final occlusal wafers.

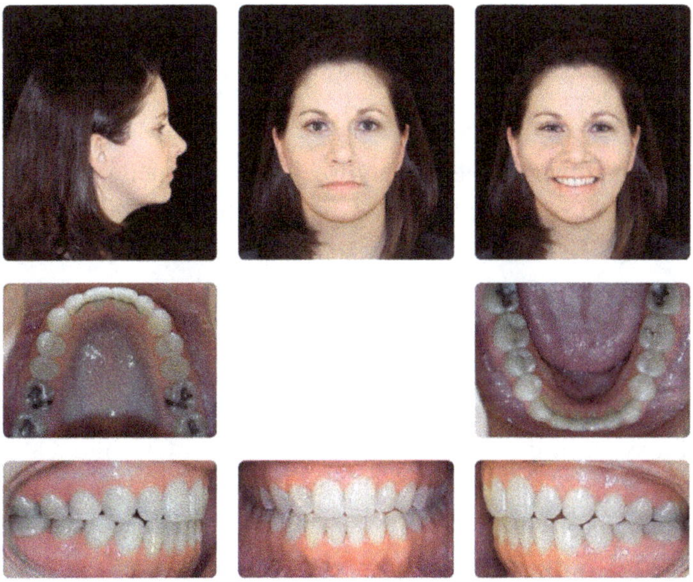

Figure 7.28 The final post-operative photographs following the removal of orthodontic appliances shows the closed anterior open bite and an aesthetic lip incisor relationship on smiling.

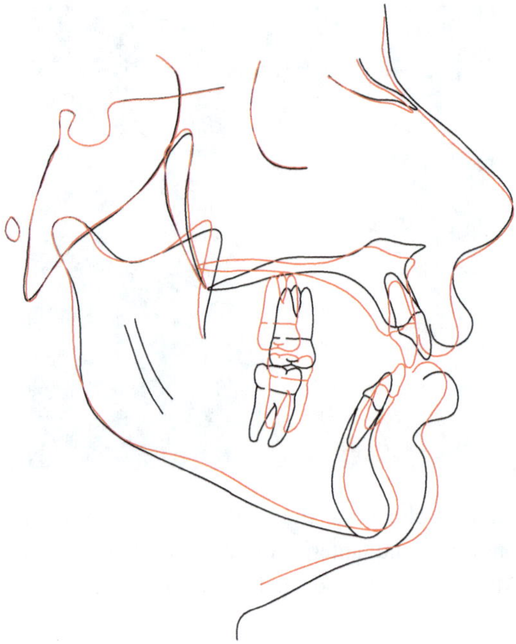

Figure 7.29 Comparison of the pre (black) and post operative (red) tracings.

Bilateral support to the mandible is maintained whilst fixation plates are applied and the caliper measurements reconfirmed.

Postoperative (Figure 7.25)

Before and after comparisons made with traditional superimposed tracing methods and cephalometric analysis are highly satisfactory although operator dependent, but unlike CASS the cephalometric data is limited to mid-sagittal plane changes. A postoperative follow up with a CBCT scan is recommended at 6 months to confirm bone union and osteotomy stability. Soft tissue changes can be monitored non-invasively with 3D photo superimposition.

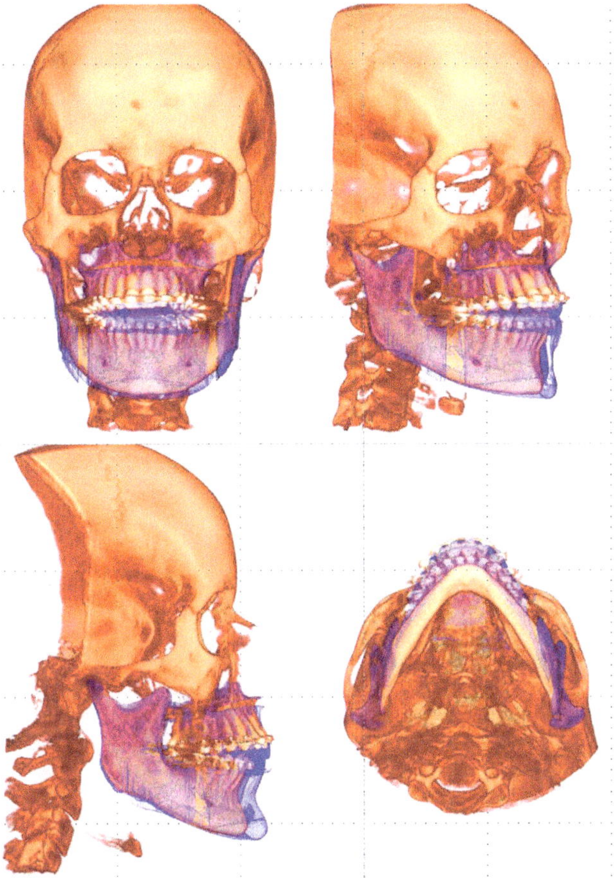

Figure 7.30 The postoperative CBCT scan has been converted to a blue mesh surface overlying the preoperative volume to visualize the surgical changes. Long-term stability can be assessed by superimposition of additional scans if desired.

Conclusions

The advantages of Computer-Aided Surgical Simulation planning are:

1. The digital planning has proved to be as accurate as the results of skilled sagittal cephalometric analysis and model surgery.

2. The opportunity to examine cranio-facial deformities in three dimensions.
3. The opportunity to explore simultaneously several surgical options and predict their virtual outcomes.
4. The creation of accurate splint and wafer prototypes by 3D rapid printing.
5. The saved time in planning procedures using CASS methods is estimated to be 7–8 hours, but this is offset by the cost of the technology.
6. However, planning is the core of the process which may anticipate surgical problems but will not solve them without surgical skills.
7. Some clinicians have advocated surgical navigation to compliment CASS, but there is little evidence to suggest increased accuracy. Furthermore the surgical navigation equipment is costly, the training and learning curve extensive and the operation and anesthesia time is increased even in the hands of the experienced.

Acknowledgements

The valuable advice of Dr Tarik Klamcha Biomedial engineer for 3D Systems.

Chapter 8

Fixation Techniques

Mohammad Anwar Bamber and Tom Walker

Introduction

The most commonly used fixation methods for orthognathic surgery are the following.

External Fixation.

- Fixed orthodontic appliances, with occlusal wafers.
- Fixed orthodontic appliances with supplementary arch wires and tubes.
- Arch bars — principally the prefabricated Erich design.
- Cortical screws for intermaxillary fixation.
- Eyelet wires are considered to be time consuming and obsolete.
- Cast metal splints are rarely used except in cleft cases.

Internal Fixation.

- Miniature titanium bone plates and cortical screws.
- Bicortical screws.
- Bioresorbable fixation plates and screws.

Most surgeons find orthodontic fixed appliance archwires with or without the addition of hooks are the most versatile and reliable method for intra- and postoperative fixation, especially when used with carefully constructed occlusal wafers. Where there has been no recent orthodontic treatment, a cortical screw placed in the buccal alveolus in each quadrant is useful for intraoperative fixation. Eyelet wires are a simple substitute but are less convenient to work with. Cast metal splints are considered to be obselete because of the clinical and laboratory complexity and are usually confined to the unstable components of a cleft case.

With the use of miniature titanium plates and screws, wire osteosynthesis is outdated except where plate systems are not available. However precise temporary intermaxillary fixation (IMF) is very important to secure the mobilised segments of the maxilla and the mandible whilst applying the internal fixation plates and screws.

Bicortical bone screws or buccal plates in mandibular procedures have totally revolutionised postoperative rehabilitation by dispensing with prolonged intermaxillary fixation. Whatever the method of fixation, it should be decided upon early so that there is adequate time for an appropriate appliance to be carefully designed and theatre time may be saved by fixation on the teeth preoperatively under local anaesthesia, with or without intravenous sedation.

The material and design of any fixation appliance must be capable of maintaining the bone fragments in the planned position until union has occurred. This is particularly important in a cleft osteotomy.

Fixed Orthodontic Appliances

Most patients require presurgical fixed appliance orthodontic treatment, these may be modified for intermaxillary fixation and segmental stabilisation with the help of rectangular wire attachments and hooks (Figure 8.1).

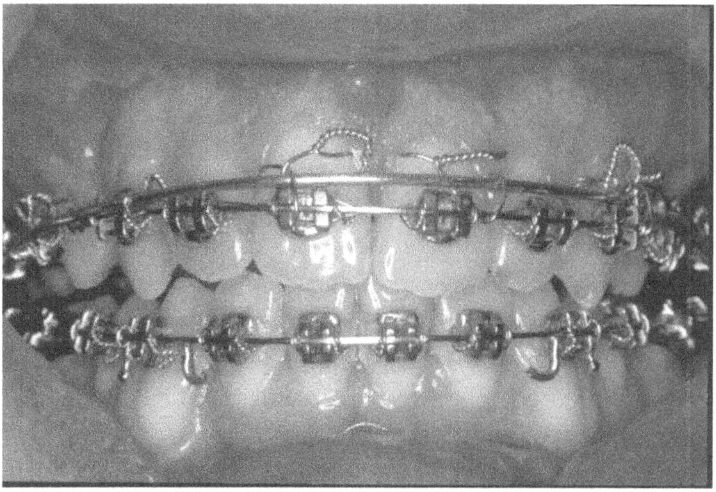

Figure 8.1 Orthodontic brackets, wires and hooks for fixation. Note the 1 mm maxillary supplemental arch wire to augment the internal fixation used to localise a divided dentoalveolar segment.

The attachments must fit well and be cemented securely to avoid dislodgement during surgery and intermaxillary fixation. The heavy rectangular wire in Edgewise brackets gives good stabilisation for fixation, and if required can be improved with the addition of crimpable steel hooks or soldered brass wires. Unfortunately it can be tedious when the hooks ensnare swabs. With segmental surgery, intra- and postoperative dentoalveolar stabilisation is essential to avoid any rotation around the internal plate fixation. Although this can be an archwire shaped on the sectioned and repositioned model used for surgical planning and which can be fitted intraoperatively by an orthodontist, it is more convenient to:

- section the arch wire at operation to facilitate the osteotomy,
- localise the segments with a wafer, and then
- stabilise by ligation to a heavy 1 mm supplemental arch wire inserted into tubes fitted on the molar bands (Figure 8.1). On the upper molars these can be the headgear tubes but in the lower arch double tubes are required.

Advantages

- Orthodontic fixation does not require laboratory facilities.
- With a rectangular arch wire every type of movement can be controlled.
- It is invaluable for intraoperative immobilisation whilst applying the plates and screws for rigid fixation.

Disadvantages

- Direct bonded attachments are occasionally lost because the cementation fails.
- It is advisable to remove any lingual attachments which may have been present during the orthodontic treatment.

Cortical Screws

These may be specifically designed for IMF and are inserted through a stab wound into the dense basal bone between the canine and first premolars. Either wire or postoperative elastics may be applied to immobilise the occlusion.

This technique is only applicable when both arches are intact.

Arch Bars

Prefabricated Flexible

Although rarely used, a prefabricated form (Erich — Dentaurum, Pforzheim) made of semi-rigid stainless steel (Figure 8.2), can be easily contoured to the arch form and ligated with stainless steel wires passed around the arch bar and the necks of the adjacent teeth. Cleats for intermaxillary fixation are also an integral part of the design. Stainless steel wire (0.5 mm) which has been prestretched by 10% is used to ligate the arch bar to the teeth, starting in the midline and working backwards.

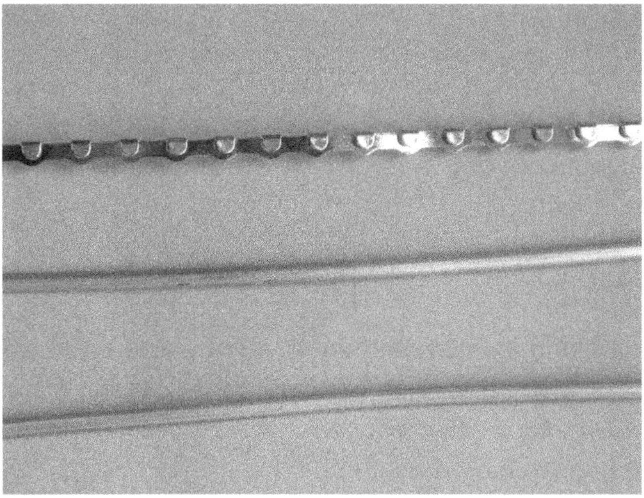

Figure 8.2 The prefabricated Erich arch bar still has clinical value but the wrought wire shown here for a custom made arch bar is rarely used.

Advantages

- These are useful where orthodontic treatment has not been used.
- No technical assistance is required for this type of fixation, and the bars can be easily adapted into the desired shape.
- Arch bars can be placed before the operation, under local anaesthesia. This reduces the time spent in the operating room.
- The occlusion can always be checked and at the end of the fixation period the arch bars can easily be removed without an anaesthetic.

Disadvantages

- An adequate number of suitable teeth are required to get rigid and reliable fixation.
- They may not be suitable in osteotomies where there are many crowns and bridges.

Ligating Arch Bars

A simple 0.5 mm wire ligature around the tooth and an arch bar is unsatisfactory and the addition of a loop around the bar creating a figure of eight between tooth and bar is essential to produce stable anchorage (Figure 8.3).

Eyelet Wires

These are used in the immobilisation of jaw fractures because of the simplicity of their fabrication and application but have been superceded by arch bars. However, they are valuable for intraoperative immobilisation with rigid fixation.

Wire of 0.5 mm is preferable to 0.35 mm as it is sturdier and easier to pass through tight contact points and gingiva without getting lost. Three metres of wire can be stretched 10% between heavy artery forceps and then cut into lengths of approximately 12 cm. Each is grasped at both ends by heavy forceps and the centre placed against a headless nail (2 mm diameter) fixed in a stable surface, or a bur shank in a vice. The wire is firmly bent around the

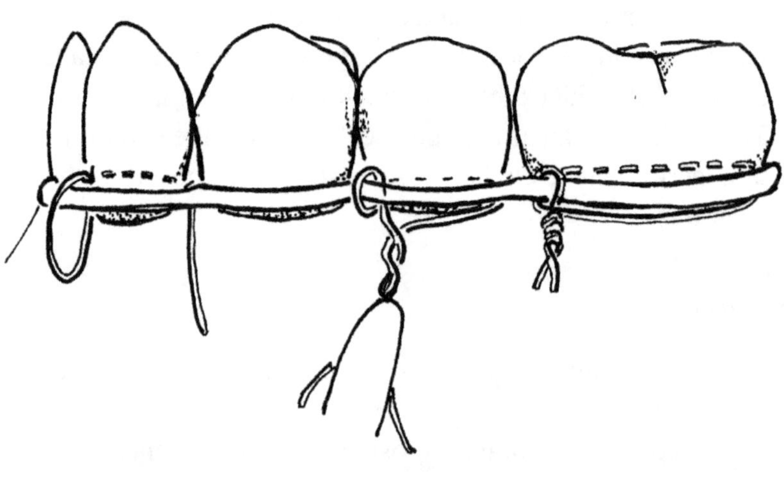

Figure 8.3 Ligation of an arch bar with 0.5 mm stretched stainless steel wire.

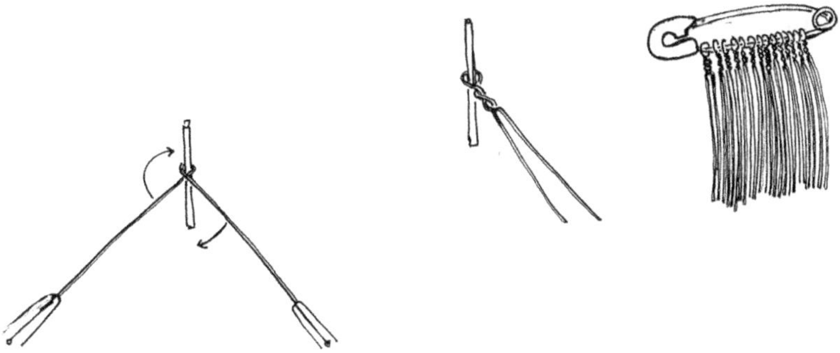

Figure 8.4 Making eyelet wires from 0.5 mm stretched stainless steel wire.

nail and then twisted twice to produce the eye. The eyelet wire is then removed and the ends are cut at 45° and trimmed (Figure 8.4).

Advantages

- The wires can be easily prepared and applied preoperatively with no technical support or dental casts (models).
- They are ideal for temporary intermaxillary fixation when rigid fixation, i.e. plates and screws are being used.

Disadvantages

- This is a time-consuming procedure where an adequate number of suitably shaped teeth are essential.
- The use of eyelet wires on crowns and bridgework intraoperatively, can produce embarrassing displacement.
- Even when used with a wafer they will not stabilise small segments.

Occlusal Wafers (See Chapter 6 which describes in detail the traditional manual wafer fabrication and also Chapter 7 for the Computerised Assisted Surgical Simulation (CASS) 3D printing technique.)

1. *The traditional manual design*: As a final step in the traditional presurgical planning, occlusal wafers are fabricated on the articulator mounted casts to establish the intermediate and postoperative positions. After surgery, the occlusal wafer can also provide a solid interdigitation of the teeth, especially in cases of mandibular advancement where the goal is a “3-point landing”. This makes it possible to defer any final orthodontic refinement of the occlusion or the replacement of crowns and bridgework until comfortable bone union has taken place.

When the dental arch is sectioned and the segments repositioned, the wafer establishes the planned position whilst securing the osteotomy site with screws and or bone plates. However the occlusal wafer alone will not prevent rotation of the dento-alveolar segments, which must be secured with an orthodontic archwire, an arch bar or a sectional splint despite the internal rigid fixation.

2. *3D printing technology for surgical guides and wafers*: The terms surgical guides, splints, or wafers are unfortunately used interchangeably but have in common their design and fabrication by rapid prototyping software and can be created by 3D printing which if done overnight saves an estimated 7–8 hours in the preoperative workup process. The design process is done with Computer Assisted Surgical Simulation (CASS) software as 3D prototypes which are printed in acrylic or epoxy-photopolymer. However this virtual surgical plan still produces an intermediate splint which relates the corrected maxilla to the unchanged mandible and a final wafer to relate the maxillary occlusion to that of the corrected mandible.

Internal Fixation

Transosseous Wiring

This is a traditional method of holding bone fragments together. Although the bone plate has superceded transosseous wiring, there are occasions when wires can be an invaluable salvage technique to hold bone fragments together. For the mandible with its rigid bone cortices cortical plates, 0.5 mm stretched, soft stainless steel wire is satisfactory. However, a finer 0.35 mm wire is essential for maxillary osteotomies to avoid pulling through the thin bone margins of the drill holes. Although the bone plate has superceded transosseous wiring there are occasions when wires can be an invaluable salvage technique.

Miniature Bone Plates and Cortical Screws

Titanium bone plates and screws,[1] are an excellent means of internal fixation. The introduction of L- and Y-shape plates should eliminate apical damage when screwing into the maxillary alveolar segment. The screw holes must be prepared with a slow, well-cooled matching drill, or a tapering tungsten carbide fissure bur (No. 101). High speeds and heavy hand pressure amplify eccentric rotation and produce a large, charred useless hole, especially in the thin maxillary wall. There are broader salvage screws available to rescue such situations. Plates provide greater security against relapse especially in cleft cases. In non-cleft osteotomies, the use of buccal plates in the maxilla and mandible or 9–13 mm bicortical screws for sagittal split osteotomies have made postoperative intermaxillary fixation unnecessary. This has dramatically simplified postoperative nursing and patient rehabilitation. Unfortunately, some plates when superficially placed submucosally give rise to irritation or become infected and have to be removed. However, when inserted with slow, gentle carefully cooled drilling of the bone, long-term incorporation is the rule rather than the exception.

Bioresorbable Fixation Plates and Screws

Resorbable plates and bicortical positioning screws have been produced from biodegradable polymers based on lactide, glycolide, and e-caprolactone which are widely used in tissue engineering and

---

[1]Gebruder Martin GmbH & Co. KG, Tuttlingen, Germany; Leibinger (QS Leibinger, Muhllheim-Stetten, Germany), Albert Waeschle, Germany.

drug delivery systems. Poly L-lactide (PLLA) is a semicrystalline polymer with a high strength modulus and a slow degradation time which is more than 24 months, whereas poly D L-lactide (PDLLA) is amorphous and has a lower modulus and a more rapid degradation time of 12 to 16 months. Depending on the product, 76% of the plate strength is retained for 2 months and 50% up to 6 months.

At the moment most are not suitable for the mandible to return to early masticatory function, as they can lose their strength within six weeks.

The breakdown products are generally inert, however some early systems have had problems with an inflammatory response. Rapid hydrolysis due to a high polyglycolide content is a suspected cause of this.

Overall resorbable plates and screws have fallen out of favour because of cost, lack of a supportive clinical evidence base and friability during screw placement.

Chapter 9

Osteotomies and Bone Grafts

Malcolm Harris

This chapter provides basic preoperative, intraoperative and postoperative instructions for surgical procedures. At first sight these may appear adequate for the correction of all deformities. However, in practice most cases have a complexity requiring the integration of several operative procedures, as described in Chapter 11.

General Preoperative Considerations

Informed consent is essential. Patients should be given an accurate although reassuring description of the immediate postoperative period. The possibility of prolonged neurapraxia of the mental or infraorbital nerves must be stressed and recorded. They should be given details of postoperative regimens for feeding and oral hygiene and also be asked to bring to hospital a small soft and medium toothbrush. All this is best done as a handout.

The patient must be fit, with a normal haemoglobin concentration. A chest radiograph is probably only necessary where a rib graft is required as a base line should there be any postoperative problem. The nasal airway must be bilaterally patent. Enlarged tonsils may create postoperative oropharyngeal obstruction when swollen, especially with maxillary osteotomies.

Emotionally unstable patients are unsuitable for surgery and find intermaxillary fixation intolerable. However this is rarely a problem with internal rigid fixation.

Preoperative Investigations

1. Haemoglobin, full blood count and blood film.
2. Urinalysis.
3. Blood group and transfusion antibody screening.
4. For major procedures especially when a bone graft is taken, cross-matching blood should be arranged at the last preoperative visit.
5. Sickling test, hepatitis B surface antigen (HBsAg) and HIV screening where appropriate.
6. Chest radiograph, if indicated by the medical history or procedure.

Blood Replacement

Loss of blood can be significantly reduced with hypotensive anaesthesia and antifibrinolytic medication. Mandibular procedures rarely require transfusion, however it is good practice to group the patient's blood and screen for transfusion antibodies but hold the serum for emergency cross-matching. With the increased concern about cross-infection, autologous blood is now being used in some centres for elective surgery.

Antibiotics

Preoperatively

Microbiologists advocate minimal regimens for non-infected surgery. The following **alternatives** are possible choices.

- A single dose of Co-amoxiclav 1000 mg/200 mg (i.e 1g amoxicillin and 200 mg clavulanic acid) is given preoperatively by intravenous injection or infusion.

- Metronidazole can be given as a 1g rectal suppository pre- and postoperatively. This is more convenient than a 500 mg slow intravenous infusion, to be followed by 400 mg orally 12-hourly for 2–3 days.
- Clindamycin 300 mg intravenously at induction and 150 mg iv. 3 hours postoperatively. This can be extended to 300 mg 6-hourly orally for 2–3 days.

Antibiotics are not required more than 3 days postoperatively unless there is evidence of wound infection or a persistent pyrexia.

Antioedema Medication

Preoperatively

Dexamethasone 8 mg is given intravenously with the anaesthetic induction agents and repeated 12 hours later.

Postoperatively

Dexamethasone 8 mg is given i.v. or i.m. 12-hourly on postoperative day 1, followed by 4–5 mg 12-hourly on day 2.

Operating Considerations

1. The patient must be anaesthetised via a nasal endotracheal tube centrally secured across the forehead. A simple low profile connector between the endotracheal and anaesthetic tubing is essential. A 12 FG nasogastric tube for postoperative aspiration should also be passed prior to the operation. Some anaesthetists will also pass a fine-bore feeding tube at the same time.
2. Clean the face and mouth with an aqueous antiseptic such as chlorhexidine or povidone-iodine.

3. Drape so that the orbital margins may be exposed for orientation. Cover the nasal tube and eyes with an adhesive drape (Steridrape — 3M, US; Opsite — Smith and Nephew, UK) (Figure 9.1).
4. If a bone graft is being taken, strip the patient, clean the hip or chest twice with iodine detergent and square drape the area with towels; cover and seal the site with a Steridrape or Opsite.
5. Check bipolar diathermy is in place. The anaesthetic machine is best placed with a long hose at the lower end of the table on the opposite side to the graft site. If used, the compressed air cylinder can also be conveniently placed at the foot end of the table so that the air drill hose may pass upwards along the long axis of the patient to the head end. This is avoided by the use of an electric drill.
6. Tilt the feet down and the head up. Lubricate the lips initially and repeatedly with 1% hydrocortisone ointment.

Instruments

The following list gives the basic osteotomy instrumentation. Most of the instruments are shown in Figures 9.2a–9.2d.

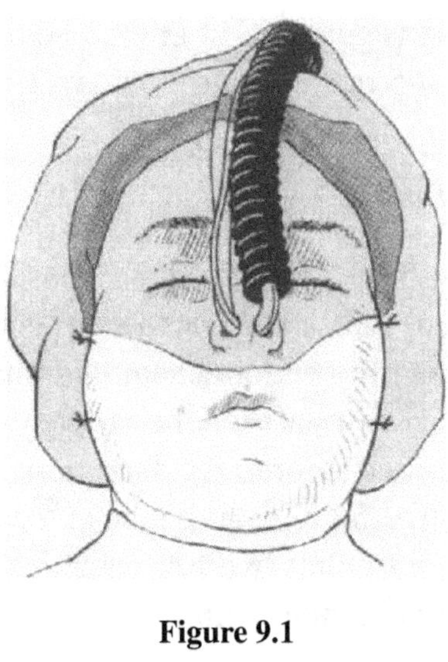

Figure 9.1

1. Ward's cheek retractor
2. Prognathism channel retractors (×2)
3. Chin holding retractor
4. Cairn's malleable retractor 17 mm
5. Cairn's malleable retractor 11 mm
6. Lac's tongue depressor — child
7. Lac's tongue depressor — adult
8. Kilner cheek retractors — insulated (×2)
9. Forked retractor 70 × 12 mm
10. Langenbeck retractors 44 × 13 mm (×2)
11. Langenbeck retractors 23 × 7 mm (×2)
12. Allis tissue forceps, 4 in 5 teeth, 15 cm (×2)
13. Halstead Mosquito artery forceps, curved 12.5 cm (×10)
14. Bachaus towel clips (×10)
15. Rampley spongeholders 24 cm (×3)
16. Dunhill artery forceps 13 cm (×10)
17. Lawson Tait artery forceps (×2)
18. Universal wire and plate shears 12 cm (×2)
19. Kocher artery forceps, straight 1 in 2 teeth 18 cm
20. Kocher artery forceps, curved 1 in 2 teeth 18 cm

(a)

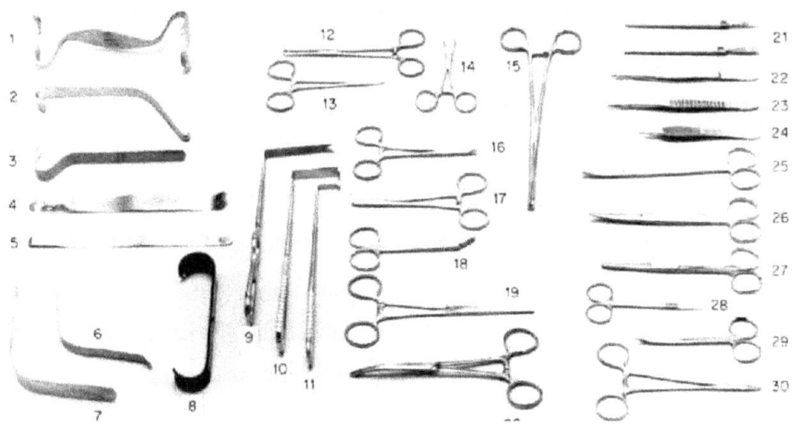

Figure 9.2 (a)

(b)

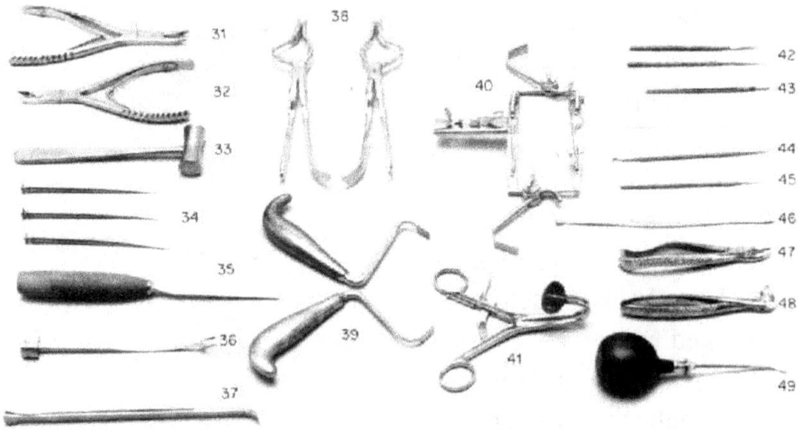

(c)

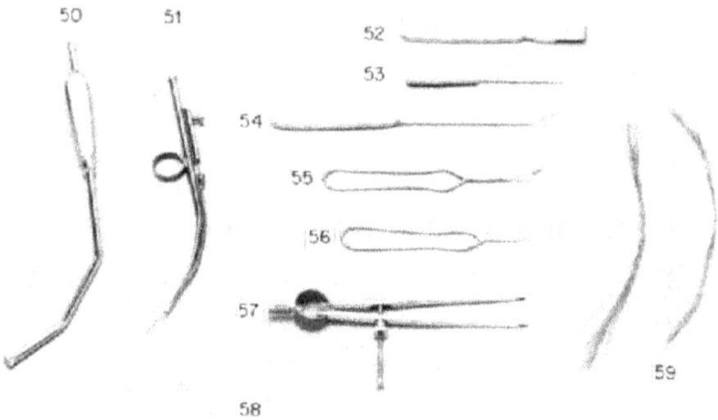

(d)

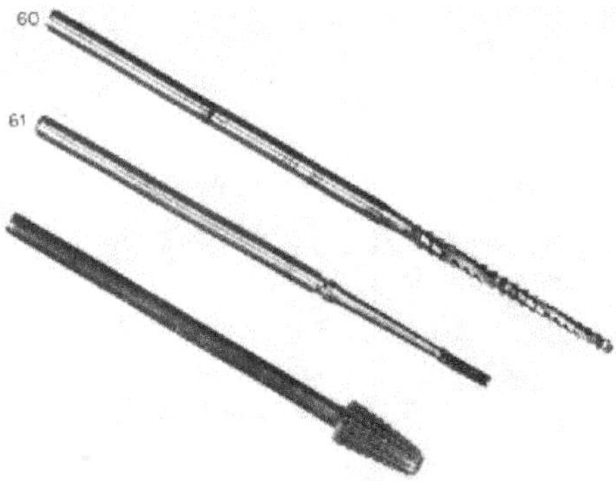

Figure 9.2 **(b)**, **(c)**, **(d)** (*Continued*)

21. Barron scalpel handles with No. 5 and 10 blades (×2)
22. McIndoe dissecting forceps 15 cm
23. Gillies dissecting forceps, toothed 15 cm
24. Adson dissecting forceps, toothed
25. McIndoe scissors T/C edge 18 cm
26. Mayo scissors T/C 17 cm
27. Blunt-ended scissors 15 cm
28. Iris scissors T/C 12 cm
29. Strabismus scissors T/C 11.5 cm marked with black tape
30. Crilewood needleholders T/C jaws 15 cm (×2)
31. Luer Jansen bone rongeur 19 cm
32. McIndoe bone cutting forceps 19 cm
33. Small mallet
34. French osteotomes 5 mm, 7 mm and 11 mm
35. Osteotomes ½" (13 mm) with round handle (×2)
36. Obwegeser nasal septal chisel
37. Pterygoid chisel
38. Rowes disimpaction forceps — right and left
39. Tessier maxillary mobilisers — right and left
40. Dingham mouth gag. Frame with cheek retractor, 3 blades S, M, L (not shown)
41. Featherstone or other self retaining mouth gag
42. Kilner skin hooks 15 cm (×2)
43. Mapping pen (with nib)
44. Mitchell trimmer
45. Dental probe No. 6
46. Howarth's nasal raspatories (periosteal elevators) (×2)
47. Dental extraction forceps 76 N
48. Dental extraction forceps 74 N
49. Chip syringes (×2)
50. Yankauer suction tube
51. Self-clearing suction tube
52. Farabeouf rougine curved 11 mm
53. Flat screwdriver

54. Obwegeser mandibular awl
55. Kelsey Fry bone awl — curved
56. Kelsey Fry bone awl — straight
57. Caliper
58. Ruler
59. 0.50 mm and 0.35 mm stainless steel tie wires (×25)
60. Long shanked Lindemann surgical bur (Meissinger)
61. Tungsten carbide surgical bur (Ash)
62. Cone shaped acrylic bur

There are an infinite number of refinements such as a coronoid stripper and coronoid forceps, and many types of periosteal elevator.

Not shown are: surgical handpieces for drills and oscillating and sagittal saws or a miniature titanium bone plating set with transfacial trocar, canullae and retractor.

Note: To ensure a harmonious operation, check the radiographs, study models with the patient the day before and the instruments, especially burs, drills and wafers *preoperatively*. A pre-admission checklist can be invaluable.

Postoperative Care

Immediate

The patient is nursed at 45° for comfort and access. A nasopharyngeal airway is left *in situ* overnight, with *strict* instructions to staff to suck out the nasopharynx every 30 minutes with a fine catheter passed through the tube. Ideally it should be humidified to prevent crusting. Some anaesthetists prefer to leave the endotracheal tube *in situ* overnight. However, it is doubtful whether suction of blood and mucus from the entire length of the tube to maintain the airway can always be guaranteed. Oxygen (40%) in air is usually administered by face mask at approximately 5 litres/min.

Hourly aspiration of accumulated blood, oral and gastric secretions, and bile from the stomach help to eliminate vomiting. As most patients are fit prior to the procedure, dedicated nursing supervision with half-hourly observations is required rather than intensive care.

Analgesics

Pain experience is variable and often absent. However repeated moderate doses of a subcutaneous or intravenous opiate, such as morphine 10 mg p.r.n. × 4 doses each 24 hours (is more useful than 10 mg 4-hourly), with an antiemetic such as metoclopromide 10 mg, should be prescribed.

An infiltration of the long-acting local analgesic 0.5% (5 mg/ml) bupivacaine hydrochloride (Marcain) with adrenaline (1:200 000) will reduce postoperative pain in addition to its intraoperative analgesic and vasoconstrictor effects. It is interesting to note that this reduced pain experience extends beyond the possible action of the drug. Up to 2 mg/kg may be used in any operative procedure.

Postoperative Care

First day; Check in particular:

1. Airway and chest clinically and if not clear, radiographically. All patients benefit from chest physiotherapy.
2. Fluid balance, i.e. blood and fluid replacement should approximate to blood and fluid loss. Note the urinary output and ensure the patient's bladder has been emptied, especially as transient retention may follow narcotic analgesics. Remember the loss via gastric aspiration, vomiting and the drains. Two litres of compound sodium lactate intravenous infusion (Hartmann's solution) should suffice in addition to any blood loss over 500 mls.

3. Occlusion and elastic fixation if used.
4. Cutaneous sensation and facial motor function.
5. Drug regimen. Antibiotics should be given intravenously or rectally, and analgesics and antiemetics intravenously. However, many patients will tolerate soluble analgesics orally or by nasogastric tube on an as required basis. A rectal non-steroidal anti-inflammatory analgesic, such as flurbiprofen 150 mg 12-hourly, is also useful to avoid continuous opiate analgesia.
6. Nutrition. During the first 24 hours continue the Hartmann's solution, 2 litres i.v., but try 100 ml/h water by mouth, then tea or orange juice, etc. as soon as the patient can tolerate feeding, using a syringe and quill, feeding cup or straw. If this is not possible use a fine-bore (Clinifeed — Roussel, UK) nasogastric tube which should be passed preoperatively to permit feeding until the patient can accept fluid and calories by mouth. If a fine-bore tube is not available, the standard Ryle's tube (12 or 14 FG) may be used. (See also Chapter 19 for postoperative feeding regimen.)
7. Oral hygiene with Chlorhexidine 0.2% solution is commenced.

Second Postoperative Day

Repeat the above but change from intravenous to an oral or nasogastric regimen, increasing the feed to a full diet.

Note: Oral fluids may be difficult for some patients up to 3 days after major procedures, especially those involving the chin, producing difficult lip control.

Discharge from hospital is determined by the nature of the procedure, the individual, and the care available at home. Most patients can be discharged on the second or third postoperative day, and on discharge should have adequate analgesics and instructions on oral hygiene, especially the use of a small tooth brush with chlorhexidine gluconate gel or mouthwash. Advice on a liquidised diet and the provision of a diet sheet is also important.

Follow-Up

The occlusion may be checked weekly or fortnightly. It is reassuring for the surgeon to assist maximal intercuspation with the final wafer and elastics. However wafers are uncomfortable and difficult to keep clean and are probably unnecessary with rigid fixation. Soluble sutures should be left or removed when they are accessible and are a source of irritation. Patients require reassurance that impaired labial or infraorbital sensation will return to normal within 6 months and that excess soft tissue will also remodel and disappear over this period.

The Operative Procedures

The Obwegeser Sagittal Split Osteotomy

Indications

This versatile operation may be used for placing the mandible backwards or forwards, but should not be used for an anterior open bite without a simultaneous maxillary impaction to reduce the posterior upper facial height.

Technique

The operation for a backward correction will be described first.

1. The jaws must be supported as widely apart as possible by a self-retaining gag which gives better access than a prop (Figure 9.3a).
2. The tissues on the lingual and buccal aspect of the ascending ramus and adjacent body of the mandible are infiltrated generously with a vasoconstrictor containing local anaesthetic, e.g. 0.5% bupivacaine with 1:200 000 adrenaline.

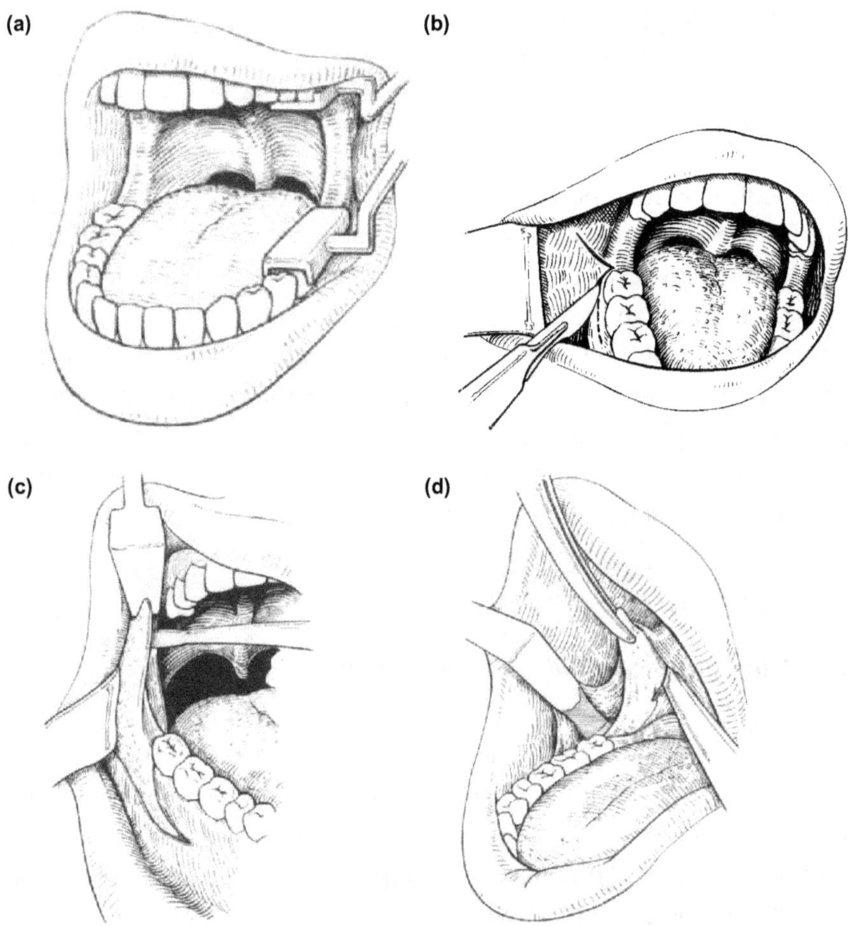

Figure 9.3 (a), (b), (c), (d)

3. The incision is a buccally based triangular flap with the apex at the back of the last standing molar (Figure 9.3b). The anterior limb should leave a generous skirt of alveolar mucoperosteum attached to the gingival margin of the first molar to assist suturing (Figure 9.3c).
4. The buccal periosteum is widely elevated, exposing the outer surface of the body and ramus of the mandible. This can be

facilitated by using the forefinger, stretching and incising the periosteal layer to produce a buccal space which helps retraction of the tissues with a channel retractor and also provides good operative access for the insertion of bone plates. Techniques recommending limited exposure are difficult to understand (Figure 9.3d).

Raise the lingual flap, with a Howarth periostal elevator, detaching the mucoperiosteum downwards and forwards from the anterior aspect of the ascending ramus to the distolingual aspect of the last molar. The inferior extent of the periosteal reflection needs to be no deeper than the mylohyoid ridge.

5. Dissect up the anterior aspect of the ramus, detaching the temporalis tendon with the sharp end of the Howarth elevator or a forked coronoid stripper. By inserting the Obwegeser coronoid retractor half way up and applying strong traction, the exposed tendon can be gradually stripped off with the elevator so that the retractor may be eventually seated comfortably on the coronoid tip. This degree of elevation greatly helps the access to the lingual aspect of the ramus (Figure 9.3c). The application of a heavy pair of curved Kocher's or coronoid forceps to the coronoid will now dispense with the forked retractor and provide a comfortable and secure alternative for the assistant.
6. Carefully raise the lingual periosteum to the level of the sigmoid notch and follow its margin until the condylar neck is reached; then smoothly detach the tissues downwards to the lingula. Care will avoid troublesome venous bleeding, which usually ceases after the channel retractor (or a reversed bent Lacs retractor) is inserted with its tip passed behind the condylar neck.
7. The horizontal cut should be made as low as possible close to the lingula where the cortices are always separated by adequate cancellous bone. The higher the cut the less chance there is of splitting the ramus cleanly. Improved access is obtained by

rotating the flat or channel retractor 45° to the vertical plane so that it lies parallel to the neurovascular bundle (Figure 9.3e).

8. The cut is made through the cortex of the bone with a long-shanked, medium-sized tapering fissure bur (Ash, Meissinger, Busch) and should be extended beyond the concave inner surface to the distal aspect of the ramus as the shorter Hunsuck modification does not always work! With maxillary impactions parallel medial cuts allow a fillet of cortex to be removed. This enables the mandible to follow the maxillary vertical displacement (Figure 9.3f).
9. The buccal channel retractor is now placed vertically opposite the mid-point of the second molar with its tip below the lower border of the mandible (Figure 9.3g).
10. Access is remarkably improved by taking out the gag and all other instruments bringing the teeth into occlusion. A line of bur holes is made parallel to the external oblique ridge, which is continued downwards onto the lateral surface of the mandible following the lateral bony prominence as it curves down on the buccal surface towards the lower border (Figure 9.3h).
11. This ensures an accurate line when they are joined together, and produces a natural continuous, lingual-buccal cortical cut. It is important to emphasise the cuts through the cortex proximally at the junction of the medial (lingual) and mid section and also antero-inferiorly through the thick cortex of the lower border to a depth of 2 mm.

    If the mandibular osteotomy is part of a bimaxillary procedure the cuts are done bilaterally, tonsil swabs inserted, and the maxillary osteotomy carried out and fixed with the intermediate wafer against the unchanged mandible.
12. The split is traditionally done with two ½ inch osteotomes which must have thick round handles enabling a firm twisting action to be used without the glove slipping. However a more controlled division can be achieved with a narrow 5 mm. osteotome tapped first distally below the horizontal medial bur line

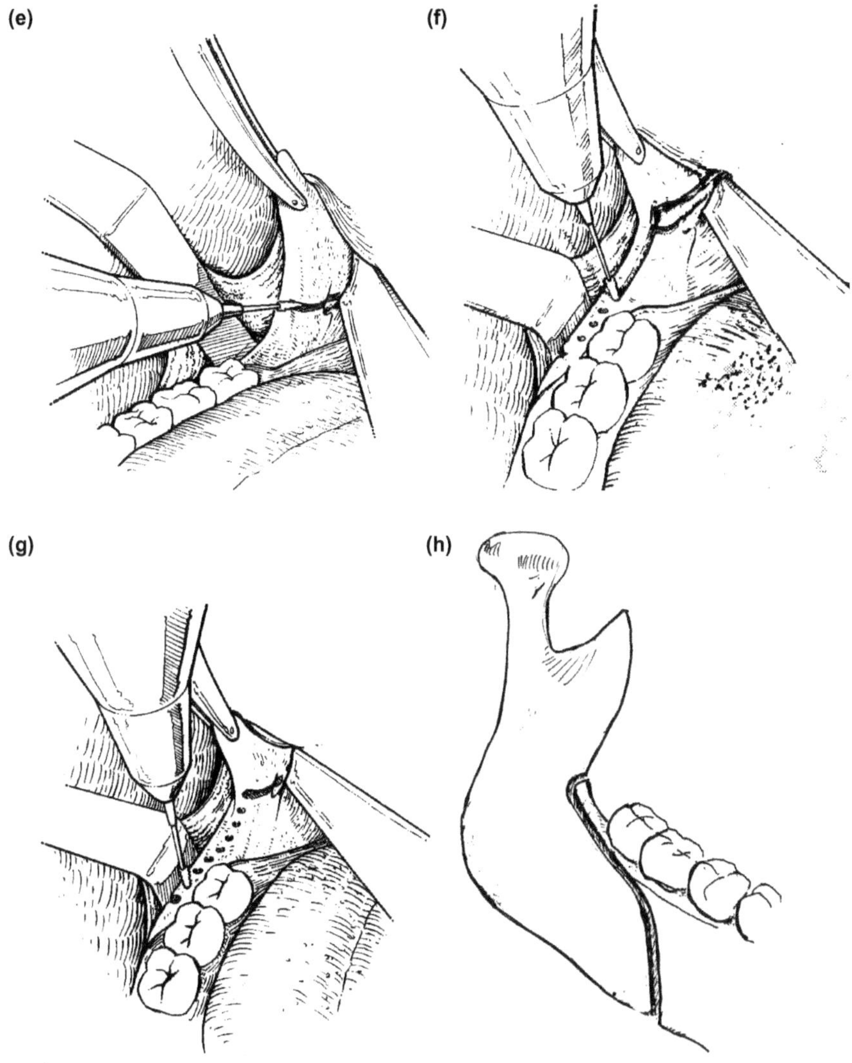

Figure 9.3 (e), (f), (g), (h)

“feeling” the inner surface of the outer cortical plate. This is repeated at least twice with an identical osteotome obliquely downwards and backwards through the buccal cut, and then downwards just within the line of the external oblique ridge which seems to be a natural plane of cleavage (Figure 9.3i).

This bone dissecting manoeuvre may produce an instant and clean split. If not the ½ inch osteotome is gently tapped into the anterior cortical cut until firm, and rotated slowly but continually until the cancellous bone begins to split. The cortical split is generated by rotating anticlockwise on the right side and clockwise on the left. Slow separation permits the neurovascular bundle to be identified if exposed and dissected from the outer fragment where it may be adherent. If a single osteotome is used, it should then moved from the anterior buccal end of the cut to the superomedial end (Figure 9.3j). The two segments must be completely separated by inserting a finger into the depths of the osteotomy cut to vigorously detach all muscular and periosteal restraints. Where the mandible is narrow or the fragments refuse to separate on twisting, the fine 5 mm osteotome can be used as just described to divide the bone by gently tapping it through to the lower and posterior borders on the inner aspect of the buccal cortex. However such resistance suggests that the cortical bur cuts are inadequate and should be repeated.

13. The estimated setback has been measured on the study models. This amount of buccal plate is held firmly in Kocher or Dingman bone-holding forceps and cut off with a Lindemann fissure bur protecting the underlying inferior dental bundle with a flat retractor (Figure 9.3k). A horizontal fillet of bone may have to be trimmed with an acrylic bar from the upper margin of the inner cut on the ascending ramus to allow a good fit, especially in cases where the maxilla has been elevated — and the mandible has to rise to maintain the occlusion.
14. The forward correction requires the buccal cortical cut to be made at the mesial aspect of the second molar. After the split, no bone is removed.
15. Internal fixation requires accurate, firm intraoperative intermaxillary fixation which is applied after the osteotomy cuts have been completed.

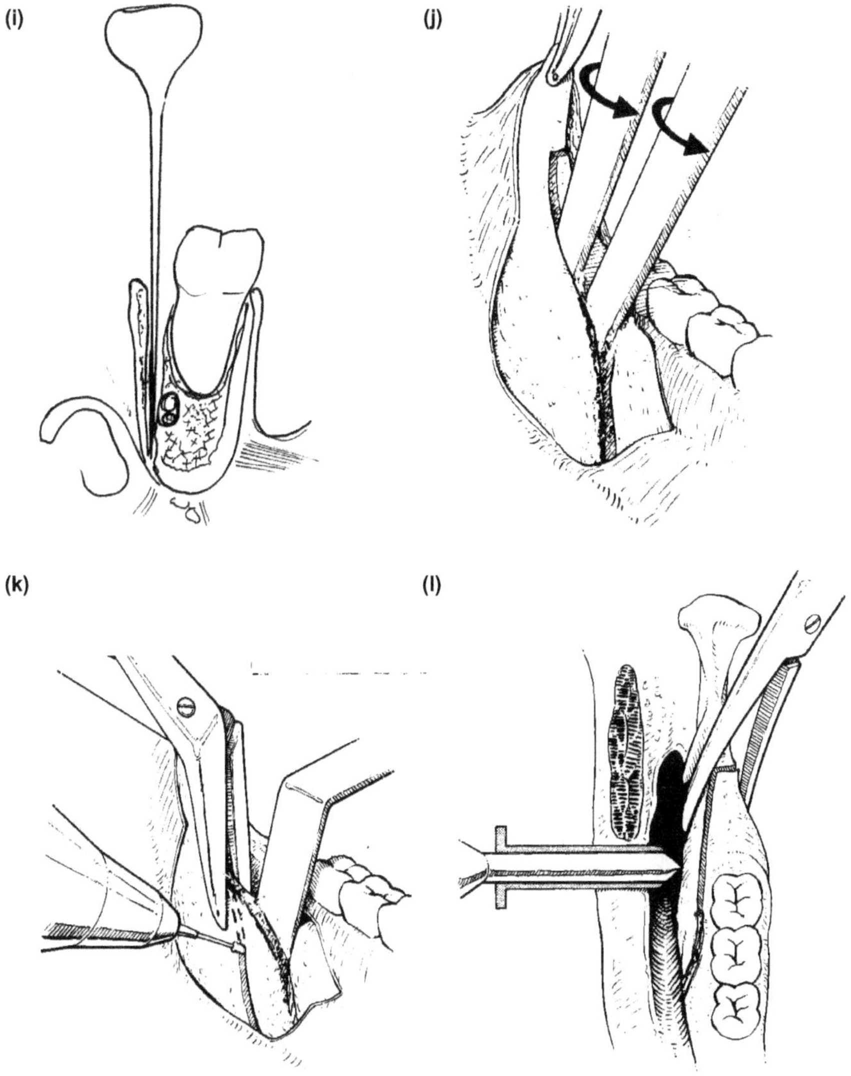

Figure 9.3 (i), (j), (k), (l)

16. A transfacial trocar, cannula and retractor are essential for bicortical screws. A short stab wound (5 mm) is made through the skin, a finger's breadth above the lower border of the mandible just anterior to the masseter muscle. Fine mosquito forceps are pushed through the tissues to enter the wound in the

mouth, opened and closed, rotated through 90°, and opened again to create an entry for the canulla.

17. The trocar and cannular sleeve are then firmly pushed through to reach the buccal plate (Figure 9.31). The trocar is removed and the cannula is attached to the extra and intraoral arms of the retractor. The design varies with the manufacturer. The cannula has a projection which helps to immobilise the buccal plate if a bone clamp is not used (Figure 9.3m).
18. The antero-posterior position of the proximal fragment (ascending ramus) is crucial Light self-retaining bone-holding or Allis forceps are used to grip the proximal fragment which is pushed back for mandibular advancements and pulled forwards for push backs. It should also be rotated downwards to lower the buccal plate just below the upper margin of the retromolar lingual cortical surface. This maintains the contour of the gonial angle which can be lost if the proximal fragment is inadvertently allowed to rotate forwards (Figure 9.3n).

    The two bone plates can then be stabilised by clamping them with an Allis until the screws have been inserted or with experience the tip of the cannula can so be used to hold them in place.
19. If there is sufficient bone beneath the neurovascular bundle the first screw hole may be drilled with the special long-shanked twist drill at this level. The drill should be applied gently as the shank is fragile and does not take kindly to torsion. A sense of give is felt when each plate is penetrated. The lingual side should be protected.
20. Screws 9–13 mm are usually adequate for bicortical fixation and are inserted with a screwholding screwdriver, which should be ready mounted to use the moment the hole is drilled. Two further screws are inserted above the bundle behind the last standing molar (Figure 9.3o). When the opposite side is complete the intermaxillary fixation is released.

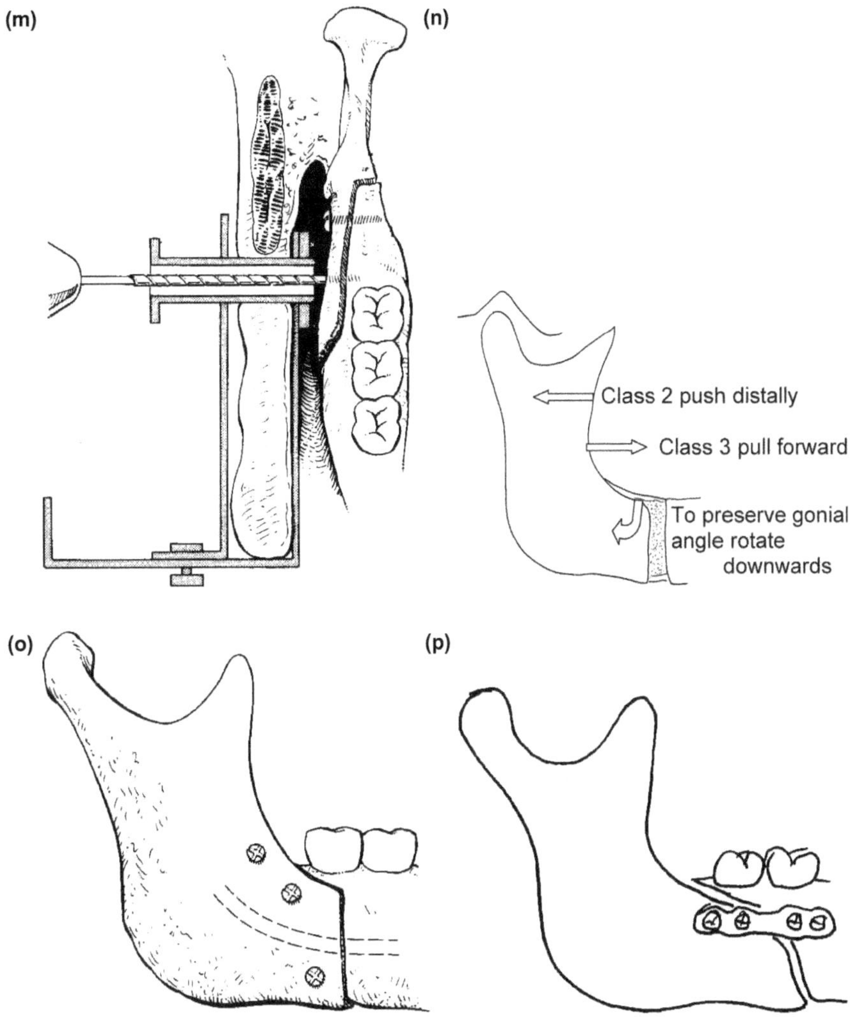

Figure 9.3 (m), (n), (o), (p)

21. The stab wounds are closed with 6/0 prolene.
22. An alternative and simpler technique of intraosseous fixation is the application of a buccal titanium plate bridging the osteotomy gap and fixed intraorally with 5 mm moncortical screws (Figure 9.3p).

23. Vacuum drains are inserted in the buccal pouches bilaterally, sutured to the skin and attached to separate bottles. There are those who do not use drains despite evidence that the subperiosteal sump gives rise to morbidity and infection without this standard practice.
24. The intra oral wounds are carefully closed with a 3/0 polyglycollate suture.
25. When all bleeding has been controlled the throat pack is removed and the pharynx carefully sucked out.
26. The wafer may be left suspended to the maxillary arch wire, but intermaxillary fixation with elastics is unnecessary and the patient is returned to the recovery area.
27. The use of the wafer and postoperative training elastics for 2 weeks is uncomfortable for the patient and of no proven value except for providing comfort for the surgeon.

Additional Notes

- As varying degrees of relapse invariably take place, especially with large movements, the planning should be based on a relaxed supine centric relation squash bite, as close as possible to the operating position. In addition overcorrection should be built into the model surgery. This should be an edge to edge incisor relationship for forward mandibular movements and a class 2 div1 relationship for mandibular setbacks.
- With major facial deformities, such as a hemifacial microsomia, the neurovascular bundle often lies superficially adjacent to the buccal cortex and can be easily severed whilst carrying out the buccal cut. With such a mandible, an extraoral subsigmoid osteotomy is recommended for vertical lengthening or an inverted L osteotomy with a bone graft for forward movements.
- Despite careful intraoperative intermaxillary fixation and a perfect immediate postoperative occlusion, occlusal discrepancies

can still mysteriously appear from 24 hours to 14 days later. The cause may be postoperative condylar recoil, intracapsular oedema or lack of muscle adaptation. This usually remits and the use of training elastics is probably unnecessary.

- If the preoperative arch co-ordination is imperfect and requires restorative or orthodontic correction, it is essential to construct a final wafer which will ensure that the midlines and incisor overjet are correct and the arch alignment is symmetrical. The underlying malocclusion can then be corrected as required.

The Subsigmoid (Subcondylar) Osteotomy

Indications

Although formerly a very popular operation and easier to perform than the sagittal split, the subsigmoid osteotomy is less versatile. It also requires elastic intermaxillary fixation unless secure plating is achieved. It can be carried out intraorally or through an external skin-crease incision, leaving a discrete scar.

The subsigmoid osteotomy is not an operation for lengthening the body of the mandible but it is useful where the mandible is narrow as in a congenital deformity, or atrophic in the older edentulous patient with unerupted wisdom teeth, when it can be used for setting back the body or lengthening or shortening the ascending ramus.

Subsigmoid Osteotomy (Extraoral)

Technique (Figure 9.4)

1. A 5 cm submandibular or retromandibular incision is marked with a pen and infiltrated with 4 ml local anaesthetic containing 1:80,000 adrenaline. This is made in a skin crease two fingers' breadth below the mandibular border to avoid the marginal

(mandibular) branch of the facial nerve. A lower crease requires a larger incision (Figure 9.4a). Note: Never mark an incision with the head rotated: this will produce unexpected changes in the surface anatomy.

2. The skin, fat and platysma are divided with a No. 15 blade. The flap margins are undermined with MacIndoe scissors or the knife to increase the elasticity of the wound margins which are carefully retracted with cat's paw retractors.
3. The deep fascia is identified, picked up with fine-tooth dissecting forceps and divided widely beyond the ends of the flap incision with a knife or scissors. Deep veins, usually the posterior facial, can be identified, divided and tied with 3/0 polyglycollate.
4. Access through the submandibular incision requires the identification of the mandibular branch of the facial nerve which lies under the deep fascia just below the lower border of the mandible. As it passes upwards on to the face it crosses the facial artery and vein. This important motor nerve may be protected by identifying the facial artery and vein as they emerge between the submandibular salivary gland and lower border of the mandible. Use scissors or Spencer Wells forceps to separate the tissues, and divide and tie these vessels, then retract and suture the distal ends upwards over the lower border of the mandible. This will carry the marginal branch of the facial nerve with them.
5. The muscle and periosteum can now be incised along the lower border with a knife and stripped upwards to the sigmoid notch and coronoid process. The Obwegeser channel or Robertson ramus retractor may be hooked over the notch to expose the ramus (Figure 9.4b).
6. A small buccal prominence is a reasonably accurate landmark of the lingula area, so a cut downwards and behind this from the midpoint of the sigmoid notch to the beginning of the curve of the angle avoids the inferior dental neurovascular bundle.

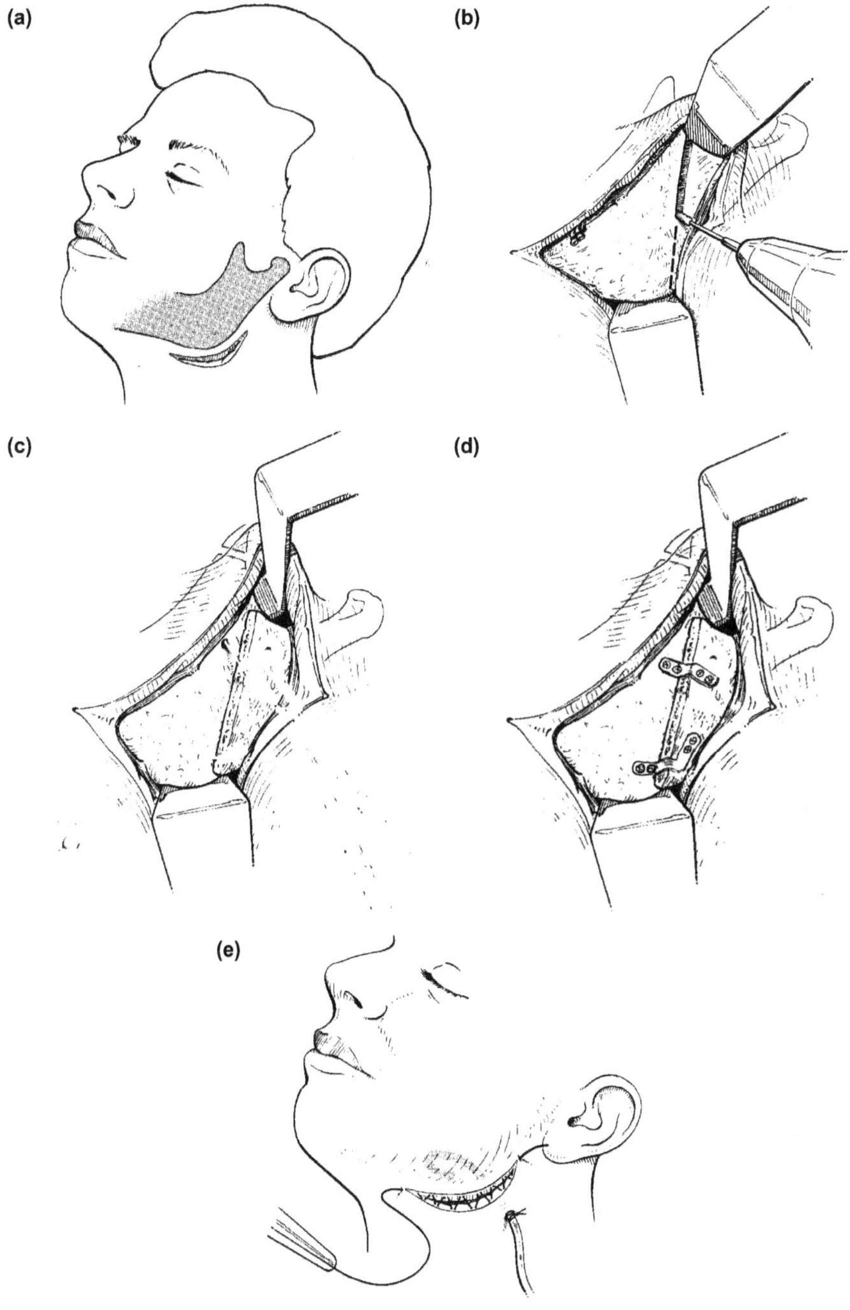

Figure 9.4 (a), (b), (c), (d), (e)

This may be done with a fissure bur or reciprocating saw. A flat retractor should be placed on the medial aspect of the ramus to protect the soft tissues.
7. Once separated, the inner cortex of the posterior narrow fragment and the outer cortex of the main segment may be bevelled with an acrylic bur to ensure good opposition.
8. For large distal displacements, i.e. greater than 0.7 cm, it is necessary to do a coronoidotomy to remove the restraining influence of the temporalis muscle (Figure 9.4c).
9. A saline-soaked tonsil swab is inserted in the wound and the procedure repeated on the opposite side.
10. With the appropriate wafer the intermaxillary wires are applied, with the teeth held in occlusion.
11. As rigid fixation is being used the cut should be as vertical as possible in order to leave a substantial posterior border. After putting on intermaxillary fixation the larger, i.e. distal, fragment should be trimmed to allow close approximation of the osteotomy margins. An L or T-shaped plate with six holes is then fashioned and screwed into the lateral aspects of the posterior and inferior borders of the mandible to bridge the bone cut firmly.
12. Vacuum drains are placed bilaterally overlying the bone surface and sutured firmly to the skin as soon as the introducer has been pulled through; ensure that at least 2 cm of non-perforated drain lies within the wound (Figure 9.4d).
13. The wound is closed by suturing the muscle and periosteum with 3/0 polyglycollate on a 22 mm half-round needle. The fascia/platysma layer and subcutaneous tissue are similarly closed, with the knots buried by suturing from deep to superficial. For a fine scar, the skin should be closed with a 3/0 continuous subcuticular monofilament [Prolene, Ethilon (Ethicon Ltd., Edinburgh, UK) or nylon] suture on a straight needle. This can also be done with a half-round non-cutting needle. Alternatively, wound closure may be achieved with 5/0 Prolene or Ethilon interrupted sutures,

or even adhesive Steri-strips (3M, US) if subcutaneous closure is satisfactory.

14. The throat pack is removed.

Intraoral Subcondylar Osteotomy

This is a relatively simple procedure and is a rapid way of treating minor displacements of the mandible, i.e. less than 7 mm, which may involve a backward or a rotational correction for asymmetry. Major movements should be accompanied by a coronoidotomy or even a horizontal ramus osteotomy because of the restraining influence of the temporalis muscle.

However neither have the great advantage of dispensing with intermaxillary fixation. The best application of this intraoral procedure is a means of salvaging a sagittal split that has not separated the condyle from the body of the mandible.

Technique

Buccal Ramus Approach (Figure 9.5).

Infiltrate the tissues on the buccal aspect of the ascending ramus with a vasoconstrictor (Figure 9.5a).

1. A buccal-based triangular incision is made with a No. 15 blade with the apex behind the last molar tooth, the upper limb stopping at the external oblique ridge halfway up the ascending ramus (Figure 9.5b).
2. The flap is elevated subperiosteally as widely as possible, using the Howarth periosteal elevator and then the forefinger to stretch the periosteum and create a generous pouch. A J-shaped periosteal elevator is useful in freeing the muscular attachment at the posterior and inferior borders. The sigmoid notch, condylar neck and angle of the mandible should be readily palpated.

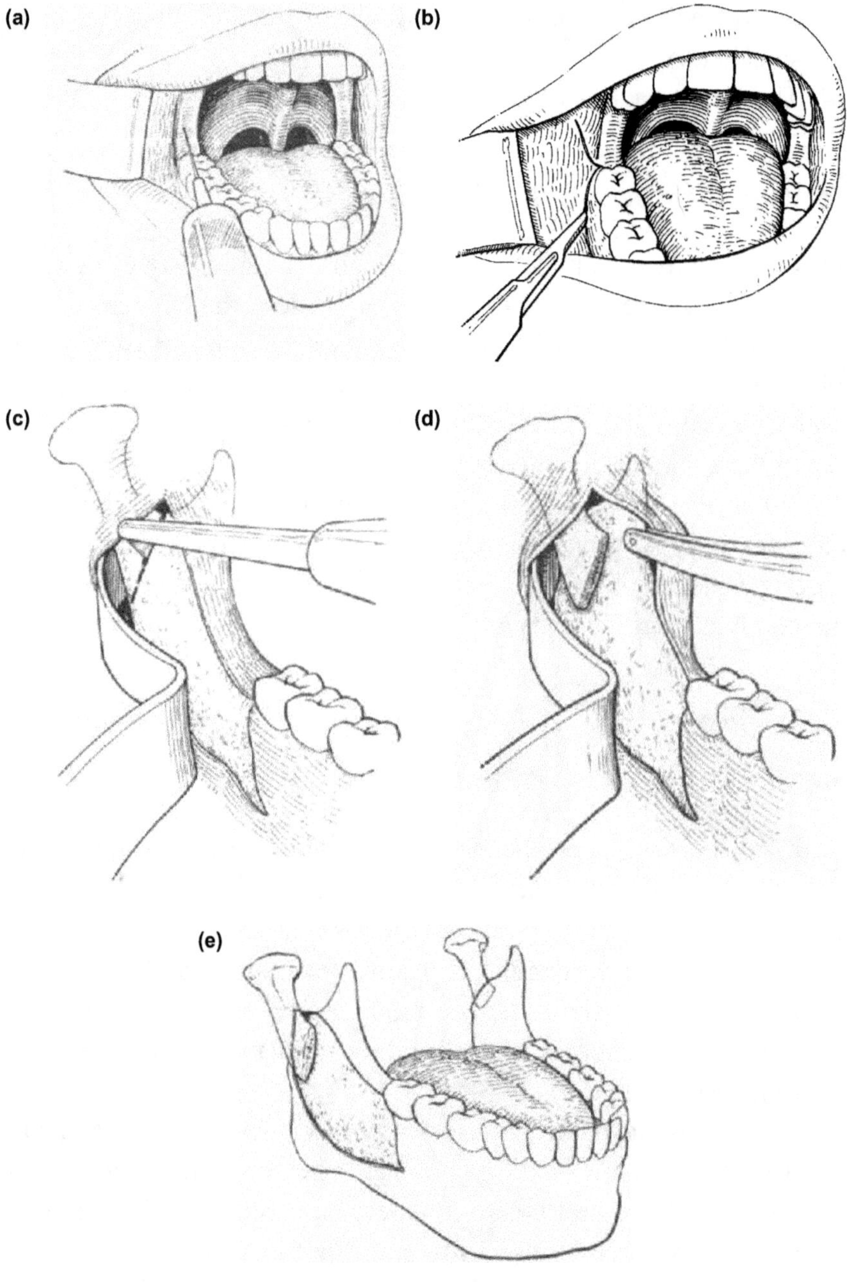

Figure 9.5 (a), (b), (c), (d), (e)

3. The Merrill or similar retractor is inserted so that the curved distal flange may be firmly placed behind the posterior border of the ascending ramus (Figure 9.5c).
4. The sigmoid notch may then be visualised and a 1.5 cm right-angled oscillating saw is used to cut downwards and backwards to 1 cm below the mid-point of the posterior border, i.e. where the condylar neck has narrowed and fused with the flat ascending ramus. It is essential to use a sharp-edged saw. Some operators prefer a blade which is 70° to the long axis of the saw.
5. Once separated, the condylar component is displaced buccally with the Howarth elevator. When both sides have been completed the mandible is displaced backwards between them (Figures 9.5d and 9.5e).
6. A vacuum drain is inserted into the wound prior to closure.
7. As this procedure does not lend itself to internal fixation elastic intermaxillary fixation is necessary.

Medial Ramus Approach (Figure 9.6)

This procedure is also useful to salvage a failed sagittal split.

1. The basic exposure is almost exactly the same as for the sagittal split technique except that only minimal stripping is required on the buccal surface of the mandible. However, with the curved Kocher's forceps gripping the coronoid process and the ramus channel retractor inserted medially just above the level of the lingula and hooked behind the posterior border of the ascending ramus, an excellent view of the sigmoid notch and posterior border is achieved form the contralateral side of the patient (Figure 9.6a).
2. With a long-shanked fissure bur and oblique cut is made through the thick posterior ramus border as low as possible, passing forwards and upwards into the sigmoid notch (Figure 9.6b).

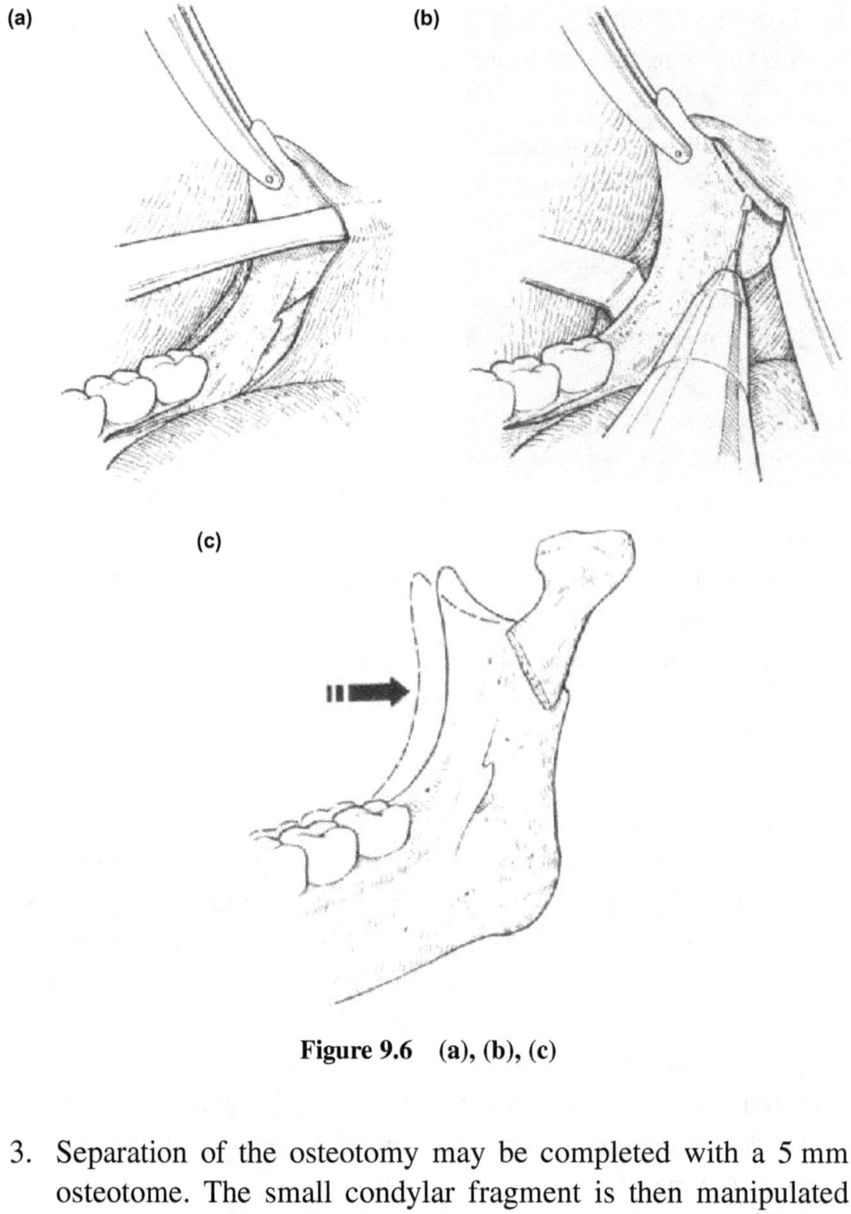

Figure 9.6 (a), (b), (c)

3. Separation of the osteotomy may be completed with a 5 mm osteotome. The small condylar fragment is then manipulated medially with the channel retractor and a periosteal elevator into the hollow medial surface of the ramus (Figure 9.6c).
4. This is repeated on the contralateral side and the mandible is placed into the planned occlusion.

5. The wounds are closed.
6. Again this procedure requires elastic intermaxillary fixation.

Note: Occasionally access is restricted where the medial aspect of the ramus is broad and concave, in which case an alternative osteotomy should be undertaken.

Body Osteotomies

This procedure is done intraorally, usually in the molar-premolar region. However, it shortens the alveolus and has not got the elegance or versatility of the sagittal split or subsigmoid procedures and requires more careful planning. For these reasons it is not considered here. The anterior mandibulotomy, in which the section is made anterior to the mental foramen, is a useful variant of this operation.

The Inverted L Osteotomy

Indications

This operation is valuable when there is a need to increase both the ramus height and body length at the same time, especially when the sagittal split osteotomy is not possible. Such cases are usually gross congenital mandibular hypoplasia or, occasionally, acquired hypoplasia following condylar fractures or when previous surgery has disturbed the bony anatomy. The operation differs in concept from the sagittal split procedure in that a bone graft is inserted to make up the deficiency.

Technique

1. The surgical approach is exactly the same as for the extraoral subsigmoid osteotomy (steps 1–6 and see Figure 9.4) except that the bone cut is made laterally from the anterior border of the ascending ramus, passing distally, to behind the estimated posi-

tion of the lingula then downwards to the lower border anterior to the angle, i.e. to the antegonial notch (Figure 9.7a).

2. With bilateral deformities the approach is repeated on the opposite side.
3. The mandible is then temporarily fixed into occlusion. Where the maxilla is normal this presents no problems. However, if there is a deformity of the maxilla this must be corrected before the inverted L and fixed with bone plates.

   Mobilising the small mandible into the desired anterior position can be difficult and is facilitated by drilling a hole bilaterally in the lower border of the mandible just anterior to the osteotomy cut and passing a 0.5 mm traction wire to be attached to heavy forceps. When anterior traction is applied, explore the deep tissues medial to the mandible with a finger to find any restraining bands of periosteum, muscle or ligament. These must be vigorously divided with the finger to ensure stability.
4. With the proximal condylar fragment confirmed to be in the fossa, the gap created can be measured, and a template formed with sterile paper or card.

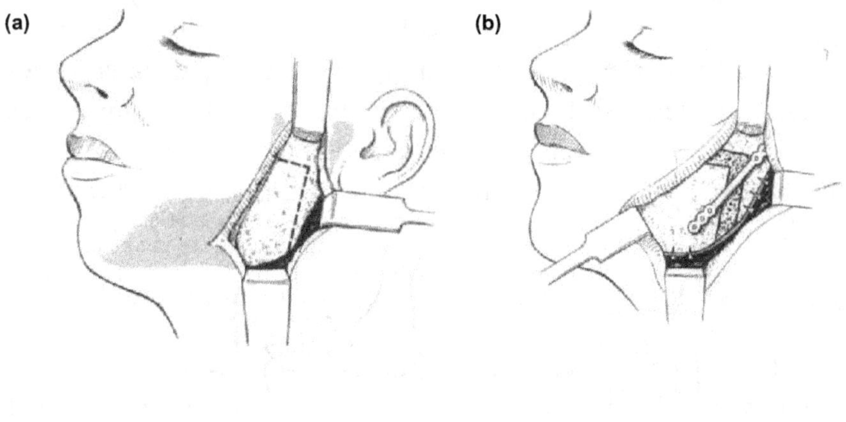

Figure 9.7 **(a), (b)**

5. An interpositional graft is now obtained. The ideal source is cortico-cancellous bone from the iliac crest. A solid cancellous graft can be used but the incorporation of one cortex provides reassuring stability. Some surgeons use split rib for the gap. Two miniature bone plates provide excellent rigidity and form (Figure 9.7b).
6. A vacuum drain is inserted and the wound is closed in layers.
7. The intermaxillary fixation is released and the pack removed.

Note: Any mandible which requires lengthening with an inverted L osteotomy also requires an augmentation genioplasty.

The Lower Labial Segmental Osteotomy (Kole Subapical Osteotomy)

Indications

Although this operation may be used to move the dentoalveolar segment in almost any direction permitted by the angulation of the teeth, it should not be used as an alternative to presurgical orthodontics and is less useful and more difficult than the anterior mandibulotomy If carried out as a single procedure, intermaxillary fixation is not required. The alveolar segments can be secured with bone plates plus:

1. An arch bar, the best being a cast chrome cobalt bar designed on the surgical planning model.
2. An orthodontic arch wire fitted intraoperatively or more readily a heavy (1 mm) supplemental arch wire fitted into distal buccal tubes and ligated to the segment and the adjacent teeth. The segments are localised by a postoperative wafer and bone plates below, which are not enough without the dental control to prevent displacement.

Where preoperative extractions are not carried out, orthodontic tooth movement is required to ensure space to facilitate the surgical cut without root damage.

Technique

Downward and posterior movements (Figure 9.8)

1. A premolar is carefully extracted bilaterally to create space for a distal movement. For vertical movements without extractions it is imperative to confirm that there is sufficient bone between the roots of the teeth. The orthodontist can achieve increased separation with a fixed appliance.
2. Whichever incision is used (see below), extend the lips, dry the mucosa, and mark it out with a pen and Bonney's blue.
3. The procedure is done with a curved incision starting below the papilla distal to the site of the vertical bone cut (Figure 9.8a) at the reflection of the sulcus mucosa. The blade is then taken very superficially through the mucosa along the inner aspect of the lip anterior to the sulcus, returning in an arc of a circle to the equivalent point on the opposite side. Finger dissection with a gauze swab will reveal the three terminal branches of the mental nerve. These must be exposed by dissecting backwards to the foramen with scissors. The anterior labial section of the incision can now be deepened with a blade obliquely downwards to bone approximately halfway between the gingival margin and lower border of the mandible. This skirt of mucosa facilitates suturing and also provides a good seal if bone chips are being inserted.
4. The mucoperiosteum is then elevated distally revealing the mental nerve at its origin. At this stage, the periosteum above and behind the foramen may be elevated and incised without fear of damaging the nerve (Figure 9.8b). If the cone of periosteum

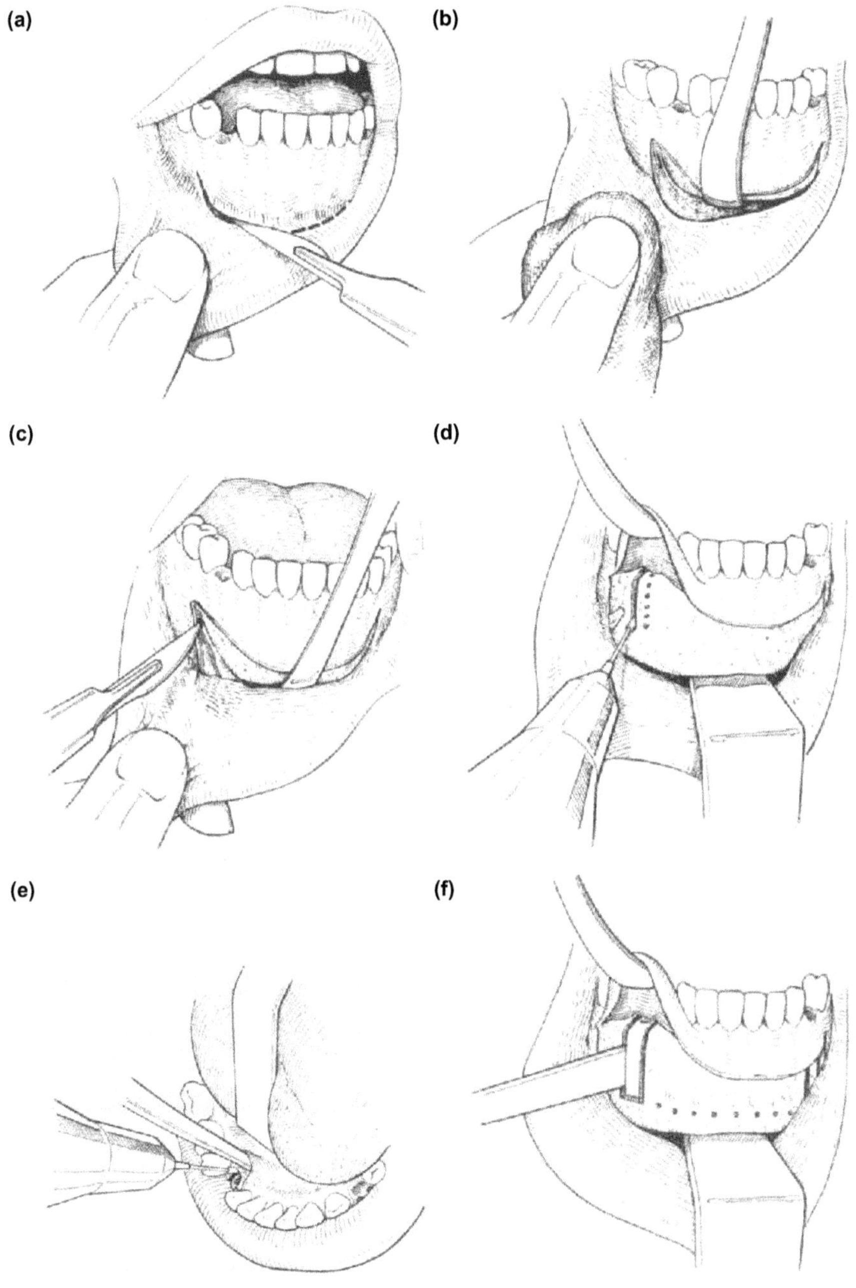

Figure 9.8 (a), (b), (c), (d), (e), (f)

around the nerve is now carefully incised with a sharp blade and the mental nerve dissected free, it becomes considerably more extensible and therefore easier to retract.

5. Using an elevator the anterior periosteum overlying the chin is then peeled firmly down to the lower border of the mandible where a Lack's or special chin (Awty, Obwegeser) retractor may be inserted to hold the flap and support the mandible (Figure 9.8c).
6. Incise along the gingival sulcus around the premolars and canines to facilitate elevation of the attached gingival flaps which will be widely undermined to form a bridge maintaining continuity of the gingiva.
7. The vertical bone cuts may be made with a narrow tungsten carbide fissure or an oscillating sagittal saw blade. If the first or second premolar has been extracted to enable the alveolar segment to be pushed backwards, the appropriate amount of bone is removed as a vertical strip (Figure 9.8d).
8. If no teeth are to be extracted the buccal cut can be made with a fine fissure bur through the outer cortex only. Then, after detaching the lingual mucoperiosteum, a cut is made vertically from above through the inner cortex. The Howarth periosteal elevator is held *in situ* to protect the mucosa (Figure 9.8e). The section is then completed between the teeth with a fine 3 mm osteotome (Figure 9.8f).
9. The horizontal cut may be completed with a bur or oscillating saw and must be placed well below the canine apices. It is useful to estimate the level of the canine apices from radiographs and the cortical contour and mark them with a bur hole on both sides. Where bone is removed for a setdown it is safer to make the upper cut first, marking it out with a series of bur holes (Figure 9.8g).
10. If there is insufficient room below the apices to remove adequate bone for the setdown, an anterior mandibulotomy must

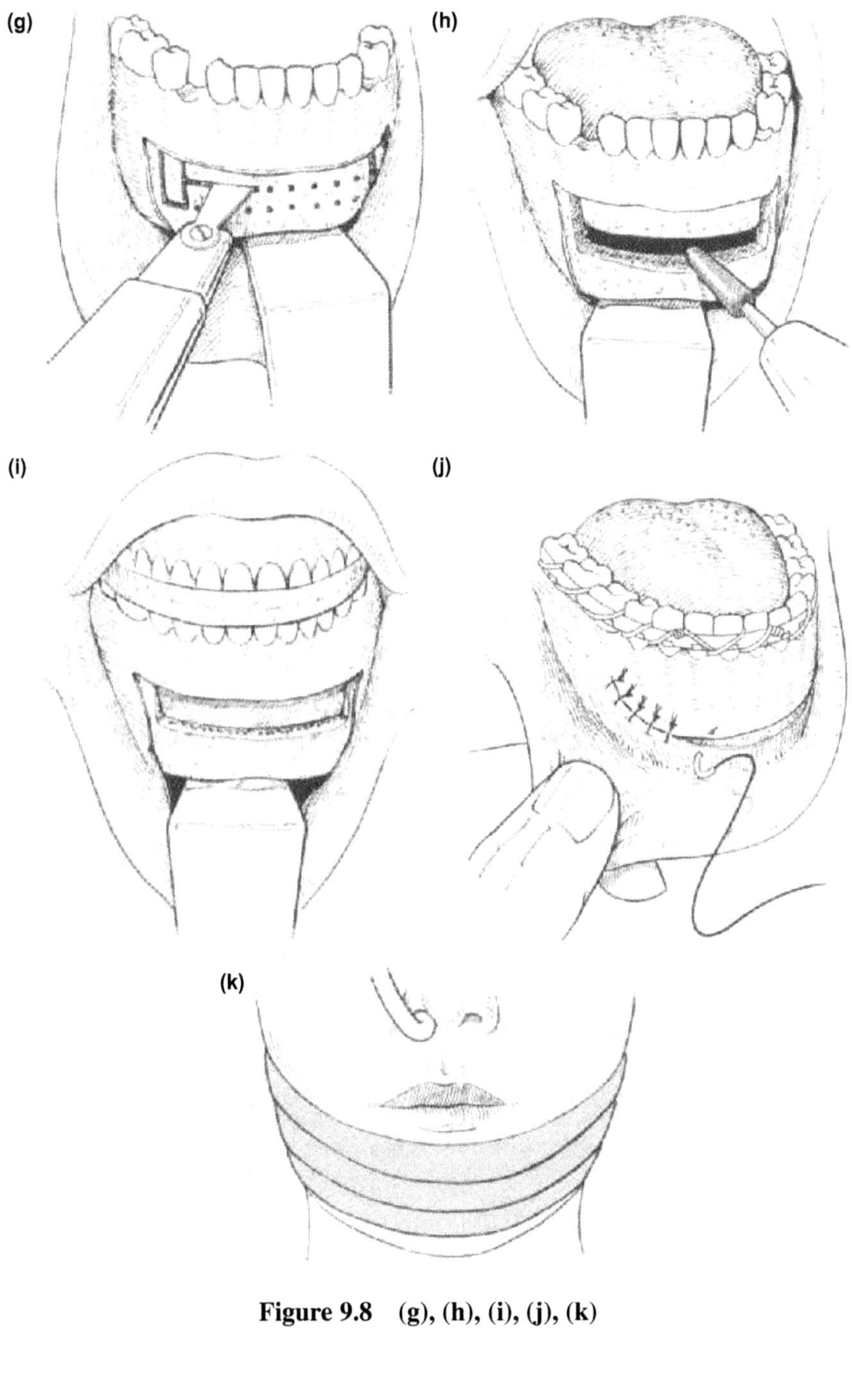

Figure 9.8 (g), (h), (i), (j), (k)

be performed. Furthermore in most situations this is a better procedure than the Kole. Save all fragments of bone in a blood-soaked swab to fill any residual dead space left after moving the segments.

11. Sometimes the mobilised segment which is pedicled on the genial muscles cannot be satisfactorily seated, in which case carefully trim off all cortical spurs, especially at the angular margins, with a well-cooled, narrow tapering acrylic bur (Figures 9.8h and 9.8i).
12. Accurate dentoalveolar localisation can be achieved by an acrylic wafer with an arch bar, heavy arch wire, or an open cast silver splint, all previously prepared on the lower model after model surgery. The splint is secured with circum-mandibular wires. The osteotomy is secured with bone plates.
13. The muscle and periosteum are closed with 3/0 polyglycollate and the mucosa is closed with a combination of simple and vertical mattress sutures (Figure 9.8j). A 2.5 cm elastic adhesive pressure dressing applied over the labiomental skin crease helps to reduce dead space and haematoma (Figure 9.8k).

Forward Movement

Occasionally a forward segmental movement is useful for correcting a Class II, division 1 deep overbite and overjet, where a sagittal split has been declined. This may be modified to include one or more of the premolars on the mobilised anterior segment, in which case the mental nerve is released from within the canal by removing the overlying cortex distally with a bur, by cutting two parallel grooves from the upper and lower edges of the mental foramen. The intervening bone can be carefully removed with a Mitchell's trimmer. The exposed neurovascular bundle is then retracted by an elastic or nylon tape held in a pair of mosquito forceps. Once the alveolar segment has been mobilised forwards and fixed by plates or a wafer and arch bars, the vertical gaps are packed with bone chips from the iliac crest and covered with a buccal mucosal flap rotated over the alveolar crest to be carefully sutured to the lingual mucosa with horizontal mattress sutures.

Upward Movement

The osteotomy is as previously described except that the space created at the subapical area by the upward movement is packed with cancellous bone chips.

The Anterior Mandibulotomy

Indications and Technique

This is anatomically a better operation than the Kole subapical procedure especially in patients with a short lower face, with little bone between the incisor apices and the lower border of the mandible and those with a deficient chin. In the former an adequate setdown cannot be achieved without damaging the apices or leaving a precariously thin strut of cortical bone. These problems can be overcome in two ways:

1. Take the vertical osteotomy cuts of the Kole down through the lower border to produce a three-part osteotomy of the mandible (Figure 9.9a). This enables a setdown which maintains or improves the lower facial height.
2. An alternative is to combine the oblique advancement genioplasty cut with the two vertical segmental cuts, producing a four-part mandibuloto-genioplasty (Figure 9.10). The anterior incisor segment is then set down and fixed as planned and will displace the genioplasty segment downwards and also allow advancement. These are not only simple solutions to anatomical difficulty but also increase the anterior inferior

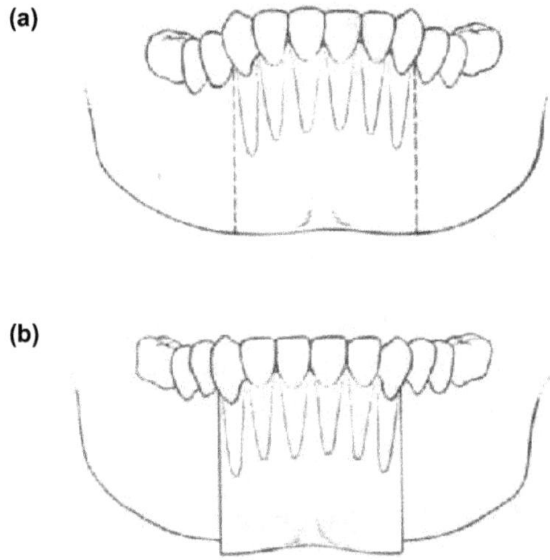

Figure 9.9 (a), (b)

dentoalveolar height and improve the lower facial proportion. However, as the mandible has been completely divided bilaterally, dentoalveolar localisation is done with a deep wafer, an arch bar or supplemental archwire in distal tubes and the lower level by bone plates.

Note: Do ensure that the osteotomy cuts at the lower border feel and look smooth prior to closure.

Genioplasty or Mentoplasty

Indications

Augmentation or reduction of the chin may be done for an isolated deficiency or combined with other osteotomies. This is also discussed in detail in Chapter 10.

Augmentation is most easily achieved with a sliding genioplasty (Figure 9.10a). A short lower face with a reduced lower anterior dentoalveolar height can also be simultaneously corrected

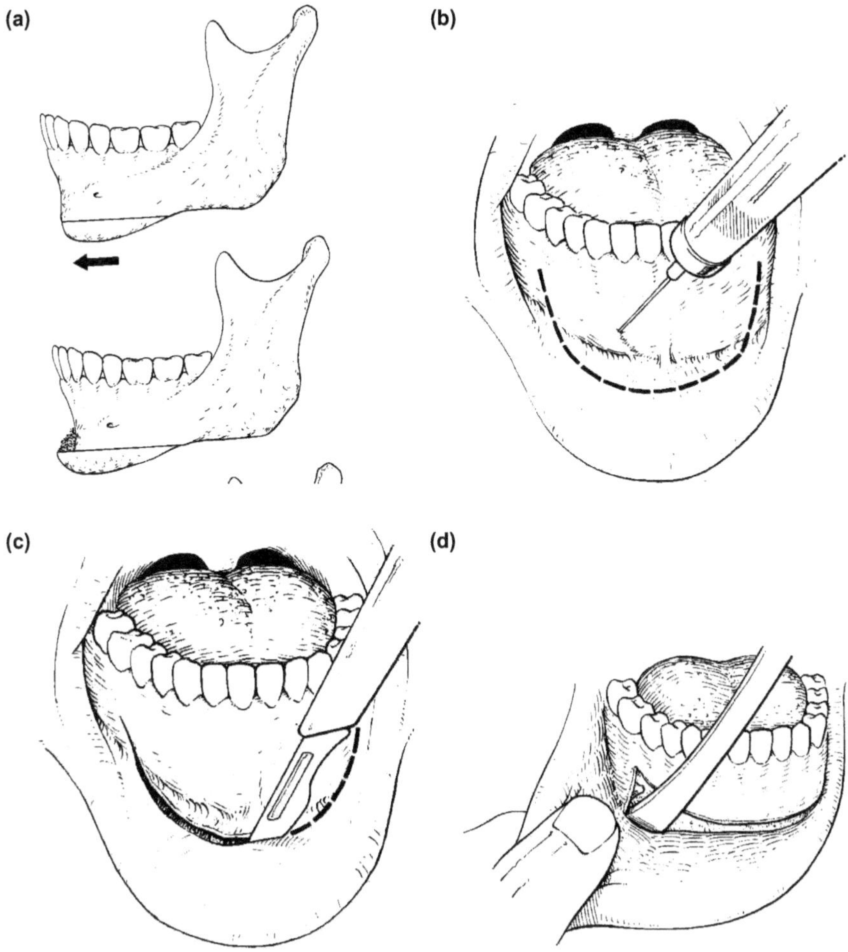

Figure 9.10 (a), (b), (c), (d)

with an interpositional bone or alloplast sandwich filling. If, however, an incisor setdown is also required to flatten the lower occlusal plane, the anterior mandibulotomy (see above), which is a combination of a segmental osteotomy and genioplasty, should be used (Figure 9.10a).

The Augmentation Genioplasty

Technique

1. Mark a U-shaped incision with Bonney's blue from 46 to 36. Start just below the attached gingiva and cross the sulcus on to the labial mucosa anterior to the canine teeth (Figure 9.10b).
2. Infiltrate the sulcus with local anaesthetic containing 1:200 000 adrenaline. The incision is made very superficially from the first molar in the unattached mucosa. This is widened anteriorly by bringing the incision out on to the inner aspect of the lip. As the knife reaches the medial aspect of the canine area the tissues may be incised down to bone but is again brought to the surface at the opposite canine. It is imperative to leave a generous skirt of unattached mucosa on the gingival side to facilitate suturing (Figure 9.10c).
3. A dry gauze swab used to displace the tissues of the divided superficial incision will reduce bleeding and also bring the three branches of the mental nerve into view. These should be further exposed by dissecting backwards with fine scissors to the mental foramen. Then incise through the periosteum with a knife in a forward arc from behind, above and in front of the nerves as they emerge from the foramen.
4. The soft tissues may then be reflected with a periosteal elevator inferiorly to deglove the mandible (Figure 9.10d). This must be done firmly and will be facilitated by carefully incising the periosteum around the origin of the mental nerves. The soft tissues can then be retracted from the lower border of the mandible with a Lack's or genioplasty retractor (Awty, Obwegeser) (Figure 9.10e).
5. It is important that the chin periosteum and overlying fascia are now vigorously stretched with the finger, incising widely any tight bands, to make a pocket to accommodate the increased bony prominence. A damp swab should be inserted in this pocket to confirm that the overlying skin looks untethered.

(e) (f) (g) (h) (i)

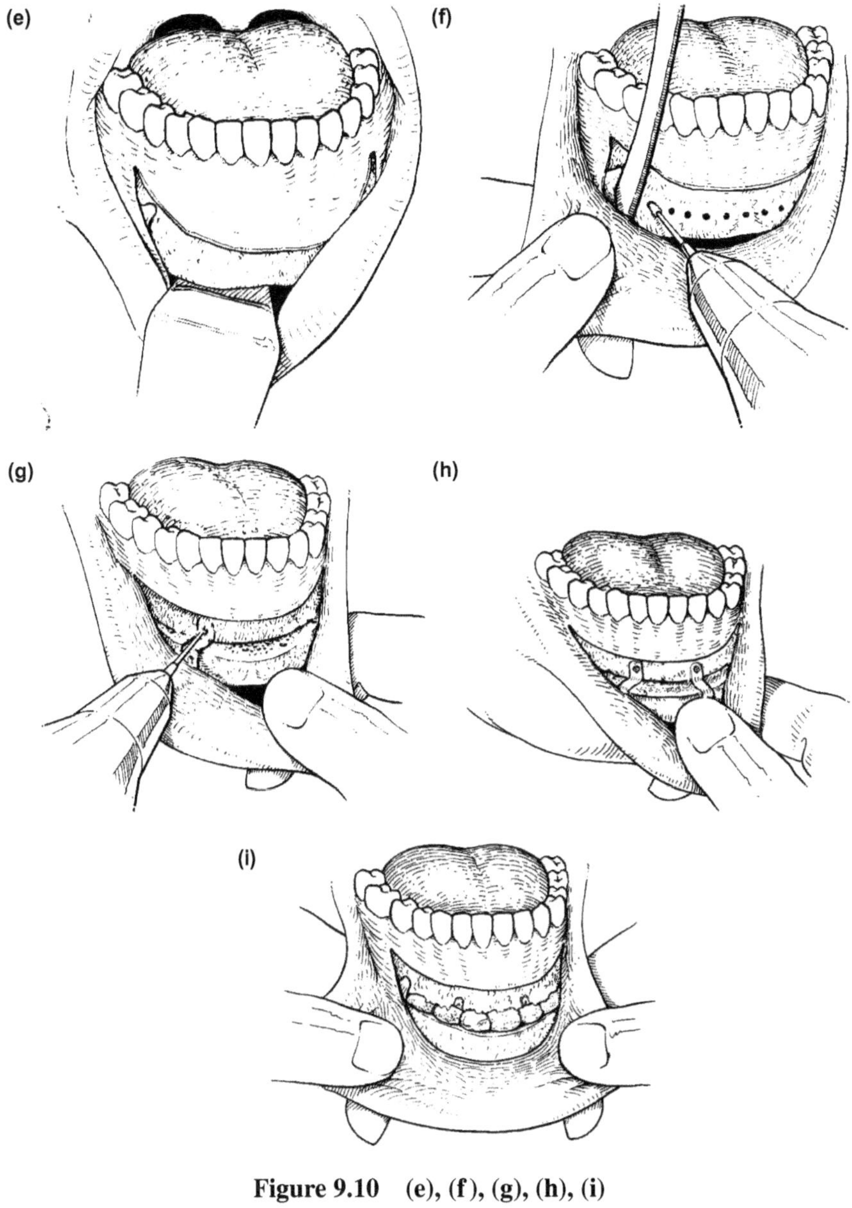

Figure 9.10 (e), (f), (g), (h), (i)

6. When cutting the bone the mental nerves must be retracted with an elastic or nylon tape and also protected with a Howarth periosteal elevator or miniature Langenbeck retractor. The bone cut

should commence at the lower border below the second premolar and come obliquely forwards and upwards on both sides. As usual, the choice lies between a tungsten carbide fissure bur or an oscillating sagittal saw, but must be carried through to divide the lingual cortex. The separation is done with a fine osteotome. It may be possible to cut two fine horizontal slices of bone which help to elongate and correct a severe retrogenia (Figure 9.10f). Leave the bone pedicled on the vascular digastric muscle behind improves the healing process. There is an approximate 15% loss of contour using this technique; this may rise to 30% if the muscle pedicle is divided.

7. A bone shelf is now created by attaching the anteriorly displaced lower border to the buccal cortex above with plates (Figures 9.10g and 9.10h). Two plates are fashioned into a three-part step with the horizontal "tread" representing a generously estimated forward move. The plates are screwed into place on the facial cortex above the section with two 5 mm screws avoiding the apices. The chin fragment is then firmly brought forward with bone holding forceps and secured with screws to the plate. Cancellous bone chips removed from the iliac crest through a short incision (the Flint Technique), fill dead space, enhance contour and promote union with large advancements (Figure 9.10i).

   An interpositional graft of bone or hydroxyapatite can be inserted at this stage to increase the lower facial height with severe deficiencies.
8. By placing the original incision well out on the labial surface, sound closure may be achieved in two layers, i.e. muscle then mucosa (Figure 9.10j).
9. An elastic adhesive pressure dressing is applied to the face to lift and compress the soft tissues overlying the enhanced chin. This prevents subsequent lip sag due to separation of the divided mentalis muscle.

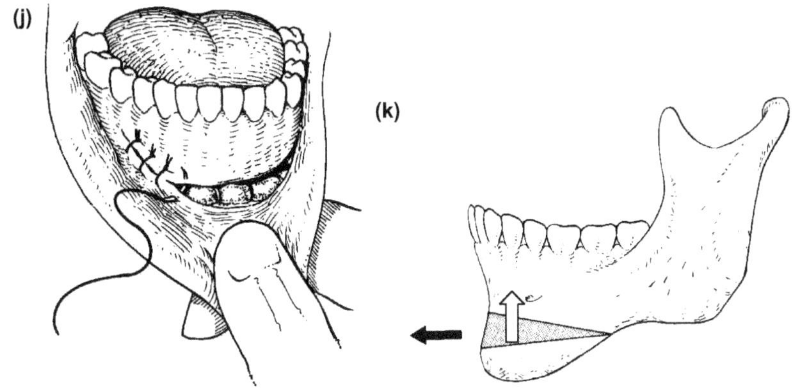

Figure 9.10 **(j), (k)**

The Reduction Genioplasty

In cases of progenia a simple technique is to deglove the chin and sculpt off the excess bone with fissure and acrylic burs. However, it is necessary to retain the concavity at the junction of the alveolus and basal bone, for the overlying labiomental fold is aesthetically important.

With the "deep mandible" (vertical chin excess) due to a markedly increased lower anterior dentoalveolar height, an intermediate wedge of bone is removed after completing the standard genioplasty oblique section (see Vertical Maxillary Excess,) but this has to be a significant wedge to make a difference externally (Figures 9.10j and 9.10k). Try not to apicect the canines. As for all genioplasty procedures, make sure the osteotomy cuts at the lower border look and feel smooth before wound closure.

Maxillary Osteotomies

The anterior segmental osteotomies, as described by Wassmund and modified by Wunderer, and the posterior segmental osteotomy of Schuchardt are rarely used compared to the more versatile Le Fort I.

Anterior dentoalveolar osteotomy (Wassmund/Wunderer)

Indications

Reduction of the overjet or localised anterior open bite. This is a simple operation but rarely achieves more than orthodontics.

Limitations

Where the upper lip is short or the dentoalveolar exposure is excessive this procedure will leave an unacceptable amount of upper incisor showing. In such cases a Le Fort I osteotomy with a vertical impaction sbould be the basis of the prescription. Also, if the maxillary first premolars have already been extracted for orthodontic reasons with forward movement of the buccal segment teeth, further extractions would leave only canines and molars. In such cases a Le Fort I osteotomy with distal movement is recommended to preserve a functional buccal occlusion.

Technique (Figure 9.11)

1. Local anaesthetic with a vasoconstrictor is infiltrated buccally and palatally on both sides (Figure 9.11a).
2. Either a first of second premolar is extracted and the gingival attachment incised from the first molar to the lateral incisor.
3. An inverted L incision is made above the apex of the tooth to be extracted, i.e. site of vertical bone cut. The gingiva is not incised but remains as a soft tissue bridge, after being carefully elevated from the alveolus from above downwards (Figure 9.11b).
4. A mucoperiosteal flap is raised forwards with the Howarth periosteal elevator, exposing the canine apex, and then extended into the pyriform fossa margin (Figure 9.11c).
5. The periosteal elevator is carefully turned through 100° and inserted submucosally along the lateral wall of the nose to protect the nasal mucosa (Figure 9.11d).

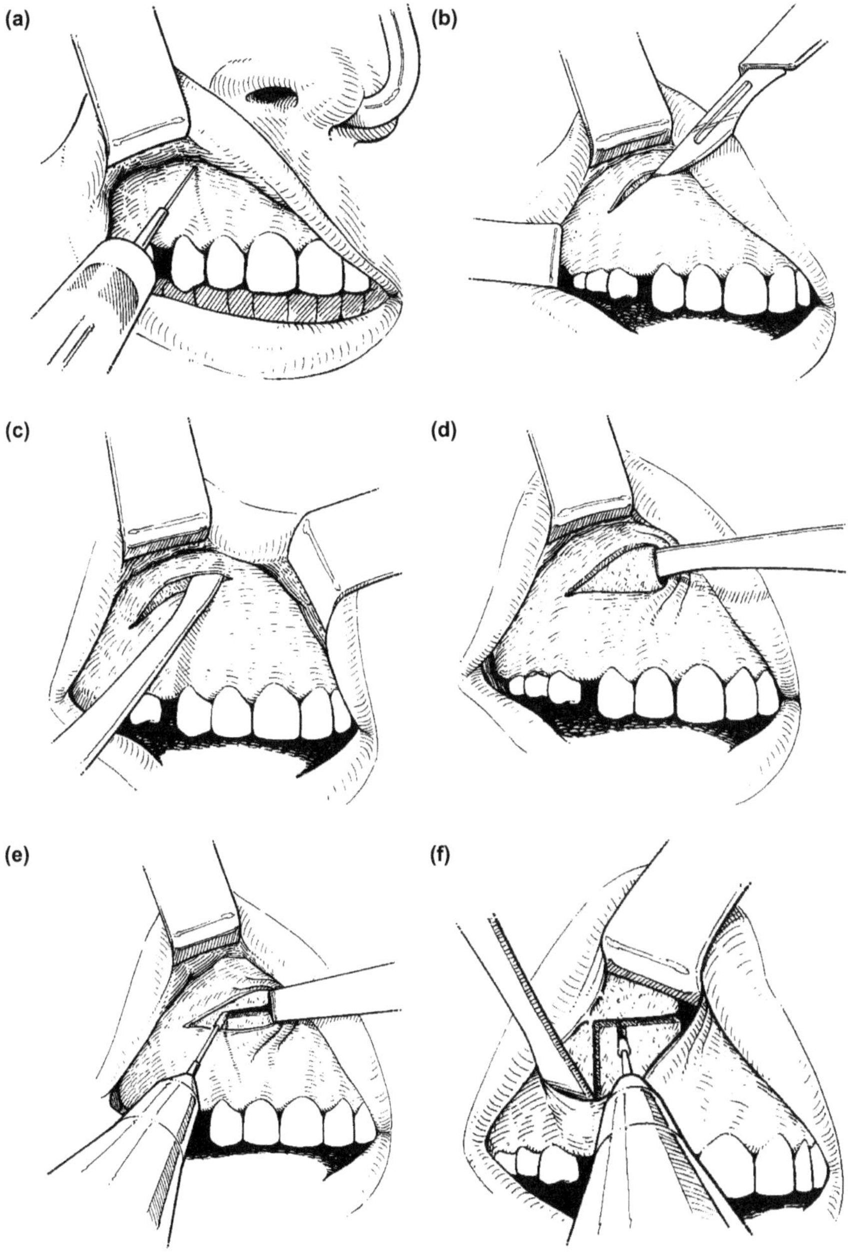

Figure 9.11 (a), (b), (c), (d), (e), (f)

6. Bone is cut with a tapering fissure bur from the pyriform fossa margin distally, parallel to and slightly above the nasal floor, then vertically downwards into the socket of the extracted tooth, i.e. a vertical fillet is outlined. The buccal gingiva is protected by the periosteal elevator (Figures 9.11e and 9.11f).
7. The palatal mucosa may be elevated and tunnelled, but this is unnecessary. A transpalatal incision planned to rest on uncut bone provides better access. This may cross from canine to canine and then be reflected backwards to expose the palatal bone. The greater palatine vessels should be tied or oversewn with polyglycollate to arrest bleeding from the posterior flap (Figures 9.11g and 9.11h).
8. The predetermined strip of palatal bone is then removed under direct vision, together with any remaining buccal plate (Figure 9.11i).
9. The buccal cuts are then made on the contralateral side.
10. Using a notched nasal septum chisel the septum is separated from the anterior fragment. This is done through a short vertical incision overlying the anterior nasal spine retracting the margins with miniature Langenbeck retractors (cat's paw) (Figure 9.11j).
11. The alveolar segment is now mobilised and repositioned. Judicious trimming with an acrylic bur, avoiding exposure of root surface, is often required to seat the segment.
12. Modifications:

    a) The intercanine width of the arch may be expanded by dividing the anterior segment in the midline through the anterior vertical incision. Start with a fine fissure bur but complete the interdental division with a narrow osteotome. This should be done before the final mobilisation (Figures 9.11k and 9.11l).
    b) Elevation of the anterior segment without distal movement can be achieved by omitting the premolar extractions and

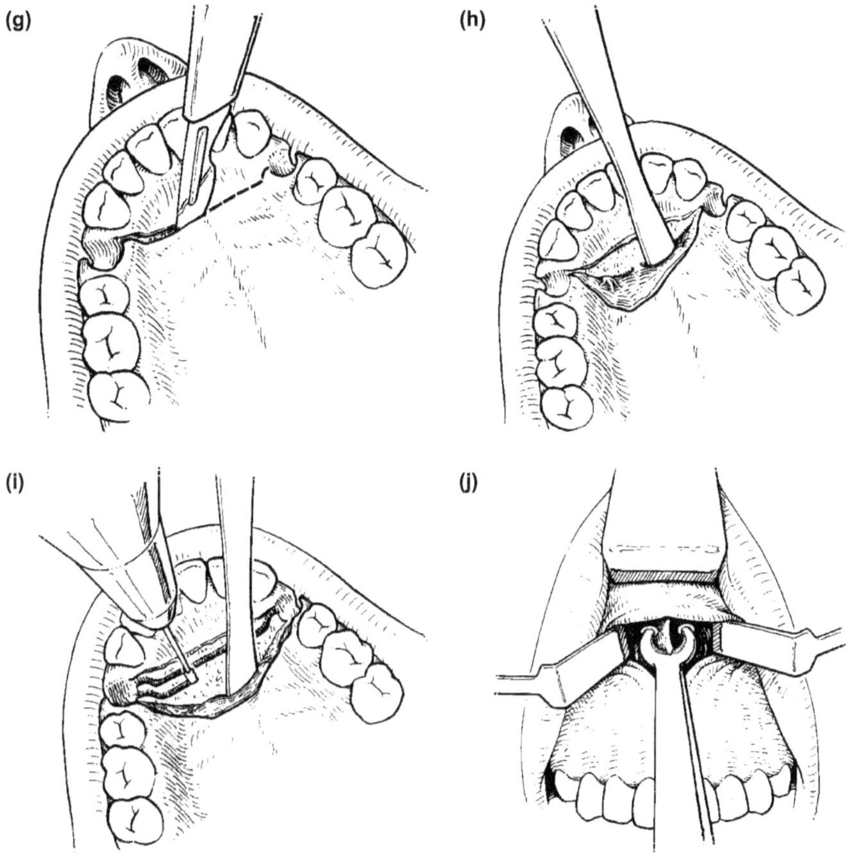

Figure 9.11 **(g), (h), (i), (j)**

removing only the overlying cortical bone. If using burs, the buccal and palatal alveolar cortices are cut and a thin 3 mm osteotome is used for the interradicular separation. Some surgeons prefer an oscillating saw.

c) The segment can only be elevated by careful submucosal trimming of the nasal septum and by cutting a V-shaped trough in the upper surface with a narrow cone-shaped acrylic bur or a large rosehead (Figure 9.11m).

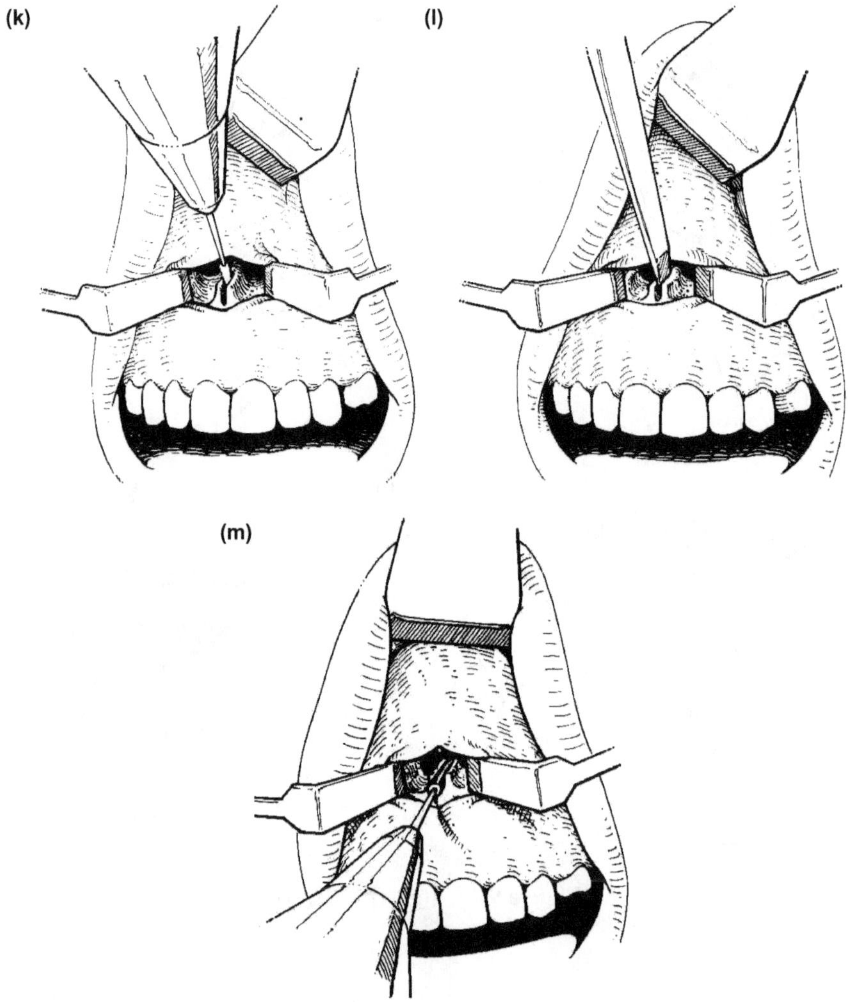

Figure 9.11 **(k), (l), (m)**

13. The final position may be confirmed with a clear acrylic splint (wafer) covering the palatal, incisal and occlusal surfaces constructed on the surgical planning model.
14. L shaped bone plates are then bent to shape and fixed with screws.

15. The splint can be wired through a series of interdental holes to the teeth to provide definitive fixation, after the flaps have been sutured. Alternative means of fixation are using a wafer for localisation and a wrought arch bar, or preformed orthodontic arch wire and brackets (see Chapter 8).
16. A compression dressing of 2.5 cm elastic adhesive tape over the lip helps reduce the swelling.

The Le Fort I Osteotomy

Indications

This is a versatile operation which can be adapted to move the whole maxillary dentoalveolar component in any direction; forwards, backwards, superiorly and inferiorly. Additional modifications can be added by segmental division from above after a down-fracture.

Remember that measured movements of the maxilla are not reflected completely by the overlying lip. The lip will be displaced only half the distance of most anterior movements. However the aesthetic outcome depends mostly on achieving a Class I incisor relationship. Approximately a quarter of an upward impaction will also be lost by elevation of the lip. Therefore, always overcorrect when planning the soft tissue changes.

Technique (Figure 9.12)

1. Infiltrate the entire buccal sulcus with local anaesthetic and a vaso-constrictor (Figure 9.12a).
2. Incise firmly down to bone with a No. 15 blade from the distal aspect of the first molar around to the opposite side. The incision must leave a generous skirt of unattached mucosa on the alveolar side for suturing (Figure 9.12b).

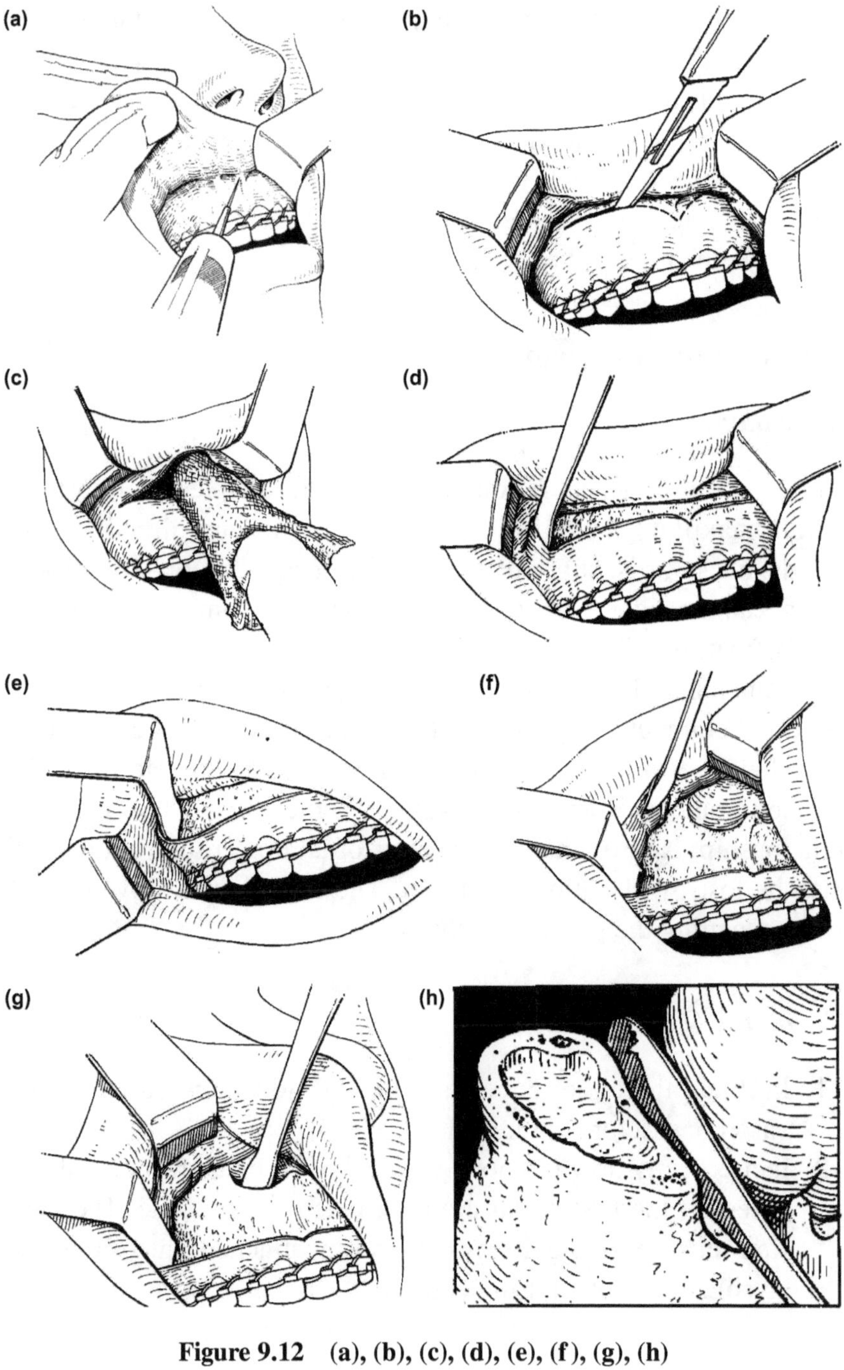

Figure 9.12 (a), (b), (c), (d), (e), (f), (g), (h)

3. Firm upward pressure with a swab will help reflect the soft tissues and periosteum as well as drying the bone surface (Figure 9.12c).
4. With a Howarth periosteal elevator carefully extend the periosteal reflection distally behind the tuberosity and then insert the curved end of a Lack's retractor behind the maxilla until it contacts the pterygoid buttress (Figures 9.12d and 9.12e).
5. Continue the reflection forwards and upwards to identify the inferior orbital foramen and neurovascular bundle, then to the margin of the pyriform fossa of the nose. Insert the Howarth's elevator submucosally distally along the lateral nasal wall to the posterior end of the hard palate; this will protect the nasal lining (Figures 9.12f to 9.12h).
6. Bone is best cut with a reciprocating sagittal saw. A tapering fissure bur is also adequate but may produce a ragged margin (Figure 9.12i).
7. The osteotomy cut is extended from the pterygomaxillary fissure behind, forwards to the margin of the pyriform fossa approximately 15 mm above the gingival margin to clear the tooth apices, especially the canine. The cut is deepened posteriorly to section the distal and medial wall of the antrum, and also anteriorly where the medial and lateral walls of the antrum meet to form the thick triangular bony canine buttress.

   A useful variation is to fashion a step-shaped osteotomy (Figure 9.12j). Start as high as possible at the pyriform fossa margin and make a horizontal cut distally, parallel to the intended direction of maxillary movement. On reaching the zygomatic buttress cut downwards, i.e. at right angles, for 5 mm, then again turn distally through to the pterygoid plates in the usual way. This technique has the advantages of allowing more precise measurements and movements and enables the use of a horizontal miniature bone plate overlying the vertical component of the step, and so avoiding the apices of the molar teeth.

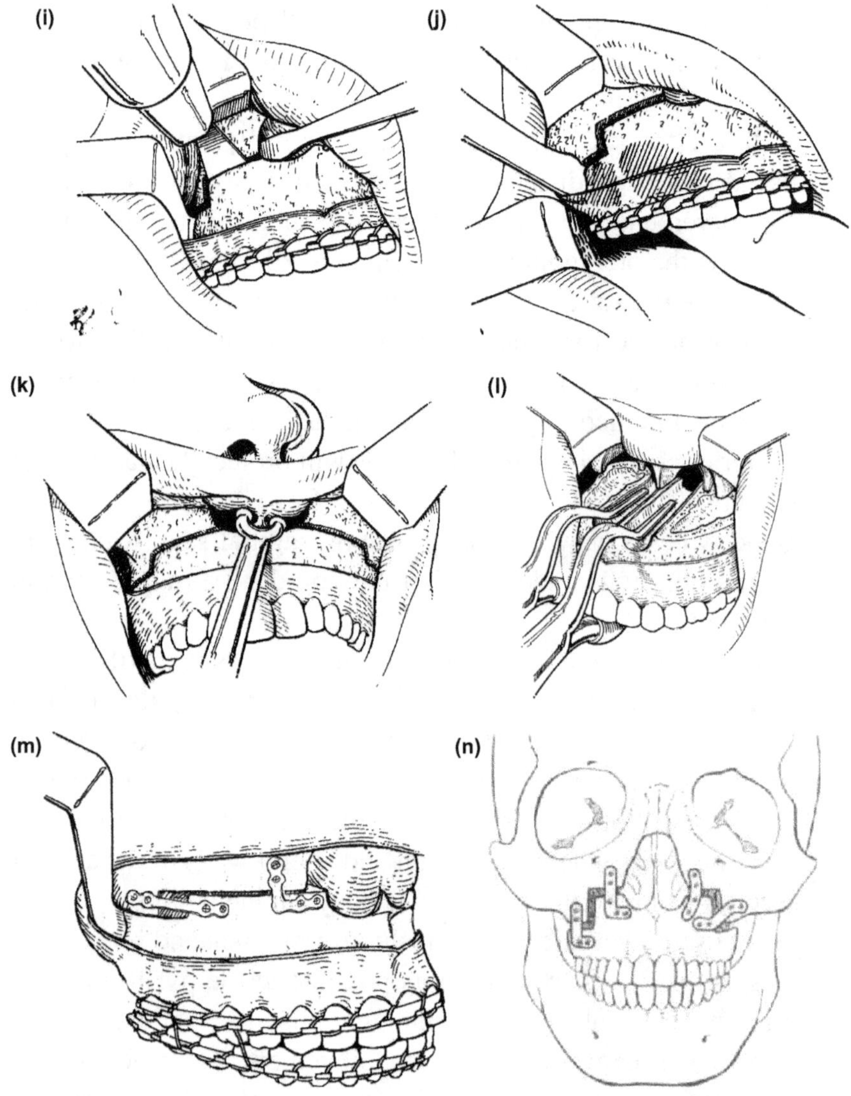

Figure 9.12 (i), (j), (k), (l), (m), (n)

8. If the maxilla is to be elevated, make two cuts the appropriate distance apart, e.g. 2–4–6 mm for minimal, moderate or significant impactions, and remove the intervening strip of bone.
9. The curved pterygoid osteotome is then inserted posteriorly between tuberosity and pterygoid plates and angled so that the

cutting edge is tapped medially with a light mallet; it may be felt protruding under the palatal mucosa with a forefinger when through the bone suture (Figure 9.12j).

10. This procedure is repeated on the opposite side.
11. The nasal septum is divided with a notched septum chisel. The Obwegeser septum chisel has a well-designed protected cutting end which prevents the chisel from straying away from the base of the septum (Figure 9.12k). Some nasal septum chisels may perforate or sever the nasotracheal tube, which produces a sudden burst of bloody bubbles. This may be prevented by passing a protective finger to the back of the soft palate.
12. The maxilla may now be fractured downwards with firm digital pressure or Rowe's disimpaction forceps. Any restraining points are divided with bone shears, saw or bur. It is imperative that the tooth-bearing component is made completely mobile, leaving it loosely pedicled on the soft palate (Figure 9.12l). If the greater palatine neurovascular bundle, which can be seen or felt at the back, restricts forward movement, it can be loosened with a forefinger. Upward displacement is usually prevented by the nasal septum at the back and the posterior wall of the antrum. Both need to be generously trimmed with bone rongeurs. Occasionally with upward or distal movements it is necessary to section the pterygoid buttress with an osteotome, and displace it backwards to enable repositioning of the maxilla satisfactorily.
13. At this stage the management will depend on the direction of the correction.

    Forward movements with an unoperated mandible. The dentoalveolar segment is placed in the planned occlusal position with temporary intermaxillary fixation. Malleable miniature bone plates are contoured and fitted across the posterior and anterior bony buttresses and screwed into place. An L-shaped plate will avoid the apices of the canine anteriorly, and a horizontal plate across the vertical cut of the posterior step osteotomy similarly preserves the molar roots (Figure 9.12m).

14. With large forward movements (e.g. >9 mm), improved stability may also be obtained by inserting cancellous bone blocks in the vertical buccal cut between the upper and lower maxillary walls (Figure 9.12m). These are secured by plates.
15. Always drill slowly with the appropriate drill or a tapering tungsten carbide fissure bur to ensure a firm bite by the screws. Rapid cutting, especially with a slightly eccentric rotation, will create a large, burnt hole. Use 5, 7 or 9 mm screws, depending on the thickness of the maxillary wall. Rescue screws are invaluable to replace loose ones.
16. With bimaxillary osteotomies the maxillary dentoalveolar segment is positioned with an intermediate occlusal wafer designed to relate its postoperative position to the unchanged mandible. By putting on temporary intermaxillary function with 0.35 mm wires, the mandible can be used to rotate the maxilla up into a stable position whilst the bone plates are placed.
17. Although at this stage it may be possible to check the lip-incisor relationship and maxillary midline by carefully displacing the anaesthetic tube to release the nose this is not reliable compared to a precise planning process and an accurate wafer.
18. **Superior positioning** simply requires the removal of a bone strip of appropriate width. However, the septum must also be generously reduced and, if necessary, a V-shaped groove made on the superior surface of the downfractured palate. Remember that, with a nasotracheal tube in place, the nose and septum are artificially elevated after the palate has been separated; this may give a false impression of adequate clearance. Inadequate septal reduction will either displace the maxilla, producing an asymmetrical malocclusion, or distort the nose itself. If ignored, both will require surgical correction. With any significant elevation, remove the inferior tubinates to prevent nasal airway obstruction. This is easily done through the anterior nares with a pair

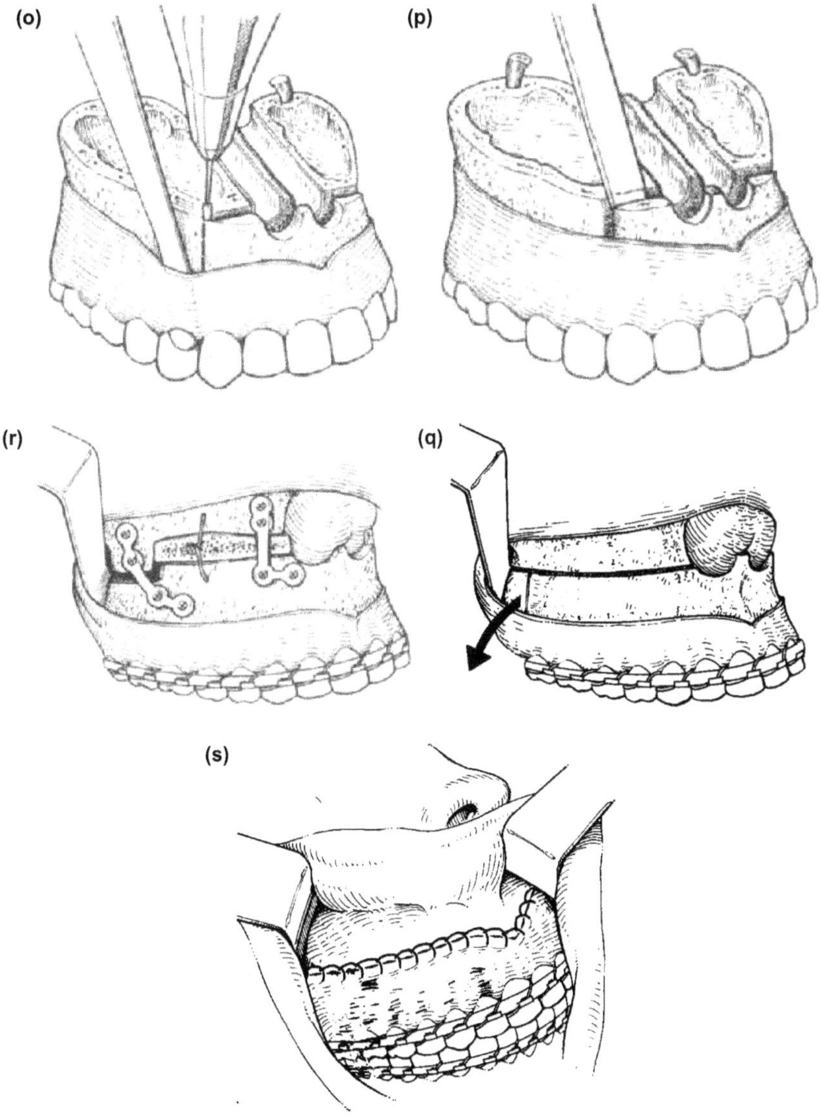

Figure 9.12 **(o), (p), (q), (r), (s)**

of heavy straight scissors, or from below after incising and opening the nasal mucosa.

19. **Segmental division** can be carried out from above with a tungsten carbide fissure bur and fine osteotome or an oscillating

sagittal saw. Care must be taken to preserve the mucosa of the hard palate beneath, which maintains the blood supply of the anterior segment. The buccal mucosa is protected by a Howarth periosteal elevator (Figures 9.12n and 9.12o).

20. **A transverse anterior** cut between the canine and first premolar is useful for levelling the occlusal plane in an anterior open-bite case with an exaggerated curve of Spee. As with all dentoalveolar osteotomies, the buccal and palate cortex are cut with a fine bur, but even if a space has been created by orthodontics or an extraction, the alveolar section must be done with a fine osteotome to avoid damaging the roots of the adjacent teeth (Figure 9.12p).
21. **A complete midline** section will enable the arch to be expanded posteriorly. Again, the anterior interincisor division must be done with a fine osteotome. Careful elevation of the underlying palatal mucoperiosteum through the palatal section from above will allow the outward expansion. If a palatal tear occurs in the midline, lateral (Langenbeck) relieving incisions will facilitate closure with a 4/0 Prolene mattress sutures.
22. **All segmental procedures require dual fixation**. The segmental components are first related with a well fitting wafer and fixation is secured with bone plates (Figure 9.12q). In addition the dental arch is accurately secured with a supplemental 1 mm arch wire which has been prepared with the model surgery.
23. **The maxilla may be lowered** by placing contoured/bent split rib overlying the cut margins of the gap in the lateral maxillary wall. Place the cancellous surface outwards to contact the overlying vascular soft tissues. Always overcorrect by 25%. This procedure will produce a downward and posterior rotation of the mandible requiring a sagittal split. Transosseous fixation with miniature bone plates gives adequate stability (Figure 9.12r). (See also The Short Face.)
24. **Posterior displacement** can be achieved by removing a triangular wedge of tuberosity sectioned through the third molar region. The tooth will, of course, be removed prior to this tuberositectomy. It is also necessary to divide the pterygoid

buttresses at their midpoint with an osteotome and displace them backwards (Figure 9.12s).

25. The wounds are sutured; but no drains are required.

The Posterior Dentoalveolar Segmental Osteotomy of Schuchardt

Indications

With the development of the Le Fort I downfracture technique allowing segmental procedures under direct vision, this operation has become obsolete.

Le Fort II Osteotomy

Indications

Nasomaxillary hypoplasia, especially where there is a deficiency at the infraorbital margins giving the appearance of a pseudoproptosis. The operation will accentuate a prominent nasal bridge, and so with a good nose a more suitable alternative operation is the Kufner modification of the Le Fort III osteotomy (see below).

The anatomical maxilla, together with the nasal bones and most of the septum, can be advanced and rotated downwards in the sagittal plane (Figure 9.13a). It is impossible to elevate the maxilla at the back with this operation and so the procedure is much less versatile than the Le Fort I osteotomy.

Technique

1. See the general preparation for bimaxillary procedures.
2. Prepare and drape the face, exposing the orbital margins and frontal area. Use a flexible armoured nasoendotracheal tube to give adaptable positioning of the anaesthetic hose. The nasal anaesthetic tube should be decontaminated with antiseptic and

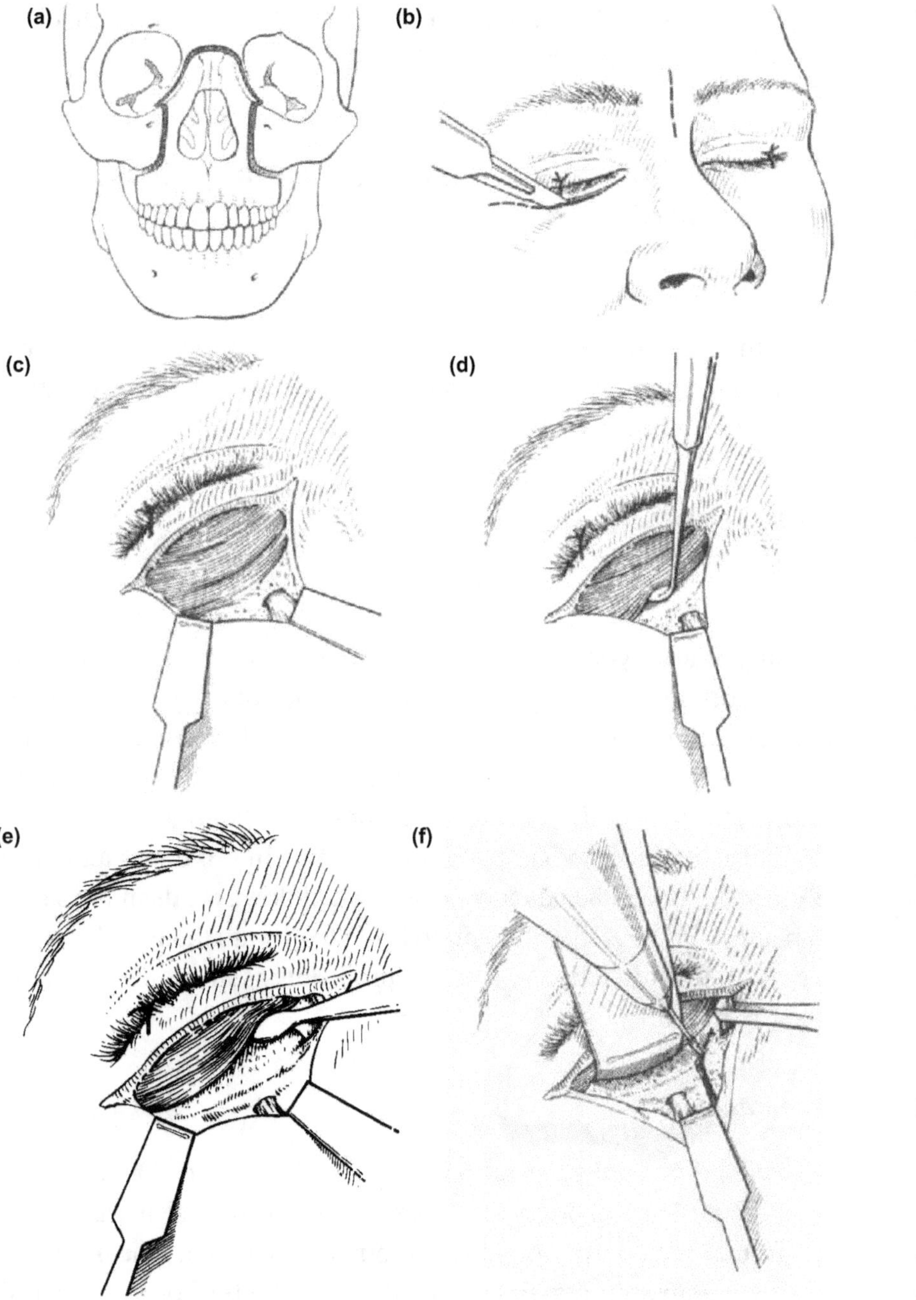

Figure 9.13 **(a), (b), (c), (d), (e), (f)**

covered with an adhesive drape (Steridrape, Opsite) to allow the surgeon access to the frontal area.

3. Insert protective coneal shells and suture the eyelids. Also suture the towels to the margins of the operative area to prevent exposure of the adjacent non-sterile surface. Hair has a habit of crawling onto the operating surface and should be fixed by brushing it away from the face with undiluted scrub detergent on a sterile scrubbing brush before towelling.
4. Mark the blephoroplasty (subciliary) and frontal incisions with a pen then infiltrate with a local anaesthetic-adrenaline (1.200,000) mixture (Figure 9.13b). A transconjunctival incision may be used as a more aesthetic approach by those who are experienced with the procedure, The coronal incision is a lot of work for a limited exposure.
5. If the operation is part of a bimaxillary procedure with:

    a) an Obwegeser osteotomy: carry out this operation up to the splitting procedure, which is left until the maxilla has been repositioned;
    b) an intraoral subsigmoid osteotomy: carry out the soft tissue surgery exposing the rami but leave the osteotomy until after the maxilla has been repositioned.

6. The blepharoplasty incision should leave no detectable scar, although occasionally there is a minor degree of ectropion, which usually resolves. The incision is made 2–3 mm below and parallel to the eyelid margin until below the outer canthus. The skin is carefully elevated with a hook or fine forceps and then, with a sharp No. 15 blade, incise obliquely downwards through the orbicularis muscle, avoiding the orbital septum, i.e. outside and parallel to the fascial layer of the lower eyelid. Any breach in the septum is announced by a bubbling protrusion of fat which should be ignored. Later the defect can be repaired with a 4/0 resorbable suture. When the bony orbital margin is palpated, a round-ended copper strip or Lack's

retractor is useful to retract the orbital contents whilst a firm clean incision through the periosteum is made.

7. Carefully raise the periosteum along the orbital margin and inferiorly down to the infraorbital foramen. This requires the detachment of the levator labii superioris alaeque nasi and the lower head of the orbicularis oculi, neither of which are recognisable (Figure 9.13c). Now extend the periosteal elevation upwards over the infraorbital margin with the spoon edge of a Mitchell's trimmer or a narrow, sharp, periosteal elevator such as a Freer or MacDonald, taking care not to breach the periosteum and release orbital fat. Elevate along the orbital floor posteriorly and then medially, supporting the orbital contents with an orbital floor retractor (Figure 9.13d).
8. Medially, the inferior orbital margin becomes narrow and sharp and is the so-called anterior lacrimal crest. Behind are the lacrimal sac and the nasolacrimal duct. Just lateral to the lacrimal sac one encounters a fine fibrovascular band which must be sacrificed in order to find the margin of the bony lacrimal fossa. The sac can be readily mobilised with a narrow dissector, first around the anterior, lateral and distal aspect, then medially around the back of the sac (Figure 9.13e). Finally extend the periosteal elevation up the frontal process of the maxilla towards the frontomaxillary suture.

   It is worth continuing the elevation at this stage, both upwards on to the down-facing convexity of the glabella and as far medially as possible on to the nasal bones. As the medial palpebral ligament is attached to the anterior lacrimal crest and the adjoining frontal process of the maxilla, this is also detached without disturbing the globe suspension.
9. The only remaining periosteal elevation is now inferiorly, passing medially and laterally to the infraorbital neurovascular bundle.
10. With a tapering tungsten carbide fissure bur cut through the inferior orbital margin, vertically downwards halfway between

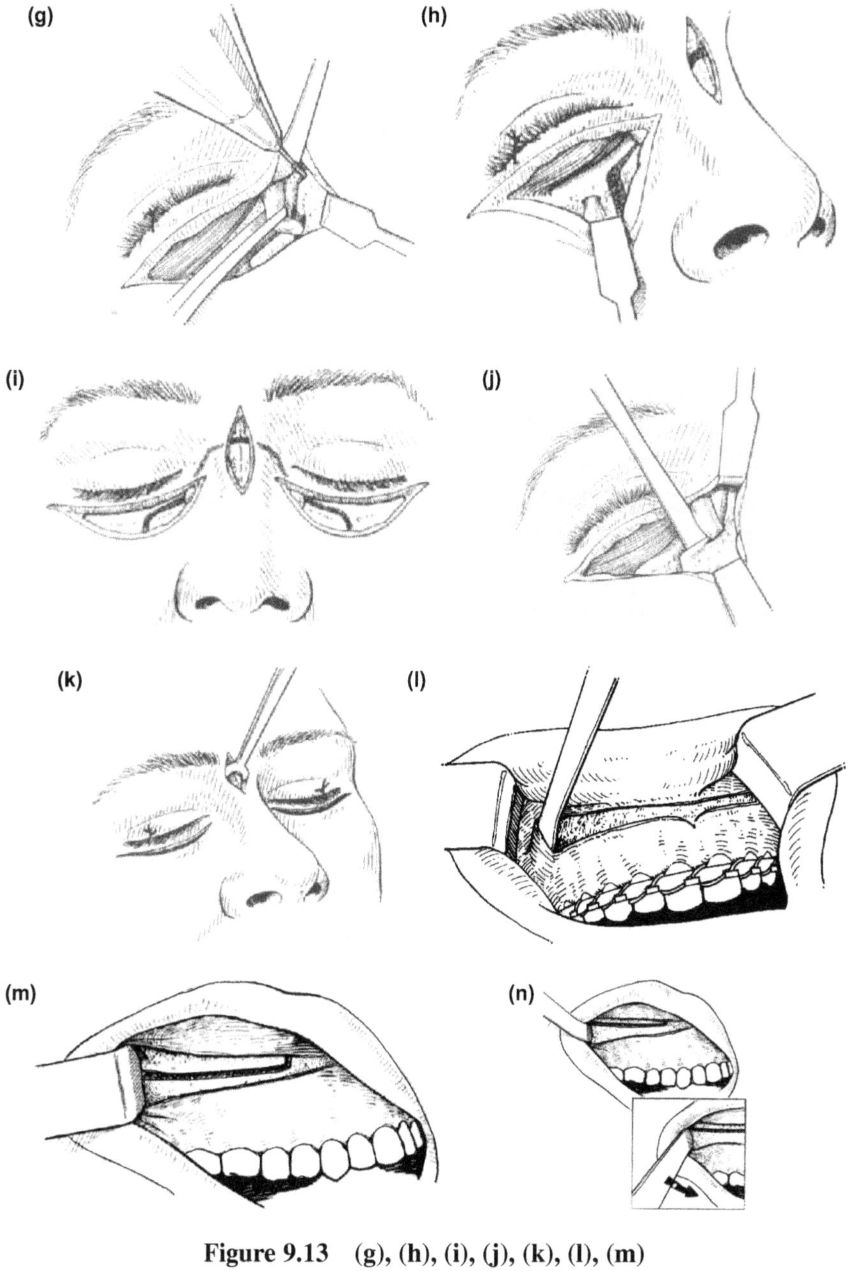

Figure 9.13 (g), (h), (i), (j), (k), (l), (m)

the nasolacrimal duct medially and the infraorbital bundle laterally. The orbital fascia and contents should be elevated and protected with a narrow, round-ended copper strip, Lac's retractor or orbital floor retractor. Extend the cut posteriorly along the orbital floor until it is distal to the lacrimal duct.

11. Now extend the cut medially behind the nasolacrimal duct, which is retracted with an elastic or nylon tape and protected with the narrow dissector (Figure 9.13f), and then continue the bur cut from the medial side of the duct (Figure 9.13g).
12. A vertical midline incision over the glabella is made down through the periosteum to bone. The tissues are firmly elevated widely, exposing the frontomaxillary suture and then passing inferiorly and laterally in the direction of the suture line into the orbit behind the lacrimal fossa.

    Using a Howarth periosteal elevator as a retractor and a tapering fissure bur, a horizontal cut is made below and parallel to the frontomaxillary suture. This suture is often the landmark of the floor of the anterior cranial fossa. The bur cut is extended posteroinferiorly into the lateral wall or the orbit behind the lacrimal sac (Figure 9.13h).
13. The two bur cuts may now be joined behind the lacrimal sac with a narrow osteotome inserted from the lateral side through the infraorbital incisions (Figure 9.13i).
14. This is repeated on the contralateral side.
15. The nasal septum is now divided through the vertical incision over the glabella. The Obwegeser nasal septum osteotome, with its convexity upwards, is inserted through the nasal bridge osteotomy cut. Once the septum can be felt firmly between the fork-like margins of the cutting edge, the osteotome is tapped diagonally downwards towards the posterior end of the hard palate, where it may be felt by the assistant's forefinger (Figure 9.13j).
16. The buccal sulcus is now infiltrated with local anaesthetic and vasoconstrictor solution and the incision made above the mucosal

(o)

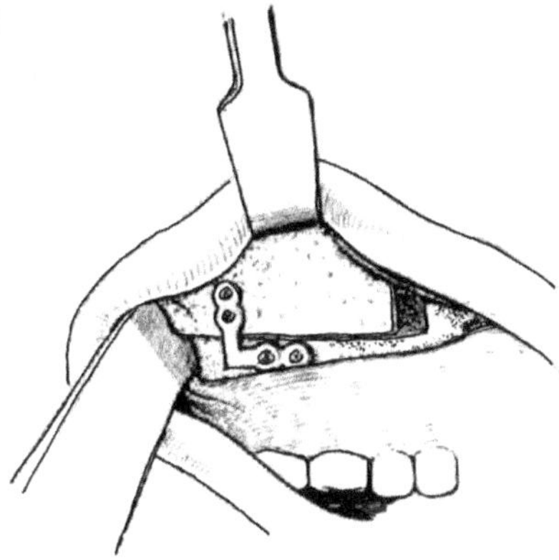

Figure 9.13 (o)

reflection from the distal aspect of the first molar around to the contralateral side (Figure 9.13k). This is reflected upwards with a dry swab and then periosteal elevator to reveal both the infraorbital neurovascular bundles and the lower ends of the osteotomy cuts medially (Figure 9.13l). The cut is extended downwards and backwards across the zygomatic buttress with a long tapering fissure bur or reciprocating sagittal saw (Figure 9.13m).

17. A flat bladed Lac's retractor will have been placed behind the posterior wall of the maxilla. As with the Le Fort I osteotomy, the cuts must be continued across to the posterior and medial wall of the antrum. Finally, the tuberosity is detached from the pterygoid plates with the curved pterygoid osteotome (Figure 9.13n).
18. Mobilisation requires firm, bilateral, extraoral traction both downwards and forwards with the Rowe maxillary disimpaction forceps and then intraoral forward displacement with the Tessier maxillary retractors (Figure 9.13o). It is necessary to insert a broad osteotome in horizontally in the cut through the zygomatic buttress and carefully rotate it to mobilise the back of the maxilla. This part of the operation must be done with vigour if it is to succeed. With marked resistance the bone cut

may need to be revised with a narrow osteotome. Gross haemorrhage can usually be controlled with hot gauze packs and tranexamic acid 1 g i.v.

19. Either during this procedure or at this stage, iliac crest bone is obtained to provide cancellous sheets to fill the osteotomy cuts. Always take too much rather than too little for a Le Fort II osteotomy.
20. The freely mobilised maxilla is repositioned and localised by relating it directly to the mandible, if it is not to be operated on, or with the intermediate wafer. Temporary intermaxillary tie wires are placed.
21. The cancellous bone is wedged between the osteotomy margins and secured with low profile plates. An inverted Y is useful at the nasal bridge. With a grossly deficient bridge a pocket can be made downwards with small blunt scissors to the nasal tip to accommodate a cortical bone strut. Minature bone plates are readily inserted inferiorly and given excellent fixation.
22. With a bimaxillary case, the temporary intermaxillary fixation is removed in order to complete the mandibular osteotomy. Insert bilateral suction drains, remove the pack and suck out the pharynx and localise the final occlusion.
23. Carefully close the skin incisions with 3/0 subcutaneous polyglycollate and 5/0 subcuticular Prolene sutures.

The Kufner Modification of the LeFort III Osteotomy

Le Fort III procedures are outside the scope of this textbook as they are more appropriate for severe craniofacial deformities. However, a useful operation for malar-maxillary advancement is the Kufner modification of the Le Fort III osteotomy. This is particularly important when the nose is prominent. As can be seen from Figure 9.14, access and therefore the instrumentation are identical to the Le Fort II procedure.

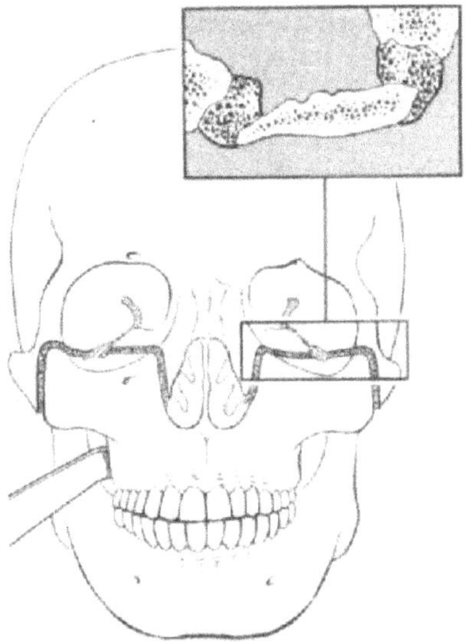

Figure 9.14

However the malar maxillary advancement may now be corrected more effectively by distraction osteogenesis.

Indications

This operation can be used for patients with mild to moderate zygomatixomaxillary hypoplasia but with a normal nose. Gross malar and infraorbital augmentation is more easily achieved with a high Le Fort I osteotomy or distraction osteogenesis.

Technique

Follow the stages described for the Le Fort II osteotomy (steps 1–8) without mobilising the lacrimal sac.

1. Elevate the periosteum and facial tissues from the orbital margin downwards and medially on the anterior surface of the maxilla until the nasal pyriform fossa margin in reached.

2. Elevate the orbital periosteum distally and laterally to expose the anterior end of the inferior orbital fissure and the lateral orbital margin.
3. Extension of the blepharoplasty incision laterally will now give surprisingly good access to the malar bone itself, which must be exposed completely.
4. The bone cuts are made (Figure 9.14) with a tapering fissure bur. This is often easier from above the patient. Take care not to damage the infraorbital neurovascular bundle which can be seen through the thin orbital floor.
5. Take the lateral osteotomy cut horizontally through the base of the lateral orbital margin. Then make a vertical cut through the zygomatic bone two-thirds of the way back from the orbital margin. This will create an inverted L-shaped separation, giving excellent access for placing a corticocancellous graft and for plating (Figure 9.14 inset).
6. Extend the medial cuts down into the pyriform margin. Repeat on the contralateral side.
7. The nasal septum and pterygoid plates are separated intraorally, as in the Le Fort I operation.
8. If distraction osteogenesis is not being used, mobilisation is carried out extraorally from above and behind the head ("slowly but strongly") with the Rowe's disimpaction forceps. Both a forward tilting and transverse rotation are required to achieve a completely mobile skeletal block. Intraoral traction with Tessier's maxillary retractors is also important.
9. Temporary intermaxillary fixation is applied, using an intermediate wafer in a bimaxillary case. The bone grafts are inserted at the osteotomy sites. The most important one is the malar cut, which is wedged open as shown in Figure 9.14 and fixed with bone plates.
10. All sharp bony margins are carefully masked with spare cancellous bone or smoothed with an acrylic bur.

11. At this stage the intermaxillary fixation is removed and, where necessary, the mandibular osteotomy completed, drains inserted and the intraoral wounds sutured.
12. The pharynx is sucked out and the pack removed.
13. The blepharoplasty wounds are closed after the insertion of miniature vacuum drains, with subcuticular 5/0 Prolene sutures.

Tongue Reduction

Indications

The enlarged tongue is an uncommon cause of anterior open bite and osteotomy failure. If it appears to be large and the incisor teeth are proclined and separated, surgical reduction is indicated and can be carried out prior to orthodontics or with segmental osteotomies.

Where there is any doubt, the patient should be informed that it may be necessary some time after the dental alignment or osteotomy, and the case is carefully followed up at 3-monthly intervals to prevent any gross relapse. This will take the form of recurrent proclination and separation of the incisors. Once this is obvious, reduction should be carried out and any dental relapse can be corrected orthodontically. The tongue should always be reduced in length and width, which can be achieved by a keyhole excision.

Technique (Figure 9.15)

1. Draw the tongue forwards with a towel clip or two heavy silk stay sutures and generously outline the tissue to be removed with a pen and Bonney's Blue.

    a) The full thickness wedge will determine the reduction in length and width at the tip (Figure 9.15a).
    b) A centrally placed ellipse overlapping the anterior wedge will reduce bulk and width, but will minimally increase the

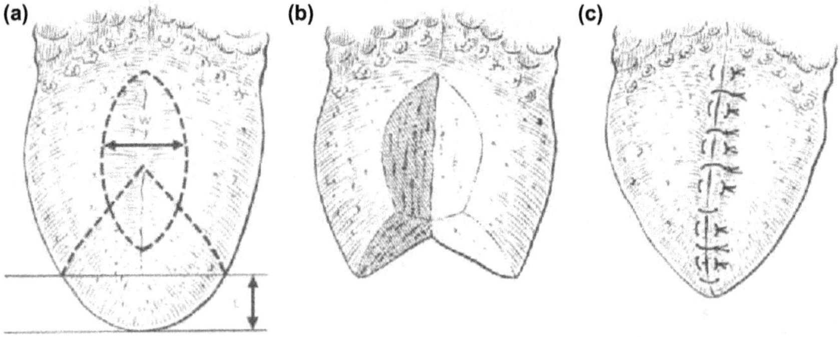

Figure 9.15 (a), (b), (c)

length. L = reduction in length. W = reduction in width (Figure 9.15b).

2. Infiltrate well with 0.5% bupivacaine and 1:200 000 adrenaline.
3. With a large blade (No. 20), first excise the anterior wedge, carefully arresting all bleeding points with mosquitoes and bipolar diathermy. Allis forceps or two heavy gauge traction sutures can be used for immobilising the tongue while the central ellipse is excised with a triangular cross-section. Again careful haemostasis is important.
4. The tongue is sutured with 3/0 polyglycollate starting at the tip and working backwards with vertical mattress sutures from the depth to the mucosal suface. Simple sutures are then placed between each of the mattress sutures from behind working forward and continuing on to the ventral surface. (Figure 9.15c)
5. The combination of careful haemostasis and anti-oedema steroids (8 mg dexamethasone, 12-hourly, × 3) should prevent any gross swelling and obstruction.
6. Generous analgesia and nasogastric nutrition will be required for at least 3 days.
7. Postoperative speech therapy is useful to re-establish comfortable diction.

Bone Grafts

Orthognathic Indications

Bone may be required for establishing continuity of a cleft palate, and for extensive maxillary osteotomies. It is used as cancellous bone chips, cancellous bone slices or corticocancellous blocks. In order of value one can use:

1. Fresh autogenous bone, which is actively osteogenic and provides the best union.
2. Decalcified lyophilised bone (either autogenous or allogenous bank bone). This is a satisfactory space filler and scaffold which induces good union but is much improved when supplemented with autogenous cancellous mush or rhBone Morphogenetic Protein 2.
3. Deep frozen or lyophilised whole autogenous bone, which may be rated only as satisfactory.

There is an increased risk of secondary infection and greater loss of graft with the stored non-vital tissues.

Where fresh bone is employed, minimal storage outside the body is desirable and the operation should therefore be planned to harvest the graft when it is needed. It should be kept in a blood-soaked swab. Immersion in saline and the application of antibiotic powders devitalise the fresh bone.

Iliac Crest

Operative autogenous harvesting, donor sites

a) open harvesting for palatal cleft cases
b) trephine harvesting: for detail and illustrations (see Chapter 12)
c) Non operative grafts.

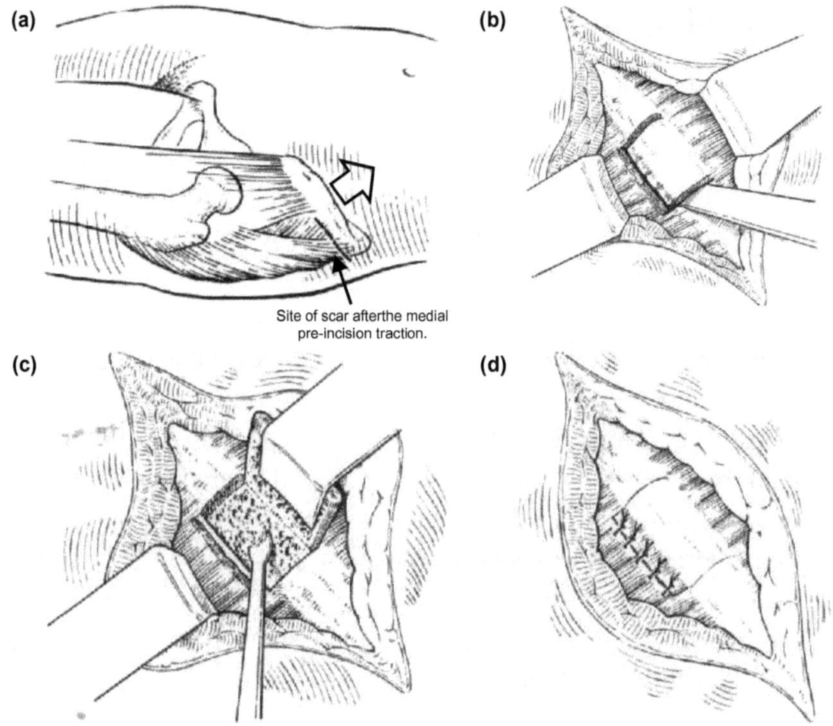

Figure 9.16 **(a), (b), (c), (d)**

1. *Open harvesting (See Figure 9.16)*

Appropriate shaving and cleansing should be carried out on the ward.

1. In orthognathic surgery and secondary cleft repair only portions of the iliac crest are required; therefore operate on the side which is most convenient. For right-handed surgeons, the left hip can be simultaneously approached by an assistant. A substantial sandbag should be placed under the buttock (ischium) to elevate the iliac crest.
2. Prepare the hip widely and carefully with a detergent-iodine solution. Square drape with 4 towels that are stitched into place

with a heavy black silk (2/0) on a straight or 30 mm curved cutting needle, cover and seal the area with an adhesive drape, i.e. Opsite, Steridrape.

Note: Ensure the anterior superior iliac spine is at the inferomedial corner of the operative area and that the crest can be palpated along its whole length to the posterosuperior corner.

3. Clean and drape the head end for the osteotomy, and then cover the the patient with a large sheet, which can be rotated downwards to reveal the donor site when ready without repreparation. The operator and assistant should change their gloves and gowns between mouth and hip.
4. For particulate cancellous bone/cancellous mush (the Flint technique).

    a) The assistant, standing on the contralateral side, pulls the skin medially so that the incision on to the iliac crest will ultimately fall elow the bony surface (Figure 9.16a).
    b) A short incision of 6 cm is made down to the iliac crest with a No. 20 blade and the margins retracted. Diathermy will be required for bleeding points and the wound is enlarged.
    c) Once the periosteum-covered bone surface has been defined with a swab and knife, a 2.5 cm osteotome is used to outline a lid 5 cm wide on the superior and lateral aspects of the crest (Figure 9.16b).
    d) This lid is elevated on its medial musculoperiosteal hinge and cancellous bone is removed using gouges and Volkmann spoon. The bone should be placed into a dry receiver and covered with a blood-soaked swab until used. Soaking fresh bone in saline kills the osteoblasts (Figure 9.16c).
    e) The lid may be sutured into place with 1/0 polyglycollate, which is also used to oppose the muscle and for deep subcutaneous closure (Figure 9.16d). A continuous subcuticular 3/0 Prolene suture on a straight needle is used for the skin.

5. For blocks and sheets.

   a) A 10 cm incision is made down to periosteum. Undermining the skin margins will give improved access. Dissection with a fresh blade will now define the periosteum-covered iliac crest.
   b) A long lid (12 cm) may be outlined with an osteotome and lifted, pedicled on the inner periosteum and muscle in the same manner as described above, and block cut from the bone beneath. By outlining a rectangle on the outer surface of the ilium with the osteotome, a lateral cortical flap may also be rotated downwards, allowing sheets of cancellous bone to be cut from the centre. Some prefer to cut a medial cortical flap in order not to disturb the origin of the gluteal fascia and muscles (Figures 9.17a and 9.17b).
   c) The cortical lids are replaced and sutured with 1/0 polyglycollate

Note: It is easier to reflect the surface periosteum with a Farabeuf periosteal elevator and simply cut out corticocancellous blocks as required.

   d) The muscle layer is closed with a 2/0 suture and a vacuum drain inserted. This ensures a marked reduction in haematoma formation and postoperative morbidity. The drain must be carefully sutured to the skin before wound closure, ensuring 2 cm of non-perforated tube within the tissues.
   e) Close the skin with a subcutaneous resorbable suture and then a continuous subcuticular 3/0 Prolene or polyglycollate and Steri-strips (Figure 9.17c). If possible, cover the wound immediately with a sterile adhesive dressing (Demacel) and then complete the osteotomy. Postoperative antibiotics are given for 5 days.

      The drain is left in until it stops draining. The Prolene skin suture is removed after 10 days; the polyglycollate suture may be left to dissolve.

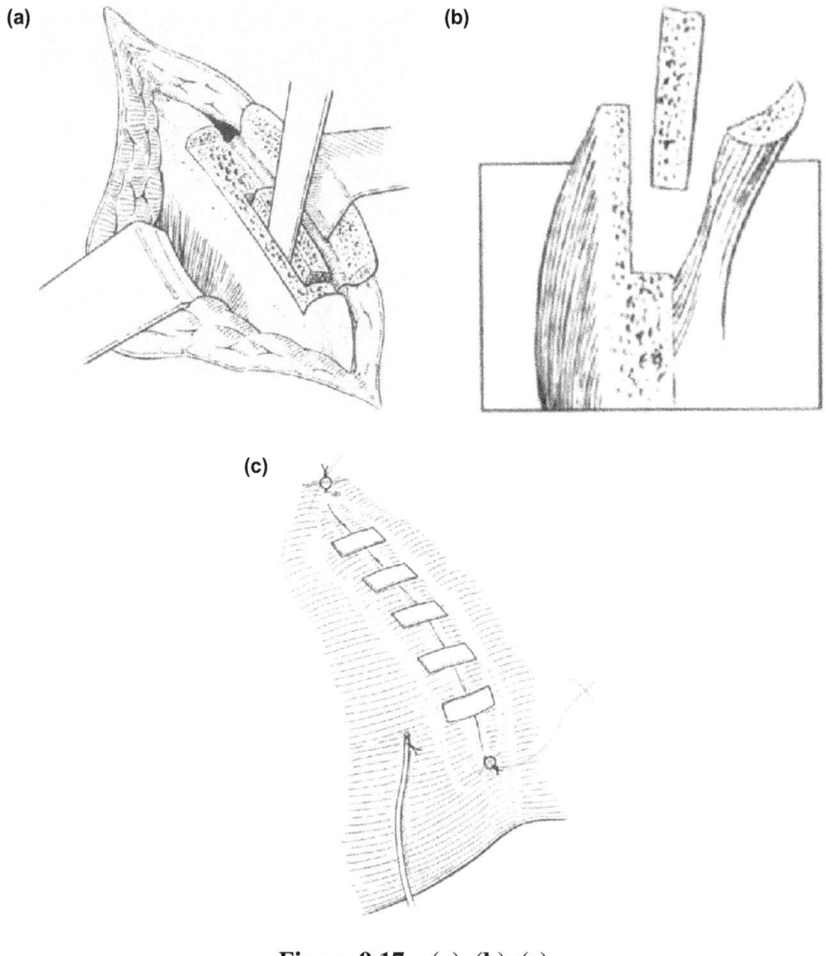

Figure 9.17 (a), (b), (c)

f) Iliac Crest Complications: The open harvesting procedure is subject to donor site pain, infection, lateral cutaneous nerve paraesthesia, hematoma formation, hernia, difficulty in walking and a residual scar. In addition at the recipient site, pain, infection, wound dehiscence, graft exposure or rejection are not uncommon. Hence there is a need to consider improved procedures especially for children with a cleft palate deformity.

2. *Trephine harvesting (See Chapter 12 for procedure details)*

Cores of autogenous bone can be harvested by a manual or power-driven trephine. The bone cores are harvested through a 1.5 cm incision on the iliac crest distal to the anterior superior iliac spine between the medial and lateral plates.

This is invaluable for the reconstruction of secondary palatal cleft repair where only modest amounts of cancellous bone are required. Trephining the iliac crest results in significantly less morbidity than the traditional open method and has overall favorourable clinical results.

3. *Non operative bone substitutes with recombinant human bone morphogenetic protein 2. (rhBMP-2)*

Osteoconductive bone substitutes such as decalcified lyophilised bone (either autogenous or allogenous bank bone) *provide a skeletal scaffold but* lack osteoinductive properties, whereas rhBMP-2 can induce adjacent pluripotential mesenchymal stem cells to differentiate into osteoblasts that will lay down new bone within the scaffold.

Freeze-dried rhBMP-2 can be reconstituted with sterile saline and applied with a bone substitute in defects as a putty or on an absorbable collagen sheet to provide a successful graft.

Complications with rhBMP-2 are minimal and are increased local oedema and trismus.

However the benefits are the elimination of the expense and complications of an additional operation.

Rib (Figure 9.18a to 9.18e)

Rib is easier to remove than iliac crest, with considerably less morbidity for the patient, but provides less bone both qualitatively and quantitatively.

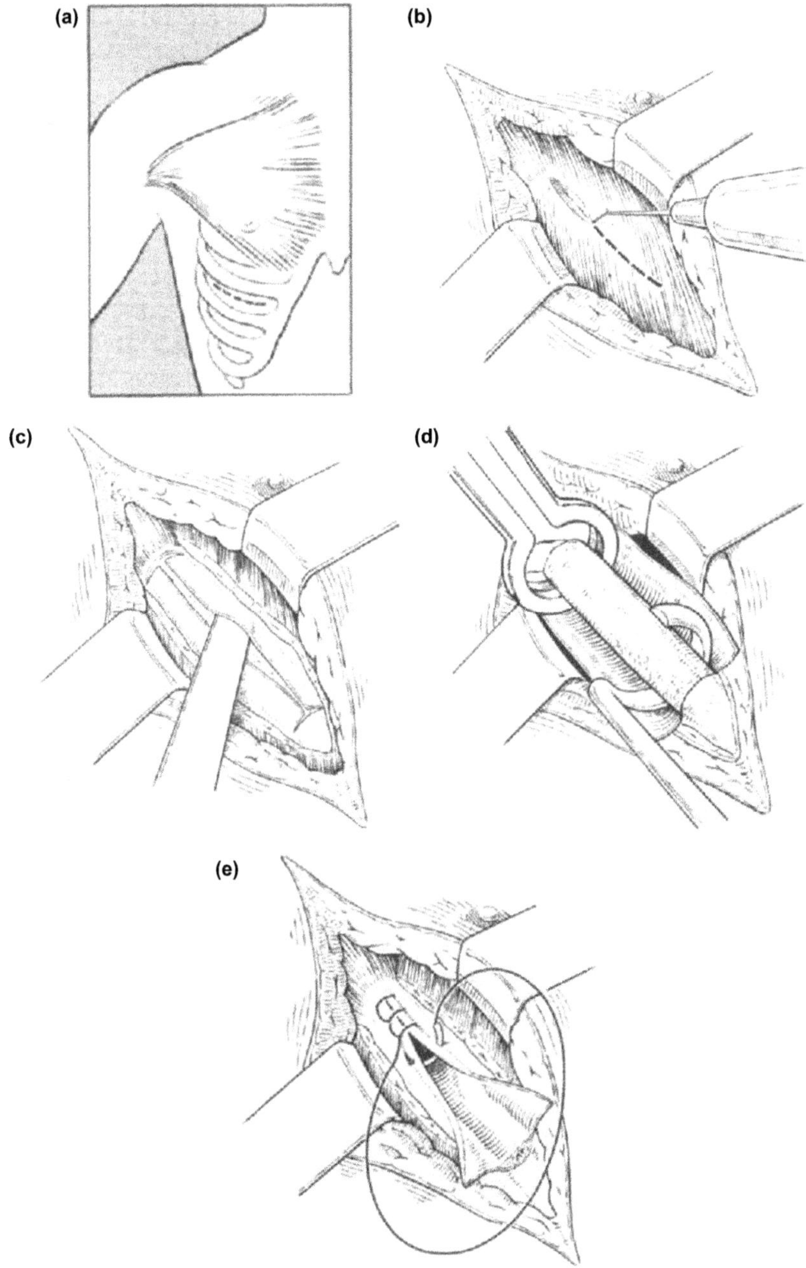

Figure 9.18 (a), (b), (c), (d), (e)

Rib may be split with an fine osteotome, separating the outer and inner cortices which are rendered pliable with Tessier rib forceps or a pair of straight extraction forceps. These strips can be laid over maxillary osteotomy cuts with the cortex facing "outwards" against the vascular soft tissues.

Technique

1. As with the hip, the chest wall must be carefully prepared with a detergent-iodine solution, dried, towelled and sealed with an adhesive drape.
2. Incisions must be planned to fall in the crease of the lower border of pectoralis major or beneath the breast. This may be done accurately using a marker pen, with the patient sitting upright, before the operation. A 6 cm incision with a No. 10 blade, once undermined, gives generous access to the 5th and 6th ribs. Coagulate bleeding vessels then incise the muscle layer, down to but not including the periosteum, with a cutting diathermy needle (Figure 9.18b).
3. The rib periosteum is incised with a fresh blade along its mid axis and then at right angles to this cut. Peel off the superficial periosteum, then carefully expose both rib margins (Figure 9.18c). The undersurface is then stripped with a curved rib rasperator (Figure 9.18d) as widely as possible and rib cutting shears are applied to cut the rib with the guillotine blade facing away from the graft to gain maximal length. It is then firmly grasped and carefully pealed off the underlying periosteum.
4. If the inner periosteum and pleura are torn, the lungs should be inflated by the anaesthetist as the defect is sutured with 3/0 Prolene or polyglycollate with a round-bodied needle. The periosteum is then closed with a continuous suture. The muscle layer and subcutaneous tissues are closed with the same needle,

and the skin with a continuous subcuticular 3/0 Prolene or polyglycollate suture (Figure 9.18e). A drain is not necessary. Cover with an adhesive dressing (e.g. Opsite), and drape a towel over the area and continue with the osteotomy.

5. The costochondral graft; a minor modification is required for a costochondral graft. A 6 cm length of rib is exposed adjacent to the costal cartilage, but the medial right angle division of the periosteum is placed so as to leave a periosteal bridge between bony rib and cartilage. The lateral bone end is cut as above and the cartilage carefully incised with a No. 15 blade protecting the undersurface with a Howarth periosteal elevator. The cartilage is then trimmed to a round condylar like surface and the graft carefully stored until used.
6. A postoperative chest X-ray is essential the following day. Not uncommonly an effusion may result, especially where large quantities of rib have been taken. However, with antibiotic cover and physiotherapy no intervention will be required. The treatment of a pneumothorax is dealt with in Chapter 15.

Chapter 10

Distraction Osteogenesis

Kieran Coghlan

Introduction

Distraction osteogenesis is an important adjunct to complex orthognathic procedures but is already too advanced to cover in a short section of this book. A palatal expansion device was first introduced in 1859 and underwent many refinements until 1968 when the Hyrax screw was introduced as a tooth-borne appliance with and without an osteotomy. At the time palatal expansion was considered to be a separation of the midline palatal suture bridged by the formation of new bone. The problem with this tooth-borne appliance is that compression of the abutment teeth against the buccal perimeter of their periodontal membranes activates the release of bone resorbing factors, so that the teeth not only tip outwardly but also lose their overlying buccal plate. This has been overcome by bone-borne expansion appliances for both the maxilla and mandible, and now many successful distraction protocols exist for craniofacial surgery.

Distraction osteogenesis is designed to lengthen and create new bone by stretching the callus at an osteotomy site by controlled tensile forces which increase the generation of immature bone laid down between the cut ends. Over time, the osteoid remodels into mature bone and the surrounding soft tissues adapt to their new volume and length. This remarkable process is made possible by the extensibility of the skin, fascia and muscle in response to gradual elongating traction. Muscle fibres have also been shown to add on sarcomeres in response to carefully controlled extension.

The Cell Biology of Distraction Osteogenesis

Preosteoblasts, osteoblasts and fibroblasts are sensitive to mechanical deformation such as the strain of osteodistraction and respond by the release of a complex soup of cellular factors. These include osteogenic cytokines such as transforming growth factor (TGF β1), bone morphogenic proteins (BMPs) such as BMP 2 and 4 and important angiogenic factors such as the basic fibroblast growth factor (BFGF). In addition osteoclastogenesis is also upregulated by the release of tumour necrosis factor-alpha (TNFα), RANKL (the Receptor Activator for Nuclear Factor Kappa beta Ligand) and interleukin 1β (IL1β) which recruit and activate osteoclasts. Both of these remodelling processes are upregulated but the balance between bone formation and resorption is probably determined by the rate of separation and vascularity of the callus. The resorption explains why teeth aggressively moved into consolidating callus (osteoid) undergo marked root resorption indicating increased cementoclast activity. The maturation process of the distracted osteoid to bone takes place during the retention phase.

The Distraction Technique

This is divided into 4 phases.

1. Osteotomy.
2. Period of latency. In the craniofacial region this is usually about 4–5 days to allow callus formation and primary wound healing.

3. Distraction phase is carried out at a constant rate (1–2 mm per day) until the desired length or volume of bone has been created. Despite this slow rate of distraction the procedure can be painful at each turn for up to 20 minutes duration and adequate analgesia is recommended on a daily basis.
4. Retention of the distracted bone is necessary to allow for calcification and remodelling of the osteoid. In the craniofacial region this will usually be a minimum of 6–8 weeks.

The Procedure

Early reports on craniofacial distraction propose corticotomies rather than osteotomies. While a corticotomy in young children with soft bone may allow mobilisation of the bone sections, it is essential to carry out a complete osteotomy in adolescents and adults. Most distraction in adults in the craniofacial region is carried out at the rate of 1 mm per day. Rates of less than 0.5 mm a day may result in ankylosis and rates of more than 3 mm a day result in non-union. Children may tolerate faster rates of distraction than 1 mm a day with the production of good quality distraction bone, however the more gradual the distraction rate the more predictable is the generation of vascular distraction osteoid. Therefore a rate of a 0.5 mm twice a day or a 0.25 mm four times a day is more effective than a single movement of 1 mm a day.

The Vector of Distraction

The vector or direction of distraction will determine where the length and volume of bone is created. The choice of the optimum vector may be estimated from plain radiographs or more accurately by 3D modelling computer programmes which simulate virtual surgery and distraction preoperatively. Simulated distraction can also be carried out for the more complicated cases prior to surgery with stereolithic models. The many distractors available can be intraoral or extraoral but require expert supervision.

Types of Distractor

The first cases were carried out using external distractors which in the oral and facial area were bulky, and produced visible scars where the fixation pins enter the skin and are moved during the distraction phase (Figures 10.1a and 10.1b). There are now many types of external and internal distractors available to suit most deformities. Multidirectional distractors allow for one or more osteotomies to be carried out simultaneously and the bone may be distracted in more than one direction. Internal distractors are more acceptable by patients. There are now a number of slim-line internal distractors with a variety of designs and sizes to accommodate most clinical situations (Figures 10.2a and 10.2b).

It was Gavril Ilizarov in 1951 who introduced his distraction technique for extending the poliomyelitis shortened limbs of children and adults with fracture malunion (Figure 10.11).

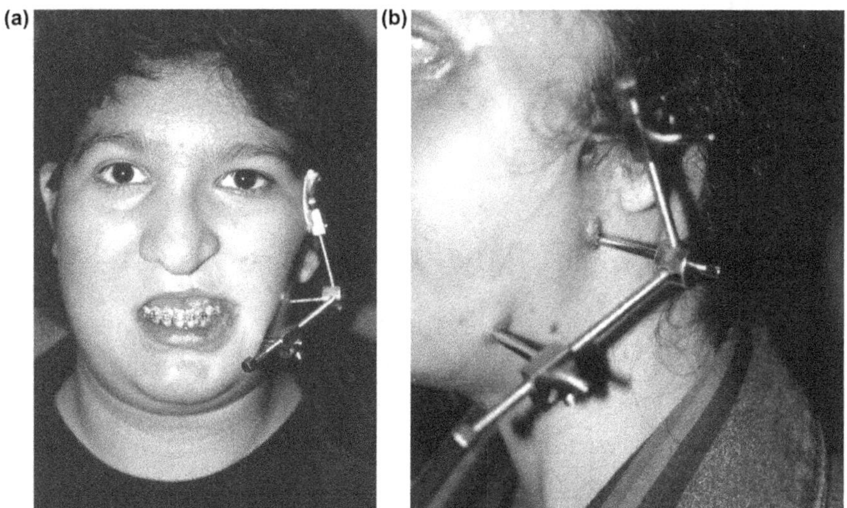

Figures 10.1 **(a)** and **(b)** An example of an older bulky distractor with scar formation.

The following applications will be presented:

- Childhood hypoplasia of the mandible
- Maxillary hypoplasias due to cleft palate surgery — see also Chapter 12
- Enlargement of the atrophic alveolus
- Dentoalveolar preparation for implant insertion
- TMJ ankylosis
- Post-maxillofacial trauma reconstruction

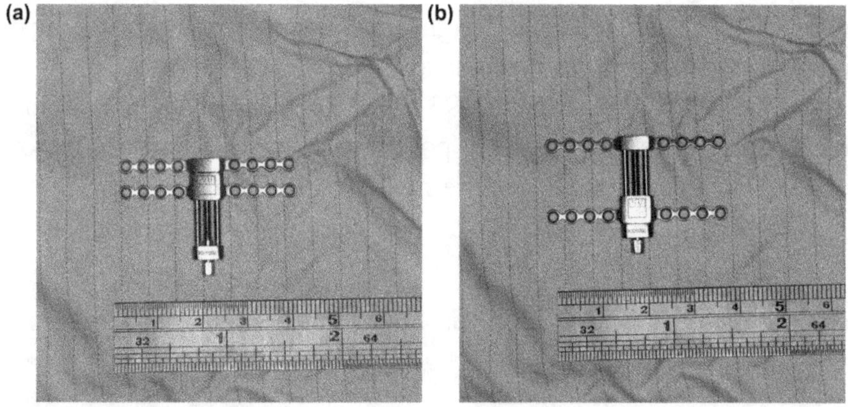

Figure 10.2 An internal distractor (**a**) closed and (**b**) open.

1. The Hypoplastic Mandible

The traditional management of a hypoplastic mandible acquired in childhood is an inverted L advancement osteotomy with a ramus bone graft and an augmentation genioplasty. An inverted L or horizontal osteotomy of the ascending ramus with internal distraction osteogenesis is a logical and assured way of achieving the same correction.

Figures 10.3a and 10.3b show a 15-year-old with mandibular hypoplasia due to the lack of condylar development attributed to early childhood trauma. The degree of hypoplasia was increasingly apparent with adolescent facial growth. Radiographs revealed a mandible which is both short in ramus height and body length (Figures 10.3a and 10.3b).

The maxilla was also deficient in posterior height possibly secondary to the mandibular hypoplasia, but it was decided to treat only the mandible at this stage.

Bilateral horizontal ramus osteotomies were carried out above the level of the lingula. This site allowed subsequent sagittal osteotomies to be carried out should the need arise when growth had ceased.

Distractors with universal joint mechanisms were used (KLS Martin) (Figures 10.3e and 10.3f).

This 15-year-old boy had an underdeveloped retrognathic mandible with short ascending rami.

Figure 10.3c shows the pre-distraction short rami and condyles.

An oblique vector was chosen to provide a downward and forward direction of distraction. This increased the vertical ramus

(a) (b)

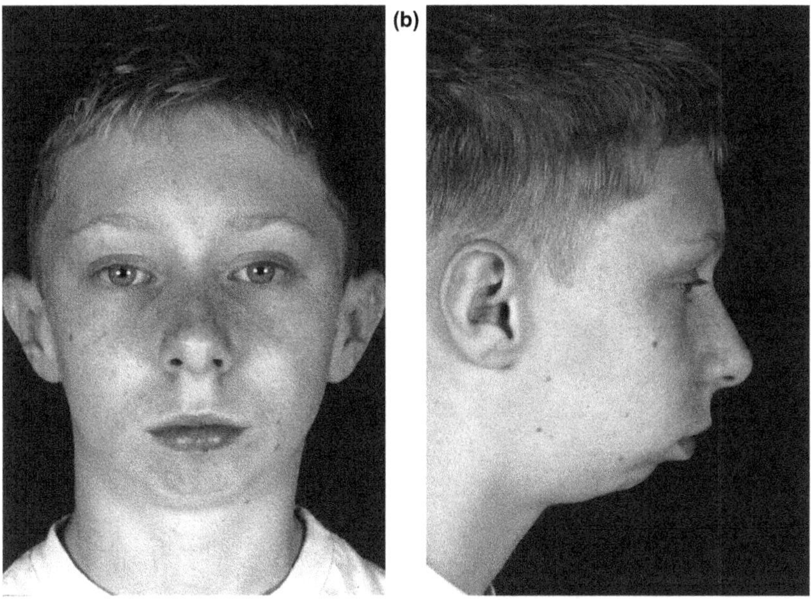

Figure 10.3 (a), (b)

(c)

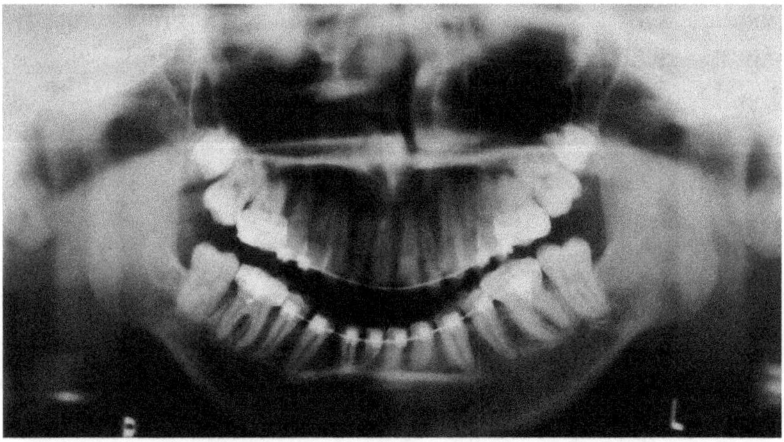

Figure 10.3 (*Continued*) **(c)**

height bilaterally and at the same time achieved forward projection of the mandible but not the chin.

Figure 10.3d shows the pre-distraction lateral skull and Figure 10.3e the ramus osteotomy with the intraoral closed distractor in place. Figure 10.3f is the OPG showing the bilateral closed distractors. Figure 10.3g shows the post-distraction OPG with separated distractor arms.

Following a post-osteotomy latency of 5 days, distraction was commenced at the rate of 1 mm per day (0.5 mm, 12-hourly) and continued for 15 days. The distractors were then maintained *in situ* for a period of 8 weeks before surgical removal (Figure 10.3g).

Figures 10.3h and 10.3i show the pre- and post-distraction lateral X-rays, the latter with the distractors fully extended and the improved lower facial height and mandibular profile.

The clinical gain can be seen in Figures 10.3j and 10.3k which illustrate the improved lower facial height and mandibular profile advancement by 11 mm.

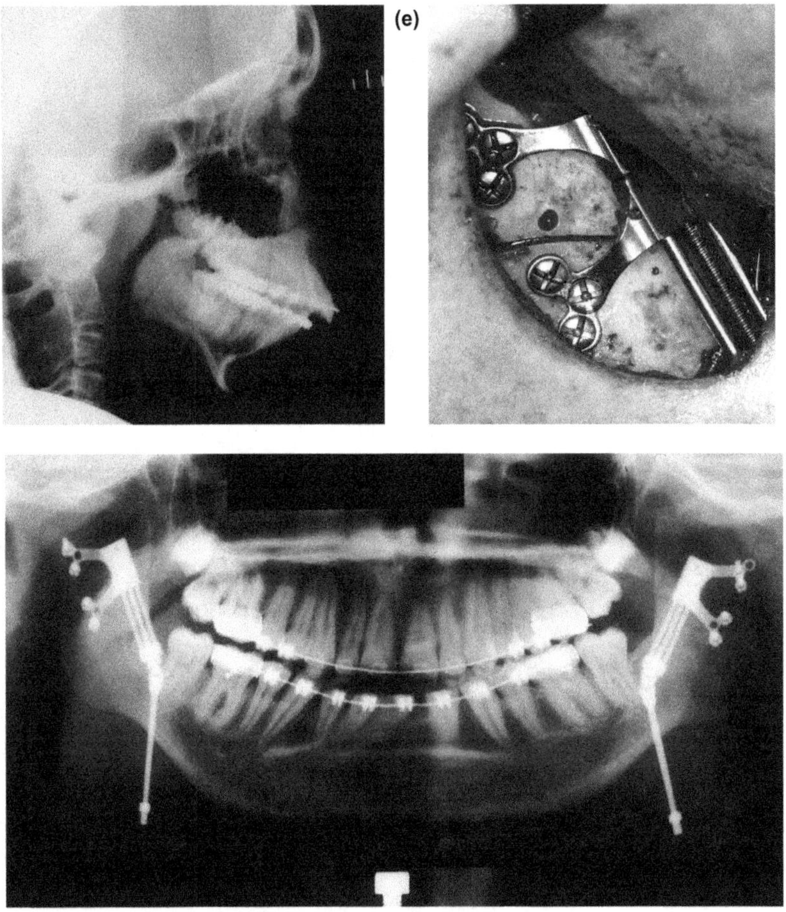

Figure 10.3 (*Continued*) **(d), (e), (f)**

Figure 10.3h shows the pre-distraction and 10.3i the post-distraction X ray profiles with advancement of the lower incisors and mandibular profile.

Figures 10.3j and 10.3k show the immediate post-distraction benefit.

The cephalometric tracing: Figure 10.3l shows that the vertical ramus height had increased 8 mm and the forward projection of the mandible increased by 11 mm.

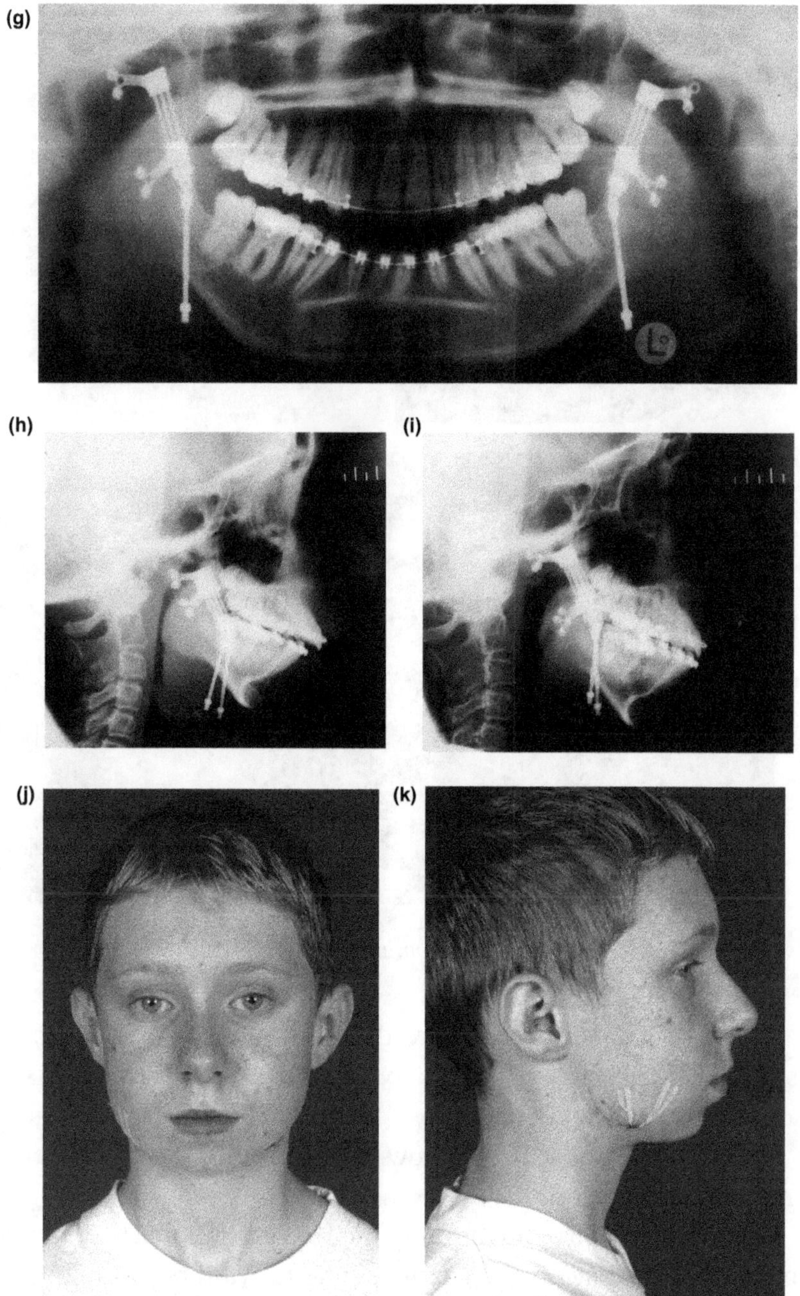

Figure 10.3 (*Continued*) **(g), (h), (i), (j), (k)**

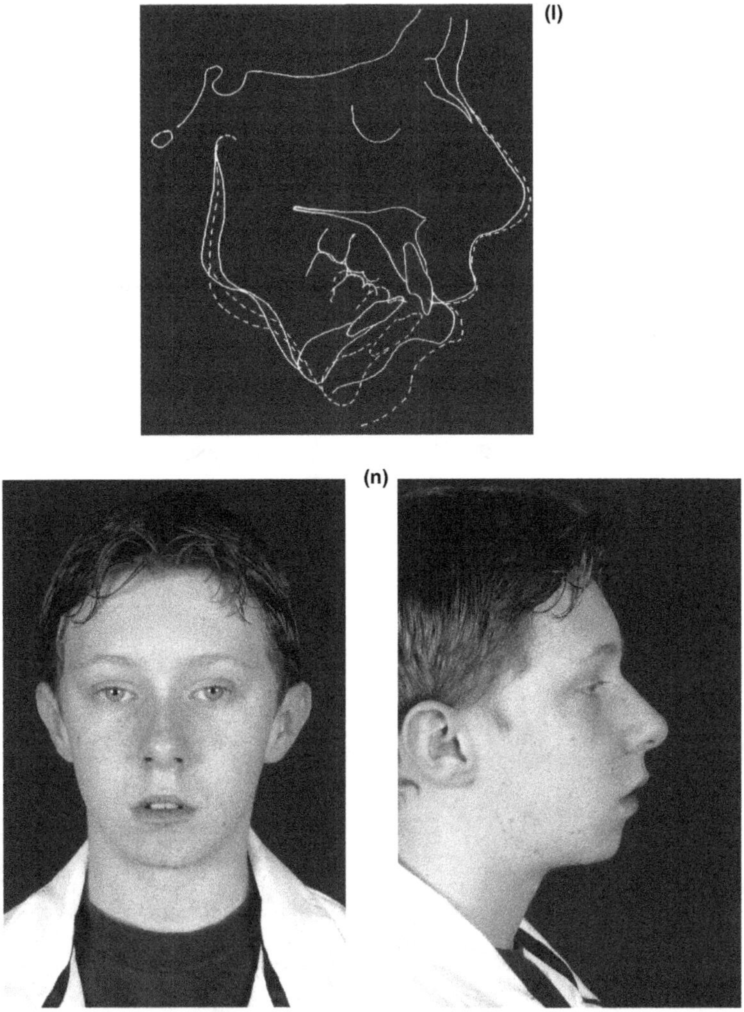

Figure 10.3 (*Continued*) **(l), (m), (n)**

The final pictures (Figures 10.3m and 10.3n) show the patient after an additional advancement genioplasty. It is essential to note that all short mandibles require a supplementary augmentation genioplasty after a lengthening procedure of the body.

Completion of osteodistraction followed by genioplasty to correct mandibular hypoplasia (Figures 10.3m and 10.3n).

2. Temporomandibular Joint (TMJ) Ankylosis (See also Chapter 13)

The established treatment of TMJ ankylosis is to divide the condylar fusion at the base of skull, create an arthroplasty with a costochondral graft as a growth centre and a temporalis myofascial interpositional flap, as a "meniscus". Bilateral coronoidotomies or coronoidectomies act as temporalis myotomies to release the restraining muscle contractures. However distraction osteogenesis has the potential to make up the growth deficiency and provide the lost ramus height and mandibular length in a more predictable way.

This patient (Figures 10.4a and 10.4b) presented with ankylosis of the right temporomandibular joint present since childhood and presumed to be due to middle ear infection. She had an intercisal opening of only 5 mm. The ankylosed right side showed the characteristic straight contour with reduced dimensions compared to the contralateral side with its distorted deviation towards the ankylosis.

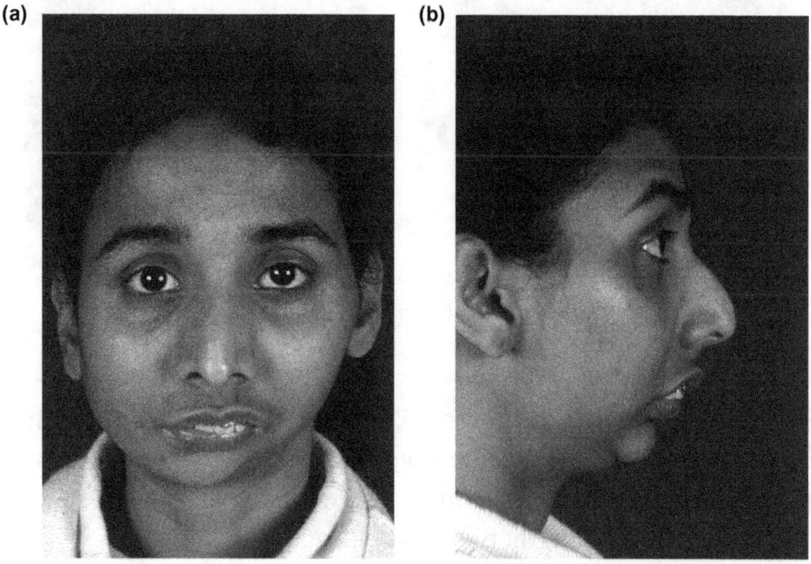

Figure 10.4 (a), (b)

There was a complete cross bite of the buccal teeth on the non ankylosed side, and with limited opening it was not possible to place a complete orthodontic appliance.

Figure 10.4a shows the paradoxical straight side of the mandible with the ankylosed joint and 10.4b shows the deviated normal left mandible.

Figures 10.4c and 10.4d with incomplete arch wire due to limited access.

Figure 10.4d also shows the limited access.

The inverted mushroom-like ankylosed condyle may be seen on the OPG (Figure 10.4e).

The axial CT scan of the base of skull shows the dense hyperostosis of the condyle-skull base fusion (Figures 10.4e and 10.4f).

(c)

(d)

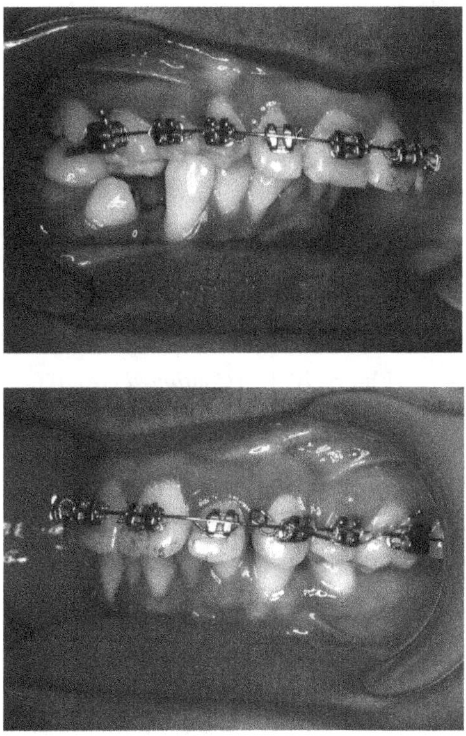

Figure 10.4 (*Continued*) **(c), (d)**

(e)

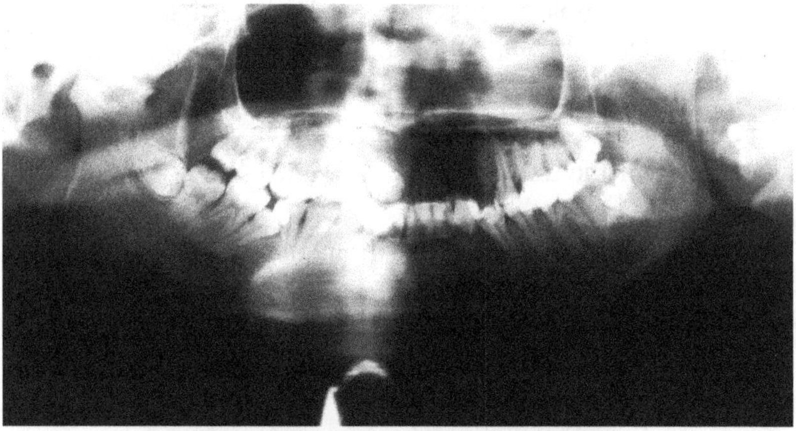

(f)

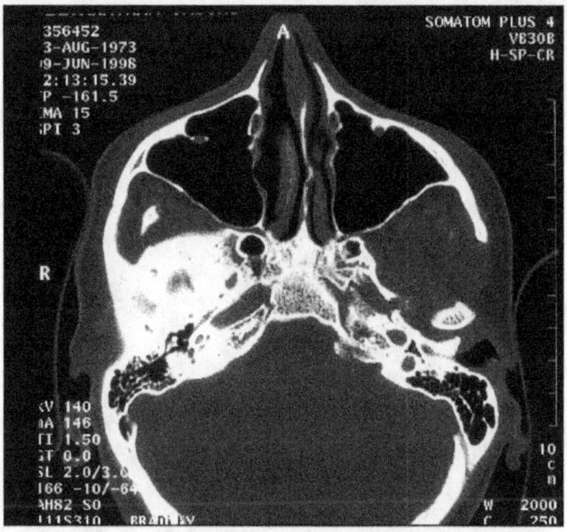

Figure 10.4 (*Continued*) **(e), (f)**

The degree of hypoplasia of the right mandible is best appreciated on the views of the 3-dimensional CT scan (Figures 10.4g and 10.4h).

Management. A simple osteotomy was first performed at the right angle of the mandible preserving the inferior dental bundle. Because of the limited opening, access required an extraoral approach and the impacted third molar was removed at the same time. The vector chosen was parallel to the lower border and a

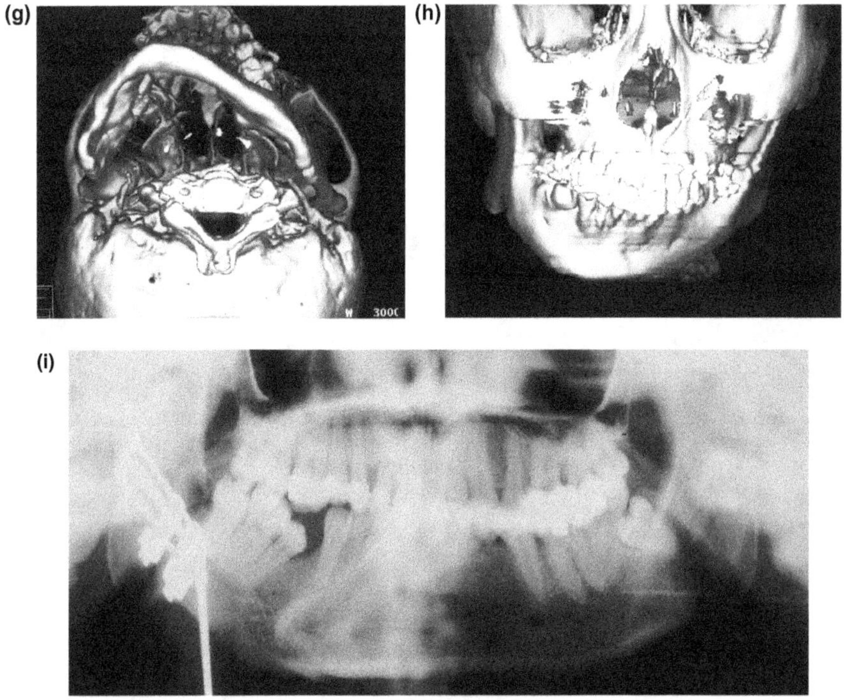

Figure 10.4 (*Continued*) (**g**), (**h**), (**i**)

15 mm distractor (Liebinger & Co.) was activated after a latent period of 5 days (Figure 10.4i).

The OPG (Figure 10.4i) shows the closed first distractor bridging the right angle osteotomy.

The OPG (Figure 10.4j) shows the open distractor which provided an interincisal opening of 20 mm and enabled access for orthodontic treatment.

Interincisal opening after the unilateral right sided distraction provided access to correct the occlusion (Figures 10.4k and 10.4l).

It was now possible to place an orthodontic appliance on the lower teeth as the buccal segment on the left side was no longer in cross bite.

Figures 10.4m and 10.4n show the moderate improvement after the first right sided distraction in facial symmetry and mandibular projection. The distractor can be seen to be *in situ*.

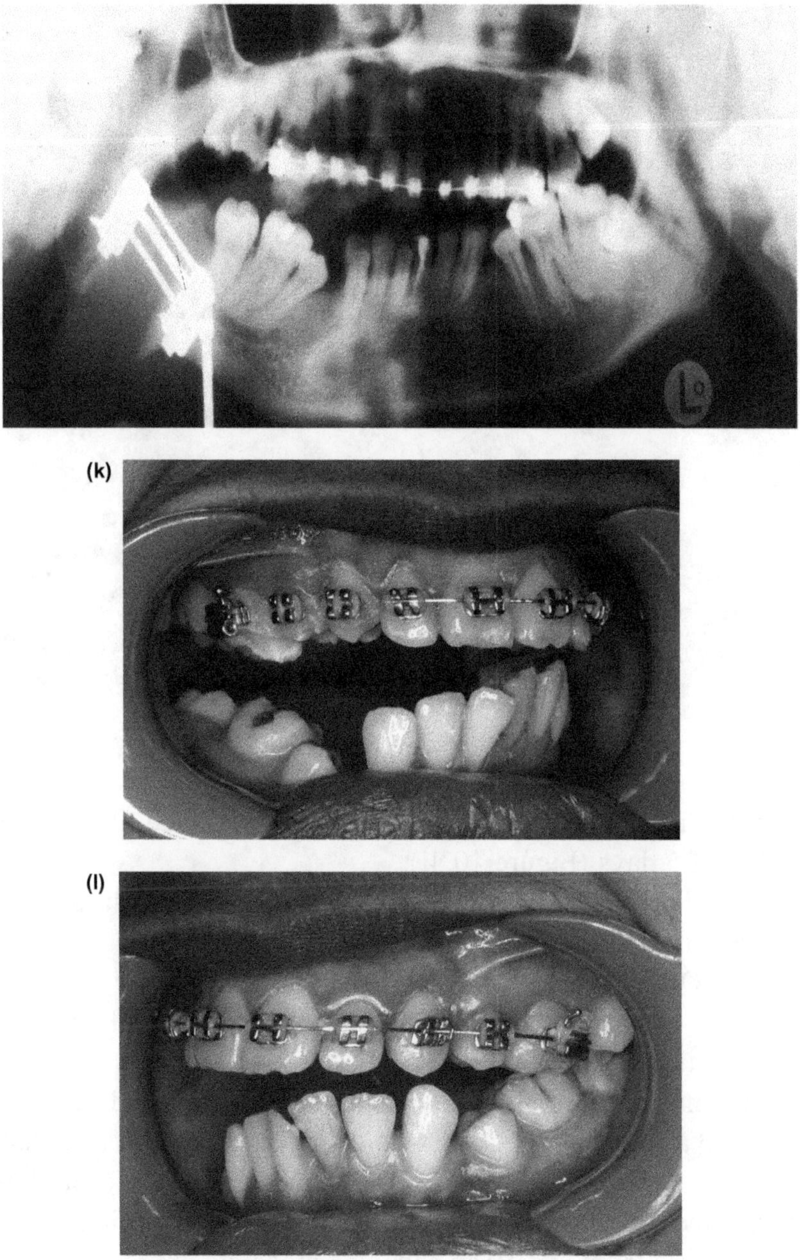

Figure 10.4 (*Continued*) **(j), (k), (l)**

A second phase of distraction used bilateral internal distractors and was carried out 3 months later to correct the marked Class II relationship.

It was now possible to place the second phase distractors from an intraoral route. The distractor on the right hand side was placed with a vector parallel to the lower border of the mandible, and the left hand distractor was placed with an oblique vector to increase mandibular height and take the posterior teeth out of premature contact. Distraction was continued for 15 days bilaterally at a rate of 1 mm per day following the latent period.

Figures 10.4o and 10.4p show the OPGs before and after the second distraction with separation of the distractor arms.

At the end of this period, the patient had an interincisal opening of 22 mm and an overcorrected edge to edge incisor occlusion to accommodate relapse as seen in Figures 10.4q and 10.4r. The final post-orthodontic views are Figures 10.4s and 10.4t.

(m) (n)

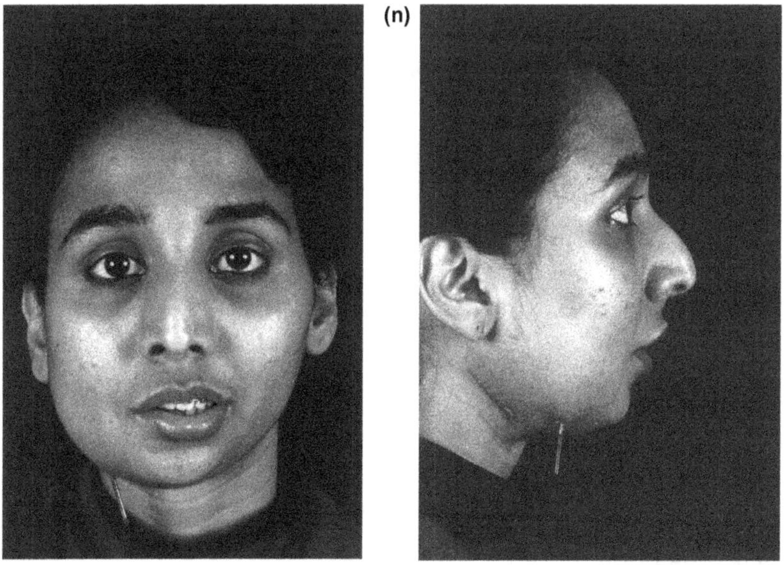

Figure 10.4 (*Continued*) **(m)**, **(n)**

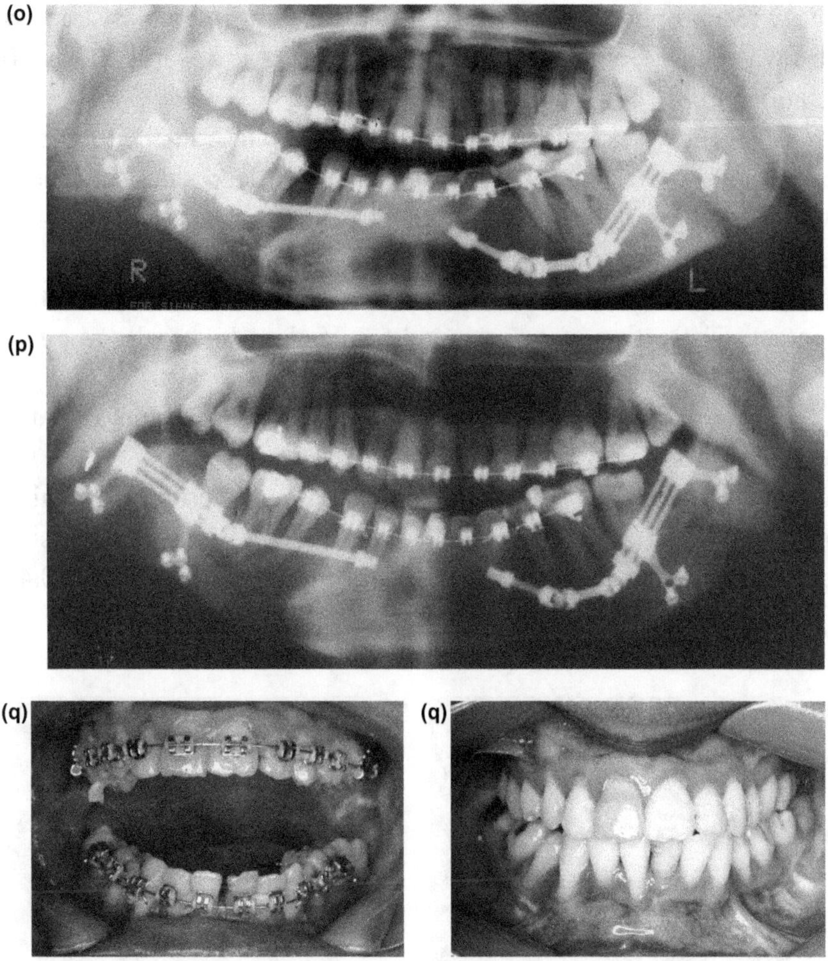

Figure 10.4 (*Continued*) **(o), (p), (q), (r)**

Figures 10.4q and 10.4r show a 22 mm opening and an aesthetic and functional occlusion.

Figures 10.4s and 10.4t show the skeletal symmetry and mandibular projection.

(s) (t)

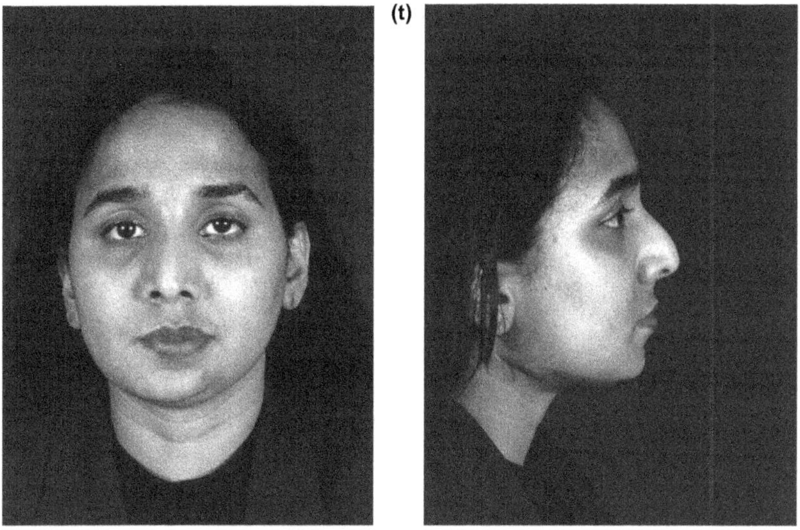

Figure 10.4 *(Continued)* **(s), (t)**

Summary and Conclusion

Ankylosis of the temporomandibular joint is the occasional outcome of joint damage combined with idiopathic bone biology and is discussed in Chapter 13. Gap arthroplasty is often unsatisfactory but improved with excision of the ankylosis bone mass to be replaced by a costochondral graft as a growth centre. Coronoidotomy releases the long standing muscle contracture to increase the interincisal opeing.

The alternative regimen to overcome the muscle and integument contracture is an inverted L ramus osteotomy with osteodistraction. In this case the affected asymmetrical right mandible was corrected by a ramus osteotomy and distraction which enabled an opening of 20 mm and orthodontic appliance fixation.

Bilateral internal distractors were then applied 3 months later to correct the marked Class II incisor relationship and profile.

The result was a sustained pseudoarthrosis at the second osteotomy sites with an inter-incisal opening of 22 mm and an excellent occlusion and profile.

3. Maxillary Hypoplasia Due to Cleft Surgery

Early surgery for the repair of the cleft palate will damage the mid face growth potential giving rise to marked hypoplasia which with scarring of the palatal muco-periosteum renders conventional surgical advancement difficult and subject to relapse. Distraction osteogenesis requires a limited osteotomy and the gradual controlled traction can overcome the restraint of the scar tissue.

This patient had a severe maxillary hypoplasia secondary to a cleft lip and palate deformity, with nasal hypoplasia due to absence of much of the septum. There was also mild mandibular elongation.

Dental radiographs confirmed the absence of the left upper central and lateral incisors. As orthodontic extractions were necessary in

(a) (b)

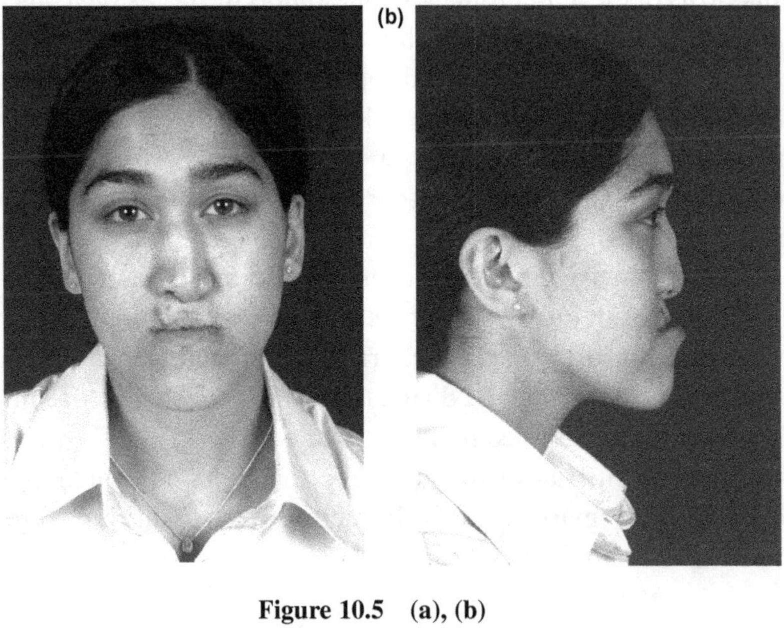

Figure 10.5 (a), (b)

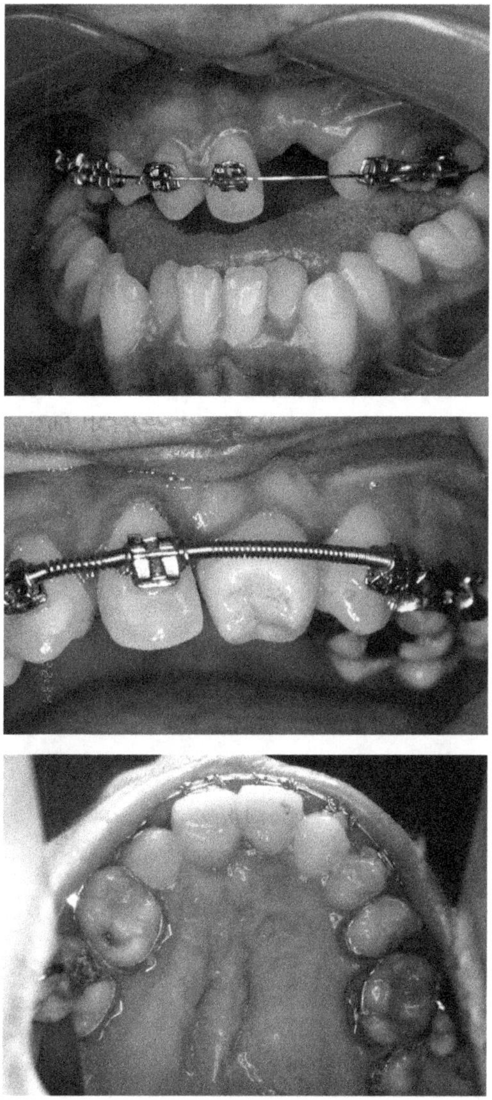

(c)

(d)

(e)

Figure 10.5 (*Continued*) **(c), (d), (e)**

the lower arch one of the lower second premolars was transplanted into the upper left central incisor alveolar region. Figures 10.5c, 10.5d and 10.5e show the presurgical orthodontics, and the transplanted premolar contoured to simulate a central incisor the upper left/1.

(f)

(g)

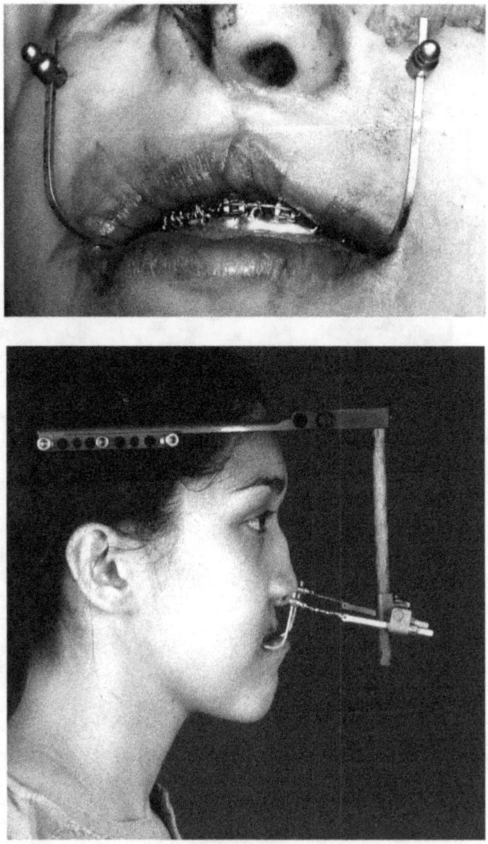

Figure 10.5 (*Continued*) **(f), (g)**

A Le Fort I osteotomy was then carried out with mobilisation, and an external halo distraction system was placed (Figures 10.5f and 10.5g) (Martin MLS/Red System). Following a latent period of 5 days, maxillary distraction was commenced at the rate of 1 mm a day and was continued for 20 days.

The halo frame was removed after a consolidation period of 6 weeks. At the time of removal sound bone regeneration at the osteotomy site was noted (Figure 10.5h).

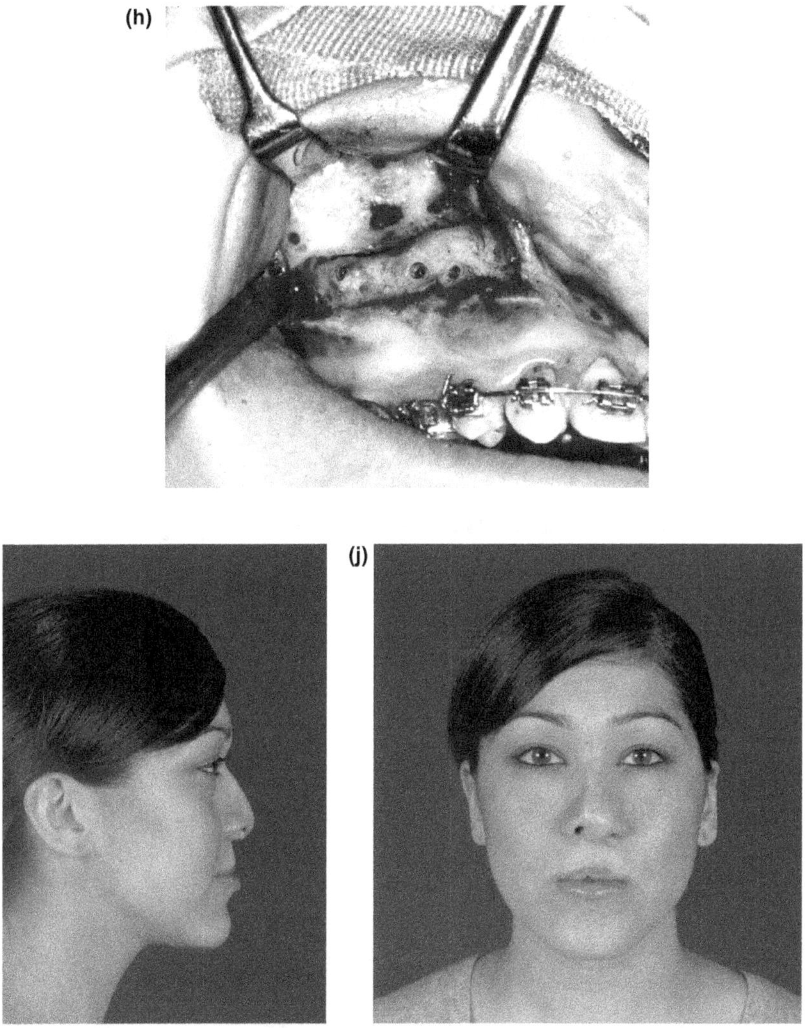

Figure 10.5 (*Continued*) **(h), (i), (j)**

These clinical photographs demonstrate the occlusion, full face and profile at the end of distraction (Figures 10.5i to 10.5l).

The patient subsequently had a rhinoplasty and a 5 mm mandibular pushback 9 months after the end of maxillary distraction.

(k)

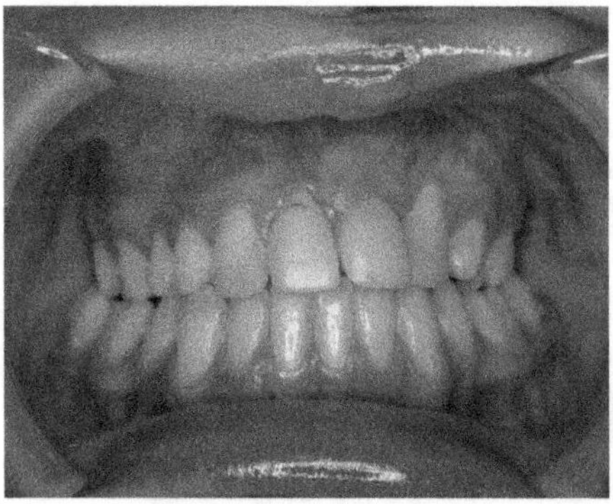

(l)

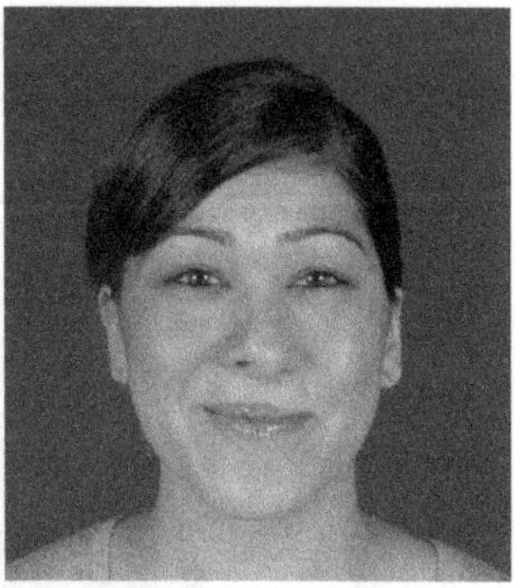

Figure 10.5 (*Continued*) **(k), (l)**

4. Distraction for Dento-Alveolar Atrophy

Augmentation of the alveolus by onlay grafting is often difficult. It will provide increased width but not height, and in very atrophic cases it is subject to failure due to mucosal dehiscence leading to the loss of the graft material.

The atrophic mandible which had an intolerable sharp residual lower alveolar ridge (Figure 10.6a).

(a)

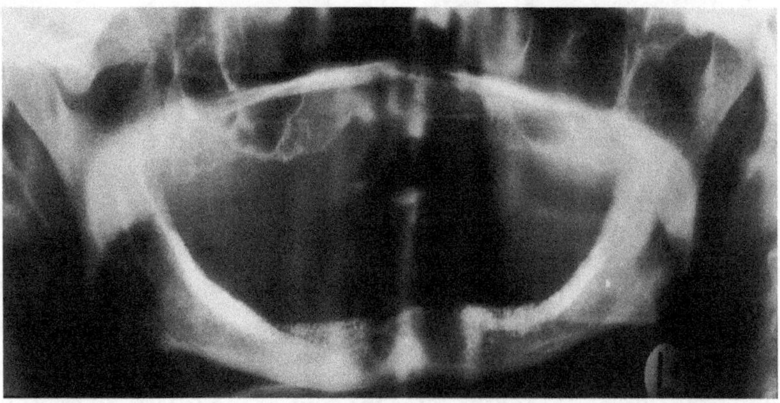

Figure 10.6 **(a)**

(b)

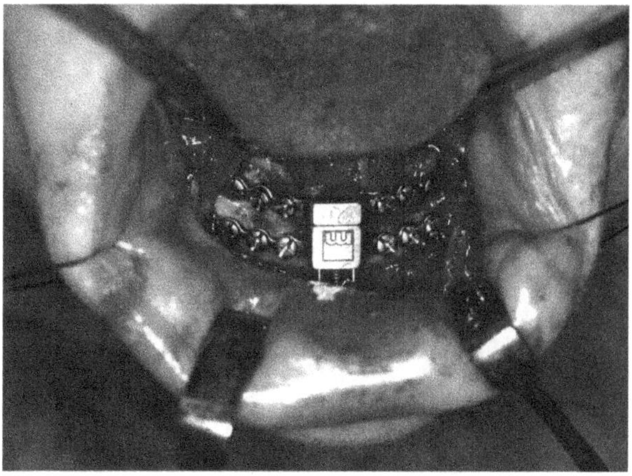

Figure 10.6 (*Continued*) (**b**)

Distractor with its unopened flanges attached to the horizontal osteotomised section of alveolar ridge and basal bone (Figure 10.6b).

The OPG shows the alveolar osteotomy and the distractor in position (Figure 10.6c).

The opened distractor exposed with intervening osteoid (Figure 10.6d).

(c)

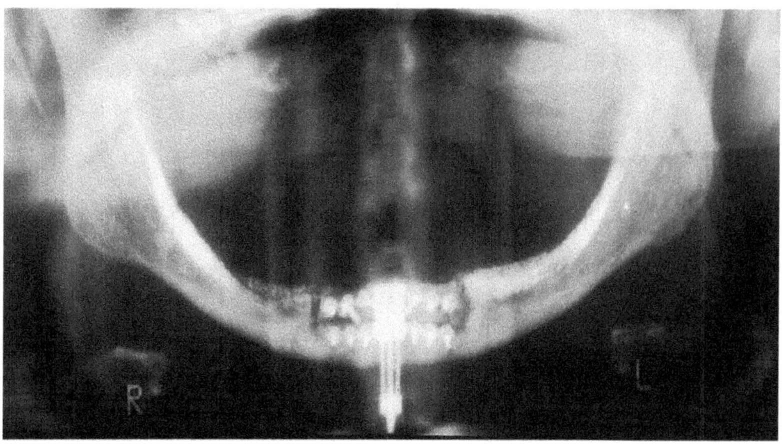

Figure 10.6 (*Continued*) (**c**)

(d)

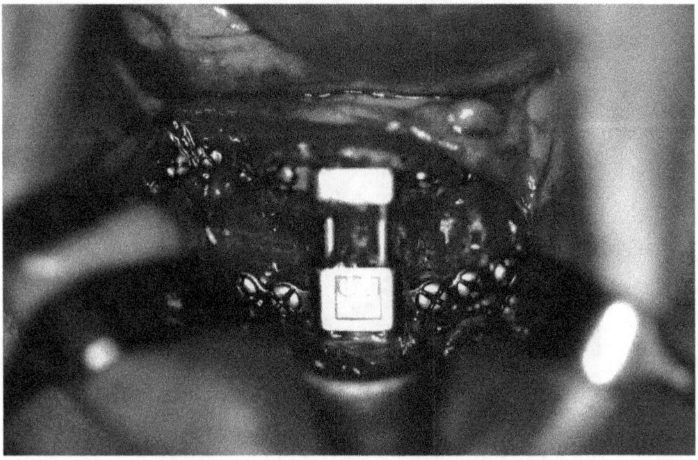

Figure 10.6 (*Continued*) **(d)**

(e)

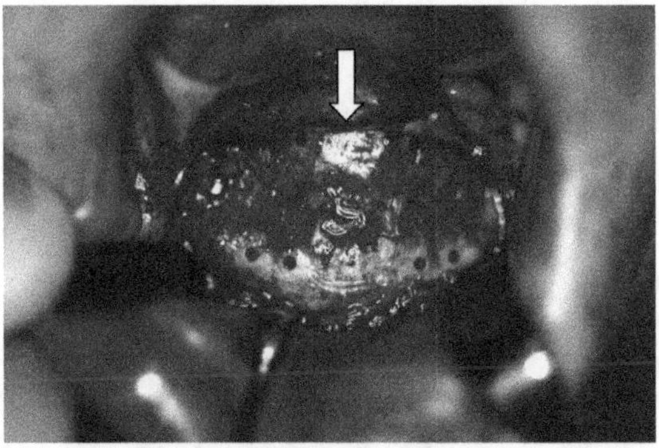

Figure 10.6 (*Continued*) **(e)**

The arrow in Figure 10.6e shows the increased height and width of the distracted alveolus knife edge ridge.

Figure 10.6f shows an OPG of the distracted area and Figure 10.6g the insertion of three implants to support and stabilise the lower denture.

Figure 10.6h shows a stable pain free implant retained denture in place.

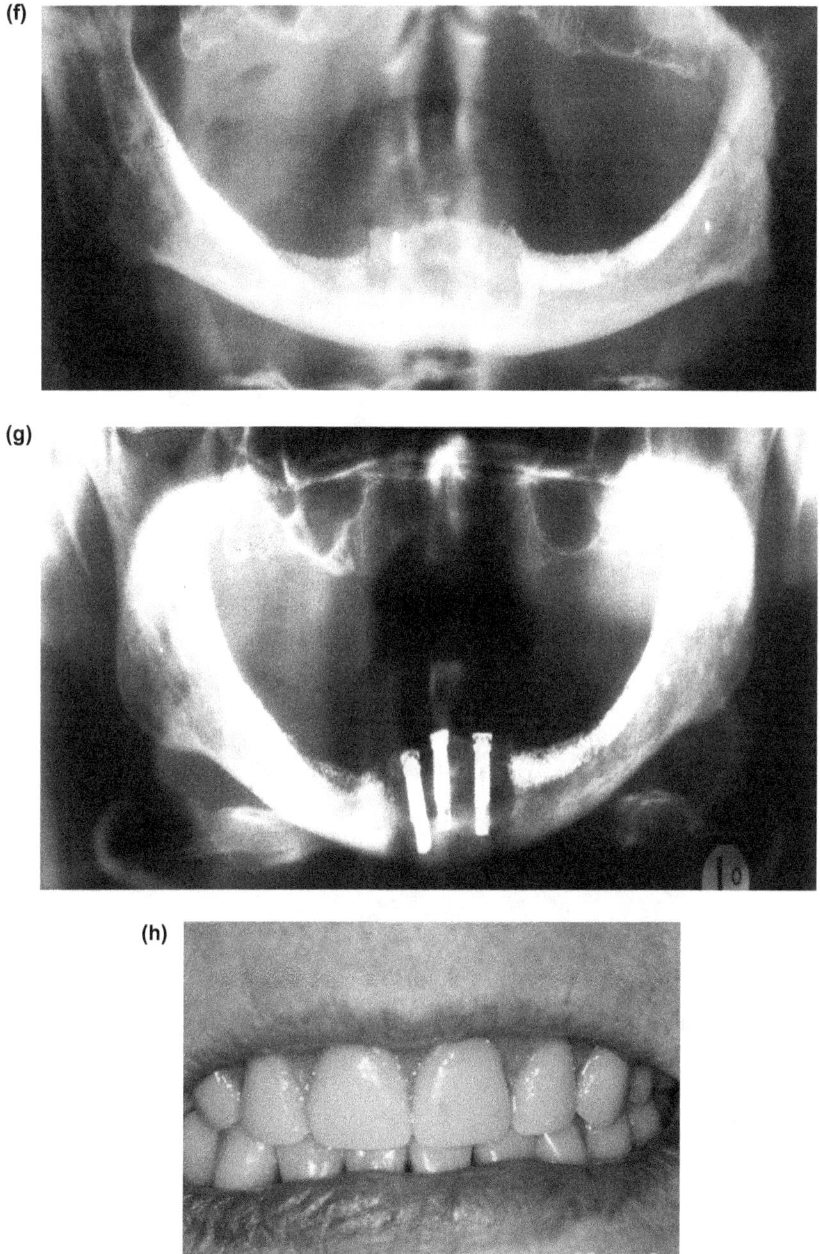

Figure 10.6 (*Continued*) **(f), (g), (h)**

5. Restoration of a Maxillofacial Trauma Defect

A 21-year-man old suffered, a comminuted Le Fort 1 maxillary fracture with the loss of alveolar bone and avulsion of the upper 21/1 incisors as the result of a road traffic accident (Figures 10.7a and 10.7b).

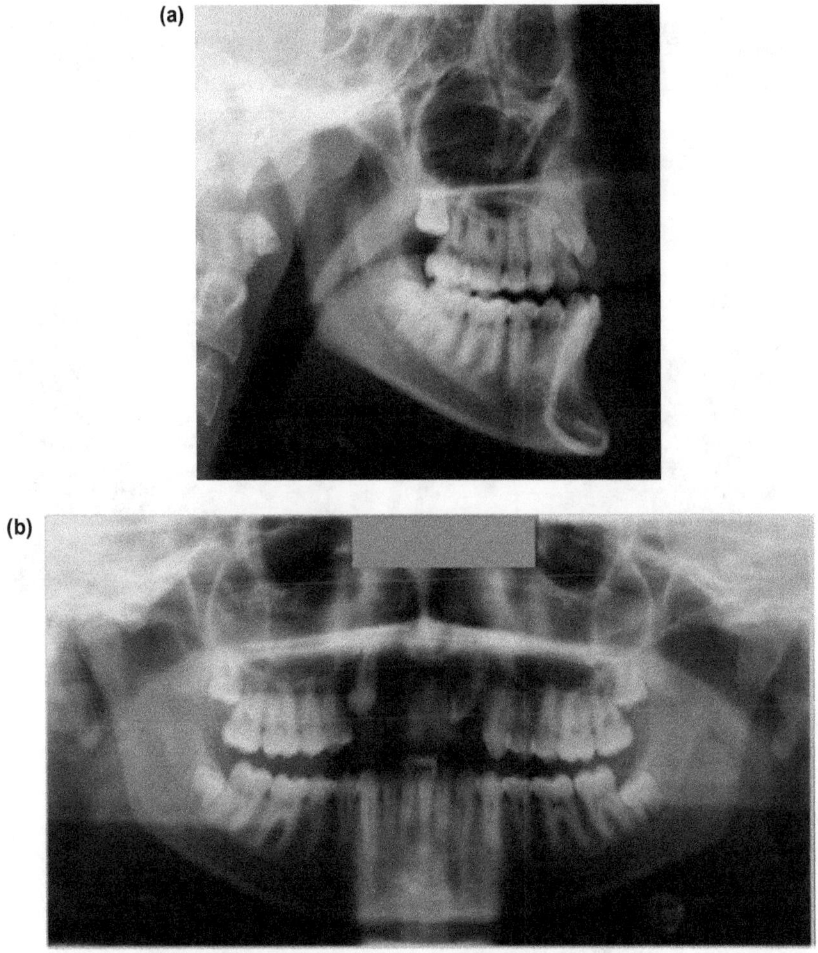

Figure 10.7 (a), (b)

Treatment plan

i. Reduce and fix the fractured maxilla.
ii. Restore the deficient alveolus by internal distraction.
iii. Insert implants to support a bridge.

The mid face impaction was corrected with a Le Fort 1 advancement. The displaced upper right canine was removed and subsequently the mobile upper left lateral incisor was also extracted (Figure 10.7c).

(c)

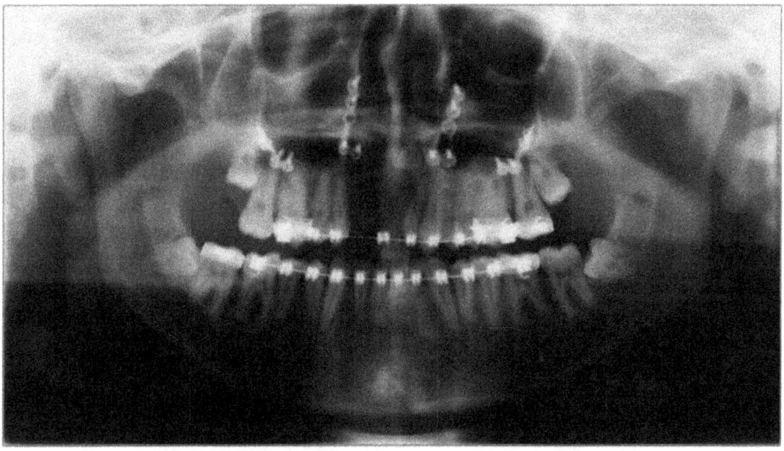

Figure 10.7 (*Continued*) **(c)**

Figure 10.7d shows the intraoral result of the Le Fort 1 reduction and internal fixation. The vertical alveolar loss left a deficiency of 8 mm of bone from the nasal floor.

Fine horizontal and vertical osteotomy cuts through the anterior alveolus enabled the insertion of a 2 cm vertical distractor (Figure 10.7e).

Figure 10.7f shows an arch wire bracketed to upper 54/345 to prevent palatal rotation of the distractor during the traction phase of 20 days.

(d)

(e)

(f)

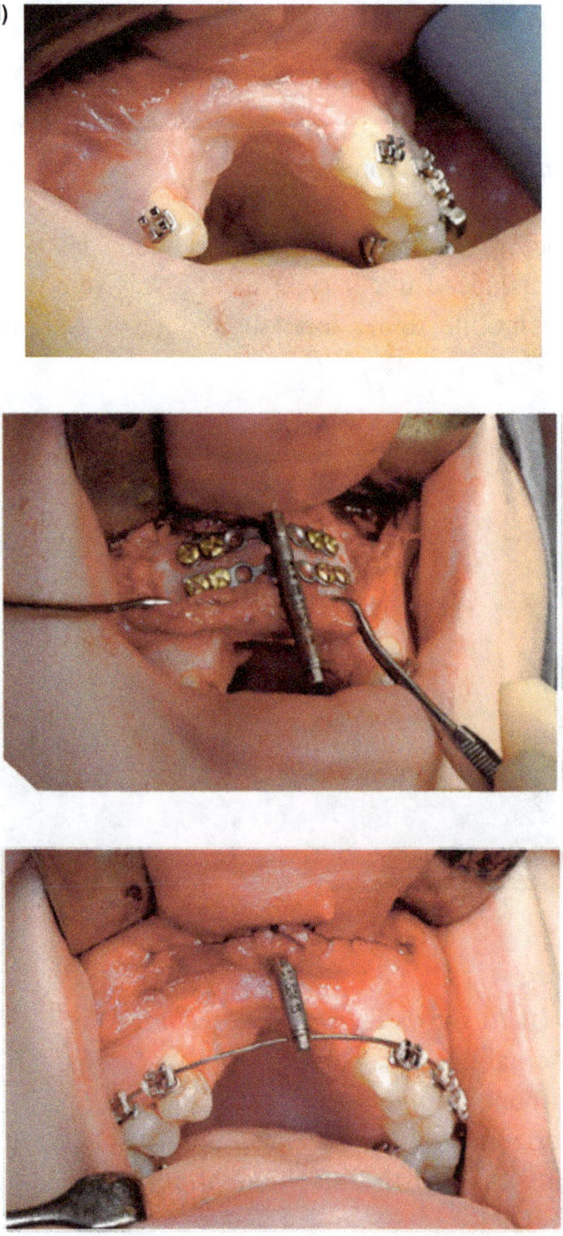

Figure 10.7 (*Continued*) **(d), (e), (f)**

(g)

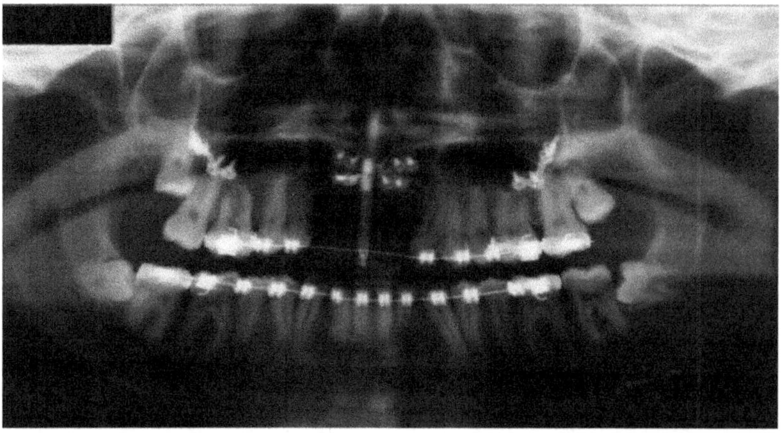

(h)

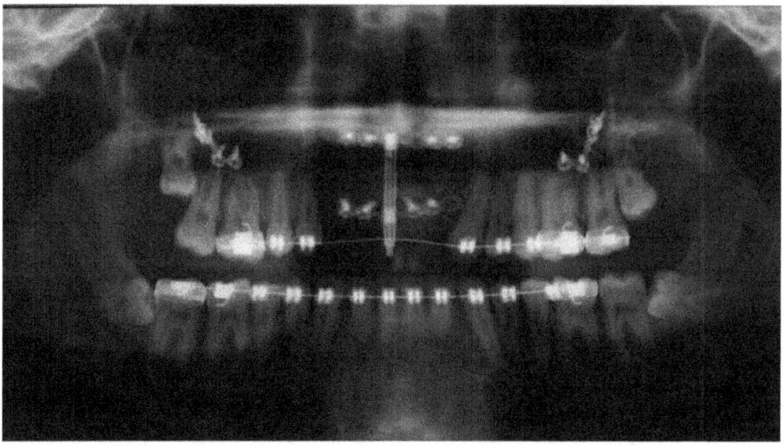

Figure 10.7 (*Continued*) **(g)**, **(h)**

Figure 10.7g OPG shows the pre-distraction and post-distraction (Figure 10.7h) position with separation of the flanges.

Figure 10.7i shows sutured mucosa covering the expanded ridge immediately after the distractor has been removed.

At the placement of the implants, a dehiscence in the buccal plates can be seen (Figure 10.7j) which was packed with bone chips shown in (Figure 10.7k).

(i)

(j)

(k)

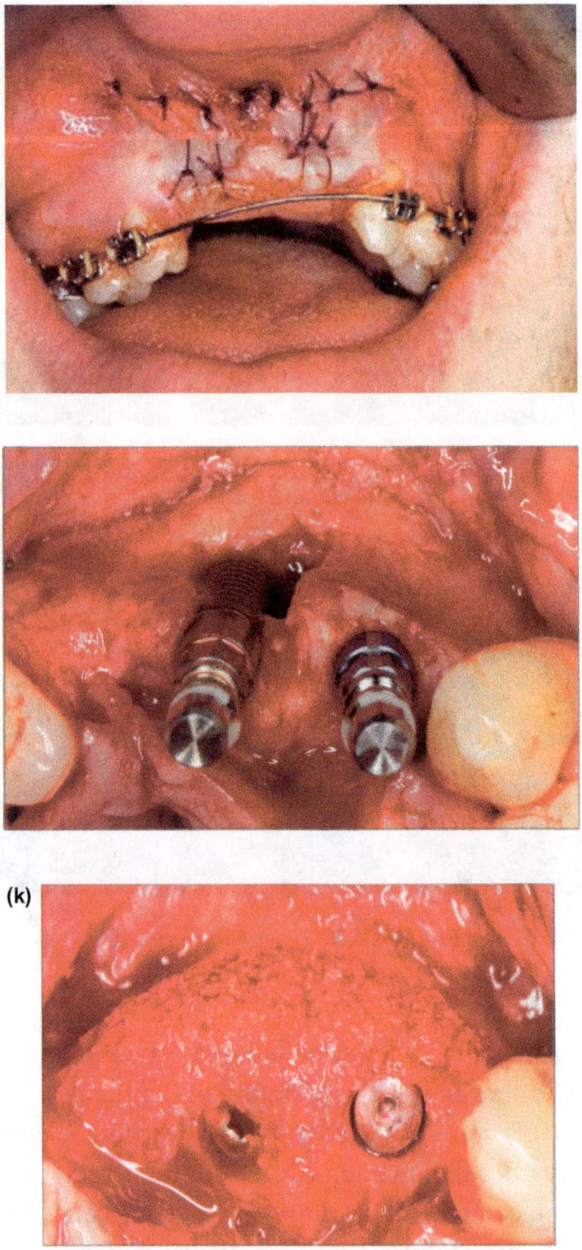

Figure 10.7 (*Continued*) **(i), (j), (k)**

Figure 10.7k shows the buccal plate dehiscence packed with bone chips, Figure 10.7l shows the healed augmented ridge, and Figure 10.7m the implant borne bridge. Figure 10.7n is the restored patient with bridge in place.

(l) (m) (n)

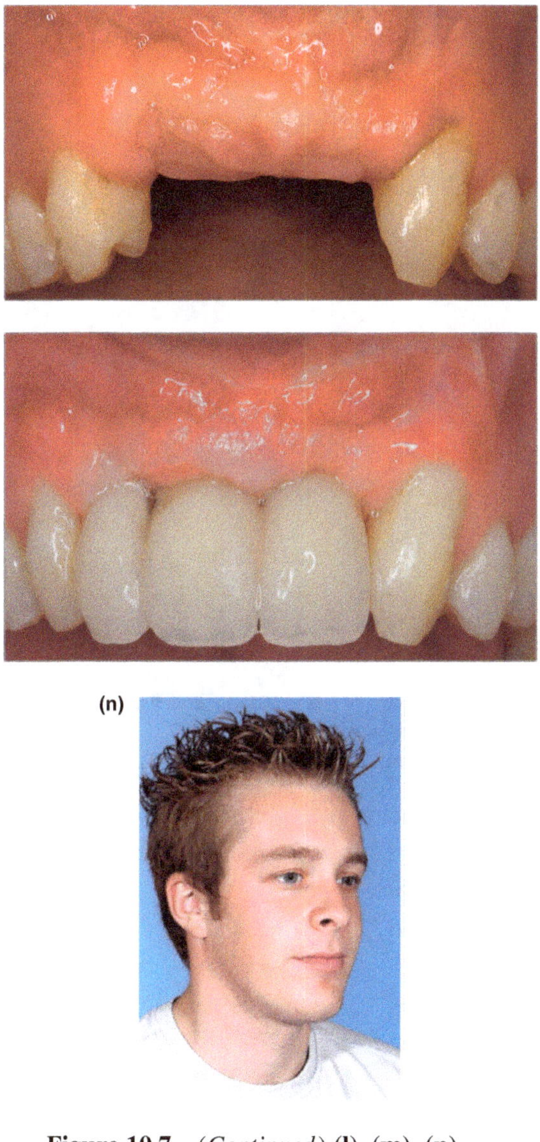

Figure 10.7 (*Continued*) **(l), (m), (n)**

Summary

Distraction osteogenesis can achieve multidimensional bone formation in situations where grafting is unsuitable or has failed. With improved mechanics the procedure will become more patient friendly and cost effective.

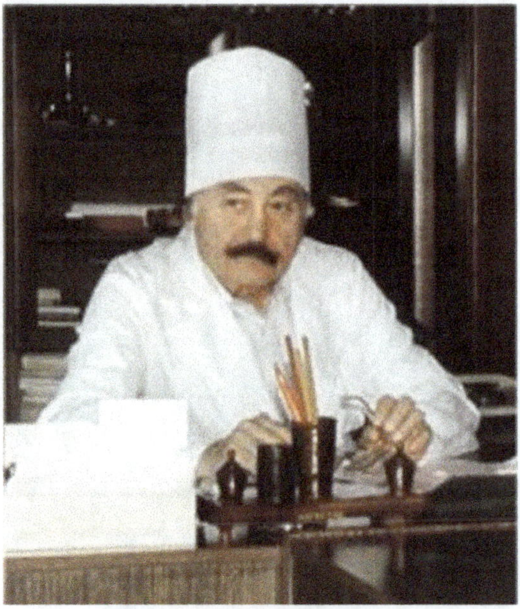

Figure 10.8. Gavril Abramovich Ilizarov: Founder of advanced distraction osteogenesis (1921–1992).

Chapter 11

The Surgical Correction of Common Deformities

Malcolm Harris

- ***Single Jaw Deformities***

  Mandibular prognathism
  Mandibular asymmetry
  Mandibular retrognathism
  The chin
  Mandibular incisor proclination
  Maxillary hypoplasia
  Nasomaxillary hypoplasia
  Malar-maxillary hypoplasia
  Maxillary prognathism

- ***Bimaxillary Deformities***

  Gross mandibular prognathism
  The deep overbite
  Bimaxillary proclination
  The long face
  The open bite (apertognathia)

The large tongue
The short face
Maxillary asymmetry

- Unfortunately, the diagnosis of a facial deformity does not always suggest an operative solution. There may be a choice of procedures or the complexity requires several simultaneous osteotomies. This chapter considers both single jaw and bimaxillary deformities. As will be seen, there is usually an overlap and what appears to be a major single jaw problem invariably requires a bimaxillary solution.
- It is also impossible to classify all cases under one treatment group. For instance, a patient with a long face may have an open bite. Both treatment sections in this chapter should therefore be consulted.
- Although it is possible to describe horizontal and vertical deformities separately, they are surgically interdependent, in that a vertical osteotomy will produce a horizontal change and *vice versa*.

Operative Timing

The choice of age for any orthognathic procedure can be difficult. The optimum age is when facial growth has finished. This is approximately 16 years for girls and 18 years for boys. Later maturation of the face can undo the benefit of a well-intentioned osteotomy. This is particularly true if the prognathic mandible is treated too early. The only exception is the rare unilateral condylar hyperplasia which may require ablation of the articular growth cartilage during adolescence to prevent a major degree of secondary deformity. As all young patients with jaw deformities require orthodontic treatment, this provides a period of scrutiny to monitor continued growth with study models and lateral skull radiographs, at yearly intervals. Wrist radiographs when considering abnormal facial growth and sequential technetium-99 m bone scans are unhelpful.

Presurgical orthodontic treatment not only simplifies the operative procedure but also improves the occlusal and profile outcome. However a decision must be made if surgery is to be the ultimate treatment of choice. The orthodontic decompensation for surgery for a jaw disproportion will be different from the pure orthodontic compensatory management to conceal the deformity, and will start later to reduce the period in appliance retention. Therefore, please read Chapter 4 (Orthodontic Preparation).

Single Jaw Deformities

Mandibular Prognathism

This is characterised by elongation of the mandible producing a negative overjet, with compensatory retroclination of the lower incisors, and proclination of the upper incisors. Both the dentition and jaws show a marked Class III relationship. Some patients also have an increased lower facial height which is automatically reduced when the mandible is displaced backwards, up an inclined occlusal plane (Figure 11.1).

Beware of seeing all negative overjets as cases of mandibular prognathism. With a mild mandibular protrusion in a man, the preferred aesthetic solution is often a forward movement of the maxilla, leaving a "strong chin". This profile correction may be predicted by padding out the upper lip with cotton wool or wax. The same cephalometric values in a female usually require a mandibular setback for aesthetic harmony. The occlusal correction is identical in both cases.

Most prognathous mandibles are associated with a degree of maxillary retrognathism with the need for a bimaxillary correction. This becomes clear after presurgical orthodontics with incisor decompensation (see below, Bimaxillary Deformities).

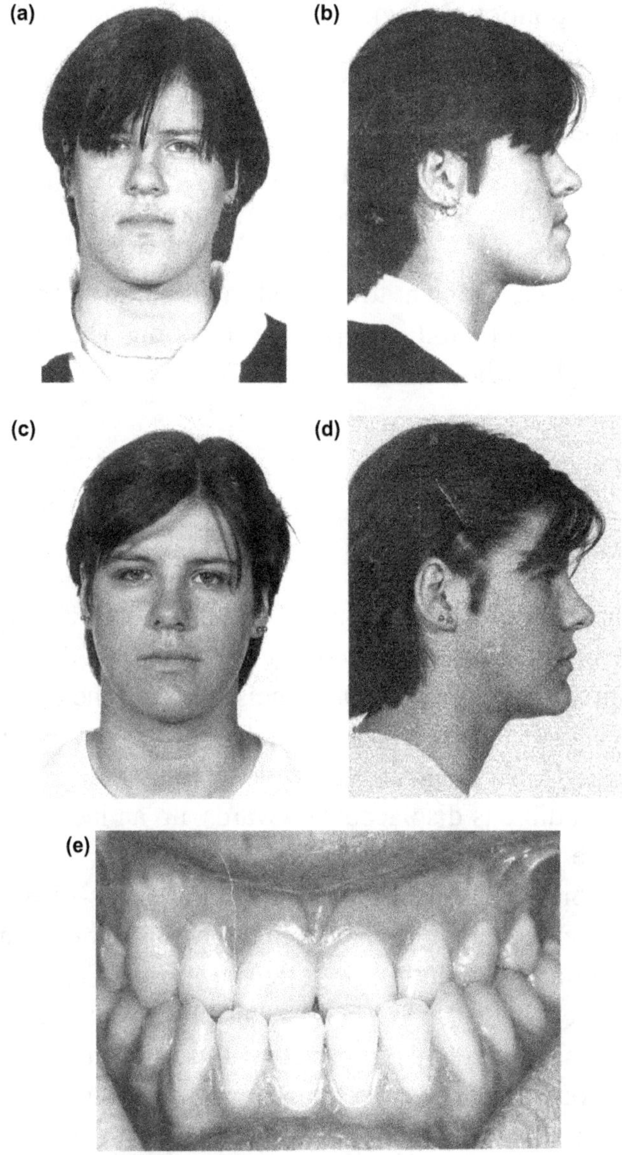

Figure 11.1 Mandibular prognathism requiring moderate orthodontic decompensation of the incisors followed by a sagittal split pushback. **(a)**, **(b)** and **(e)** Preoperative. **(c)**, **(d)** and **(f)** Postoperative.

(f)

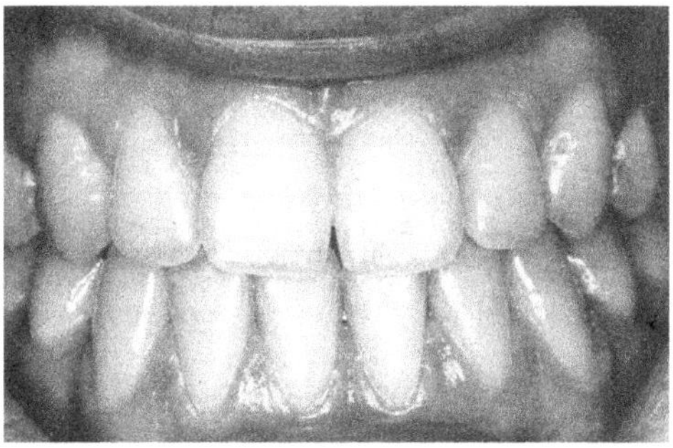

Figure 11.1 (*Continued*)

Treatment

Presurgical orthodontics will be required to correct arch size discrepancy, overcrowding and to decompensate the incisors. Posterior displacement of the mandible can be achieved by a:

1. sagittal split osteotomy,
   and less commonly,
2. oblique subcondylar (subsigmoid) osteotomy
   a) extraoral,
   b) intraoral (buccal approach), and
   c) intraoral (medial approach).

Mandibular Asymmetry (Unilateral Hyperplasia and Hypoplasia of the Mandible)

Introduction

There are two distinct types of asymmetrical overgrowth, but hybrid forms are occasionally found with both abnormalities merged on one side or even one of each deformity on opposite sides. Each deformity is frequently attributed to condylar hyperplasia. However, in both types the increased dimension arises beyond the accepted localised area of condylar growth.

Unilateral hypoplasias will be treated in the same manner as mandibular retrognathism, except when part of a hemifacial microsomia deformity, which will require additional attention to the difficult problem of soft tissue deficiency.

Beware of diagnosing asymmetry where a malocclusion is really causing a unilateral displacement of the mandible on closure.

Hemimandibular Elongation

This asymmetry presents with an increased ascending ramus width and length of the body on the affected side, with deviation of the dental and jaw midline to the contralateral side and a crossbite (Figure 11.2). The condylar head may be minimally enlarged compared with the normal side but the neck is elongated. The occlusal plane is undisturbed. Surgical correction should be delayed until the end of adolescent growth particualrly as some cases "creep on" to the end of the second decade.

Treatment

Presurgical Orthodontics

Insufficient maxillary intercanine width to accommodate the lower arch is not uncommon. Surgery should therefore be preceded by maxillary expansion. Where there is a gross discrepancy between the arches the maxillary arch may be expanded with a quadhelix appliance, which increases the width from behind forwards over a period of three to five months. However in such cases, tipping of the molars may relapse postoperatively and produce an anterior open bite. For this reason with large discrepancies surgical expansion of the maxilla may be the treatment of choice or distraction osteogenesis with a bone borne expansion appliance.

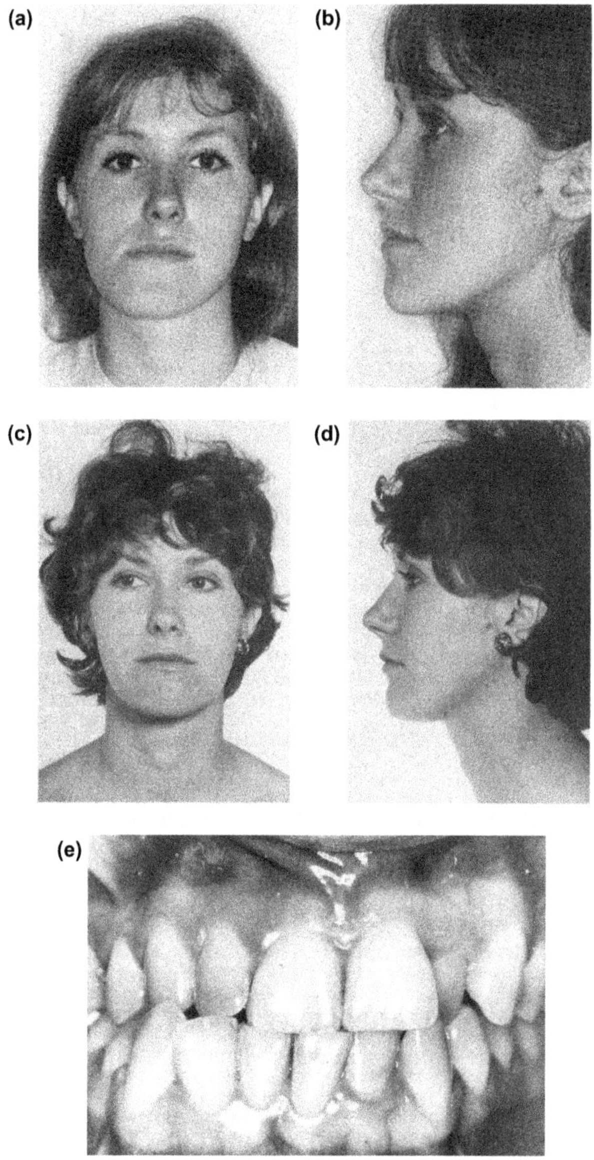

Figure 11.2 Left hemi-mandibular elongation with prognathism and deviation of the midline to the right, corrected by a bilateral sagittal split osteotomy. (**a**), (**b**) and (**e**) Preoperative. (**c**), (**d**) and (**f**) Postoperative.

(f)

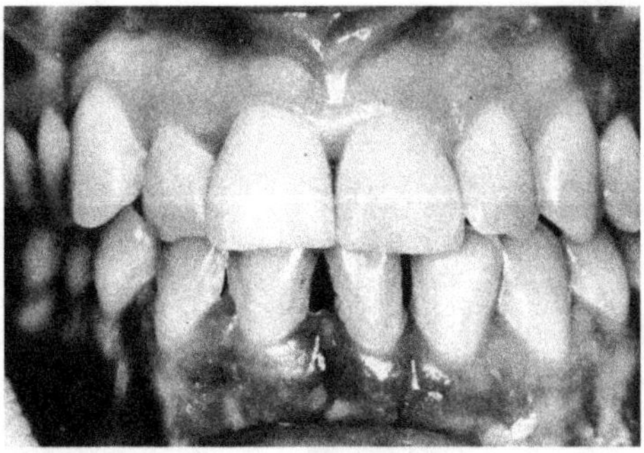

Figure 11.2 (*Continued*)

Surgery

Asymmetry, with or without prognathism, can be corrected by a bilateral ramus osteotomy, such as the sagittal split, which shortens the affected side and allows rotation at the contralateral angle.

Although correction of the bony deformity produces a marked improvement in appearance by eliminating both the unilateral deviation and prognathism, there is often a persistent asymmetry of the face in movement.

Recurrent growth creates a difficult decision and will require a careful high condylar shave preserving the meniscus.

Hemimandibular Hyperplasia

This type of mandibular asymmetry often starts dramatically with the pubertal growth spurt, although it is detectable earlier. Other cases appear to develop insidiously during adolescence. Another enigma is the principal site of overgrowth. Although often considered to be a condylar hyperplasia, there is, in addition to the considerably enlarged condylar head and ascending ramus, a convex downward growth of the lower border of the mandibular body which extends as far forward as the midline. Initially this creates an ipsilateral lateral open bite followed by secondary maxillary

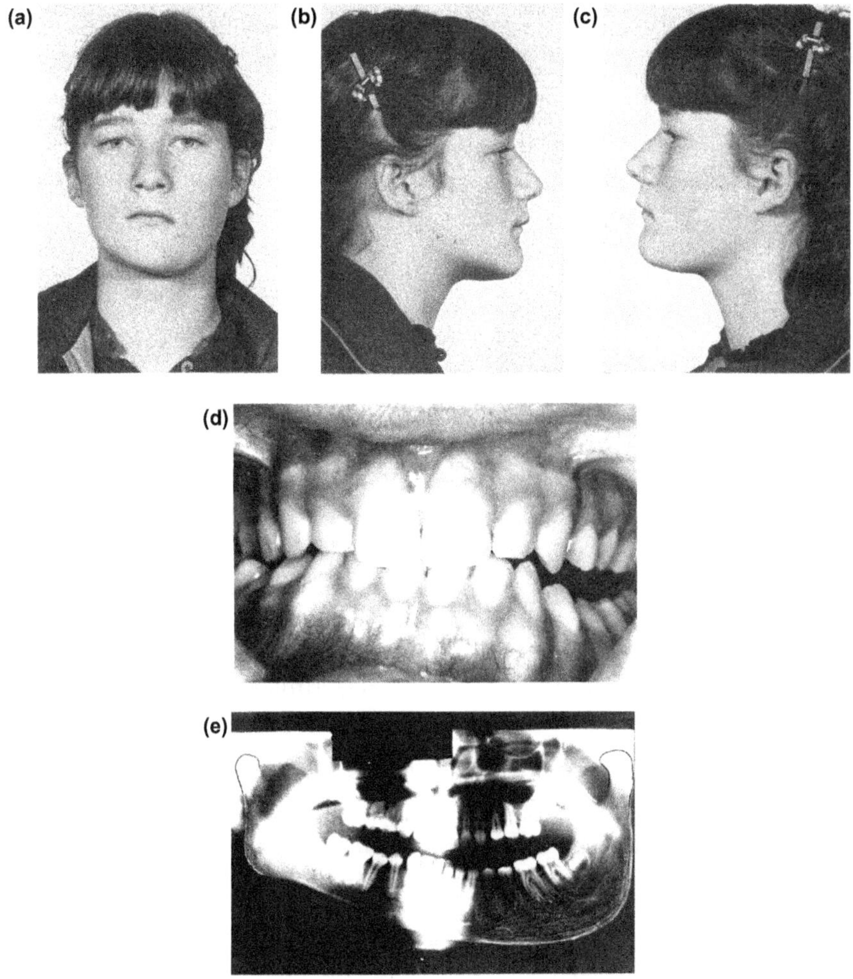

Figure 11.3 (**a**) to (**e**) This left hemi-mandibular hyperplasia dramatically occurred over 6 months at the onset of puberty. There is no horizontal displacement of the lower midline despite the increase in vertical dimensions producing a lateral open bite.

alveolar growth. When all mandibular growth is complete, there is an overall hemimandibular hyperplasia and an occlusal cant down to the affected side but no deviation of the midline (Figure 11.3). The inferior dental neurovascular bundle is carried downwards with this growth. This seems to be associated with hyperplasia of the associated mylohyoid muscle in the same way as masseteric hyperplasia produces an enlarged square gonial angle. Excess growth appears to cease in most cases at the end of puberty. It is interesting to see the ipsilateral antral floor is also lower due to remodelling following the alveolar downgrowth.

Treatment

Early

When seen early, the aim of surgery is to reduce ramus height before the secondary alveolar growth creates a permanent asymmetry with an oblique cant of the occlusal plane. It is tempting to remove part or all of the condyle to ablate the growth centre, i.e. a partial condylectomy. However, not only does the excess growth take place throughout the hemimandible beyond the influence of the condylar growth area, but it has usually finished by the time the deformity is diagnosed. Therefore, at this stage, surgical damage to the joint mechanism would seem unwarranted. A simple approach is a subsigmoid osteotomy, either intraorally or extraorally, to bring the teeth into occlusion. Later the increased depth of the body of the mandible can be corrected with trimming of the lower border and this can be done extraorally through a skin crease incision (see below) or if access permits, intraorally. However the displaced neurovascular bundle must be protected.

Late

Where compensatory alveolar growth has taken place, bringing the separated buccal segment teeth into occlusion, the most economical correction is simply reducing the lower border convexity. This improves the facial appearance and corrects the obliquity of the mouth, but not the occlusal plane (Figure 11.4). However, if desired,

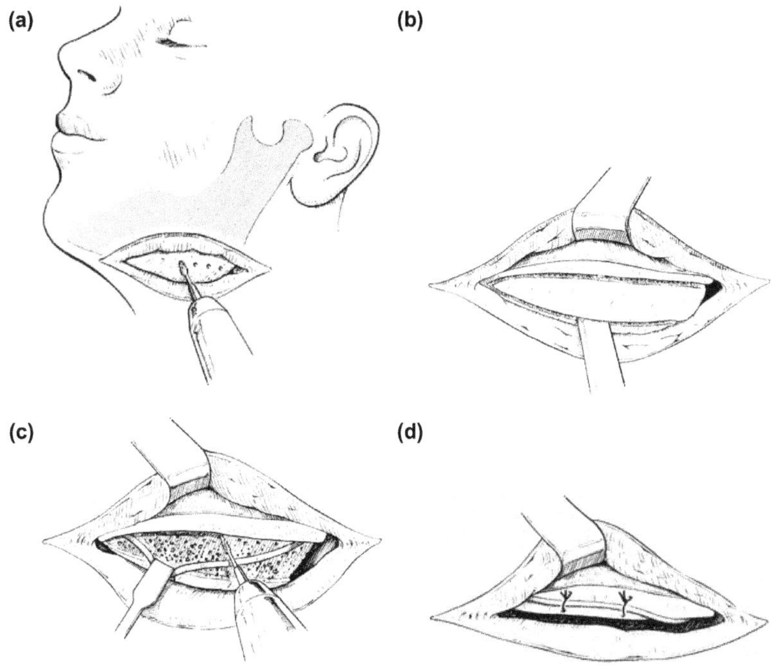

Figure 11.4 Lower border cortical split to expose and preserve the neurovascular bundle prior to trimming the excess depth of mandible. (**a**) The outer cortical plate is removed. (**b**) If the neurovascular bundle is found within the hyperplastic lower border, it is dissected from its canal and retracted prior to resection of the inner cortical plate (**c**) and (**d**). An adult left-sided hemimandibular hyperplasia where the lateral open bite has closed spontaneously leaving an ipsilateral downward slope of the occlusal plane. The external deformity has been corrected by trimming the lower border of the mandible through an external approach. (**e**) and (**f**) Preoperative. (**g**) to (**i**) Postoperative.

the downward tilt of the occlusal plane can be corrected with a bimaxillary procedure elevating the maxilla with a Le Fort I osteotomy (see Maxillary Asymmetry) and the mandible must then be adjusted to this horizontal occlusal plane, either by a sagittal split or subcondylar osteotomy. Finally, the convex lower border will still need to be trimmed. This is sometimes possible intraorally but is more easily achieved in conjunction with an external subcondylar osteotomy through the same skin incision.

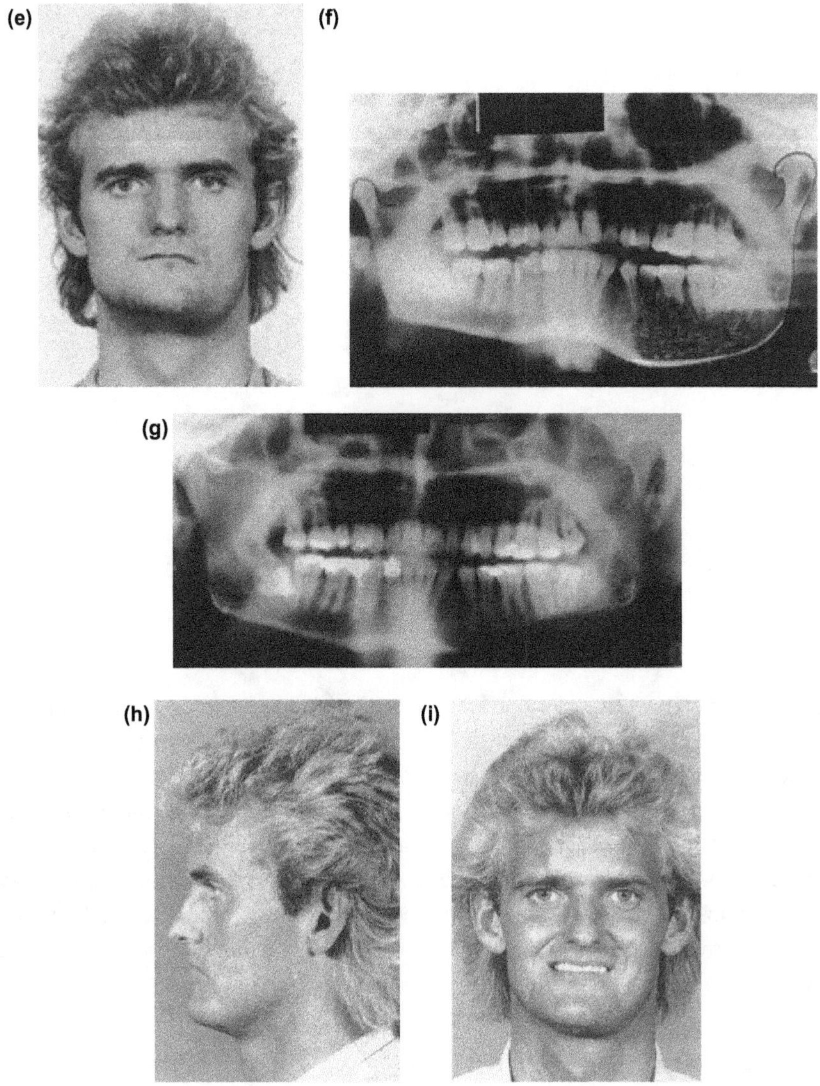

Figure 11.4 (*Continued*)

Rarely, when all growth seems to have ceased and the deformity has been corrected, the condylar cartilage may suddenly spring to life again. This justifies a condylar cartilage trimming procedure with careful preservation of the meniscus.

Trimming the convex mandibular lower border (Figure 11.4).

1. An aesthetic incision is made in a low skin increase, or where a crease might be anticipated. The mandible is exposed subperiosteally.
2. The lower border excess is outlined with bur holes, using the normal side for comparison (Figure 11.4a).
3. These holes are then joined together, cutting only through the outer cortex so as not to damage the inferior dental neurovascular bundle, which is invariably near the lower border.
4. A similar cortical bur cut is then made along the lower and posterior border and the excess outer cortex can then be split off with an osteotome, which is inserted in the lower cut, and rotated (Figure 11.4b).
5. This allows the neurovascular bundle to be exposed by carefully trimming off its overlying shell of compact bone.
6. The bundle is retracted and the excess lingual plate is trimmed off and the margins smoothed (Figures 11.4c and 11.4d). The neurovascular bundle is then left loosely sutured above the new lower border.
7. The wound is drained and closed in layers after loosely suturing the neurovascular bundle into the deep aspects of the wound. The skin is sutured with a continuous subcuticular 3/0 Prolene suture.

Figures 11.4e–11.4i shows such a case.

Condylar Hypoplasia

Occasionally it can be difficult to decide whether the asymmetry is the result of unilateral overgrowth or contralateral deficiency. Most unilateral hypoplasias appear to follow neonatal or childhood condylar damage with preservation of the meniscus. In addition to deviation of the chin to the affected side, the condyle is usually short, flattened or deformed. An exaggerated antegonial notch is present on the affected side. As the deficiency in ramus height gives rise to a secondary restriction in maxillary growth, the asymmetry is also reflected in the transverse occlusal plane. This is tilted downwards towards the normal side. Loss of the meniscus through a fracture displacement or destruction by infection or juvenile arthritis may lead to joint ankylosis and an even greater asymmetry due to the lack of functional stimulation to the growing mandible. Such cases require reconstruction of the joint with a costochondral graft (see Chapter 14).

Treatment

Moderate degrees of hypoplasia may be treated like an asymmetrical hyperplasia, with a bilateral sagittal split osteotomy. This will lengthen the affected side and provide a rotation adjustment on the normal side. However, the maxillary occlusal plane has to be levelled first. In adolescence this can be achieved orthodontically after the mandibular surgery by creating a lateral open bite intraoperatively with a unilateral thickened occlusal wafer or splint. The lateral space to be created may be estimated by examining the models mounted with a face-bow on an anatomical articulator. In most cases, a little excess is desirable. Following the sagittal split osteotomy the buccal teeth are brought into occlusion orthodontically (Figure 11.5).

With a large unilateral deficiency, or where there has been previous ramus surgery, the downward and forward mandibular reconstruction can only be achieved with an inverted L osteotomy and interpositional bone graft or distraction osteogenesis (see Chapter 9). Again, the maxillary occlusal plane will also require correction.If the patient is an adult, a Le Fort I osteotomy will be necessary to level the transverse occlusal tilt, and precedes the mandibular correction as part of a bimaxillary operation (see also Maxillary Asymmetry).

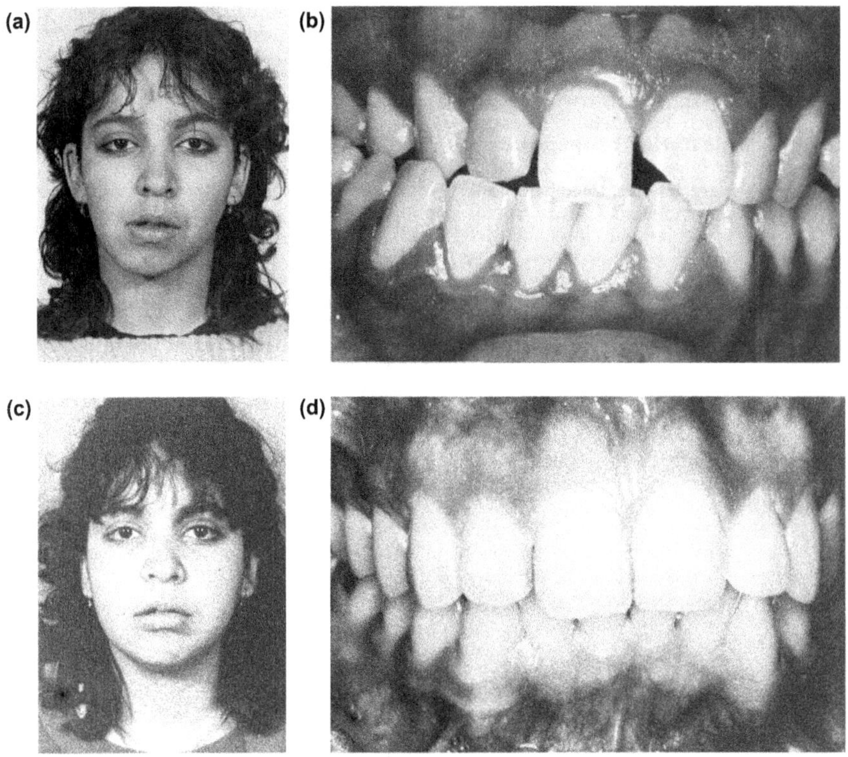

Figure 11.5 Post-traumatic right condylar hypoplasia treated with an inverted L bone graft to increase ramus height and correct the midline deviation. Postoperative orthodontics is used to achieve a horizontal occlusal plane. (**a**) and (**b**) Preoperative. (**c**) and (**d**) Postoperative.

Mandibular Retrognathism or Hypoplasia

The retrognathic mandible is either too small, i.e. a short Go-Pg, or set too far back with an increased saddle angle (NSAr) or a combination of both.

These cases may be classified as mild to marked skeletal Class II division 1 malocclusions. However, as with unilateral hypoplasias, there are both congenital and acquired forms of this deformity. The more severe, "bird face" deformity can be inherited, or acquired *in utero* as in the congenital Robin syndrome. One of the common features of this inherited form is a beak-shaped nose, which may also require reduction. In all cases the lower lip and tongue produce a secondary deformity of the maxilla, with dentoalveolar proclination and a narrow arch.

The severe acquired form follows bilateral loss of the condylar growth centres and is usually due to childhood trauma, in which case the condyles are small with no neck, and stigma of a submental scar may be found (Figure 11.6). Occasionally, the patient may have suffered juvenile rheumatoid arthritis (Still's disease).

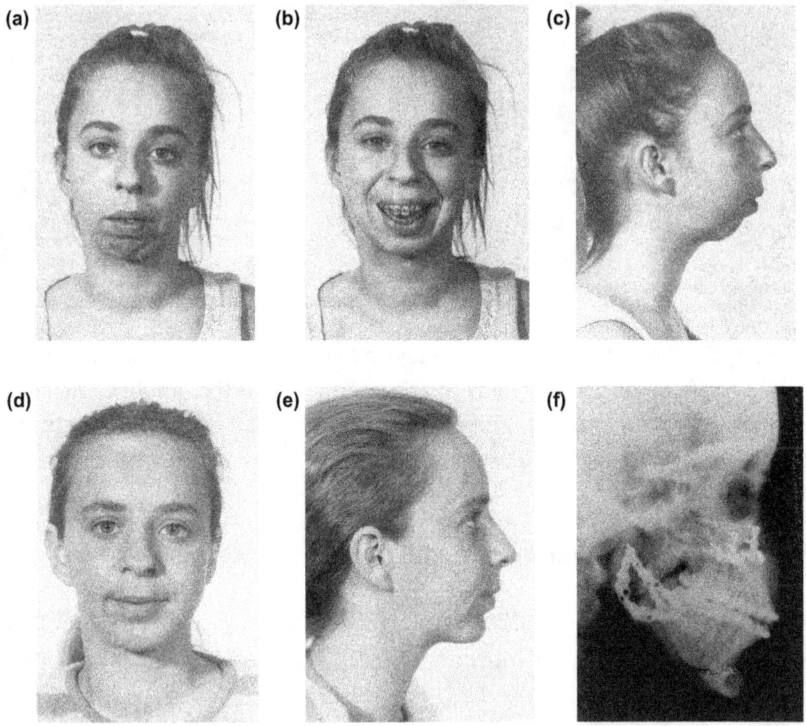

Figure 11.6 Marked retrognathia and an anterior open bite due to bilateral condylar damage in childhood (**a**), (**b**) and (**c**). Correction by a combination of a Le Fort I posterior impaction to close the open bite, and a bilateral inverted L advancement with interpositional bone grafts. The augmentation genioplasty was carried out simultaneously (**d**), (**e**) and (**f**).

Ankylosis only occurs when the meniscus is also displaced or destroyed, allowing the condyle to proliferate against the surface of the condylar fossa. In such cases the lack of function leads to a greater loss of mandibular development. The management of temporomandibular joint ankylosis will be discussed in Chapter 14.

Clinically there is an increased overjet which is usually exaggerated by the lower lip being trapped behind the upper incisors, increasing their proclination and spacing (Figure 11.7). Externally this is seen as an everted lower lip exaggerating the labiomental groove.

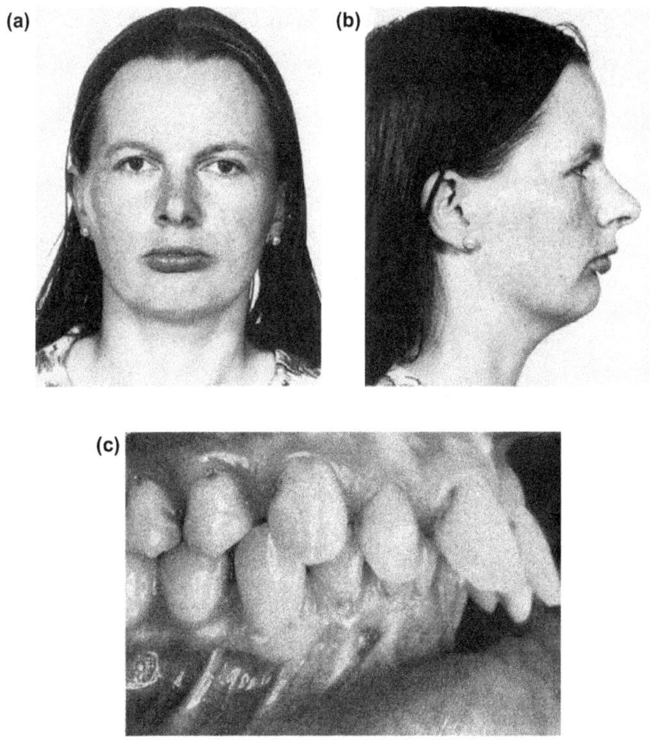

Figure 11.7 Surgical correction of mandibular retrognathism by a sagittal split advancement, after orthodontic incisor retroclination and levelling of the occlusal plane. Note to dramatic improvement of the lower lip contour as well as the skeletal profile. **(a)** to **(c)** Preoperative and preorthodontic therapy. **(d)** to **(f)** Postorthodontic therapy and surgery.

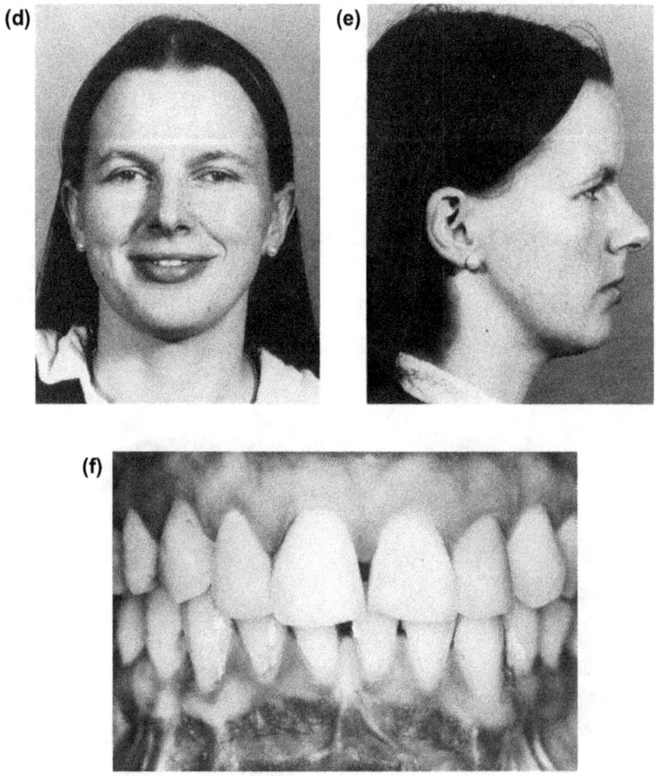

Figure 11.7 (*Continued*)

With unopposed occlusal drift (overeruption) of the lower incisors, the overbite is also increased.

The reduced lower facial height is a secondary aesthetic defect which may be self-correcting with the forward repositioning of the mandible.

A simple means of visualising the surgical correction is to study the face and profile before and after protruding the mandible. Before protrusion the chin will be set back and there will be a relatively low anterior facial height. With forward movement, not only does the profile improve but there is also an aesthetic gain from the increased lower facial height as the mandible moves downwards and forwards on the occlusal plane.

Treatment

The Occlusion

1. As will be seen clinically and on the study models, the over erupted lower incisors will prevent the mandible being moved forward into a satisfactory relationship without a lateral open bite. In adults this lateral open bite will not be self-corrected by postoperative compensatory eruption of the molars and premolars. Some means of levelling the occlusal plane orthodontically pre- or postoperatively, or surgically will be necessary. Orthodontic depression of the incisors with the associated eruption of the posterior segments may not be possible to achieve preoperatively in adults without the lower incisors being proclined through the alveolar labial cortex.

   The choices are:

   a) Decompensation of the incisors and a forward osteotomy of the mandible to an overcorrected edge to edge incisor relationship, giving a three-point contact occlusion, i.e. incisors and distal molars, followed by orthodontic closure of the lateral open bites. However, this is only possible if there is sufficient interdental space in the buccal segments to allow the premolars and molars to erupt from the perimeter of a curve into the shorter horizontal straight line.
   b) Separate orthodontic levelling of the canine and incisors, and the buccal segments. This will be followed by a lower anterior mandibulotomy setdown carried out at the same time as the mandibular lengthening procedure. This has the advantage of providing an additional supplement to the lower facial height. Figure 11.8 shows the increase in lower facial height and improved lip and chin profile after forward repositioning of the mandible with a lower incisor setdown achieved by an anterior mandibulotomy.

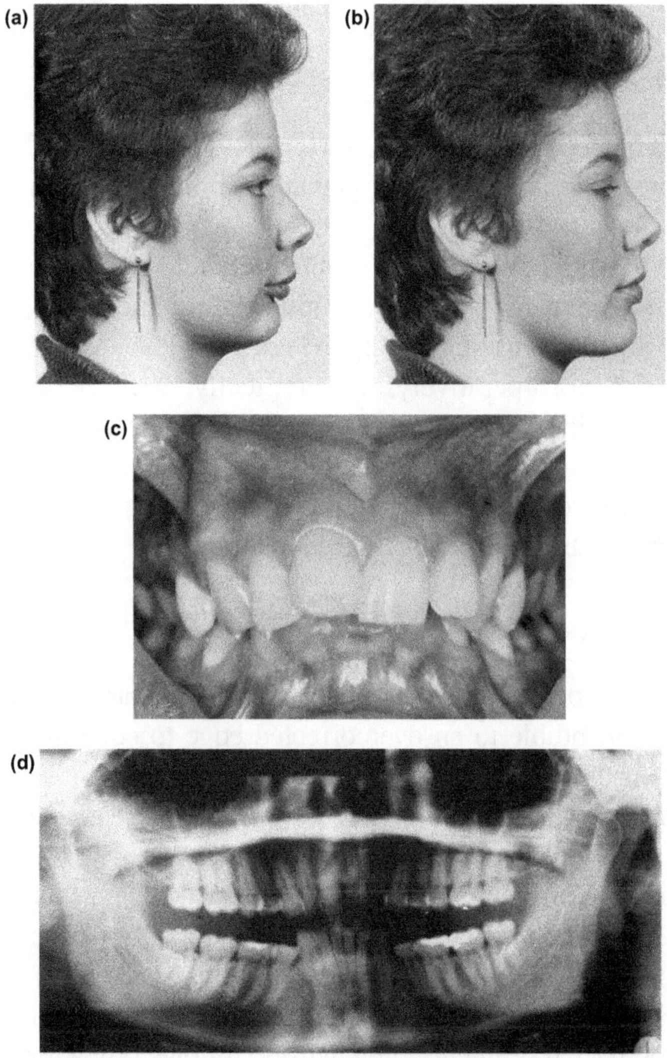

Figure 11.8 An anterior mandibulotomy combined with a forward osteotomy not only flattens the occlusal plane but also increases the chin depth. (**a**) Shows the preoperative profile in occlusion and (**b**) with the mandible postured forwards stimulating the surgical advancement. (**c**) to (**e**) The preoperative occlusion and radiographs before orthodontics and (**f**) after levelling the incisor and buccal segments independently. (**g**) to (**k**) Postoperative results. (**k**) The immediate postoperative orthopantomogram which shows the mandibulotomy cuts and set down.

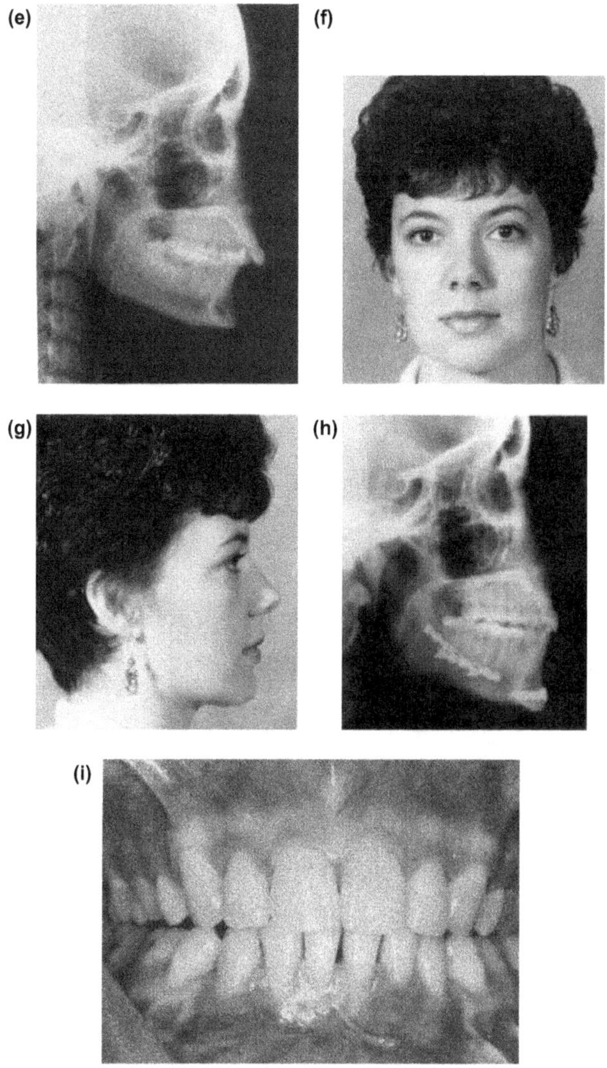

Figure 11.8 (*Continued*)

2. In all cases, preoperative orthodontic decompensation, coordination of the arches and closure of any spaces, is essential preparation for surgery (Figure 11.7). This may reveal an unsatisfactory upper lip incisor relationship requiring a Le Fort I impaction.

(j)

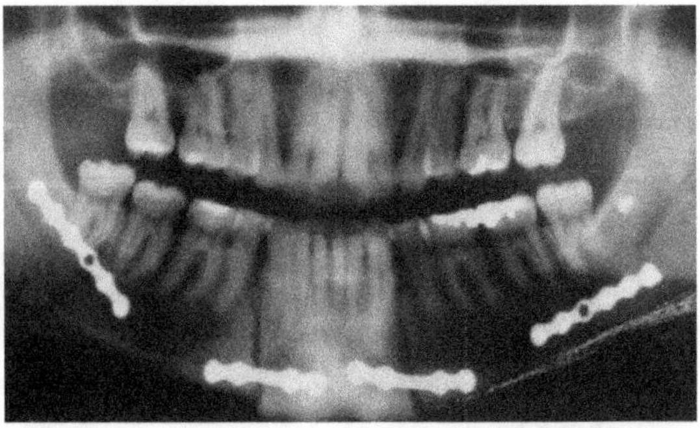

Figure 11.8 (*Continued*)

Lengthening the Mandible and the Chin

Most marked Class II division 1 cases require not only a forward repositioning of the mandible to an overcorrected edge to edge incisor relationship by a sagittal split but also a sliding augmentation genioplasty. Always resist the temptation to wait and see if a genioplasty is also required — it is! (Figure 11.9).

The Chin

As described earlier there are aesthetic and ethnic variations in the profile. In most cases the chin point, i.e. the soft tissue pogonion (Pg), should lie within 6 mm of a vertical drawn downwards from subnasale at right angles to the Frankfort horizontal plane (Figure 11.10). Retrogenia is a receding chin and must be differentiated from the more common retrognathia, where the mandible is set too far back and is too short. The increased overjet of retrognathia is not usually found in pure retrogenia.

The chin depth (anterior inferior dentoalveolar height) from the incisor edge to the bony menton is 40 ± 2 mm for women and 44 ± 2 mm for men. This usually equals the distance of the lower lip margin to the soft tissue menton. Chin depth is often overlooked and may also require augmentation or reduction.

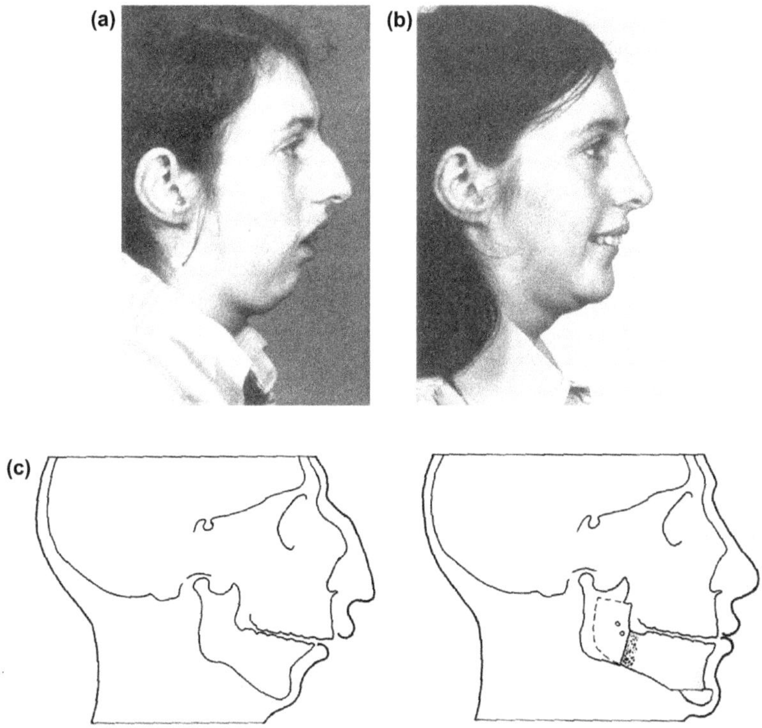

Figure 11.9 Severe "bird face" retrognathism corrected with a forward sagittal split osteotomy and genioplasty followed by a rhinoplasty. (**a**) Preoperative (**b**) postoperative, and (**c**) diagrammatic representation of change.

Unfortunately these estimations will be complicated by changes brought about by other osteotomies. For instance:

- after a Le Fort I elevation the chin will advance with the forward autorotation of the mandible, simultaneously reducing the apparent chin depth;
- forward movements of the mandible will have a predictable effect on the chin point (Po), but will simultaneously increase the lower facial height as the mandible moves down the occlusal plane;
- with backward correction of a prognathous mandible the distalisation of the chin is usually desirable, but occasionally it may require a paradoxical augmentation foreward slide;

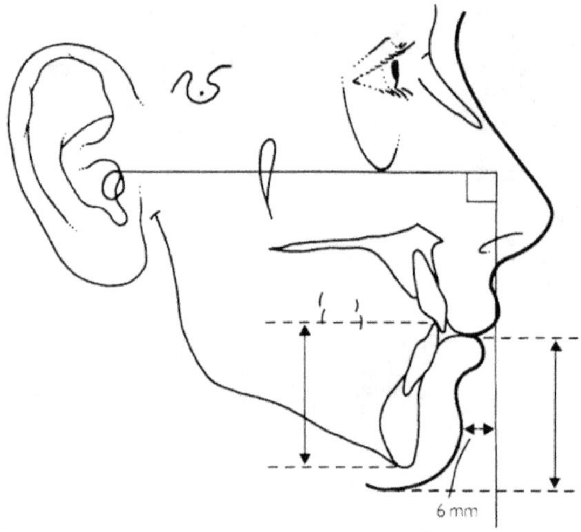

Figure 11.10 The vertical and horizontal parameters of the chin in relation to the vertical from the Frankfort mandibular plane (see text).

- bimaxillary osteotomies will also influence the chin profile if the occlusal plane is altered. By increasing the occlusal plane angle, the chin will rotate backwards and downwards. With a decreased occlusal plane, the chin will rotate forwards and become more prominent.

In all these cases a planning tracing on which the mandibular outline may be moved in the anticipated direction will enable the outcome to be predicted. Only in this way can any supplementary surgical addition or subtraction of the chin be confirmed.

Figure 11.11 shows the result of augmentation with a sliding genioplasty. Reduction and augmentation of chin depth will be discussed with the Long Face, and the Short Face.

Lower Lip Sag: A Warning

With some cases of augmentation genioplasty, especially when carried out with a Le Fort I elevation (upward impaction), the lower incisor occlusal plane rises above the lower lip line. Poor adaptation of the

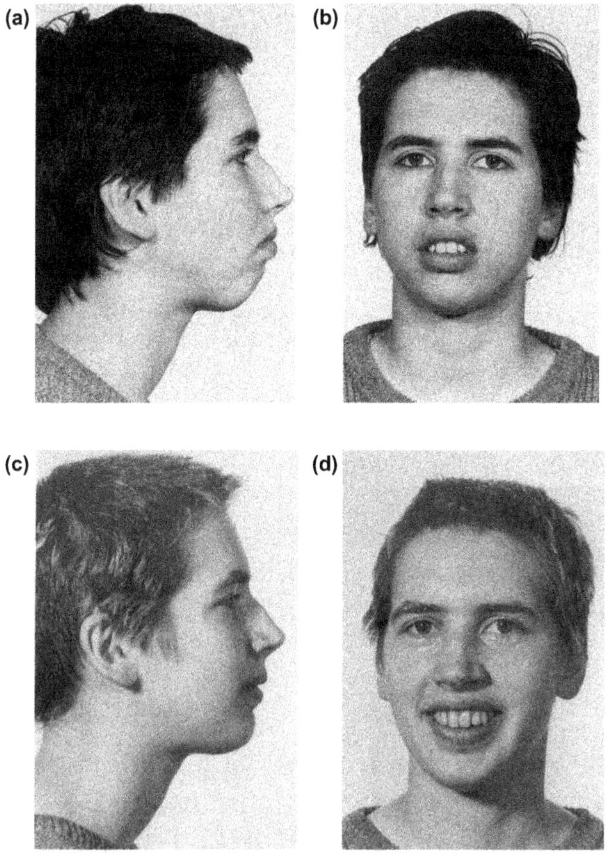

Figure 11.11 Retrogenia treated with a sliding genioplasty. (**a**) and (**b**) Preoperative. (**c**) and (**d**) Postoperative.

soft tissue and mentalis function leaves an unsightly display of lower incisor and gingival margin (Figure 11.12). This may be avoided by

1. Extensive undermining of the soft tissues of the neck to accommodate the advanced chin,
2. Careful suturing of the divided origin of the mentalis to the depths of the periosteal aspect of the degloved chin.
3. External elevation by an adhesive pressure dressing for a week, followed by active "upward" lip exercises by the patient to restore upward muscle tone.

(a) (b)

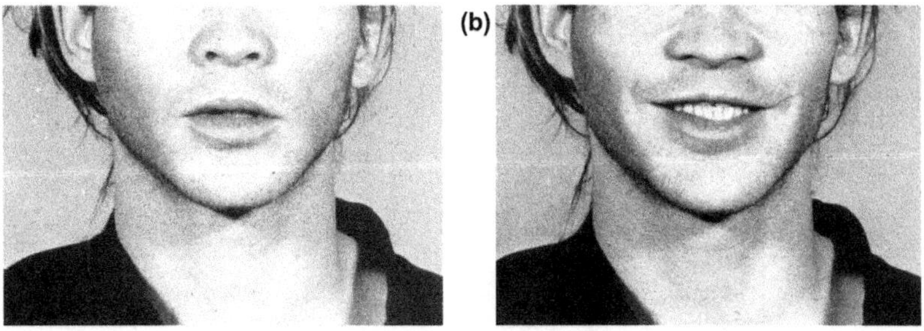

Figure 11.12 Lower lip sag following augmentation genioplasty. (**a**) at rest. (**b**) smiling.

Mandibular Incisor Proclination

Proclination of the lower incisors with a normal jaw-base relationship is an uncommon deformity. The incisors are usually spaced, suggesting the tongue as the cause of the problem.

Treatment (see Figure 11.13)

- Where orthodontic retraction is not practicable, the first premolars can be extracted and the canine-incisor segment brought backwards with a Kole subapical (labial segmental) osteotomy.
- If the tongue looks large, reduce it with the osteotomy. If there is any doubt, warn the patient that should incisor proclination relapse occur, tongue reduction may be necessary (see also Bimaxillary Proclination).

The Maxilla

Maxillary Hypoplasia

- Although one would expect to recognise a maxillary deficiency, many cases are diagnosed and operated on as a mandibular prognathism. The result is a flat face, which is more noticeable

(a) (b) (c) (d) (e) (f)

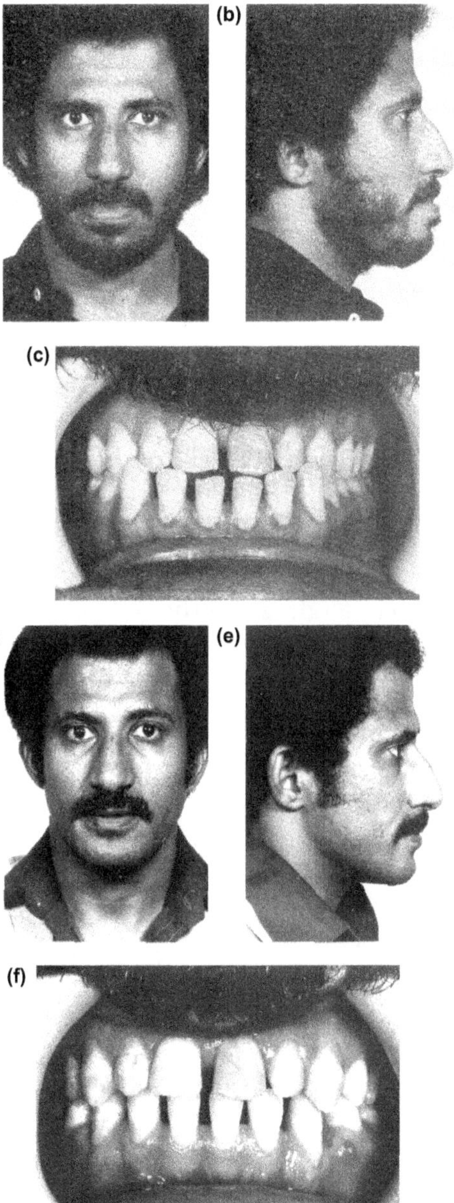

Figure 11.13 Segmental setback of lower incisors and canines. (**a**) to (**c**) Preoperative. (**d**) to (**f**) Postoperative.

in a man than a woman. This is particularly likely to occur if the SNA is artificially high, i.e. more than 82°, due to a high sella or a short cranial base, i.e. a short SN.

- Cleft cases require special consideration. One important factor is the misconception that the cleft hypoplastic maxilla is associated with an enlarged mandible. Cleft patients often have a small mandible, which rarely may be elongated with the maxilla advancement for an ideal correction of the profile.

Treatment

The treatment of choice is a Le Fort I osteotomy with a forward movement of 3, 6, or 9 mm. Depending on the degree of deficiency. (Figure 11.14). In addition to correcting the occlusion, the maxillary forward movement will elevate the nasal tip but does not usually decrease the nasolabial angle. A narrow intercanine width will have to be increased orthodontically (Figure 11.14) or surgically at operation after the down-fracture (Figure 11.15).

Where there is marked hypoplasia of the inferior orbital margins a Le Fort II osteotomy is necessary or a high Le Fort I with a bone onlay (see below). However, with a good nose the Kufner modification of the Le Fort III osteotomy produces an advancement of the malar bones and infraorbital margins (see Malar-maxillary Hypoplasia).

Major movements, i.e. more than 9 mm, require carefully sited plates with bone grafting of the osteotomy gaps. However, where significant movements appear necessary, especially in non-cleft cases, a bimaxillary procedure is needed. This will divide the distance between the two jaws (see Bimaxillary Deformities).

Nasomaxillary Hypoplasia

With nasomaxillary hypoplasia, especially with a deficiency of the infraorbital margins, a Le Fort II osteotomy is required. There may

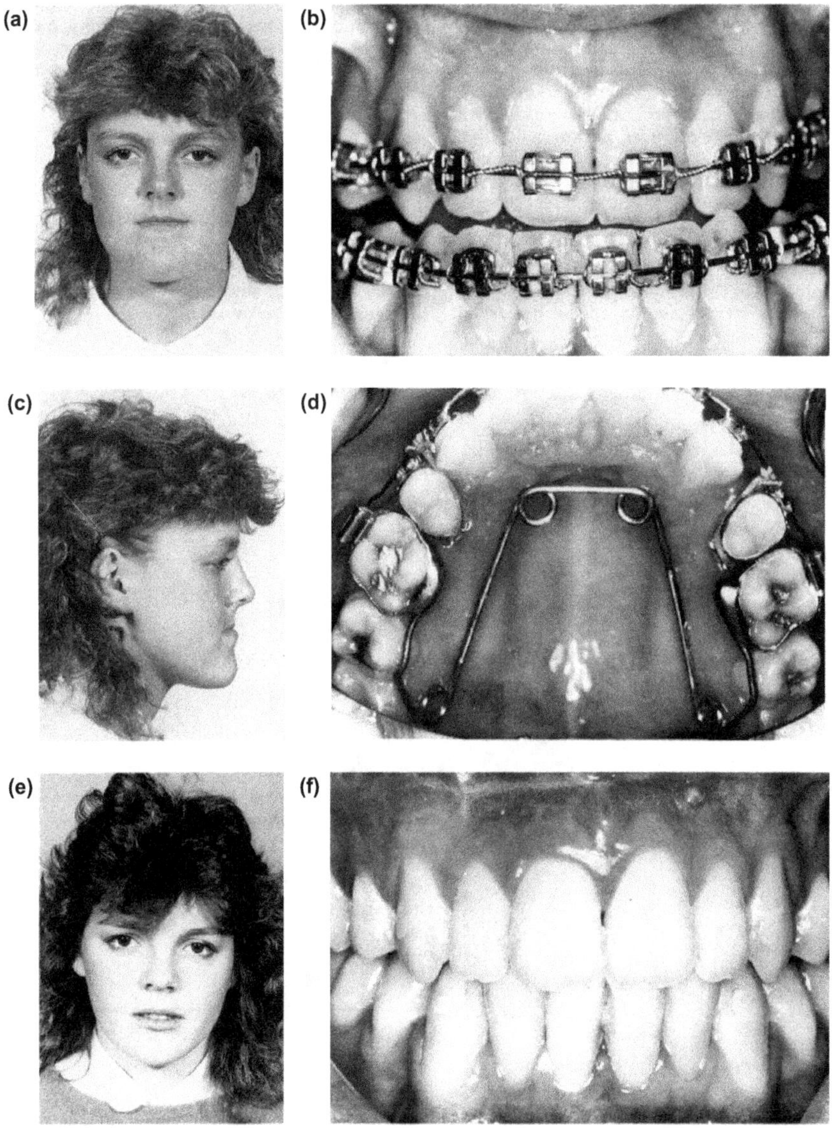

Figure 11.14 Maxillary retrusion corrected by a Le Fort I advancement. This was facilitated by preoperative upper arch expansion with a quadhelix appliance. **(a)** to **(d)** Preoperative. **(e)** to **(g)** Postoperative.

(g)

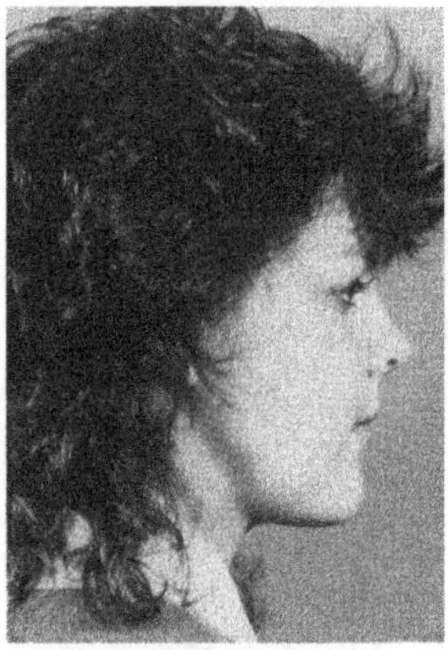

Figure 11.14 (*Continued*)

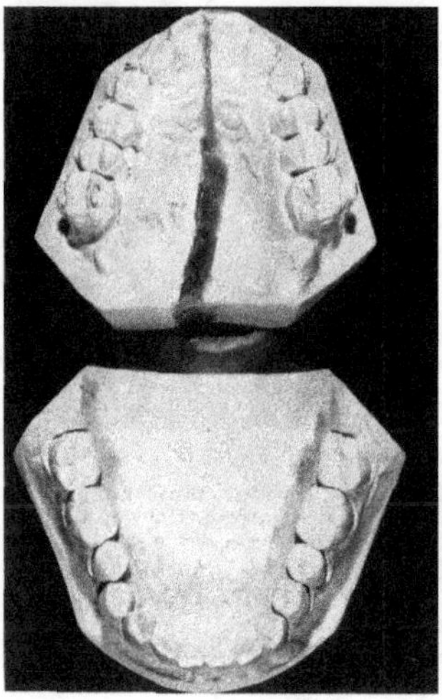

Figure 11.15 Planning model for surgical expansion of maxillary arch.

be a noticeable band of white sclera below the limbus of the iris, and in profile there is some degree of pseudoproptosis, i.e. the globe protrudes more than 2–3 mm beyond the infraorbital margin. Figure 11.16 shows the result of a combined Le Fort II advancement and mandibular pushback.

(a) (b) (c) (d)

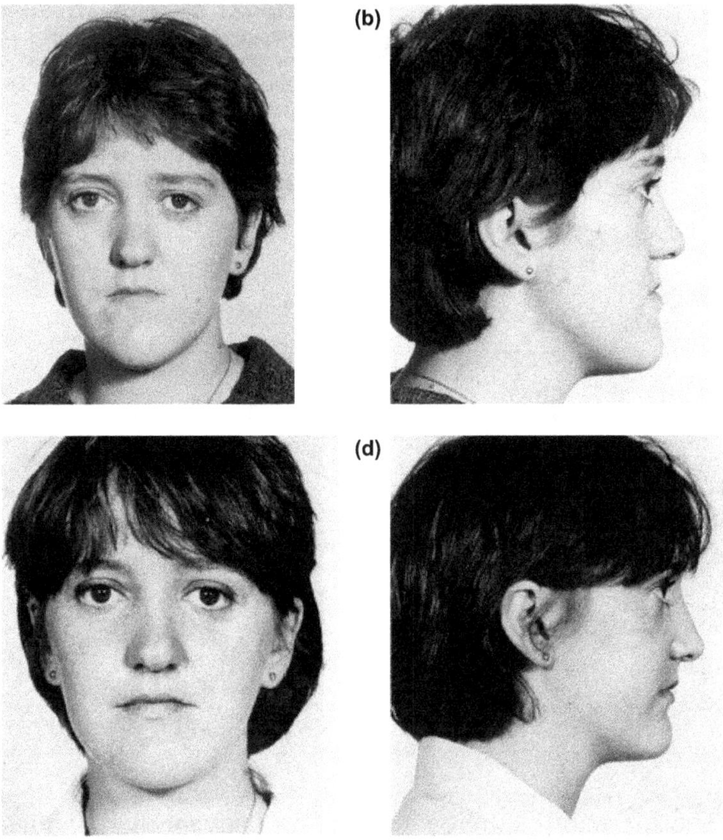

Figure 11.16 Nasomaxillary hypoplasia and mandibular prognathism corrected with a Le Fort II advancement and mandibular setback. (**a**), (**b**) and (**e**) Preoperative. (**c**), (**d**) and (**f**) Postoperative.

Malar-Maxillary Hypoplasia

The presentation is very similar to the previous case, requiring a Le Fort II correction, except that the nose is either good or prominent. Here, the treatment of choice is:

i) A malar-maxillary advancement, leaving the nose undisturbed. This procedure is the Kufner modification of the Le Fort III osteotomy (Figure 11.17).

(e)

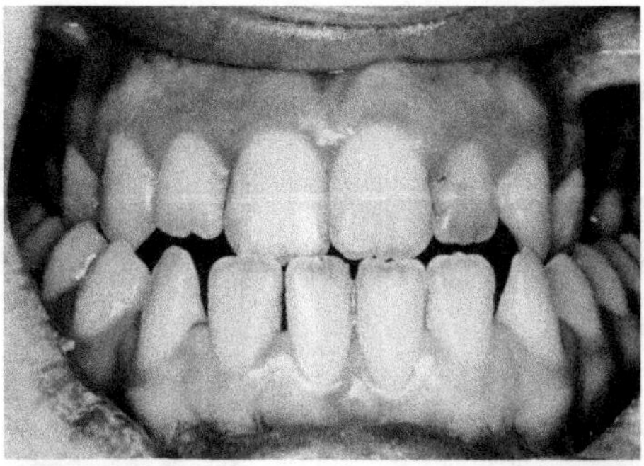

(f)

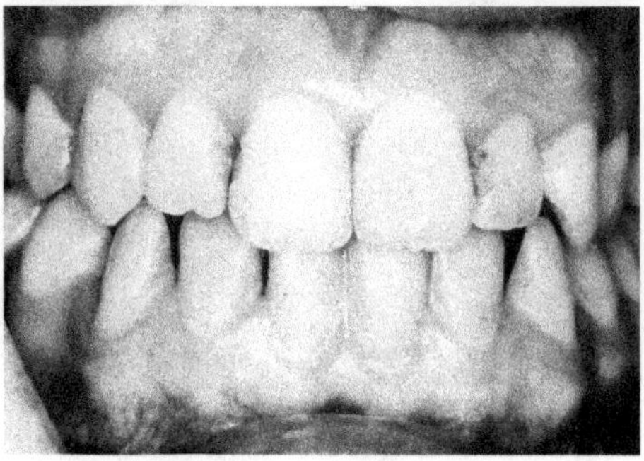

Figure 11.16 (*Continued*)

ii) The alternative solution is a Le Fort I advancement with simultaneous alloplastic malar onlays.
iii) The Kufner osteotomy followed by distraction osteogenesis.

Maxillary Protrusion

Patients with this deformity are usually severe Class II division 1 cases that have had failed orthodontics or refuse orthodontic treatment. As they also present with deep overbite problems, they are discussed in detail in the next section. Occasionally the uncomplicated maxillary prognathism may be treated with an anterior segmental osteotomy (Wassmund/Wunderer). This is usually an adult patient who is unwilling to undergo orthodontic treatment (Figure 11.18). The canine-incisor segment is set back after extraction of the first

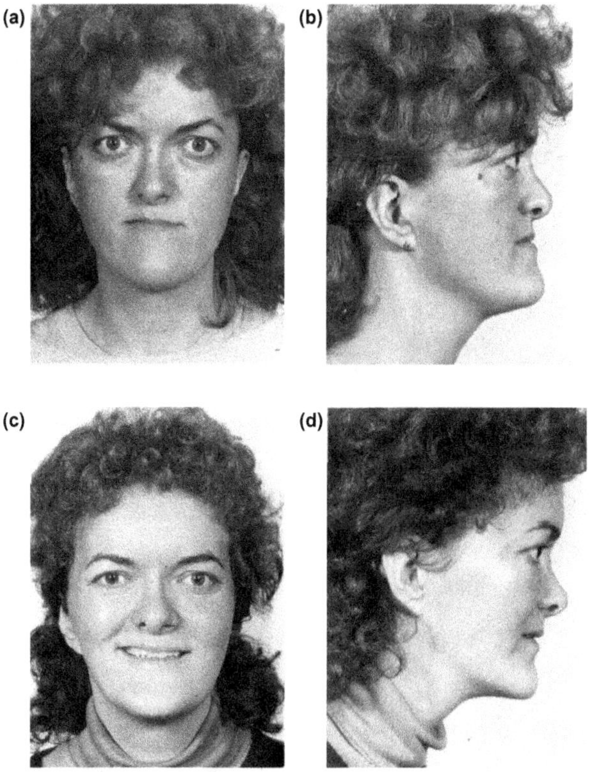

Figure 11.17 Malar-maxillary hypoplasia and mandibular prognathism corrected by a Kufner modification of the Le Fort III osteotomy and a mandibular setback. (**a**) and (**b**) Preoperative. (**c**) and (**d**) Postoperative.

premolars. A midline split is necessary to maintain a natural dentoalveolar arch. Where premolar extractions have shortened the buccal segments the best approach to achieve optimum aesthetics and occlusion is to correct with a Le Fort I setback.

Bimaxillary Deformities

There is a natural temptation to treat most deformities with an operation on one jaw, but this often produces an acceptable occlusion and a poor profile. Where a single jaw procedure requires a

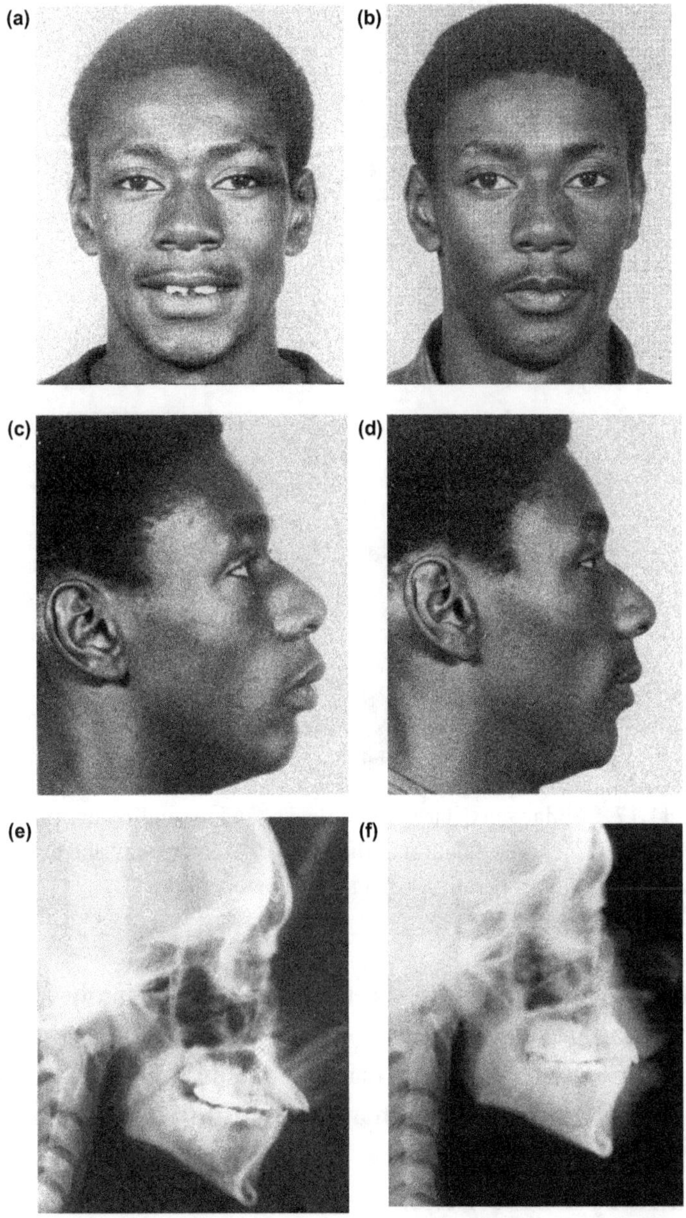

Figure 11.18 Maxillary prognathism with increased overjet and proclined incisors corrected with an anterior segmental setback. **(a)**, **(c)** and **(e)** Preoperative. **(b)**, **(d)**, **(f)** and **(g)** Postoperative.

(g)

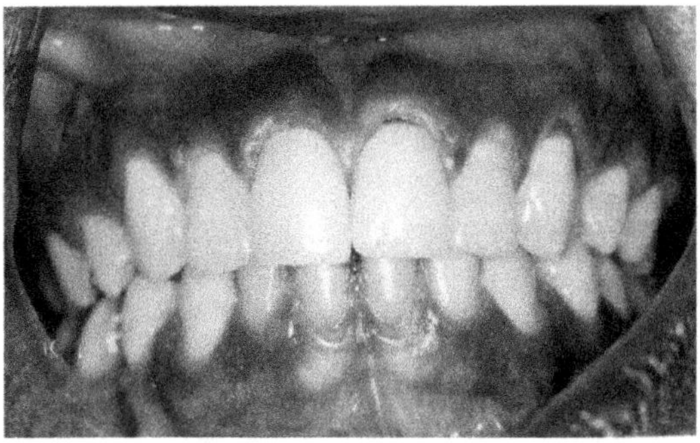

Figure 11.18 *(Continued)*

large dentoalveolar displacement of 6 mm or more, one should always reconsider the case as a bimaxillary deformity. By dividing the displacement into two complementary components, a stable result with a better profile will be achieved.

Figure 11.19 shows how a small maxilla, with an SNA of 72° and a large negative overjet (SNB = 90°), has been "successfully" treated with a large mandibular pushback. Unfortunately, this has created a flat mid-face with an obtuse nasolabial angle. The surgery of choice should have been a combination of a forward Le Fort I and a mandibular setback procedure (see below). Furthermore, before this is done, orthodontic decompensation of the incisors with arch coordination, provides a considerably better postoperative dental occlusion and profile. Incisor decompensation always reveals the true discrepancy between the upper and lower arches and facilitates greater surgical movement and the best profile.

With all bimaxillary osteotomies, care should be taken to maintain or achieve a normal occlusal plane which is 8 ± 4° to the Frankfort plane. This will ensure:

- a good chin profile
- optimum function, and
- occlusal stability.

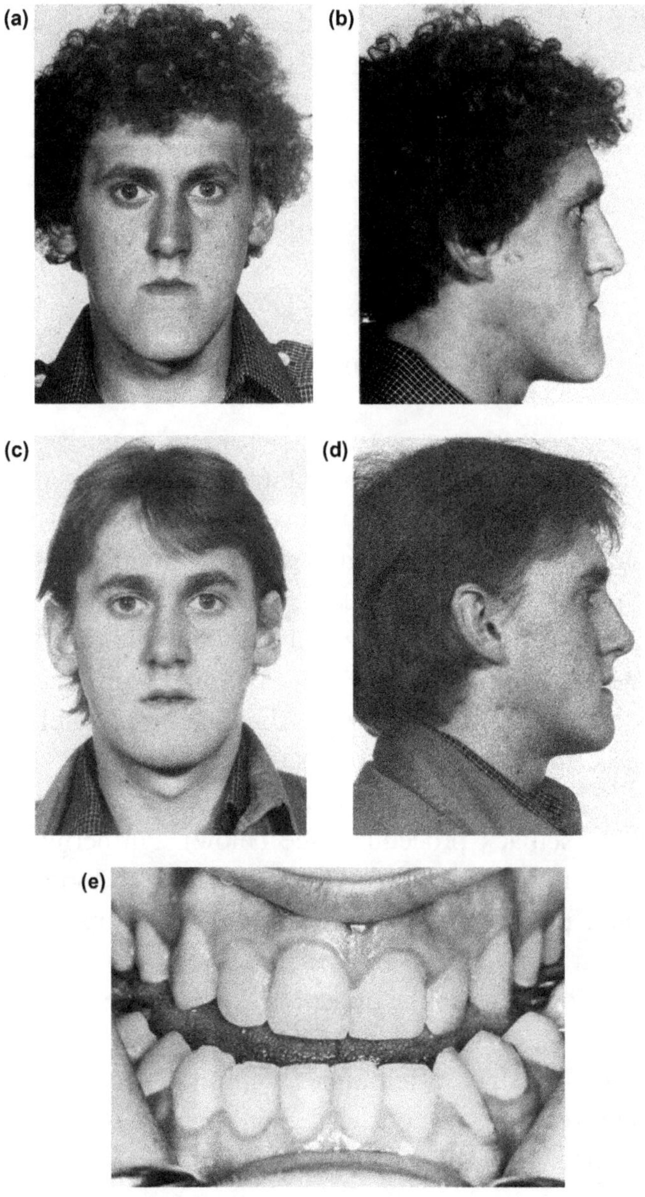

Figure 11.19 Marked mandibular prognathism treated with a pushback osteotomy but no orthodontic decompensation produced a satisfactory occlusion, but an unsatisfactory flat profile. **(a)**, **(b)** and **(e)** Preoperative. **(c)**, **(d)** and **(f)** Postoperative.

(f)
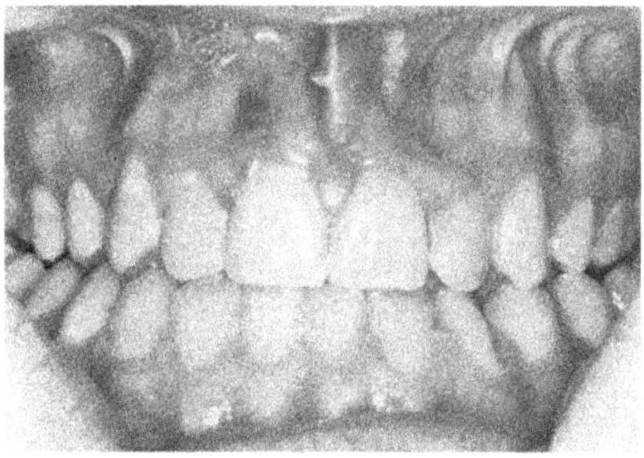

Figure 11.19 (*Continued*)

Gross Mandibular Prognathism

As stated all cases of gross mandibular prognathism have an element of maxillary hypoplasia (Figure 11.19) which should be defined in order to plan an advancement in addition to the mandibular setback. This can only be achieved by presurgical orthodontic treatment decompensating the incisors and arch coordination.

The surgery is done as one combined procedure in the following way.

1. The sagittal split osteotomy cuts are carried out as far as, but not including, the ramus split.
2. The maxillary osteotomy, which is usually a Le Fort I, is completed and positioned with an intermediate occlusal wafer designed to relate the forward movement of the repositioned maxilla to the unchanged mandible. Bone plates provide stable fixation both during and after the mandibular surgery.
3. The mandibular osteotomy is completed and repositioned distally to the planned overcorrected postosteotomy occlusion with the maxilla.

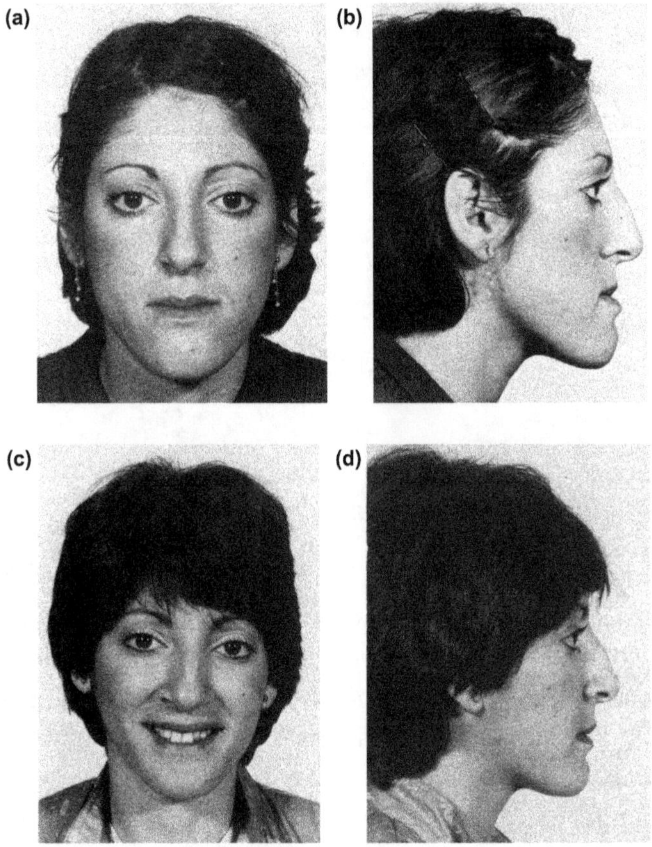

Figure 11.20 Combination of maxillary hypoplasia and mandibular prognathism treated with a Le Fort I advancement and an intraoral subcondylar pushback. Note how the prominence of the nose dimishes with the corrected facial drape. (**a**) and (**b**) Preoperative. (**c**) and (**d**) Postoperative.

Operating time can be reduced by using one of the intraoral subsigmoid osteotomies. The operative sequence, including a subsigmoid osteotomy, is as follows (see Figure 11.20):

i) A medial (or lateral) intraoral subsigmoid osteotomy is performed, cutting only the posterior border of the mandible.
ii) The maxillary osteotomy is carried out and repositioned with the intermediate wafer designed to relate the postosteotomy maxillary position with the unchanged mandible.

iii) The intraoral subsigmoid osteotomy is completed and the final occlusal relationship determined and fixed with elastics.

Unfortunately this loses all the advantages of internal fixation with the elimination of intermaxillary fixation and immediate rehabilitation.

The Deep Overbite

Patients with a deep overbite are neglected because they do not usually complain of an aesthetic deformity. Their problem consists of incisor attrition damaging the opposing mucosal surface, leading to bone and tooth loss. The lower incisor over eruption also leads to premature loss with the onset of periodontal disease. Conventional solutions are an overlay or bite guard, or extractions with the provision of a denture. Orthodontics and orthognathic surgery can readily eliminate these problems without a prosthesis and with preservation of the dentition.

The patients fall into the two Angle Class II groups, each with subgroups.

Class II Division 1

Here the damage is on the palatal aspect of the upper incisors, leading to increased proclination and separation with progressive bone loss.

Treatment

1. With a poor profile, consisting of a retrognathic mandible, reduced lower facial height and the lower lip trapped behind the upper incisors (Figure 11.21), treatment comprises orthodontic decompensation of the incisors followed by a combination of a lower anterior dentoalveolar setdown with an anterior mandibulotomy, and a sagittal split osteotomy to bring the whole mandible forward to an overcorrected edge to edge incisor relationship.

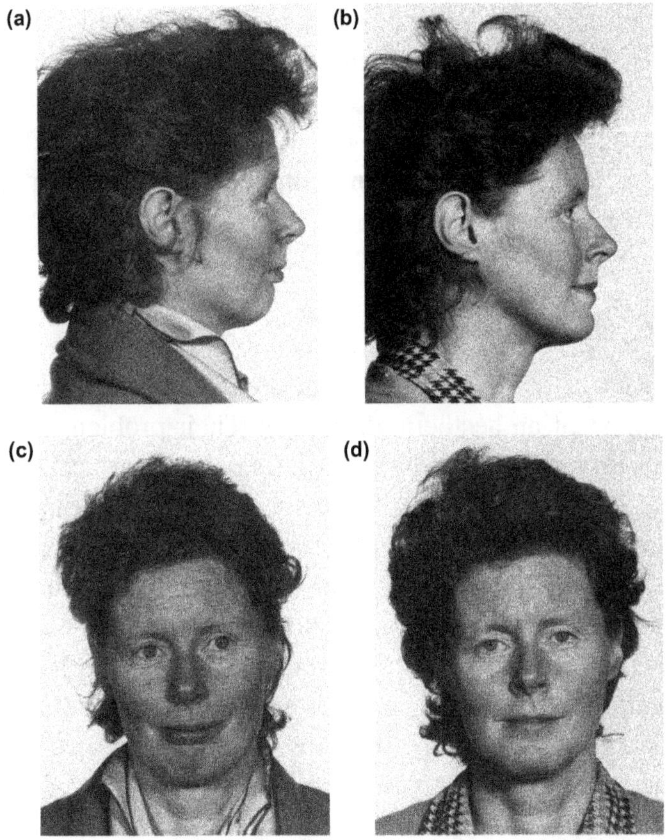

Figure 11.21 A forward sagittal split osteotomy combined with an anterior segmental setdown to correct a marked Class II, division 1 skeletal disproportion. The spaced proclined maxillary incisors were aligned preoperatively. **(a)**, **(c)** and **(e)** Preoperative. **(b)**, **(d)** and **(f)** Postoperative.

If a satisfactory upper incisor lip relationships cannot be corrected orthodontically it will also be necessary to elevate the maxilla with a Le Fort I osteotomy. The operative sequence will be:

a) The sagittal split cuts, but without splitting.
b) The maxillary Le Fort I impaction osteotomy with rigid fixation.

(e)

(f)

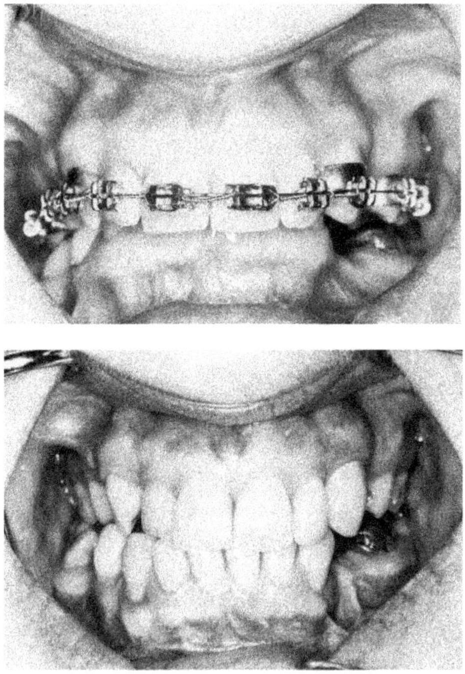

Figure 11.21 *(Continued)*

c) The lower anterior segmental setdown with an anterior mandibulotomy. A Kole subapical osteotomy is more challenging and reduces the chin depth which may not be aesthetically desirable.
d) Completion of the sagittal split and anterior movement to an overcorrected edge to edge incisor relationship. Relapse is a natural tendency and is avoided by the forward overcorrection.

The Class II Division 2

Here the incisor trauma affects both the buccal and palatal gingivae leading to loss of the lower incisor bony support and secondary periodontal disease. Cases may be divided into two groups:

1. Uncommon patients with a satisfactory profile and upper incisor inclination. Relief of the traumatic occlusion may be achieved by a lower segmental setdown alone. For stability, an edge-to-edge relationship must be established (Figure 11.22).
2. The majority of cases have retroclined upper incisors and orthodontic proclination must precede the surgery. This converts the case into a Class II division 1 problem over a period of 18 months. It is then treated surgically, as described above for the poor

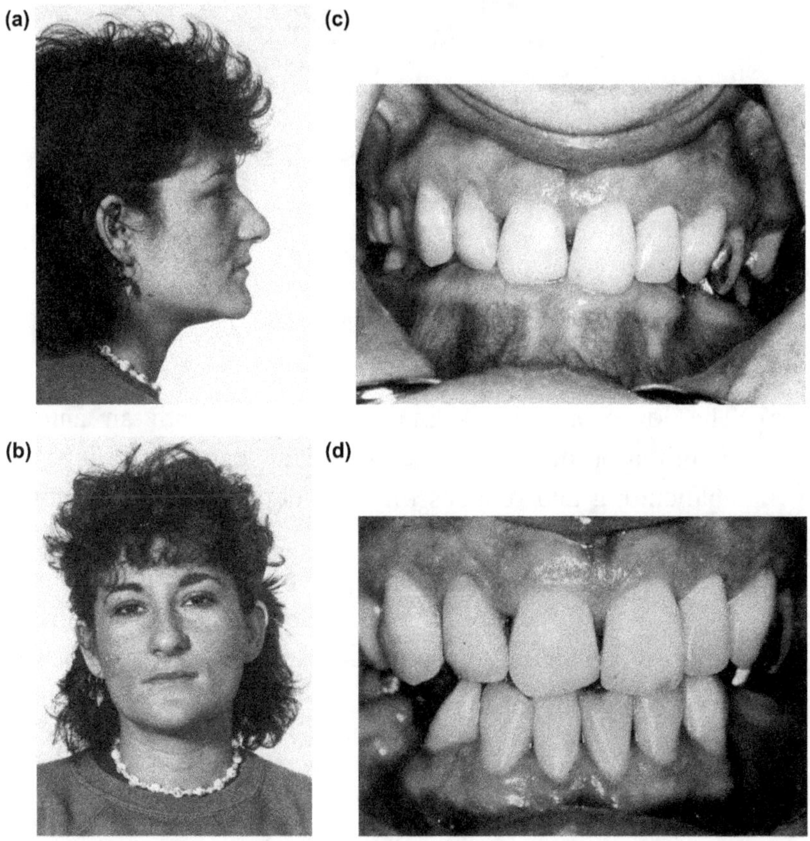

Figure 11.22 Elimination of a deep class II division 2 overbite by a lower segmental setdown. (**a**) to (**c**) Preoperative. (**d**) Immediate postoperative. (**e**) Note the lower incisor eruption and imbrication two years after operation. (**f**) The final restoration with fixed bridgework.

(e)

(f)

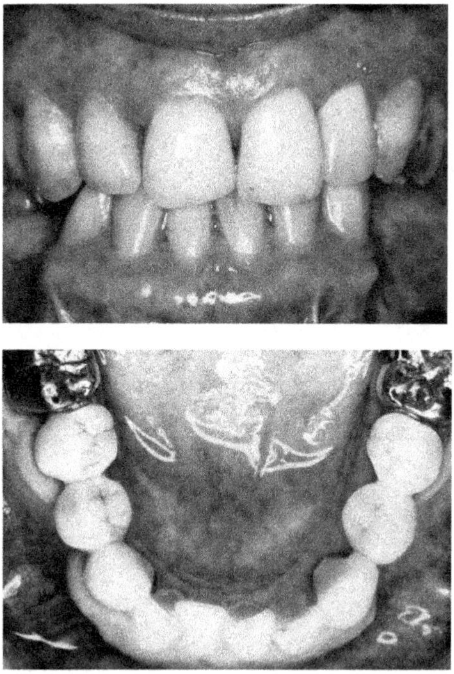

Figure 11.22 *(Continued)*

profile Class II division 1 deep overbite, i.e. (a) the upper lip-incisor relationship correction, (b) a lower anterior setdown, and (c) a forward slide mandibular osteotomy (Figure 11.23).

The Long Face Syndrome ("Vertical Maxillary and Chin Excess")

Although the mean facial heights for males and females are quoted as 130 mm and 120 mm respectively, the standard deviation of 8 mm, i.e. a range of 32 mm, indicates a very wide normal variation. However, in terms of vertical facial aesthetics, the most important diagnostic factors are:

1. labial competence at rest,
2. the upper lip-incisor relationship, and
3. the upper/lower facial proportions.

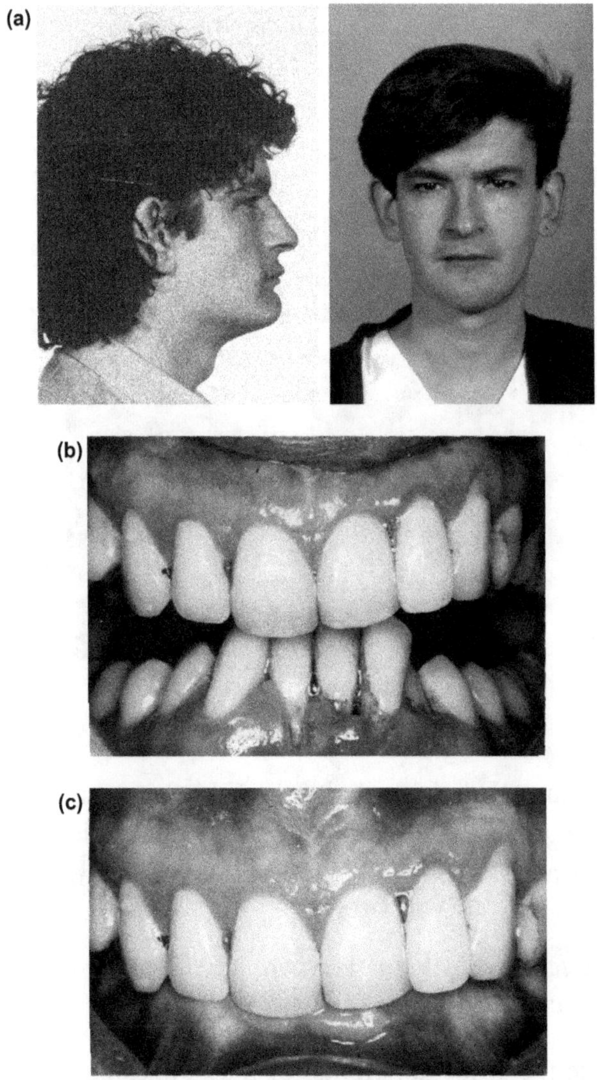

Figure 11.23 Class II, division 2 deep overbite with marked periodontal breakdown due to gingival trauma and poor oral hygiene. **(a)** to **(c)** Preoperative. Models show orthodontic "conversion" to Class II, division 1, **(d)** and **(e)**, which was then treated surgically with a lower segmental setdown and a mandibular advancement. **(f)** to **(h)** Postoperative. Note the increase in the postoperative lower facial height seen on the profile, and the marked change in the interincisal occlusion.

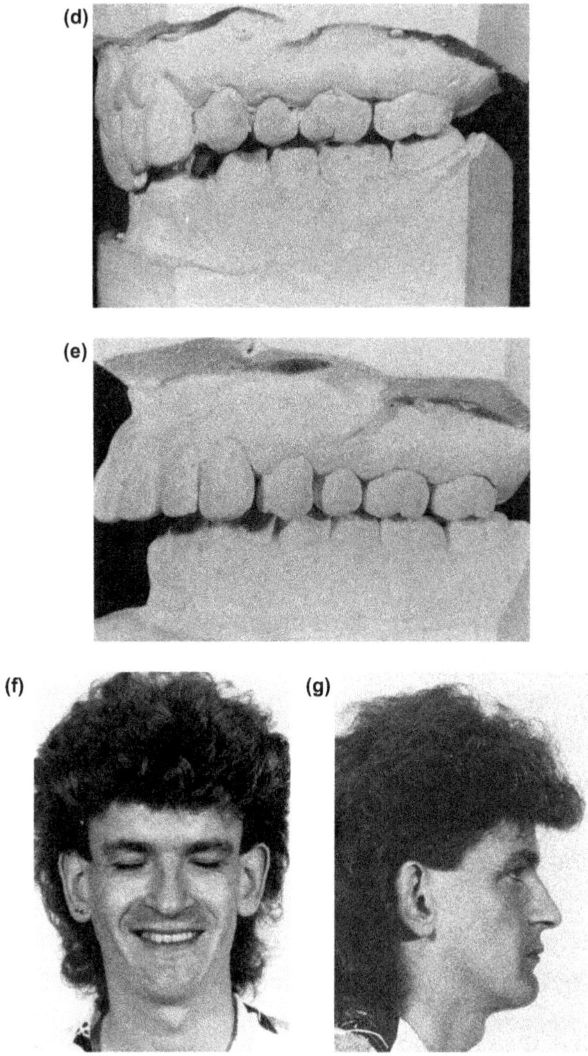

Figure 11.23 (*Continued*)

The soft tissue profile can be roughly divided into thirds from hairline to nasion, nasion to subnasale, i.e. the junction of philtrum and columella, and then to the lower border of the chin. The lower facial height can also be subdivided into a third and

(h)

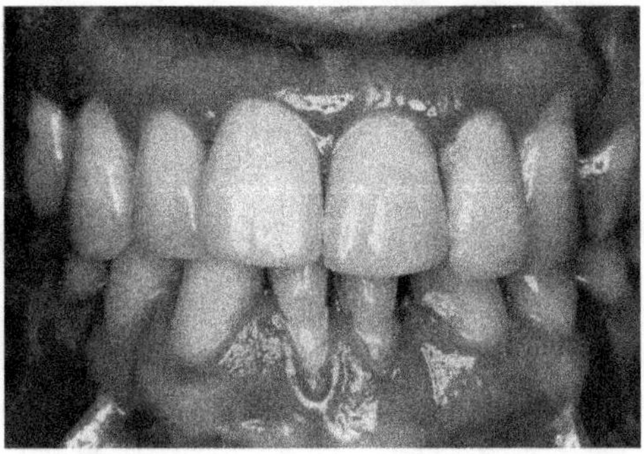

Figure 11.23 (*Continued*)

two thirds by the line of labial contact, the one third being the upper lip, which is 20 ± 2 mm in females and 22 ± 2 mm in males. However for surgical planning, the best guide is the underlying skeletal ratio of 45:55 between the upper facial height (N to ANS) and the lower facial height (ANS to Me).

Patients with long faces exhibit a variety of growth disturbances which are principally, but not exclusively, in the vertical plane (Figure 11.24). It is obviously important to identify the true vertical maxillary excess (VME) case. Clinically this will present as labial incompetence with a poor incisor-lip relationship, i.e. an excess of incisor showing at rest. This will be exaggerated on smiling, revealing excess gingiva. Be sure that such a discrepancy is not due to a short upper lip. If this is misinterpreted as VME and treated exclusively with a superior maxillary impaction, the end result will be a short mid face. Therefore any maxillary impaction must be proportional to lip length. The longer the lip length, the greater the upward impaction and *vice versa*. Standard cephalometry will help to clarify the skeletal proportions, and a template such as the Jacobson or Bolton Standard will also show whether there are discrepancies in the levels of the maxillary (palatal) and occlusal planes.

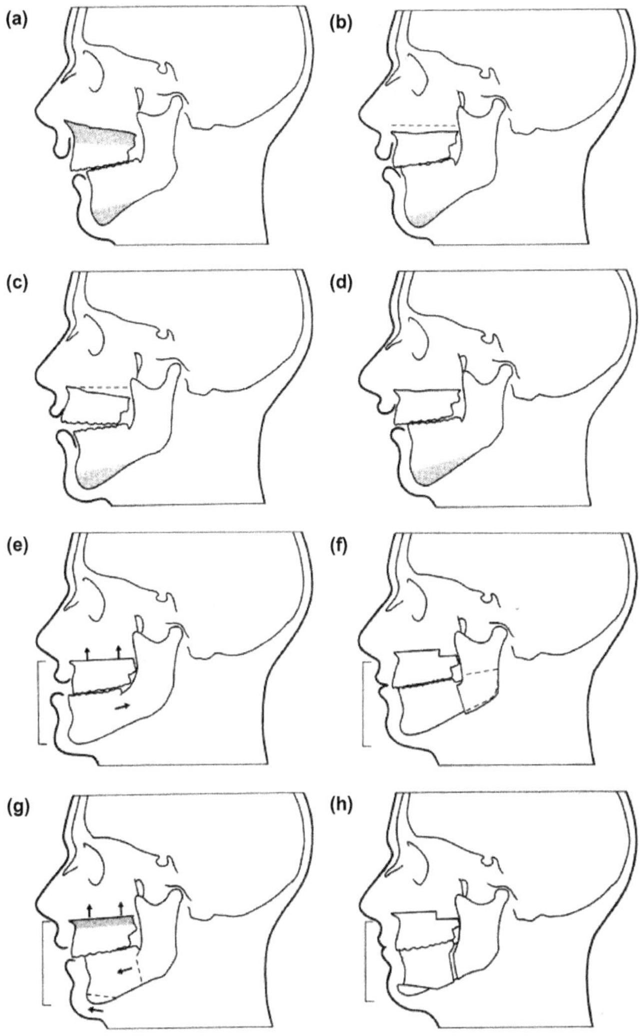

Figure 11.24 The four basic varieties of a long face. The shaded areas indicate skeletal excess. Each form of vertical maxillary excess may co-exist with a vertical chin excess. (**a**) Vertical maxillary excess. (**b**) A low maxilla. (**c**) A tilted maxillary oclussal plane producing an anterior open bite. (**d**) A short upper lip simulating vertical maxillary excess. All VME is treated by a Le Fort I impaction, which allows a forward autorotation of the mandible. This will eliminate minor degrees of vertical chin excess. (**e**) Here impaction creates a prognathous mandible requiring a push back. (**f**) (**g**) and (**h**) A forward mandibular movement with an augmentation genioplasty.

This will reveal an increased alveolar depth with (a) a normal maxillary plane, whereas the rest have (b) a low, or (c) postero-inferior tilted maxillary planes with or without alveolar overgrowth.

Many VME cases also have a degree of vertical chin excess (VCE). In men, the anterior inferior dentoalveolar height measured from lower incisor tip to bony menton is 44 ± 4 mm and in women 40 ± 4 mm. Note that this is remarkably similar to the lower lip margin to soft tissue menton depth.

An important 25% of patients with a long face have a normal maxilla but vertical chin excess, or an anterior open bite (or both).

The four basic varieties of a long face are shown in Figure 11.24 where the shaded areas indicate skeletal excess. Each form of vertical maxillary excess may co-exist with vertical chin excess.

a) Vertical maxillary excess with vertical chin excess.
b) A low maxilla with plus vertical chin excess.
c) A postero-inferior tilted maxillary occlusal plane producing an anterior open bite (plus vertical chin excess).
d) A short upper lip simulates vertical maxillary excess which may be exaggerated by vertical chin excess.

The surgical management of VME cases is the reduction of maxillary height with a Le Fort I vertical impaction, which is determined by the upper lip-incisor relationship. It is essential to measure the unaesthetic tooth excess at rest with dividers and a ruler and record it in the planning notes. Remember any maxillary impaction will tend to shorten the upper lip by up to 25% and some overcorrection is therefore desirable.

Treatment Planning

As maxillary elevation produces a forward rotation of the mandible it reduces chin depth. It is also necessary to decide whether the final occlusion and profile will be satisfactory or will also require a mandibular osteotomy. The two simple ways of making a decision are (a) by a planning tracing and (b) by precise model surgery using an anatomical articulator. The study models will also indicate whether the dental arches match or require modification by orthodontic therapy or additional segmental surgery.

a) Draw the repositioned maxilla on the lateral skull tracing and, with dividers, rotate from the lower incisor tip around the centre of the condyle into the new occlusion. In this way it is possible to see if on autorotation, the mandible will

1. find a satisfactory anteroposterior occlusion (Figures 11.24a–11.24d),
2. require a setback because of an acquired prognathic relationship (Figures 11.24e and 11.24f), or
3. require a forward mandibular slide and genioplasty to improve the incisor relationship and profile (Figures 11.24g and 11.24h).

Minor discrepancies (<3mm) in the postoperative occlusion can be resolved by a forward or backward movement of the maxilla which must be planned on the articulator to provide the appropriate intermediate wafer. This will confine the surgery to one jaw. However most cases need a mandibular osteotomy. P.T.O.

Figures 11.25a and 11.25b show a moderate degree of vertical maxillary excess with incompetent upper lip and marked incisor exposure. The maxillary impaction corrected the vertical height, labial contact and autorotation improved the chin profile.

The combination of vertical maxillary excess with a vertical chin excess requires careful consideration especially with a degree of mandibular retrognathism.

The correction requires a Le Fort I elevation, together with a mandibular advancement and a combination of vertical chin reduction with an anterior advancement genioplasty (Figures 11.26a to 11.26h).

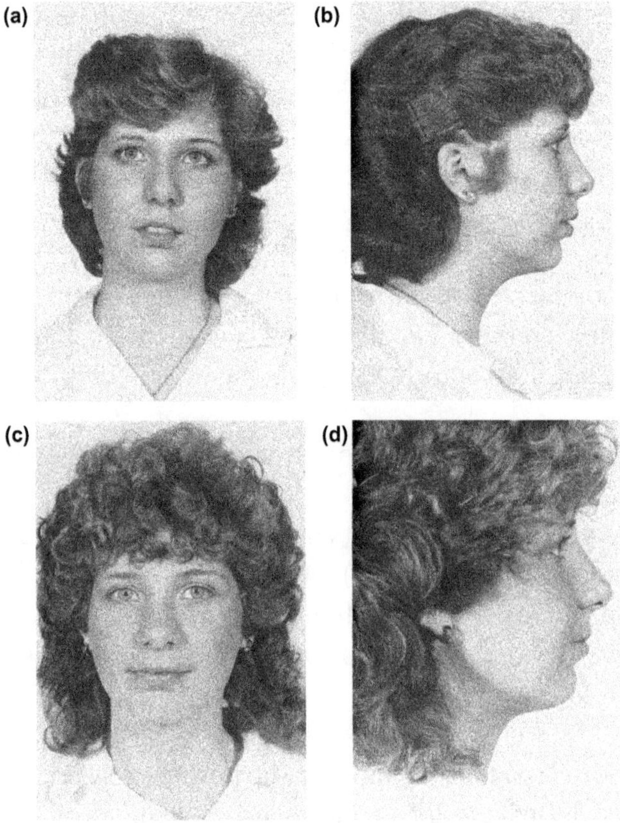

Figure 11.25 (**a**) and (**b**) Moderate vertical maxillary excess with incompetent long upper lip and marked incisor exposure. Maxillary impaction corrected the vertical height, labial contact and autorotation improved the chin profile.

Vertical Chin Excess (VCE)

If this is not great and is associated with VME, treat the maxilla and leave the chin alone as the forward autorotation of the mandible or an associated mandibular setback procedure invariably reduces the vertical chin profile.

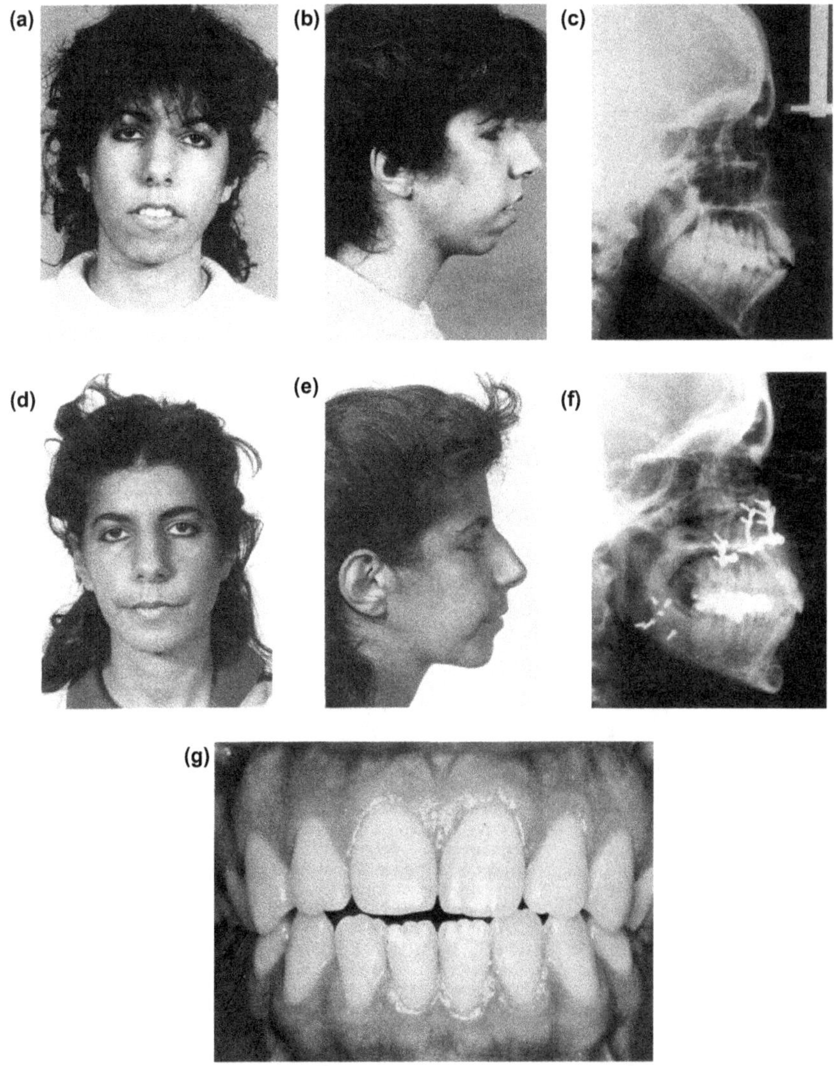

Figure 11.26 Vertical maxillary excess with a vertical chin excess but mandibular retrognathism. Hence the correction requires a Le Fort I elevation, together with a mandibular advancement and a vertical chin reduction but with an anterior augmentation genioplasty. **(a)** to **(c)** and **(g)** Preoperative. **(d)** to **(f)** and **(h)** Postoperative.

(h)

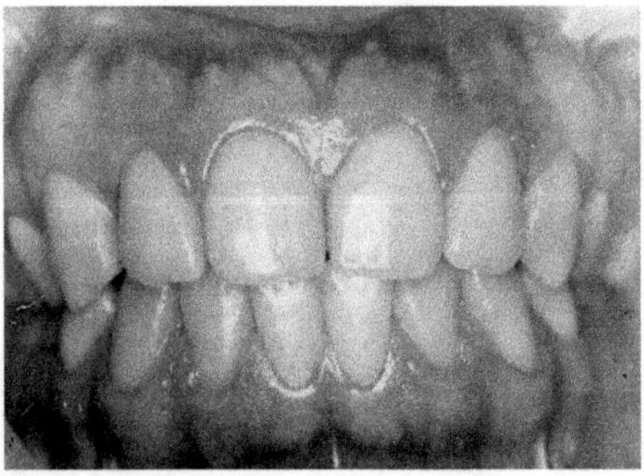

Figure 11.26 (*Continued*)

If VCE is significant or is the principal cause of the long face, a wedge reduction genioplasty is the treatment of choice (Figure 11.27). Do warn all patients that the excess facial soft tissue may take 6–12 months to remodel after a large maxillary elevation.

Long faces with an anterior open bite are discussed in the next section.

Bimaxillary Proclination

Bimaxillary proclination is often well within the acceptable aesthetic norm for Africans and Asians. Whereas the mean interincisal angle for Caucasians is 135°, this falls to 125° for these racial groups. Therefore the need for correction will not only depend on the cephalometric analysis but also the patient's aesthetic expectations.

The more problematic presentation is a bimaxillary proclination in combination with an anterior open bite and incompetent lips which is discussed later (see Figure 11.31).

Treatment

Where the dental bases are normally related and the vertical facial proportions acceptable, the treatment of choice is orthodontic retroclination with fixed appliance therapy closing any interincisal

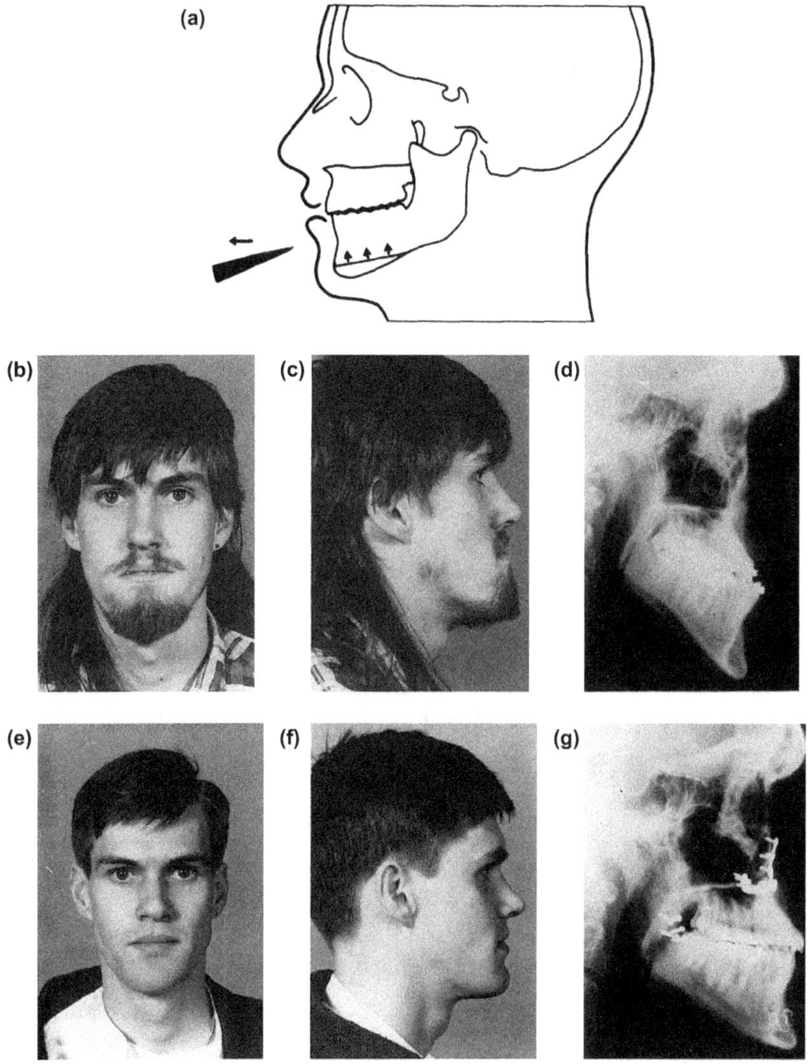

Figure 11.27 (**a**) Vertical chin excess is treated by a wedge reduction genioplasty preserving the lower border. (**b**) to (**d**) Preoperative vertical maxillary excess combined with a vertical chin excess which is camouflaged with a beard. The vertical chin excess was reduced by the removal of a wedge of bone, in addition to a mandibular pushback. The Le Fort I elevation corrected the vertical maxillary excess. (**e**) to (**g**) Postoperative.

spacing. If the patient will not accept this, the alternative management consists of upper and lower anterior segmental osteotomies utilising space from the extraction of all four first premolars.

If the deformity includes an anterior open bite this can be closed surgically but if related to an enlarged tongue, a tongue reduction is carried out at the same time (see Figure 11.31). Unfortunately the all-surgical solution may create two problems.

i) Model surgery may show that with markedly proclined incisors the rotation required to correct the interincisal angle will produce distally inclined upper canines, and in the lower alveolus a step defect between the canines and second premolars. This is an obvious indication for orthodontics rather than a surgical correction.
ii) Anterior segmental osteotomies in patients with an increased facial height and an excessive upper incisor show can be very unsatisfactory. If there is initially an excess of dentoalveolar exposure on smiling, this will be exaggerated by segmental surgery without a Le Fort I upward impaction. This problem will be reviewed in the next section.

The Open Bite Deformity (Apertognathia)

Of all the dentofacial deformities the anterior open bite can be the most challenging. Relapse is well recognised but has become less of a problem with the Le Fort I osteotomy with its segmental modifications and rigid fixation.

Open bite is commonly classified as dental (acquired) or skeletal (congenital). This classification is not wholly reliable.

The dental open bite has been considered an acquired deformity because it primarily affects the anterior teeth and is usually attributed to childhood habits such as thumb sucking, with perpetuation of the gap by a tongue thrust to close an inadequate lip seal. However, not all so called dental open bites can be associated with such habits and not infrequently the incompetent lip seal is due to an increased lower facial height. In other words, the problem, although localised, can be a congenital skeletal deformity or rarely secondary to an enlarged tongue (see Figure 11.32). The principal diagnostic feature of the true acquired open bite is a normal maxillary-mandibular plane angle of 27 ± 5°.

The Skeletal Open Bite

The skeletal open bite has an increased maxillary-mandibular plane angle (>35°) and may be localised or extend posteriorly into the molar region (see Figure 11.33).

A similar deformity may arise from a loss of ramus height due to a variety of causes, including bilateral condylar fractures, degenerative arthopathies, idiopathic condylysis or following resorptive condylar remodelling in neuromuscular disturbances of the face.

There are two principal types of skeletal open bite with important surgical implications.

i) Class II (Figure 11.28). Here the mandible appears to be rotated backwards and may be small. The maxillary occlusal plane is usually tilted upwards and forwards with an increased posterior superior dentoalveolar height. Some patients also appear to have a reduced anterior maxillary dentoalveolar height. The overall appearance is that of a skeletal Class II jaw relationship with a long lower face.
ii) Class III (Figure 11.29). Here the mandible is large with a normal maxilla. The posterior inferior facial height is in excess of 44% of the total posterior facial height. The overall appearance is a skeletal Class III with a long lower face.

Therefore a more useful open bite classification would be:

1. Dentoalveolar open bite: where the deformity is a localised dentoalveolar defect with normal facial proportions.

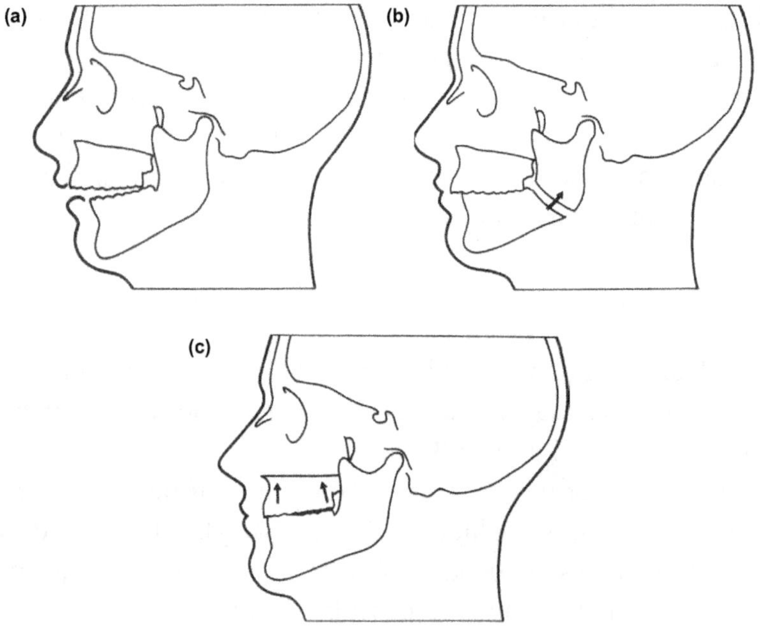

Figure 11.28 (**a**) Any attempt to correct a marked class I or class II anterior open bite with a ramus osteotomy which stretches the 'pterygomasseteric sling' will lead to a relapse. (**b**) The arrow indicates the strong musculofascial relapsing force. (**c**) A Le Fort I elevation with a posterior upward rotation allows the entire mandible to autorotate forwards and close the open bite within musculofascial constraints of the posterior facial height.

a) Congenital.
b) Acquired, e.g. sucking habits, alveolar trauma, enlarged tongue (including lymphangioma, haemangioma), and neuromuscular disturbances.

2. Skeletal open bite: where the dentoalveolar separation may be localised or extensive and is associated with an increased lower facial height and maxillary-mandibular plane angle. The two principal groups are:

   (a) Congenital.

   Class I, II or III.

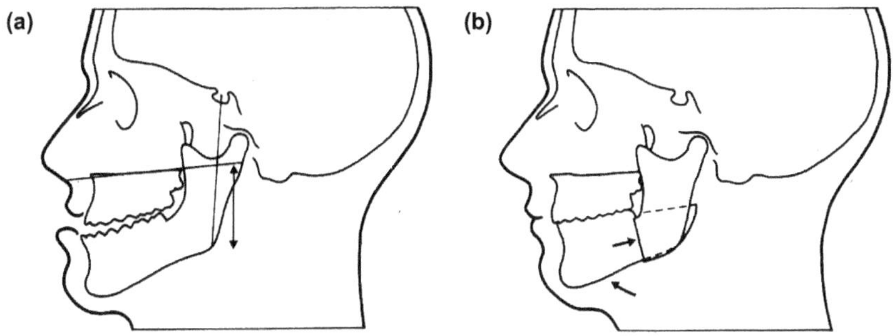

Figure 11.29 (**a**) and (**b**) The rare pure Class III open bite with a large ascending ramus may be corrected by a mandibular pushback procedure without relapse. Here, with the increased posterior inferior facial height (i.e. in excess of 44% of the total posterior facial height (S-Go) the pushback and rotation osteotomy do not stretch the "pterygomasseteric sling". See Case Figure 11.35 (p. 301).

(b) Acquired.

Bilateral condylar fractures, malunited untreated maxillary fractures, destructive arthopathies, idiopathic condylysis, condylar remodelling due to muscular dysfunction, acromegaly.

The Dento-Alveolar Open Bite

Treatment

Open bite deformities restricted to the anterior dentoalveolar segment with a normal facial height and proportions, can be successfully corrected with either orthodontics or segmental surgery, rotating the upper incisors downwards (Wassmund) and elevating the lower incisor segment (Kole) (Figure 11.31). However, this will only be successful if, on completion

a) the lip seal is competent and relaxed;
b) there is no excessive display of the upper incisors especially on smiling; and
c) the tongue is not enlarged.

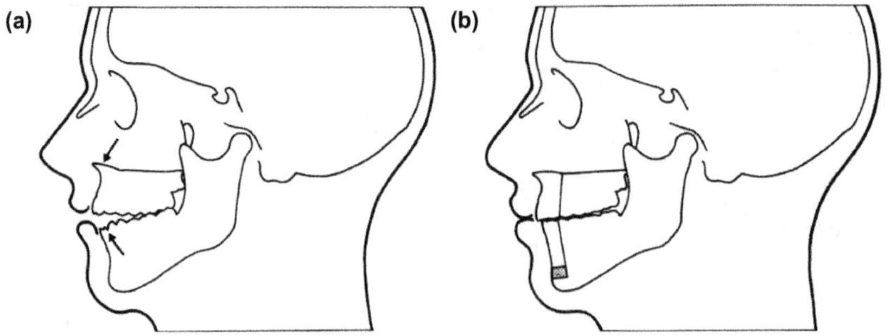

Figure 11.30 (**a**) and (**b**) An anterior (dentoalveolar) open bite with appropriate orthodontic preparation can be closed with bimaxillary anterior segmental osteotomies. The preoperative dentoalveolar open bite is treated by levelling of the upper incisors orthodontically and raising the lower incisors surgically. See Figure 11.31.

The choice of surgery will be determined by the height of the gap and the length of the upper lip. Minor degrees of incisor open bite may be corrected with a maxillary anterior segmental osteotomy (Wassmund/Wunderer). Where the separation is larger it is necessary to close part of the gap with an additional lower segmental osteotomy (Kole) (Figure 11.31). The lower incisor segment may be rotated or elevated with an interpositional graft. The graft material may be rib or iliac crest, or an alloplastic material such as hydroxyapatite.

However be sure that

i) its closure would not expose more than 4 mm of tooth below the upper lip margin and would therefore be better treated as a skeletal open bite incorporating a Le Fort I impaction.
ii) the patient does not require a tongue reduction, The treatment of a large tongue combined with an anterior open bite is shown in Figure 11.32.

The Skeletal Open Bite: Classes I and II

Attempts to treat these cases with operations on the mandible alone invariably gave rise to relapse, regardless of the procedure and the period of fixation (see Figures 11.28 and 11.32).

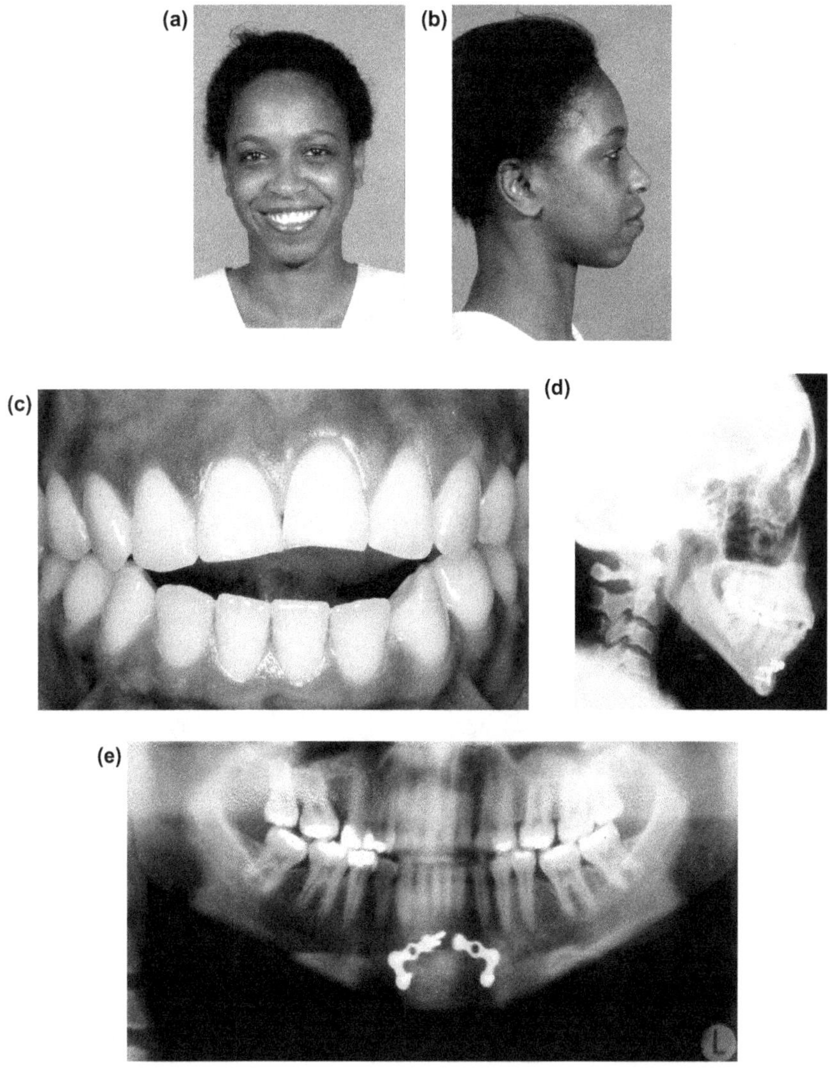

Figure 11.31 Dental anterior open bite treated with a combination of orthodontics and surgery.

The anatomical problem is that of rotating a retroplaced mandible upwards and forwards around the fulcrum created by the second or third molar teeth. This overextends the pterygomasseteric musculofascial sling. Unfortunately no surgical ingenuity can beat this

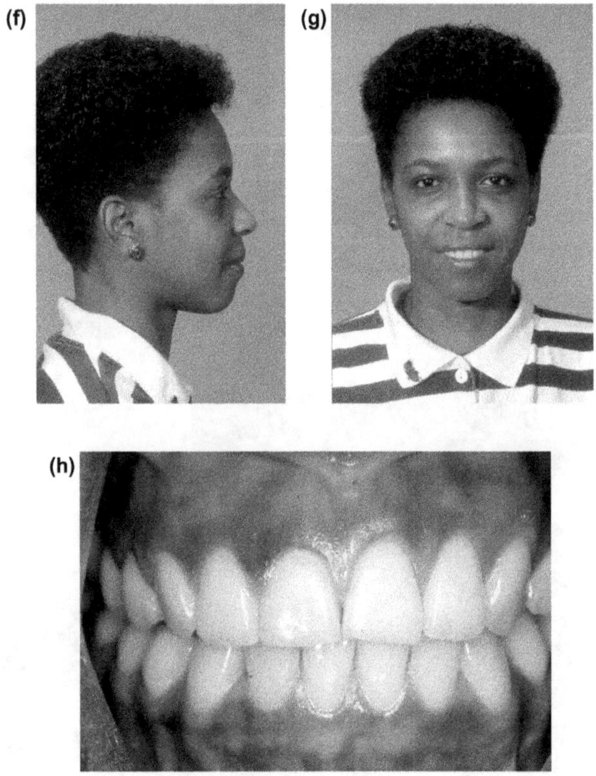

Figure 11.31 (*Continued*)

restraining force (Figure 11.33). If however the maxillary occlusal plane is normal, minor to moderate degrees of open bite can be treated with a sagittal split osteotomy and robust rigid fixation.

Treatment

The aims of the surgery are to produce a normal maxillary occlusal plane by reducing the posterior facial height with a Le Fort I impaction. This allows the mandible to rotate forwards and close the open bite. As always the starting point is the upper incisor-lip relationship. If it is satisfactory and the articulated study models show that the maxillary

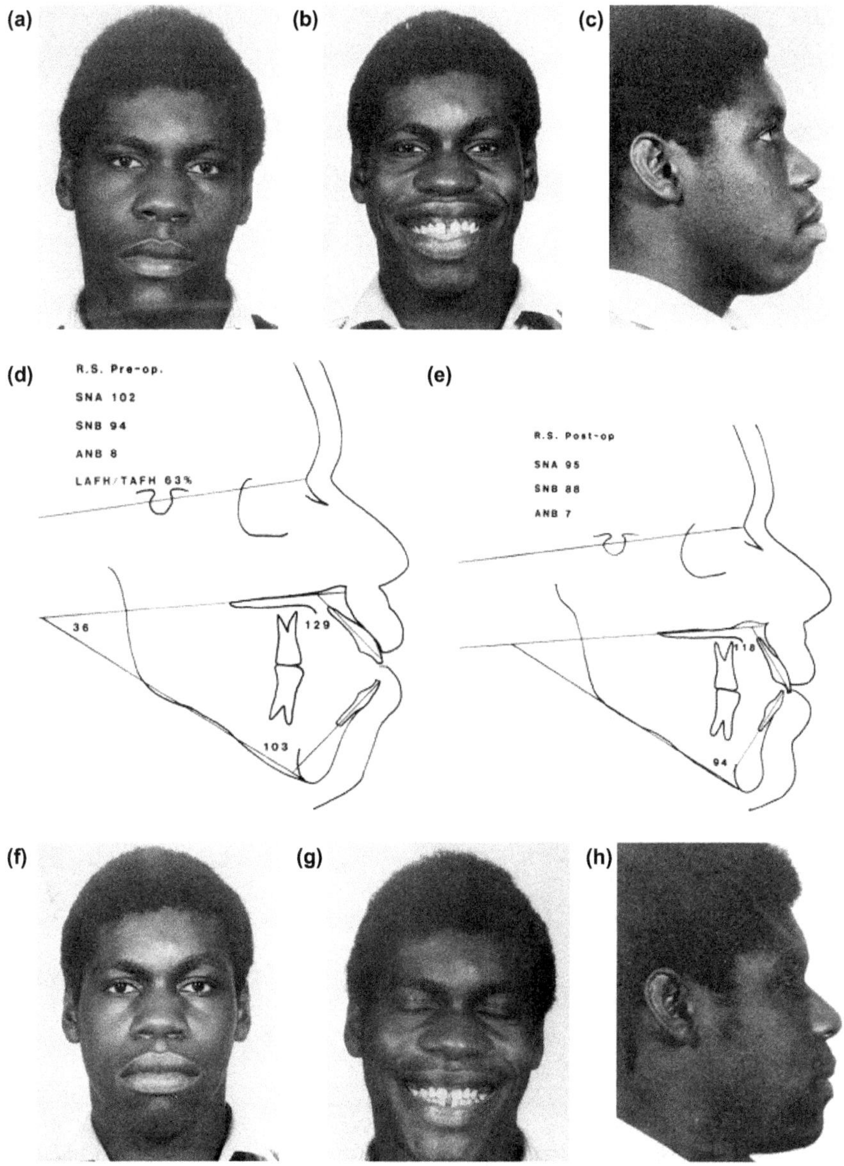

Figure 11.32 The combination of large tongue and anterior open bite treated by tongue reduction and segmental surgery. (**a**) to (**d**) Preoperative. (**b**) The tongue-incisor relationship with the molars in occlusion. (**f**) to (**h**) Postoperative.

(a) (b) (c) (d)

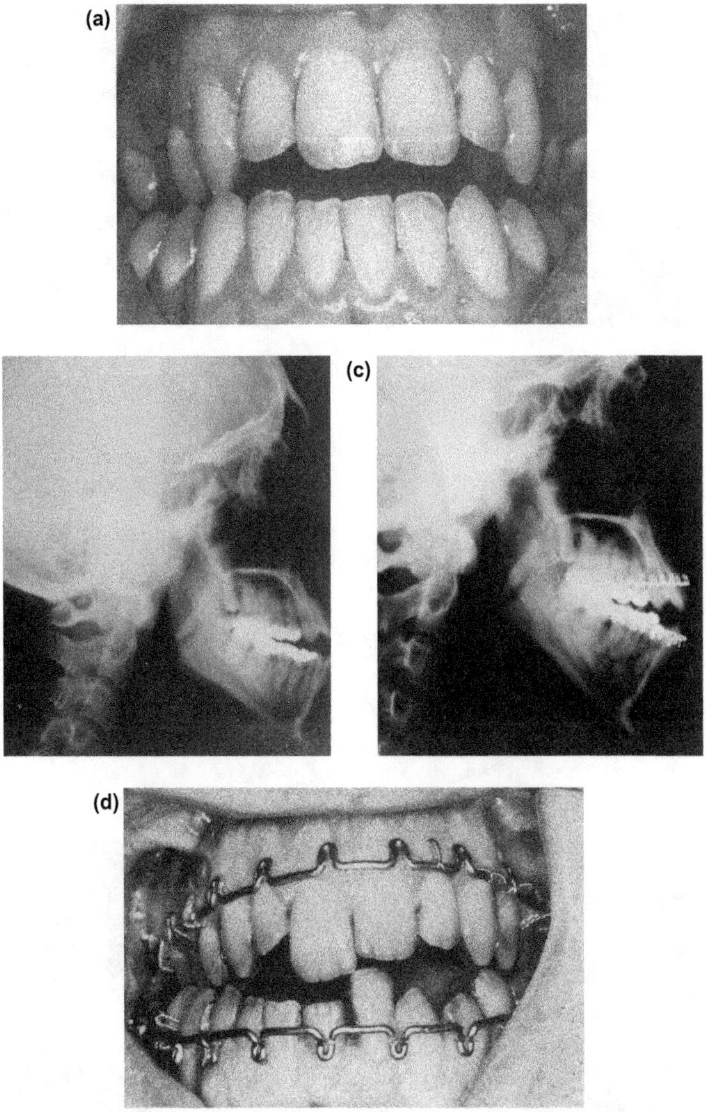

Figure 11.33 An attempt was made to close this skeletal Class I open bite **(a)** and **(b)** with a sagittal split osteotomy, interosseous wiring and arch bar intermaxillary fixation. The postoperative illustrations **(c)** and **(d)** show the arch bars after the removal of the IMF. Note that the relapsing force was able to extrude several incisor teeth despite the intermaxillary fixation.

occlusal plane will occlude with the autorotated mandibular teeth, surgery may be limited to a Le Fort I osteotomy with removal of a posterior maxillary wedge This wedge will equal the anterior open bite as measured in millimetres between the incisal edges (Figure 11.34).

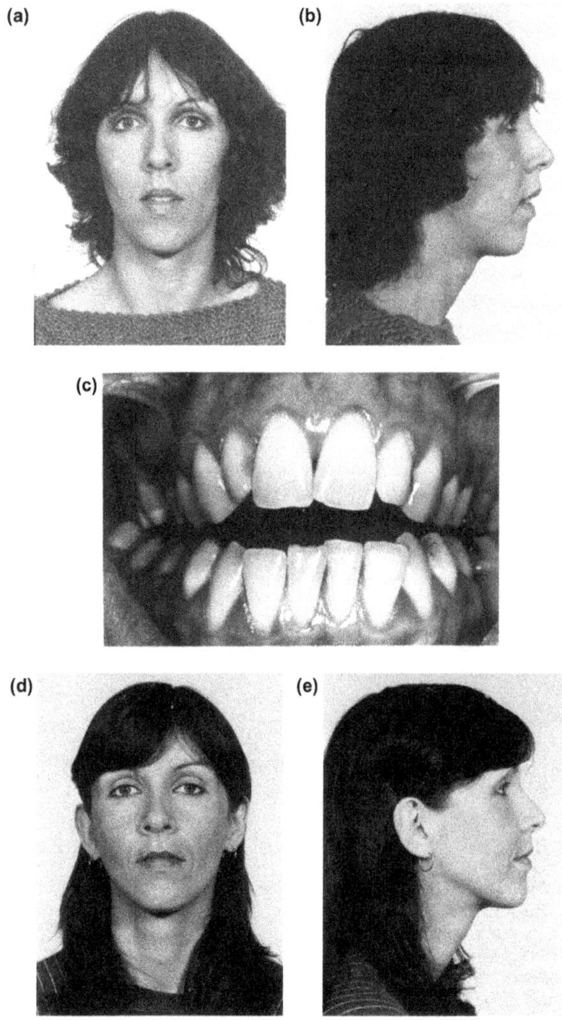

Figure 11.34 Long face with incompetent lips, narrow alar width and anterior open bite corrected with a posterior Le Fort I elevation. **(a)** to **(d)** Preoperative. **(e)** to **(h)** Postoperative.

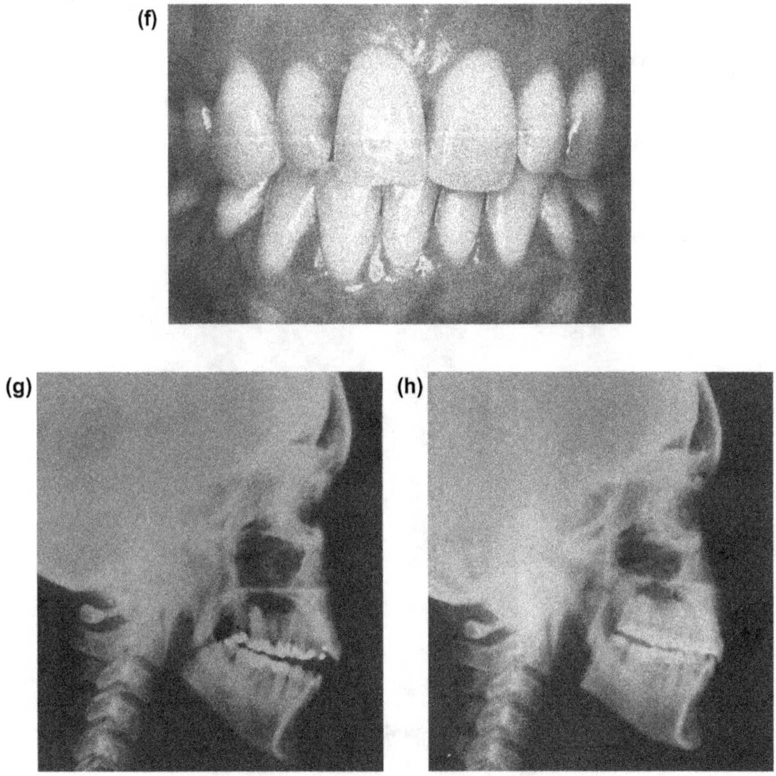

Figure 11.34 (*Continued*)

Where there is an element of vertical maxillary excess identified clinically by an increased anterior alveolus and incisor exposure, then a differential Le Fort I vertical impaction osteotomy designed to include the remove of bone both posteriorly and anteriorly, but with more from the back than front.

Variations

1. Where both occlusal planes have exaggerated curves of Spee they will require flattening either orthodontically or surgically. Orthodontic levelling of the maxillary and mandibular

occlusal planes is done with fixed appliances, but in severe cases it is impossible to produce matching occlusal tables. In this case the incisor and canines are levelled independently of the buccal segments requiring segmental surgery to achieve flat interdigitating occlusal planes. The surgical protocol will be:

i) In the maxilla, an anterior segmental section is carried out between the canine and premolars from above after the down-fracture. This allows a downward rotation of the incisor segment flattening the maxillary occlusal plane.
ii) The maxilla is then elevated as a whole.
iii) In the mandible a segmental elevation or anterior mandibulotomy may also be necessary (Figure 11.35).

2. The maxillary arch may have to be widened orthodontically or surgically to accommodate the lower dentition. In the latter case a midline section from above is required.
3. Where Class II retrognathism is marked, the maxillary elevation is carried out with a forward movement of the mandible by a sagittal split osteotomy with an augmentation genioplasty.

The Skeletal Open Bite Class III

Treatment

1. a) Where there is no VME and the maxillary occlusal plane is normally inclined, but the mandibular ramus and body length are increased (which can be confirmed by the posterior lower facial height being in excess of 44% of the total posterior facial height), a sagittal split osteotomy is performed to displace the mandibular body upwards and backwards to occlude with the maxillary teeth

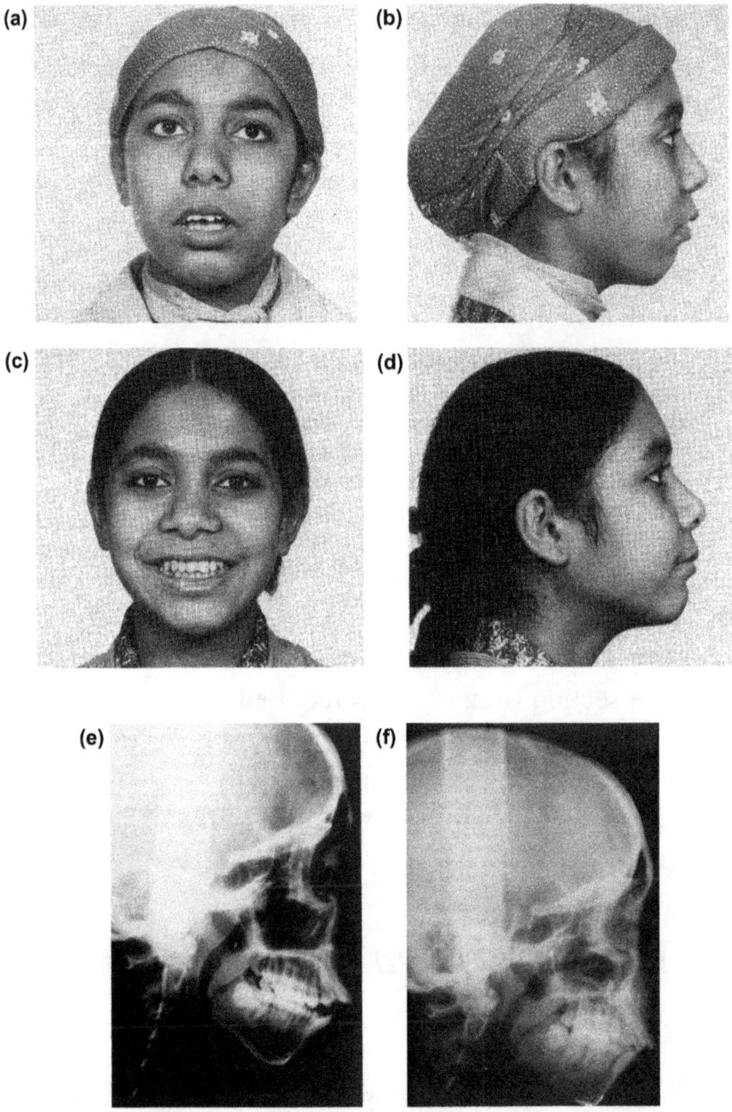

Figure 11.35 Orthodontic preparation was not possible for this patient with diphenyl hydantoin gingival hyperplasia, vertical maxillary excess, an anterior open bite and a marked curve of Spee. Therefore a Le Fort I elevation was combined with an anterior segmental osteotomy to level the occlusal plane and correct the incision lip relationship. The mandible autorotated to close the open bite. **(a)** to **(c)** Preoperative. **(d)** to **(f)** Postoperative.

(Figures 11.29 and 11.36). Bicortical screws or well placed buccal bone plates will provide end result stability.

b) Where there is an associated degree of maxillary retrusion this can be corrected by a Le Fort I forward movement which will reduce the open bite and mandibular setback.

2. In the more common, mixed case, consisting of a prognathous mandible with a VME, a Le Fort I elevation of the maxilla will be essential. This will increase the degree of mandibular prognathism and therefore the pushback (Figure 11.37).

The Large Tongue

This is an area of some uncertainty. Most of the tongue lies in the oropharynx, where it is paradoxically called the posterior "third". The anterior two-thirds is a very adaptive and mobile organ which cannot be easily assessed anatomically or functionally. Tongue reduction was formerly carried out on theoretical grounds to prevent a relapse following the reduction in oral volume by a body ostectomy procedure for prognathism. The custom ceased with the introduction of the sagittal split osteotomy with its increased stability because it was assumed that the tongue moved backwards with the mandible. As tongue position is determined by the hyoid bone, which is not affected by this operation, surgical tongue reduction was correctly discarded for the wrong reason.

However, some patients do present with proclined incisors, a localised anterior open bite and a clinically large tongue. The management of such a case should be as follows:

1. Reduce the tongue at the same operation as the open bite segmental osteotomies. With careful haemostasis, antiodema steroidal cover, and careful postoperative nursing, this presents no great problem.

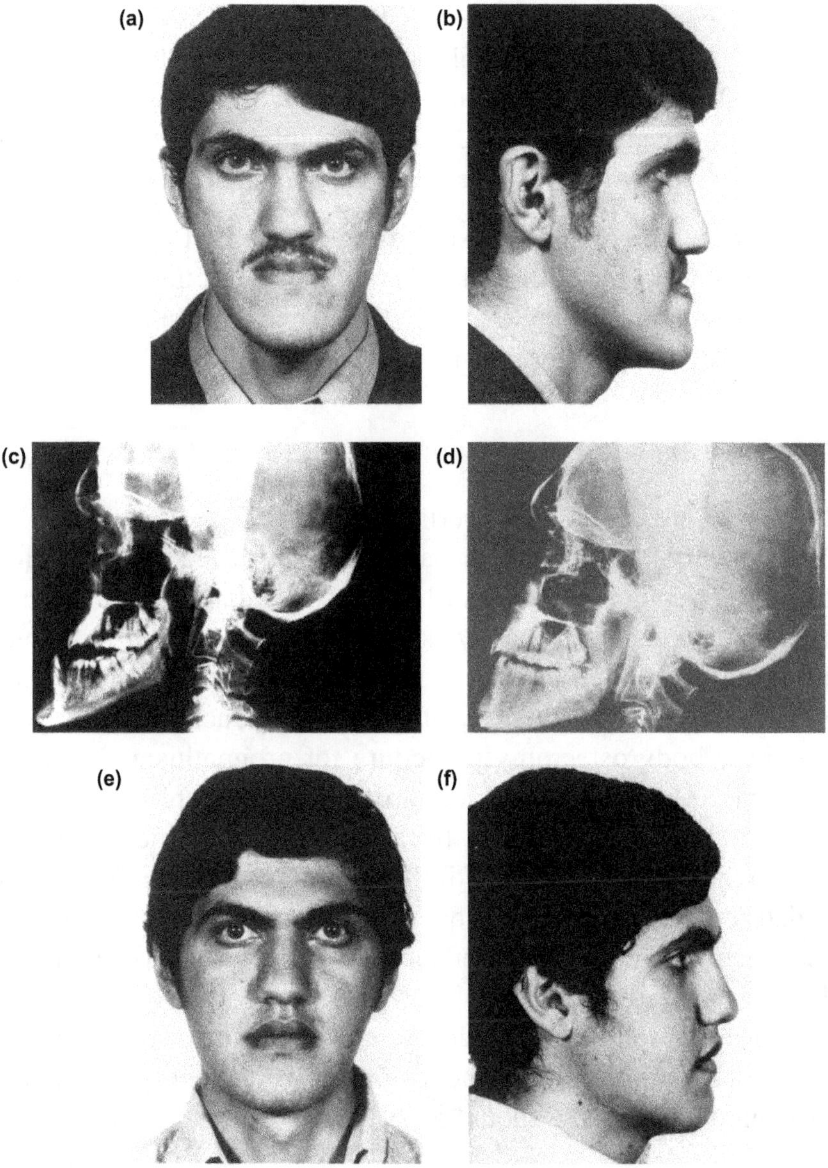

Figure 11.36 An non-decompensated Class III skeletal open bite which was treated only by a mandibular setback and trimming of the chin point. (**a**) to (**c**) Preoperative. (**d**) to (**f**) Postoperative.

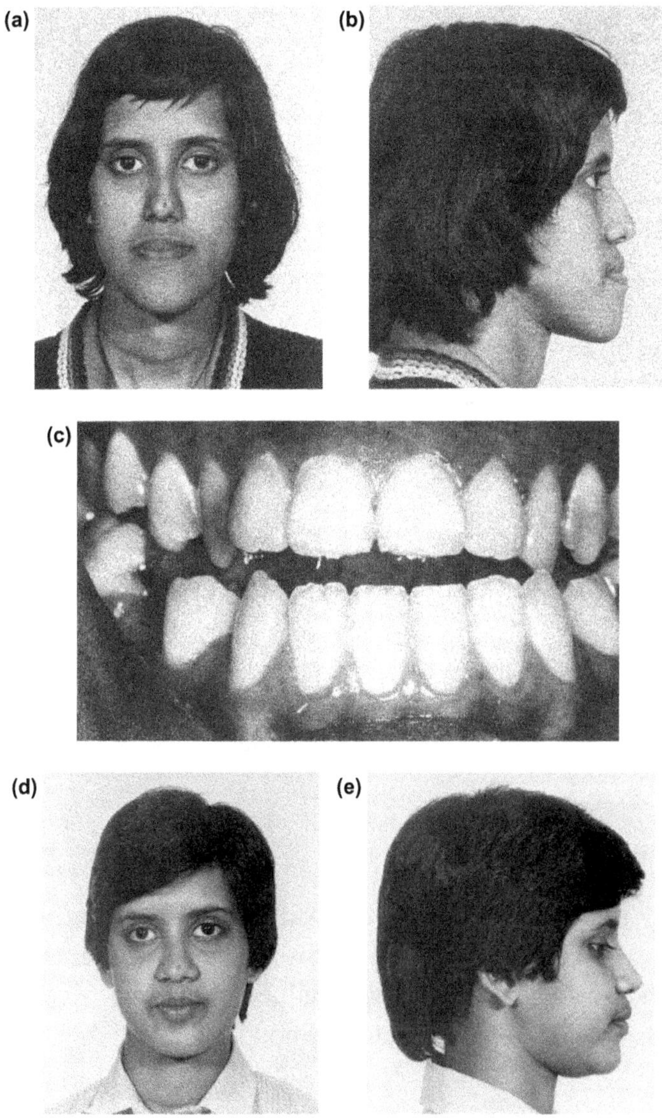

Figure 11.37 A non-decompensated combination of vertical maxillary excess, mandibular prognathism and an open bite **(a)** to **(d)**. This was corrected by a Le Fort I elevation and a mandibular setback **(e)** to **(h)**. Note the postoperative facial soft tissue excess which has remodelled over the subsequent 4 years; **(i)** shows the stable result 4 years later.

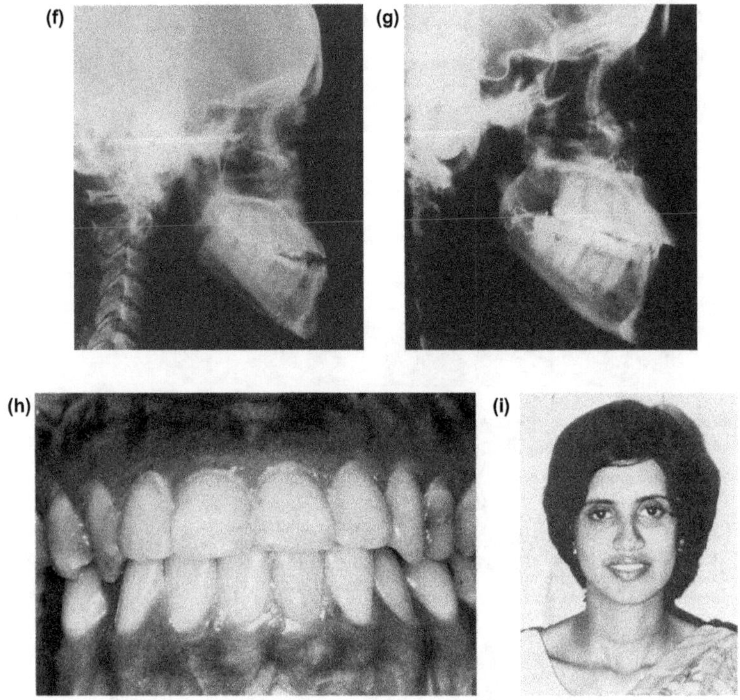

Figure 11.37 (*Continued*)

Or, if in doubt:

2. Carry out the osteotomies but warn the patient that if a relapse becomes obvious, particularly with recurrent proclination of the lower incisors, then a tongue reduction will be necessary. The relapse can then be corrected orthodontically.

The Short Face

This is uncommon in non-cleft patients and, as usual, can present in three forms:

1. Where the shortage is essentially in the lower face. This is the marked Class II division 1 mandible with a small anterior

dentoalveolar height and an everted lower lip. The mid-face is normal or acceptable (Figure 11.8).

2. Where there is a decrease in middle facial height, occasionally with a small alveolar process and small teeth in both jaws (Figure 11.38). As cleft patients present with additional problems, they will be dealt with separately in Chapter 12.
3. A combination of both.

Treatment

1. Lower face deficiency

There is usually over-eruption of the incisors, producing a marked curve of Spee. Therefore the choice is between:

i) a) Preoperative orthodontic levelling of the occlusal plane.
   b) A mandibular advancement. Bone can also be inserted as a vertical augmentation sandwich genioplasty (Figure 11.38).

ii) a) Orthodontic levelling of the occlusal plane at two levels.
   b) An anterior mandibulotomy which will flatten the occlusal plane and simultaneously increase the lower facial height.
   c) A mandibular advancement (Figure 11.38).

2. Mid-face deficiency

Treatment is by a Le Fort I osteotomy with an interpositional bone graft to lower the maxilla (Figure 11.39).

Preoperatively an estimate must be made of the required increase in facial height. This may be determined clinically by inserting wax wafers of increasing thickness between the teeth until the desired profile "in occlusion" with the lips at rest is achieved. Add 25% to give the immediate postoperative vertical separation of the jaws and height of the interpositional graft. This is measured and recorded.

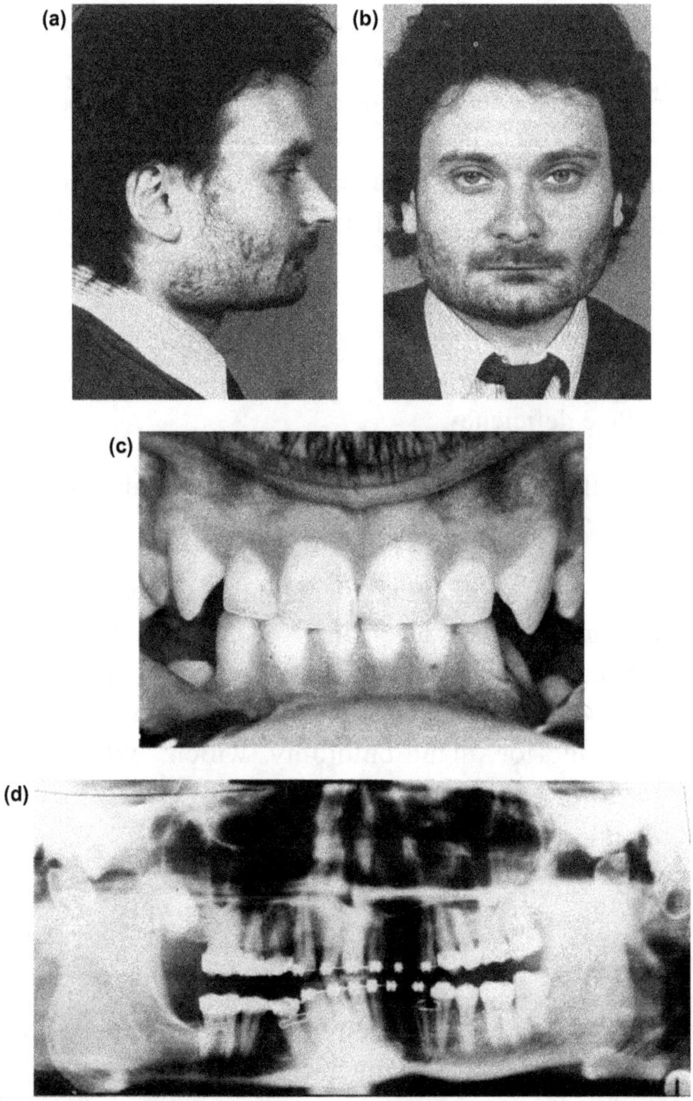

Figure 11.38 (**a**) to (**m**) A short face with vertical maxillary deficiency and also a marked lack of mandibular vertical height. This is an acquired developmental defect due to prolonged wearing of a Milwaukee brace to correct scoliosis in childhood. Preoperative (**a**) to (**d**). Presurgical orthodontics levelled the incisor and buccal occlusal planes independently. The maxilla has been lowered by a Le Fort I osteotomy with split rib interpositional grafts fixed with bone plates. The mandible

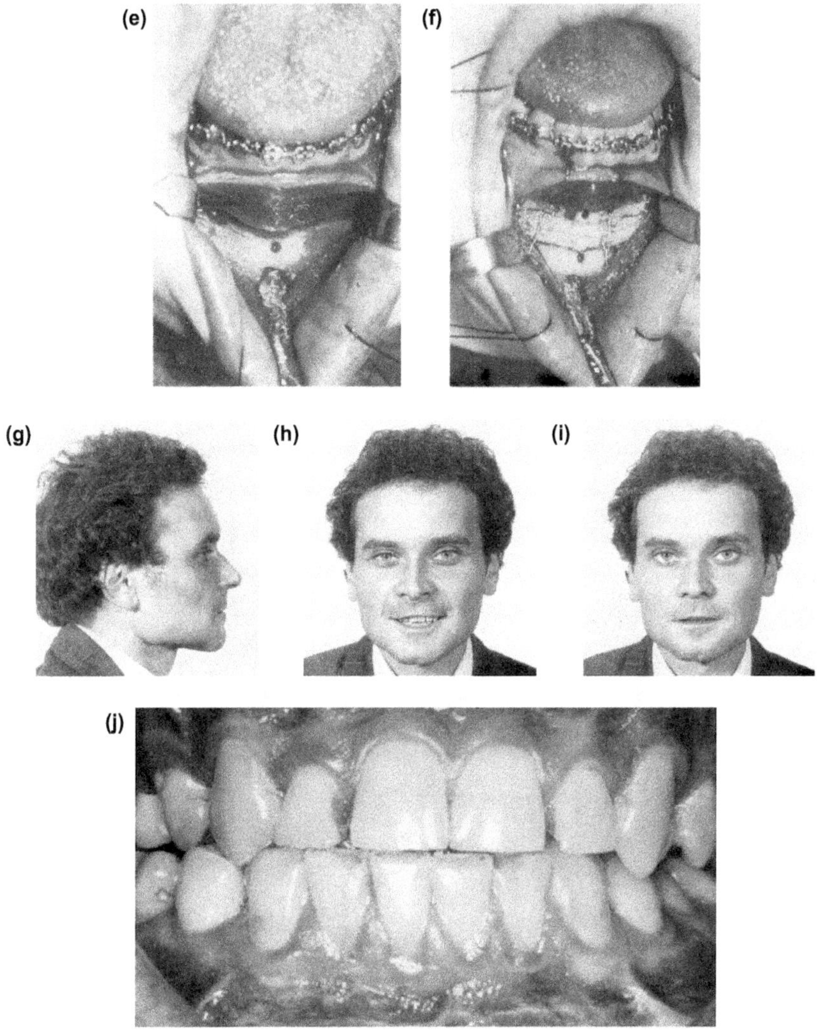

Figure 11.38 (*Continued*) has been advanced to correct the retrognathism. The underdeveloped anterior inferior dentoalveolar height has been corrected by a combination of a segmental mandibulotomy set down with a Proplast interpositional graft. The mandibulotomy also flattens the occlusal place **(e)** to **(i)**. Genioplasty section before **(j)** and after insertion of a alloplast wedge **(k)**. Preoperative **(l)** and postoperative **(m)** lateral skull radiographs.

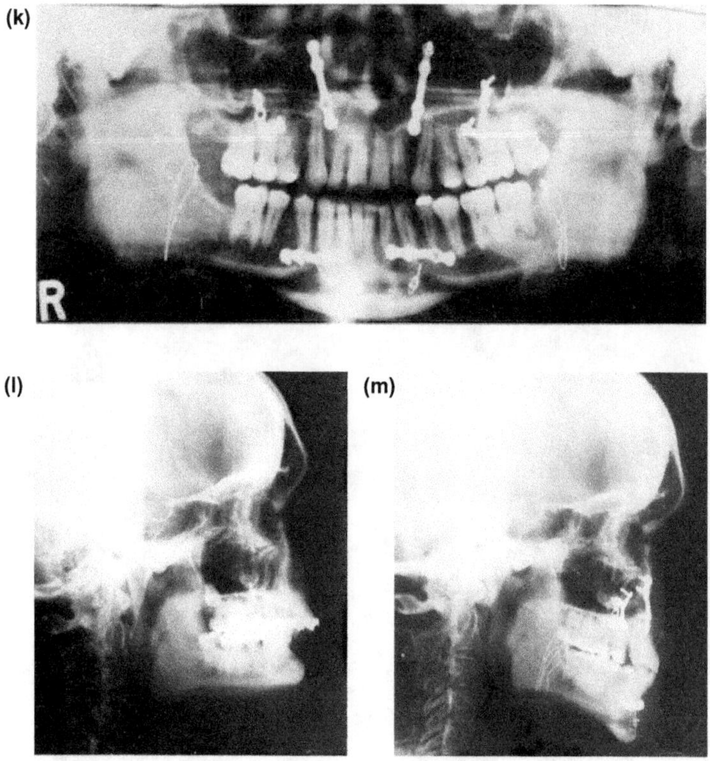

Figure 11.38 (*Continued*)

Operative Procedure

1. The cuts of the sagittal split are made but not separated.
2. A Le Fort I osteotomy is carried out, with the maxilla well separated from the pterygoid plates. The maxilla is then wired temporarily to the unchanged mandible using an intermediate wafer.
3. Using dividers and ruler to confirm the planned separation (i.e. increased facial height) measured from the canine tips to the inner canthi, bone plates are screwed to the upper border of the maxillary osteotomy, and then the split rib or iliac crest cancellous bone blocks are wedged between the bone cuts and

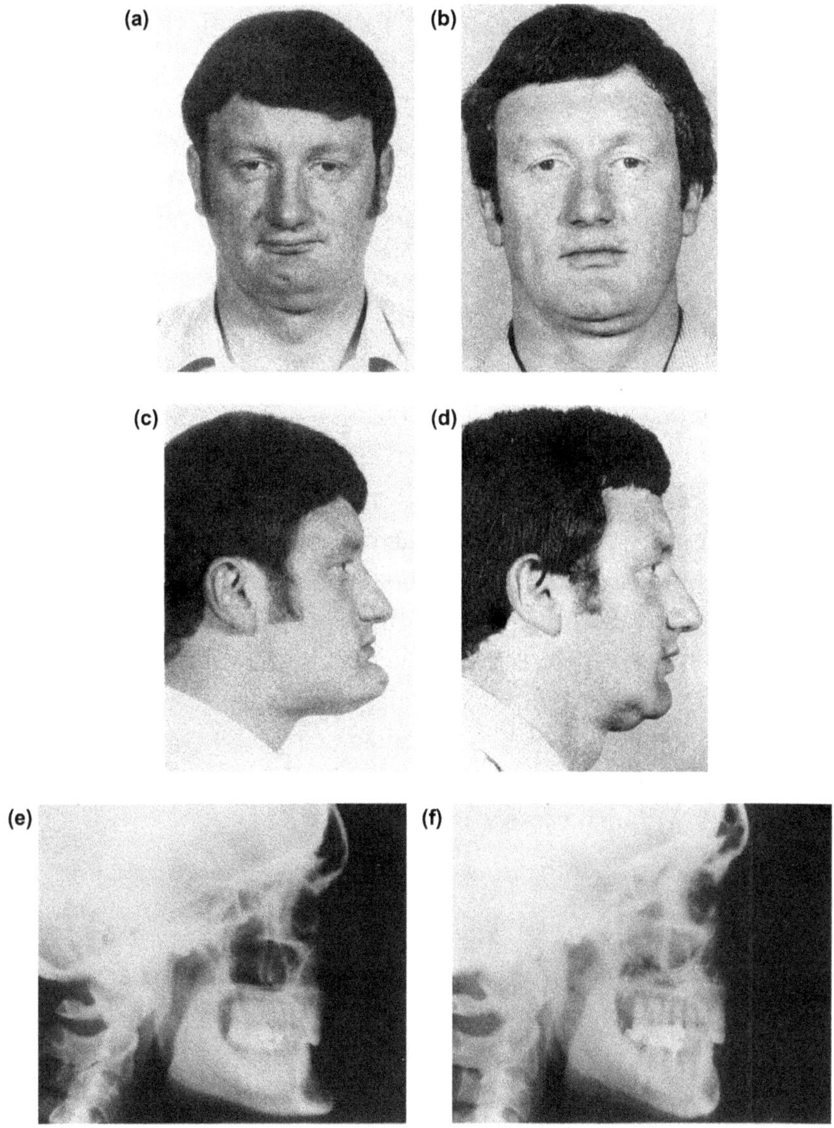

Figure 11.39 A short face due to a maxillary vertical deficiency with dentoalveolar hypoplasia. The maxilla was set down 1cm with iliac crest interpositional bone grafts and the mandible repositioned with sagittal split osteotomy. (**a**) to (**c**) Preoperative. (**d**) to (**f**) Postoperative.

secured with screws. Face the medullary surface of the split rib outwards against the periosteum to ensure the best opportunity for graft vascularisation (see Bone Grafts).
4. Intermaxillary fixation is released, the mandible is split and fixed using the final wafer.
5. The throat pack is removed and the nasopharynx and hypopharynx carefully aspirated.

Maxillary Asymmetry

Maxillary asymmetry may be:

i) Primary and associated with deformity of the whole facial skeleton. In mild disturbances it can be difficult to decide whether one side is reduced in height or the other increased. However, in primary deformities, in addition to the coronal tilt in the occlusal plane, there is usually a cant in the orbital plane.
ii) The late presentation of a secondary maxillary alveolar response to the lateral open bite in a unilateral mandibular hyperplasia. Fibrous dysplasia of the maxilla and slowly-growing benign tumours will also present in the same way.

Treatment

- Minor degrees of orbital asymmetry are acceptable and therefore the surgery only consists of levelling the occlusal plane by a Le Fort I osteotomy, removing bone on the long side.
- If the difference in height is split between the two sides the coronal ipsilateral upward rotation, creates a horizontal deficiency on the short side. This deficiency may be closed by inserting the removed bone fragments into the defect stabilised with screws and plates. A sagittal split or subsigmoid osteotomy will be required to rotate the mandible into occlusion with the repositioned maxilla (Figure 11.40).

(a) (b) (c) (d)

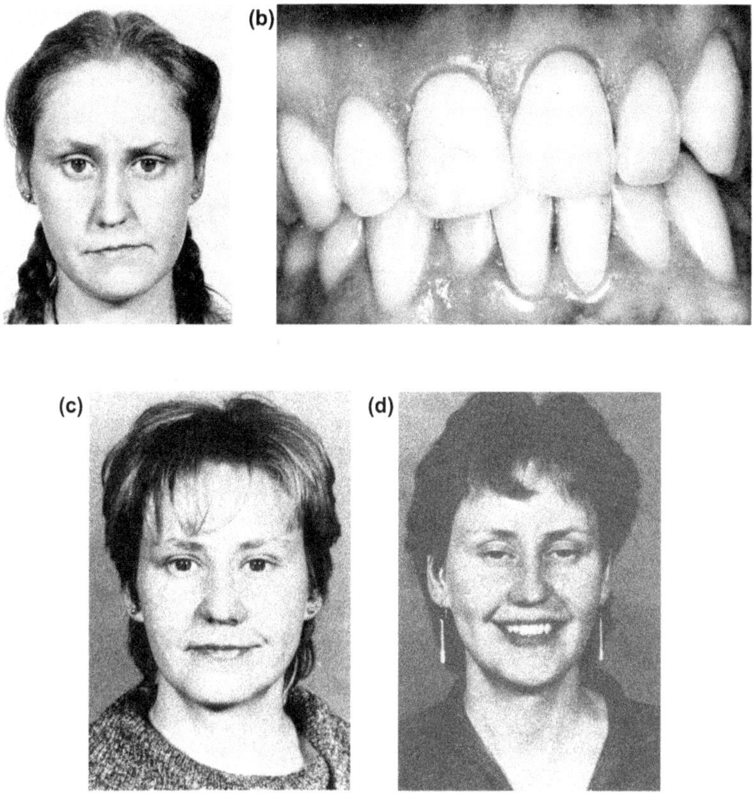

Figure 11.40 Maxillary asymmetry with a marked slope of the occlusal plane. This was corrected by bimaxillary osteotomies rotating the maxilla upwards on the right side, and bringing the mandible into occlusion with a bilateral sagittal split both jaws. A fillet of bone should be removed on the inner aspect of the right ascending ramus to allow it to rise in the coronal plane and occlude with the maxilla. (**a**) and (**b**) Preoperative. (**c**) and (**d**) Postoperative.

- With a unilateral maxillary fibrous dysplasia, a Le Fort I down-fracture allows the solid dysplastic tissue to be radically removed from orbital floor to antral floor, leaving the periosteum to regenerate the facial antral wall.

Encapsulated tumours, such as ossifying fibromas, may be removed in the same way.

Chapter 12

Secondary Cleft Lip and Palate Deformities

Peter Ayliffe and Tom Walker

Introduction

Cleft lip and palate deformities are the most common congenital deformities of the facial region. This chapter will focus on the secondary correction of cleft-related deformity.

The management of secondary deformity must involve the surgeon, orthodontist and speech pathologist working closely with the paediatrician, ear nose and throat surgeon, plastic surgeon, and clinical psychologist when appropriate.

The clinical problem depends on the type and severity of the cleft and on the type and quality of the primary surgery and any revisions of these "primary procedures". Compromises between function, aesthetics and growth have to be made which determine the timing of surgery. For instance the timing of palate repair is a balance between enabling speech development and optimum facial growth. What ever the compromise the number of operations must be kept to the minimum.

Important Factors

1. The amount of tissue in the original embryological defect (Figure 12.1).

   Although structures may be displaced, the amount of soft tissue is not usually deficient in the unrepaired unilateral or bilateral cleft deformity (Figures 12.2a and 12.2d). Impaired growth and development usually arise from subsequent surgery rather than inherent differences in growth potential. The exception is in some bilateral cases where the premaxilla and prolabial segment can be relatively small before surgical intervention (Figures 12.3a and 12.3b). True aplasia of tissue is uncommon although can be seen in cases of mid line clefting.
2. The nature and quality of the primary surgery.

   Facial deformity will develop as a consequence of scar contraction following surgery especially in the palate (Figures 12.4a and 12.4c).

   Patients with similar clefts repaired in different ways may exhibit different patterns of facial growth. Figures 12.5a and 12.5h illustrate two brothers, both with complete right side

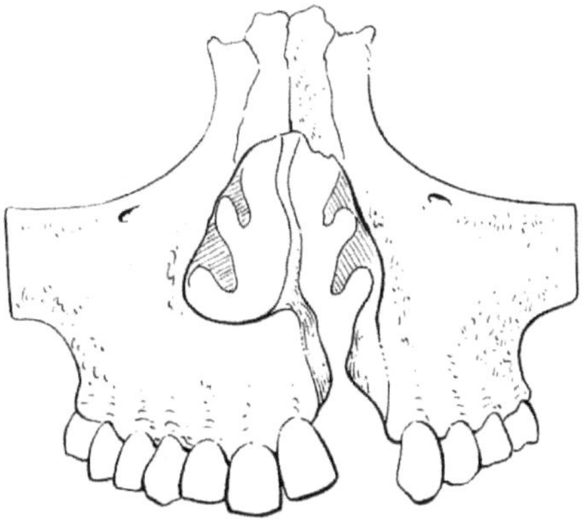

Figure 12.1 A complete cleft of the lip and palate through the alveolus in the region of the left lateral incisor with or without fistula extending into the nose.

unilateral cleft lip and palate operated using different palatal techniques demonstrating different mid facial growth.

3. Also important is the preservation of tissue. Tissue removal should be avoided whenever possible.

The surgical correction of skeletal cleft deformity presents a greater challenge than most orthognathic procedures. A variety of programmes for treating these cases is possible. Unfortunately the selection of operation is usually dictated by the surgeon's preference rather than objectively compared data.

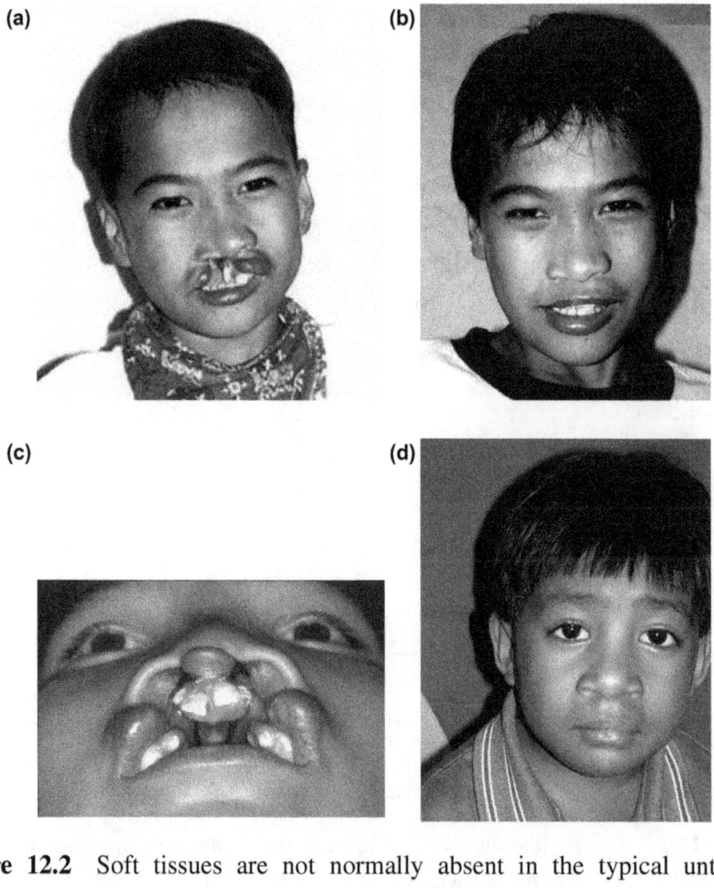

Figure 12.2 Soft tissues are not normally absent in the typical untreated unilateral or bilateral cleft **(a)**, **(c)** preoperatively, and **(b)**, **(d)** postoperatively.

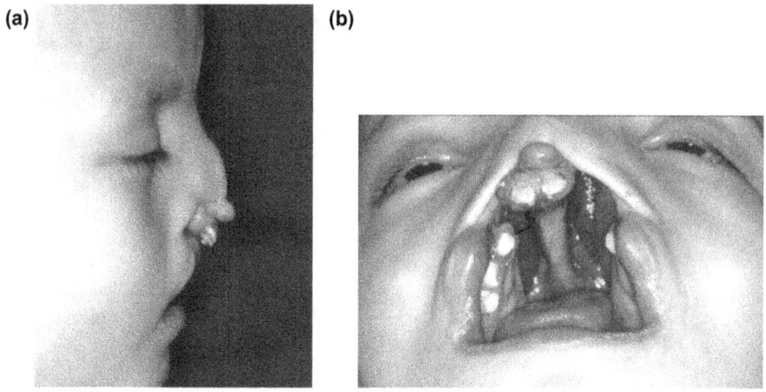

Figure 12.3 Hypoplasia may occur in bilateral cases — particularly of the premaxilla and prolabial segments.

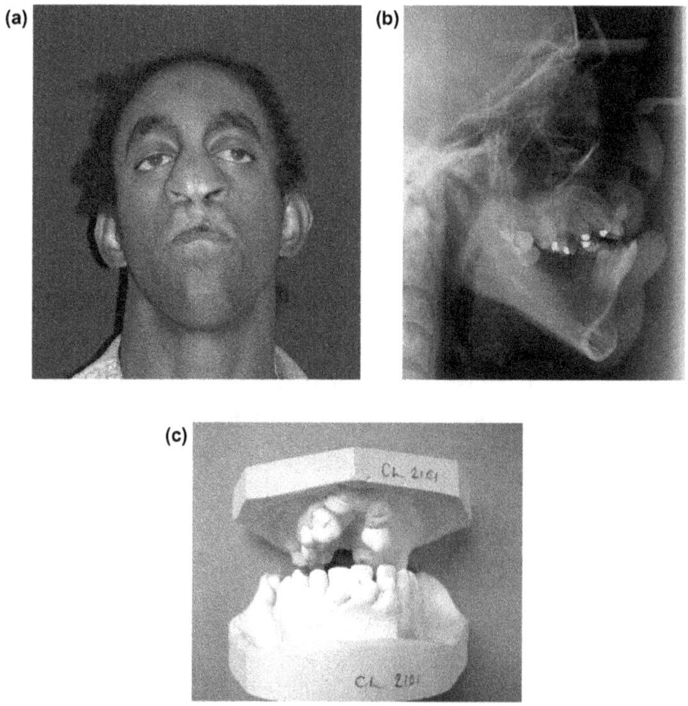

Figure 12.4 Surgery, particularly to the palate can cause secondary changes resulting in marked deformity of the mid-face.

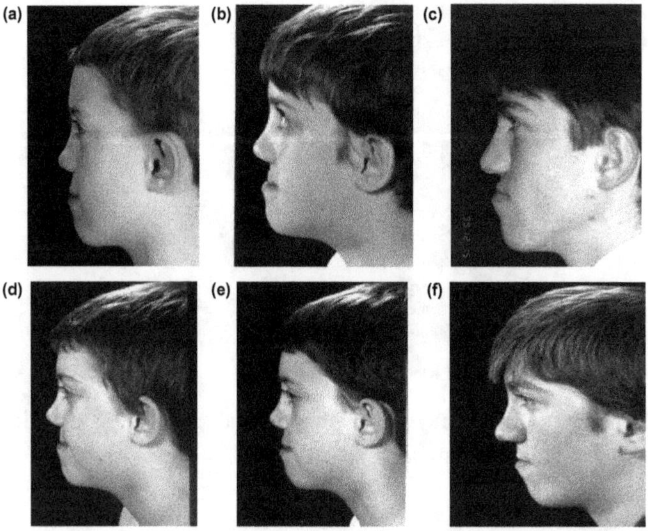

Figure 12.5 These photographs show the contrast in facial development of two brothers from 5 to 20 years of age. They had similar clefts but very dissimilar outcomes due to differing surgical corrections. The results show brother "**(a)** to **(c)**". would benefit from a bimaxillary correction of his relative mandibular prognathism, and brother "**(d)** to **(f)**" an augmention genioplasty.

Surgical Instrumentation

Intra-oral access is possible with a Mushin dental prop but this can be distracting at crucial moments. A self-retaining gag such as a Featherstone is better, but for ultimate ease one should use a cleft palate gag such as the Sommerlad modification of the Dott gag, which also provides simultaneous retraction.

The choice of needles is crucial, and include the 5/8 25 mm (Denys Browne), a 16 mm slim blade needle or the small J shaped compound curved needle mounted with 4/0 or 5/0 Vicryl Rapide (Ethicon). Children require fine soluble sutures. Small needles demand a fine-tipped ratchet needle holder, e.g. Stille Converse, and very fine dissecting forceps, e.g. Adsons. Subperiosteal flap dissection within a cleft also requires a small sharp periosteal elevator such as the McDonald, Friers pattern or even a Mitchell's trimmer.

Table 12.1 Pathways of care

Early stages of treatment

Aims:

1. Reconstruction of the labial sphincter and restoration of an acceptable appearance.
2. Reconstruction of the soft palate to allow speech development.
3. Avoid unnecessary surgery and enable optimal facial growth.
4. Ensure normal psychosocial development.

Means:

1. Lip repair within first 6 months.
2. Soft palate repair at one year of age.
3. Speech therapy and hearing assessment at 18 months, 3 years and 5 years.
4. Secondary hard palate surgery should be delayed as long as possible. Usually until 12 months.

Treatment in the mixed dentition

Aims:

1. Orthodontic alignment of the developing dentition.
2. Reconstruction of the alveolar cleft and dental arch form.
3. Oronasal fistula closure.
4. Restore normal symmetrical maxillary bony contour.
5. Stabilisation of the dentoalveolar segments.
6. Maintenance of a healthy adult dentition.

Means:

1. Orthodontics essential for surgery.
2. Alveolar reconstruction with bone grafting.
3. Segmental alveolar distraction osteogenesis where appropriate.
4. Fistula closure.
5. Preventative and restorative dental care.

Treatment in adolescence and early adulthood

Aims:

1. Correction of any disturbance of facial growth and skeletal imbalance.

(Continued)

Table 12.1 (*Continued*)

2. Reconstruction of nasal deformity.
3. Correction of any soft tissue deformity.
4. Correction of any occlusal disturbances.
5. Provision of an aesthetically pleasing smile.

Means:

1. Presurgical orthodontic treatment.
2. Malar maxillary distraction osteogenesis where appropriate.
3. Orthognathic surgery to correct secondary skeletal deformities.
4. Post-orthognathic orthodontics.
5. Residual fistula closure.
6. Dental reconstruction.
7. Definitive nose and lip correction.

The Surgical Procedures

Bone grafting is required to establish continuity of the cleft alveolus for the following reasons.

- The optimum time for alveolar bone grafting is between 7 and 12 years, before the permanent canine on the cleft side erupts and when half to two thirds of its root has formed.
- At this age, anteroposterior and transverse maxillary growth is practically complete apart from the alveolar development of the erupting permanent teeth. Hence grafting at this time does not affect mid face growth but provides the all important bone support for the erupting canines.
- The bone also enables orthodontic positioning of the canines.
- Creates a one piece maxilla for orthognathic surgery.
- Provides stabilisation for any prosthetic replacement.
- It is also possible to simultaneously graft the alar base.

Prior to grafting, presurgical orthodontics will have expanded the maxillary arch to restore the arch form between the major and lesser segments. The teeth adjacent to the cleft will have been aligned providing there is sufficient bone around their roots and a good periodontal attachment to accommodate the alignment.

If the premaxillary segment has been surgically repositioned forwards or orthodontic arch expansion has been used to facilitate the grafting procedure, a retaining appliance is essential to prevent collapse before consolidation of the bone graft.

Harvesting the alveolar bone graft

i. **Open harvesting** from the anterior iliac crest between the anterior superior spine and the adjacent curved crest. Before the incision, the integument is manually drawn superioromedially so the healed scar will lie infero-laterally and not over the crest. For children, access is achieved by a 5 cm. incision made through the skin, muscle and periosteum.
ii. **Harvesting cancellous bone using the Ayliffe trephine**.
iii. **Without donor site surgery**; The maxillary bone defects can be obturated with a mixture of demineralised bank bone and recombinant human morphogenetic protein (rhBMP2). This method eliminates the cost and complications of an additional operation.

The Problems

- A unilateral alveolar defect.
- Anterior oronasal fistula.
- Alar-base asymmetry.

Surgical Management

1. Instruments should comprise a basic intraoral surgical set with the addition of a fine periosteal elevator, such as a McDonald, Frier or Mitchell's trimmer, and skin hooks. Access may be gained with a Sommerlad modification of the Dott mouth gag.

2. The incision is made down to bone around the margin of the anterior fistula, except where the fistula lies high in the anterior vestibule beneath the upper lip. At this point there is no underlying bone and the incision is through mucosa only (Figures 12.7a).

   Figure 12.7b shows how the narrow strip at the cervical margin of the tooth is sliced to create as wide a band of de-epithelialised tissue as possible.

   The initial incision can be extended safely along the buccal sulcus overlying the lesser segment unless a segmental osteotomy is required.

   If the fistula or alveolar defect extends into the palate a palatal flap will need to be raised (Figure 12.7c).

   Subperiosteal dissection is directed into the fistula and the liberated soft tissues are pushed up towards the nasal cavity. Much of this tissue becomes redundant and can be cut away leaving just sufficient to form a nasal layer.
3. Where the soft tissues bridge the cleft, i.e. in the buccal sulcus and behind on the palate, two layers are created by sharp dissection.
4. If the fistula is wide enough the nasal layer can be closed with resorbable sutures on a very small needle (Figure 12.7d). If the bone defect is too narrow to insert a suture in the nasal layer (Figure 12.7e), a piece of oxidised cellulose (Surgicel, Ethicon Ltd, Edinburgh, UK) or acellular submucosal matrix can be inserted to seal the nasal surface of the cleft (Figure 12.7f). Any supernumerary teeth are extracted and cancellous bone chips are packed into the whole defect.

   Cancellous bone chips are obtained from the iliac crest and packed firmly into the bone cleft. The location of the scar needs to be considered. Stretching skin that would normally hide beneath underwear over the iliac crest can lead to the normscar being invisible when dressed. This scar can be stretched by the weight of the skin and poor support from the fascia underneath.

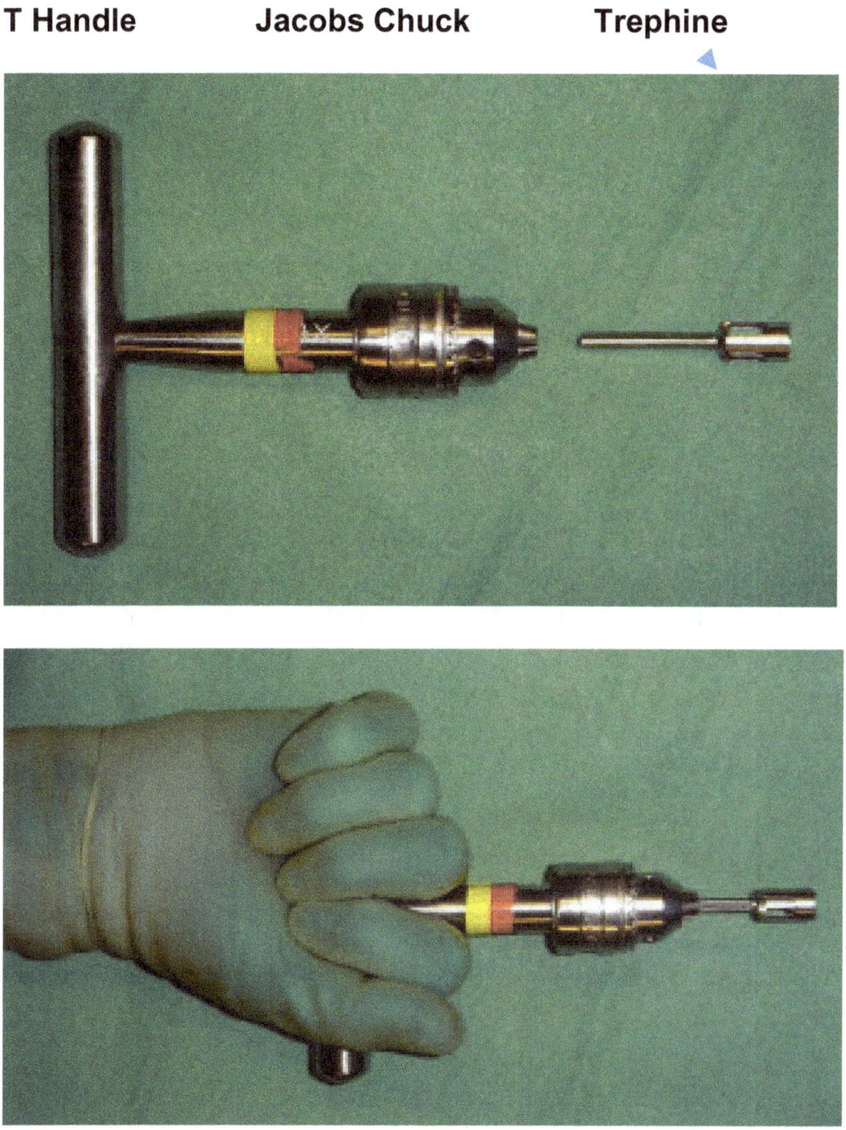

Figure 12.6 Alveolar bone grafting with simultaneous repair of oral and nasal mucosal layers. The rotator finger flap (**g** and **h**) is seldom used in current practice. (**i**) The Ayliffe DTR Medical Trephine has fine teeth and a wide shaft with a window in the casing to retrieve the bone.

A scar directly over the iliac crest can be visible but heals much better. Eminence to avoid a stretched scar.

Numerous techniques exist for harvesting bone and there is evidence that trephination reduces site problems, operative time and post-operative stay.

Trephination cores are cut in the iliac crest. The cancellous bone is used, with the cartilage cap, and any cortical bone is used for the nasal floor. A substantial amount may be required as it is particularly important to pack bone up under the lateral part of the alar cartilage to create a nasal sill (Figure 12.7g).

5. An oral defect remains at the site of the original incision. These margins cannot be brought together as they are largely attached gingiva.
6. A mucogigival transposition flap pedicled superiorly in the sulcus is raised and mobilised by dividing the inelastic periosteum with a sharp blade. When rotated into position it leaves a bare area of buccal alveolus distally, which will epithelialise spontaneously. This technique is most useful after bone grafting in the patient with a mixed dentition. In these cases the oral defect is narrow and the transposition flap is taken from the gingival margins of the deciduous molars, which are usually extracted at the same time (Figures 12.8a–12.8c).
7. The flap is rotated over the bone graft and sutured to the margins of the fistula with 5/0 Vicryl on a 16 mm slim blade needle. This must be done meticulously with multiple fine sutures to produce a watertight edge-to-edge closure.
8. The palatal flap from the greater segment is not always required in small defects.
9. Figures 12.8d to 12.8f show the alveolar defect before and after grafting and the erupting canine.
10. A resorbable porcine collagen membrane impregnated with antibiotic can be used for guided bone regeneration, although

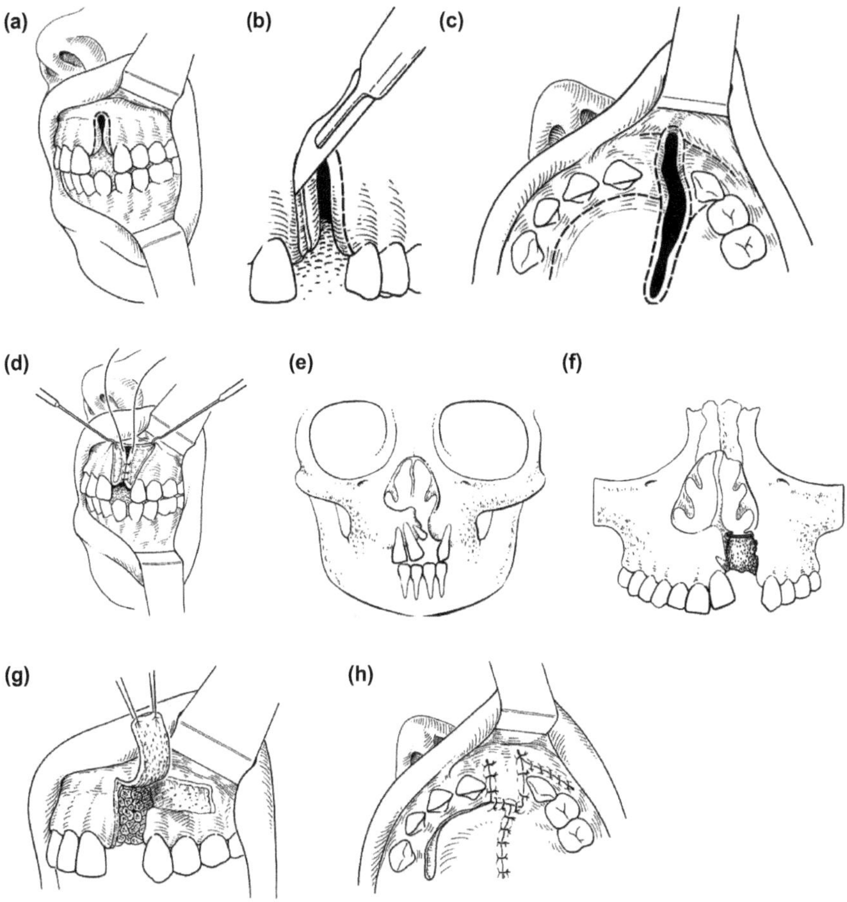

Figure 12.7 Alveolar bone grafting with simultaneous repair of oral and nasal mucosal layers. The rotator finger flap (**g** and **h**) is seldom used in current practice.

the antibiotic Impregnation has unproven value. A resorbable porcine collagen membrane impregnated with antibiotic can be used for guided bone regeneration, although the antibiotic Impregnation has unproven value.

(a) (b) (c) (d) (e) (f)

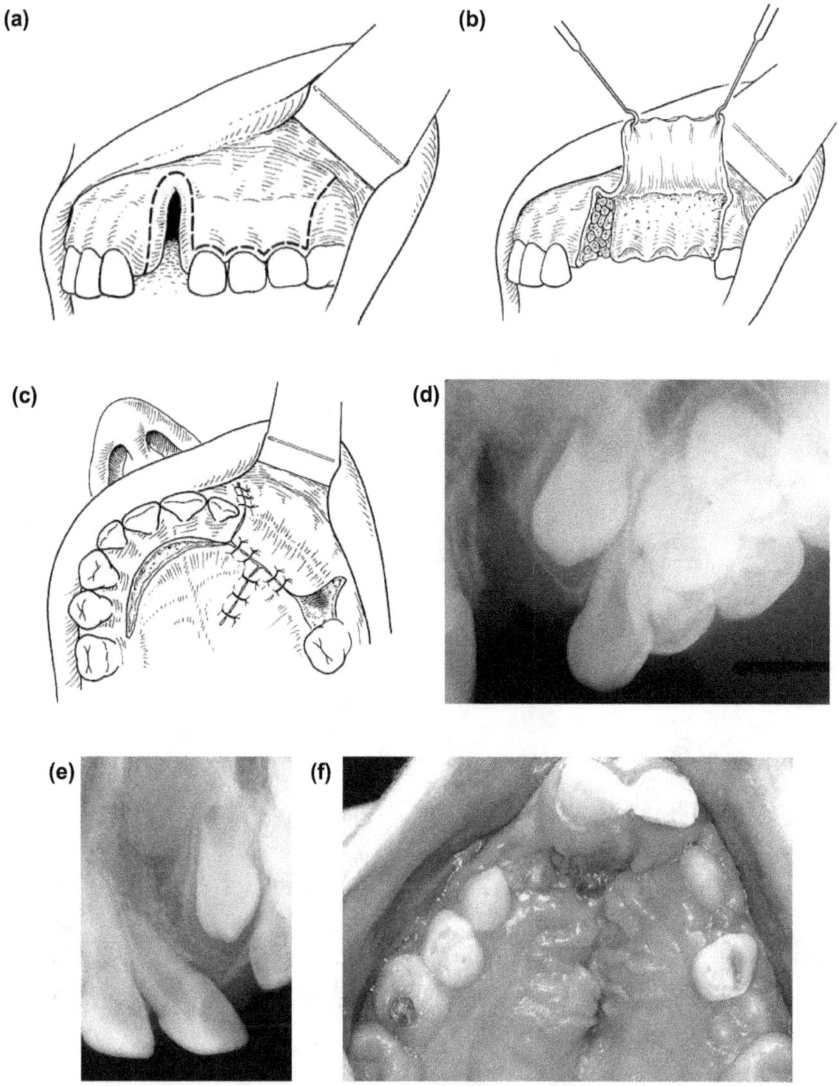

Figure 12.8 (**c**) Raising and rotating a buccal transposition flat. (**d**) Ungrafted cleft. (**e** and **f**) Canine erupting through consolidated bone graft.

Postoperative care

Intraoral bone grafts in cleft patients require meticulous postoperative care. The following precautions are recommended:

1. Preoperative intravenous antibiotics should be administered and then postoperative prophylactic antibiotics given orally for 5 days based on the weight of the child.
2. Maintain scrupulous oral hygiene. The patient is given a semi-solid diet by mouth and chlorhexidine gluconate mouthwashes.
3. Analgesia — Children undergoing cleft surgery are successfully managed with intraoperative 0.25% laevo-bupivacaine administered as follows:

    Cleft Lip Repair: Intraoperative infra-orbital nerve block.
    Cleft Palate Surgery: Local infiltration or palatine nerve block.

    Harvesting iliac crest for an alveolar bone graft: Infiltration of 10 mls. 0.25% laevobupivacaine both subcutaniosly and into the the crest area. Some use the subcutaneous placement of a bupivacaine soaked absorbable sponge.

    The local anaesthetic is followed by postoperative NSAID's such a ibuprofen or paracetamol.

    The paracetamol regimen for 6–12 years is 250 to 500 mg maximum 4 doses in 24 hours.

    Over 12 years 0.5–1.0 g 4 hourly maximum × 4 in 24 hours.

    The NSAIDs do not appear to prolong peri-operative bleeding.

    Consult the paediatric BNF for the occasional need of low dose pethidine or fentanyl which significantly prolong the duration of the local anaesthetic blocks.

Segmental Surgery

Segmental surgery is now rarely required at the time of alveolar bone grafting, as orthodontic preparation or distraction osteogenesis will usually align the segments. It should be avoided because

a) fixation is problematic and
b) bone grafts do not unite with mobile segments.

However, the local dentoalveolar relationship may be improved by combining the alveolar bone graft with an osteotomy to the lesser segment or premaxilla. The most common indications are:

1. Adequate vertical and anterior growth of the greater alveolar segment but vertical deficiency of the lesser segment. This may be associated with dental arch collapse and recession with asymmetry of the nasal base.
2. The fistula is too large to close for bone grafting, and soft tissue coverage is not possible.
3. Orthodontic expansion of the arch has not been possible as the lesser segment may be trapped palatally.
4. Distraction osteogenesis is not available.

The Problems

- A unilateral alveolar defect.
- Anterior fistula and nasal base asymmetry.
- Deficient vertical growth of the lesser segment and collapse of the maxillary dental arch.

The Surgical Treatment

- Osteotomy to reposition the lesser segment.
- Bone graft to the alveolar defect and osteotomy site.
- Closure of the anterior oronasal fistula.

1. The initial incision is made around the intraoral margin of the fistula, as before. A horizontal sulcus incision can be made at this stage to improve access but this incision should now be made along the line of the greater segment (Figure 12.9a).

2. The lesser segment osteotomy is carried out at the LeFort I level from the buccal side by inserting a suitably protected bur or the narrow blade of a reciprocating power saw. The horizontal cut is carried through until the blade action can be palpated beneath the attached palatal mucosa (Figure 12.9b).
3. The lesser segment is still not free posteriorly. In cleft patients the anatomy of the tuberosity-pterygoid plate junction is frequently distorted and the bone may be very dense in this area. In order to free the segment, a 1 cm transverse mucosal incision is made behind the tuberosity and a 7 or 10 mm thin osteotome directed vertically (Figure 12.9c).
4. The freed lesser segment is now further mobilised by blunt dissection until it can be aligned according to the preoperative plan.
5. If the dental arch is expanded to any extent it will open up the cleft of the hard palate. This can only be made good by lifting and rotating the mucoperiosteum covering the palatal aspect of the greater segment and suturing it to the freshened edge of the palatal mucosa covering the lesser segment. The palatal mucosa covering the lesser segment should remain attached to maximise the blood supply to the segment. In practice, nasal layer closure is not found to be a problem, even after surgical expansion of the maxillary arch.
6. Cancellous bone chips and sheets of cancellous bone obtained from the iliac crest or by trephining the tibia, are used to fill the alveolar defect and to pack the osteotomy site on the lesser segment.
7. The lesser osteotomised segment is immobilised by attachment to the greater segment using a preformed arch bar (Figure 12.9d) ligated with 0.35 mm prestretched soft stainless steel wire.
8. There remains the oral mucosal defect on the buccal and alveolar aspect of the cleft. It is not advisable to raise an anteriorly based finger flap or buccal mucogingival transposition flap. If there is concern over blood supply to the osteotomised segment, a finger flap should be avoided. It is associated with more

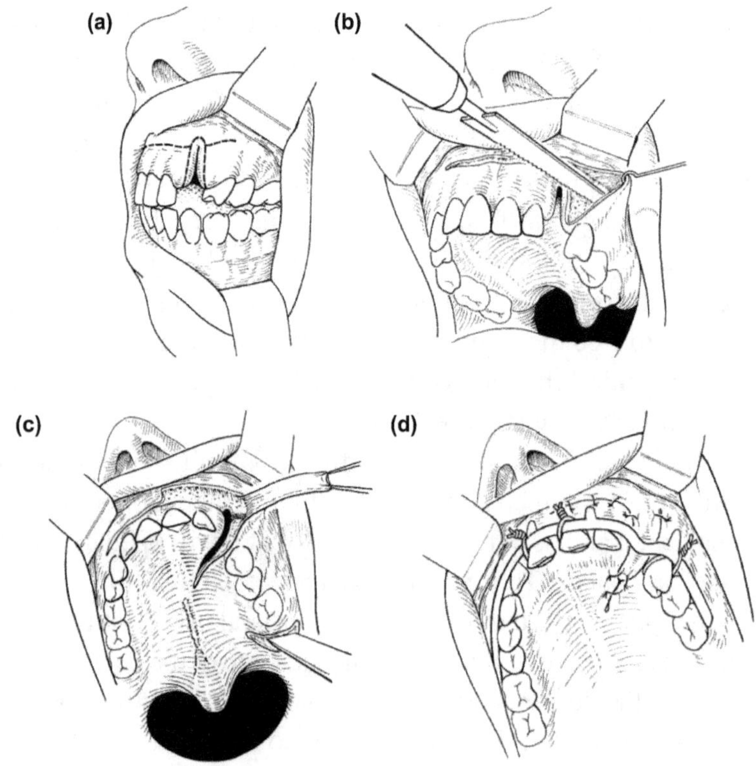

Figure 12.9 Lesser segment of alveolar osteotomy at the time of alveolar bone grafting.

scarring, and teeth erupting through keratinised mucosa that will lead to periodontal problems and ultimately tooth loss. Further more, sutures may end up over the grafted bone, which can lead to failure of the graft. Ideally a muco-periosteal advancement flap should be made with periosteal scoring to length the flap. The vestibular finger flap is therefore based posteriorly and raised from the mucosa and submucosa of the buccal sulcus between the anterior part of the greater segment and the lip, as shown in Figures 12.9c and 12.9d.

9. Suturing and postoperative care are as already described above.

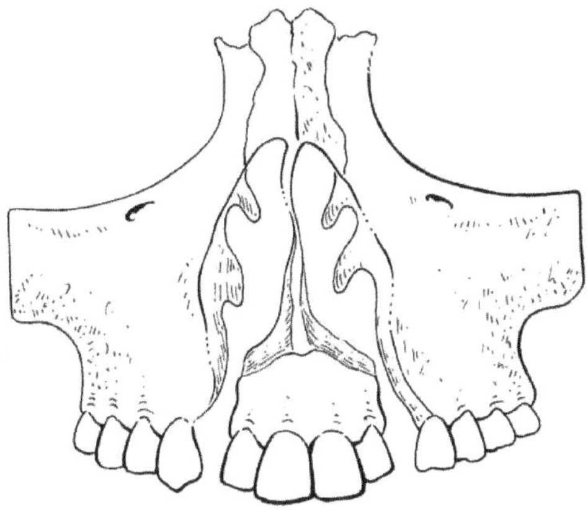

Figure 12.10 Care must be taken not to compromise the blood supply of the premaxillary segment in bilateral cleft cases.

Bilateral Clefts (Figure 12.10)

Orthognathic surgery for bilateral clefts is very difficult and should only be attempted by experienced surgeons. Three presentations will be considered. However all cases are complicated by:

i) scarring of the prolabium indicating poor vascularity,
ii) multiple previous operations,
iii) a large anterior palatal fistulae extending bilaterally through the alveolus, and
iv) marked asymmetry.

Presentation 1 — The Problems

- A large anterior palatal fistulae extending bilaterally through the alveolus.
- Recession of the nasal tip.
- Shortening of the columella.
- Symmetrical flaring of the alar bases.

The Surgical Treatment

Closure of the anterior fistulae with bone grafts to the alveolar defects.

- Reconstruction of the nasal sills providing bony support to the alar bases.
- Lengthening of the columella, and forward repositioning of the alar cartilages with narrowing of the nasal tip.
- Rotation of the alar bases inwards towards the mid line.
- Narrowing of the nasal bridge (see Rhinoplasty).

1. Orthodontic expansion of the maxillary arch must precede surgery. Rapid maxillary expansion may be employed if the scarred palatal tissues are later mobilised surgically. However too much expansion may increase the volume of the alveolar defect and make soft tissue closure precarious.
2. If the maxillary arch alignment and forward development is adequate, surgical dissection of the anterior fistulae and alveolar defects can proceed as in the unilateral case, duplicating the surgery for each of the two clefts (see previously).
3. Teeth in the premaxillary segment adjacent to the cleft alveolus on each side may be found to be denuded of bone. This applies particularly to any remaining lateral incisors. In order to achieve a successful bone graft such teeth must be removed.
4. Care needs to be taken when raising the healthy mucoperiosteal flap from the palatal aspect of the premaxillary segment which can be sutured to the scarred palate mucosa and the buccal flaps which are rotated inwards to cover the bone graft. A Mitchell's trimmer and using the alveolar cleft for access can make this easier.

   It is therefore better to confine the autogenous grafts to the higher and buccal parts of the alveolar defect and to make no attempt to achieve a bridge of bone across the anterior part of the hard palate.

Presentation 2 — The Problems

- Retroposition of the premaxilla with collapse of the maxillary arch, but satisfactory vertical growth of the bilateral posterior segments.
- Nasal deformity as above, but more severe.

The Surgical Treatment

- Osteotomy of the premaxilla in severe cases.
- Bone graft to the alveolar defects with closure of anterior fistulae.
- Rhinoplasty.

1. If the orthodontic expansion is satisfactory and produces a satisfactory alignment of each segment, surgical closure of the anterior fistula can proceed as in point 1 above.
2. Frequently, expansion of the lateral segments is achieved but the premaxilla remains retroposed (Figure 12.11a). In this case, an osteotomy of the premaxilla alone is necessary at the time of the alveolar grafting.
3. Retropositioning of the premaxilla also prevents surgical dissection of the clefts from a buccal approach. The premaxilla is held back by a solid spur of bone extending forward from the anterior part of the base of the vomer, the vomerine-premaxillary spur, VMS (Figure 12.11b). Figure 12.11c shows the sagittal section of a bilateral cleft to illustrate the vomerine-premaxillary spur of bone. This spur may have a cartilaginous section behind the premaxilla in some cases but is too dense to be fractured by manipulation alone.

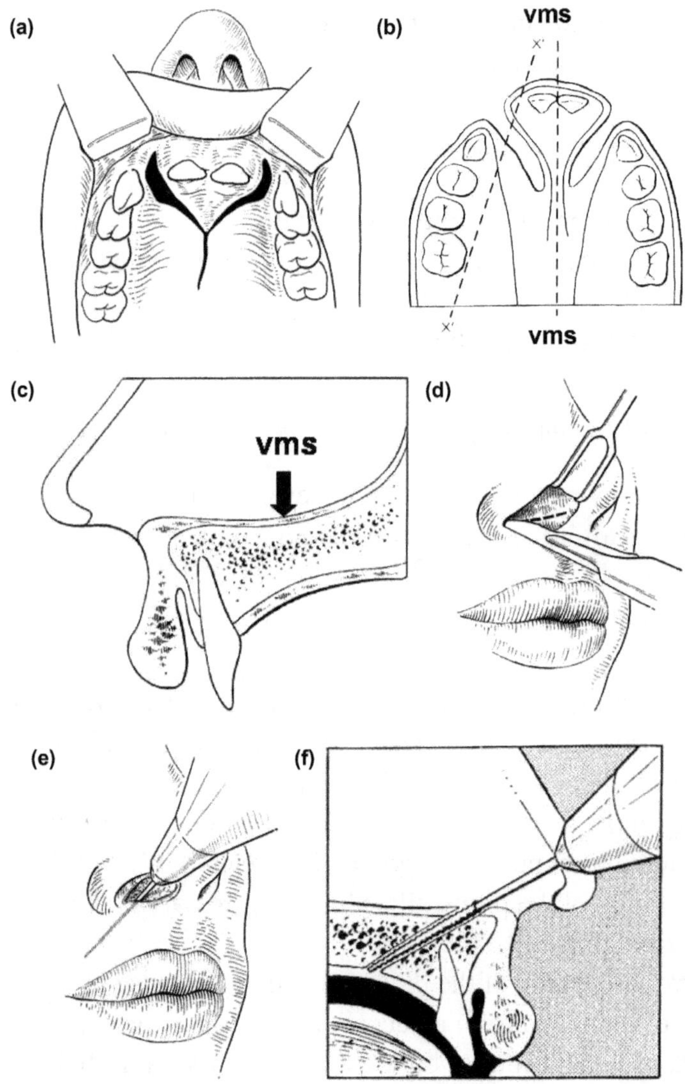

Figure 12.11 Osteotomy of the retroposed premaxillary segement in the bilateral case by sectioning of the vomerine-premaxillary spur (vms). Once displaced forwards the mucosa is carefully raised to provide cleft closure **(g–l)**.

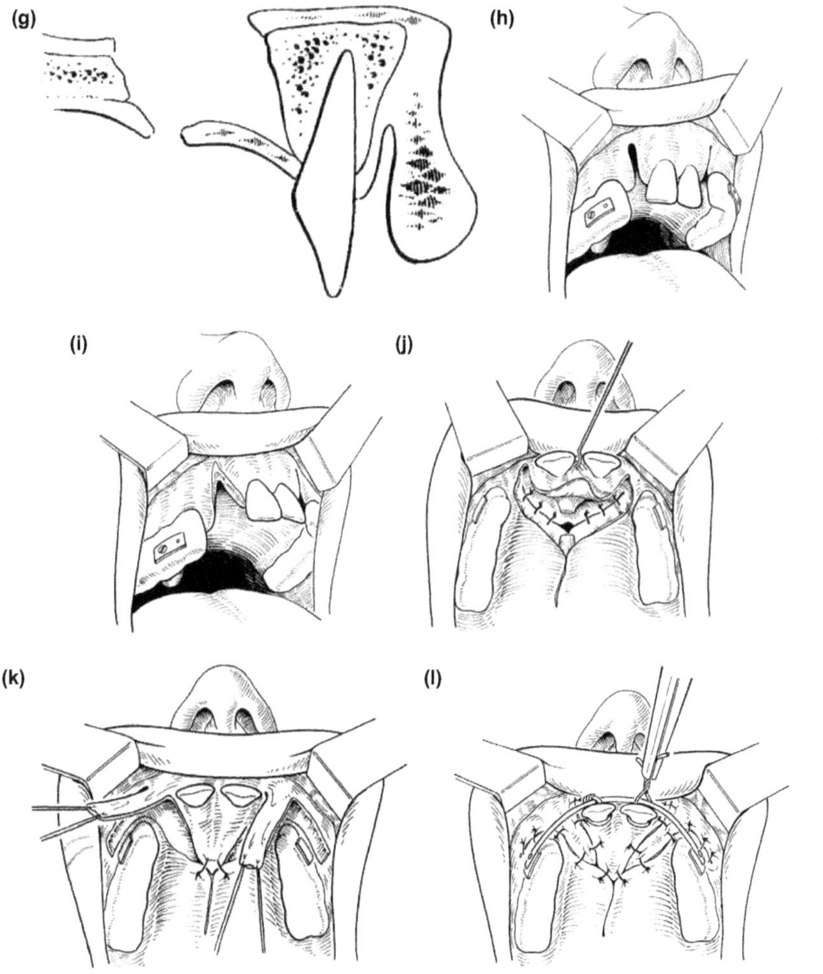

Figure 12.11 (*Continued*)

4. The surgical exposure of this spur of bone can be achieved via the nose. Horizontal incisions are made in the nasal mucosa overlying the anterior part of the base of the septum (Figures 12.11d and 12.11e).

   The mucosa is raised by sharp dissection on each side of the septal base in a downwards and backwards direction towards the oral cavity just behind the premaxilla. In this way the vomerine-premaxillary spur is dissected free of its overlying mucoperiosteal cover without penetrating the mucosa on the nasal and oral aspect. The spur is cut with a surgical fissure bur at which point the premaxilla can be swung forwards, opening up the cleft on each side with its mucoperiosteum still attached (Figures 12.11h and 12.11i).

5. Dissection of each side of the cleft can now take place as in the unilateral case and bone grafts inserted. Stabilisation of the pre- maxillary segment is important as a mobile bone graft will fail. Note the preservation of the mucosa on the back of the premaxillary segment to assist palatal closure together with the anteriorly based vestibular flaps (Figures 12.11j to 12.11l).
6. Figure 12.11j illustrates the amount of palatal mucosal which needs to be carefully raised from the back of the premaxillary segment to achieve oral closure after the premaxilla has been repositioned.
7. The premaxilla is immobilised by means of a preformed arch bar. Cap splints may be previously applied to the lateral segments but the premaxilla itself is best retained by gentle 0.35 mm ligatures to a preformed arch bar screwed to locking plates on each of the two cap splints on the lateral segments (Figure 12.11l).
8. Rhinoplasty is carried out as a secondary procedure.

Presentation 3 — The Problems

- A retropositioned premaxilla with a collapsed maxillary arch.
- Inadequate vertical growth of the lateral segments.
- Mid facial retrusion.
- Severe nasal tip recession.

The Surgical Treatment

This presentation would benefit from distraction osteogenesis. However if not available surgical correction can be performed in two stages separated by 6 weeks. It is impossible to carry out, with consistent success, segmental osteotomies, grafting of alveolar defects, closure of fistulae and total maxillary repositioning in one operation.

1. Orthodontic expansion of the lateral segments is usually required.
2. The premaxillary osteotomy and grafting is performed as in point 2 above. In this case it is frequently necessary to reposition the premaxilla upward to align with the lateral segments, in which case part of the nasal septum may have to be cut away to accommodate the segment.
3. A simultaneous segmental osteotomy of one or other lateral segment may be required to achieve satisfactory total arch alignment. If the lateral segments have been expanded orthodontically against resistance from the scarred palatal tissues, the palatal mucoperiosteum must be mobilised surgically at this stage to prevent relapse.
4. After at least 9 months, and preferably 1 year, a standard Le Fort I osteotomy with down-fracture can be undertaken in those cases where alveolar reconstruction has been successful. The repositioned maxilla no longer requires extraoral craniomaxillary fixation in addition to miniplate internal fixation.
5. Rhinoplasty is carried out after the maxilla has been shown to be stable for 1 year.

Lesser Segment Alveolar Distraction (*See also Chapter 10 "Distraction Osteogenesis"*)

Segmental alveolar distraction may overcome the technical difficulties of dividing and fixing small osteotomy segments. By slowly moving the lesser segment at one millimetre per day towards the cleft, the size of the alveolar and dental gap is reduced. This decreases the size of both the graft and the flaps raised to close the fistula. It may even eliminate the need for an autogenous bone graft.

- Segmental distraction is only possible in patients with erupted teeth on which brackets and tubes can be applied to enable a rigid wire to guide the distraction forward and around the arch form.
- Care must be taken to preserve the vascular supply to the osteotomised bony fragment and so a tunnelling approach is used buccally and palatally in order to perform the osteotomy cuts.
- The segment of alveolus chosen to be distracted will determine the site of the interdental osteotomy cut.
- This site requires the provision of space by the orthodontist, and a rigid archwire is fitted before surgery to guide the distraction.

The Surgical Preparation for Distraction

1. A horizontal incision is made through the buccal mucosa and the flap is raised to provide access for the horizontal segmental cut and a vertical interdental cut which is started buccally with a fine surgical bur (Figures 12.12a and 12.12b). Interdental space has been made orthodontically. The adjacent palatal mucoperiosteum is also raised with a fine elevator such as a Frier or a MacDonald exposing only sufficient bone to make the equivalent vertical cut through the palatal alveolus.
2. The palatal horizontal cut is now made by a tunnelling approach through the anterior cleft margin with a periosteal elevator (Figure 12.12a) and then the distal interproximal bone is divided with a fine osteotome.
3. The distractor is placed buccally across the vertical osteotomy site. The clover leaf plate on each side of the division is secured with three 5 mm screws and a trial distraction is carried out to

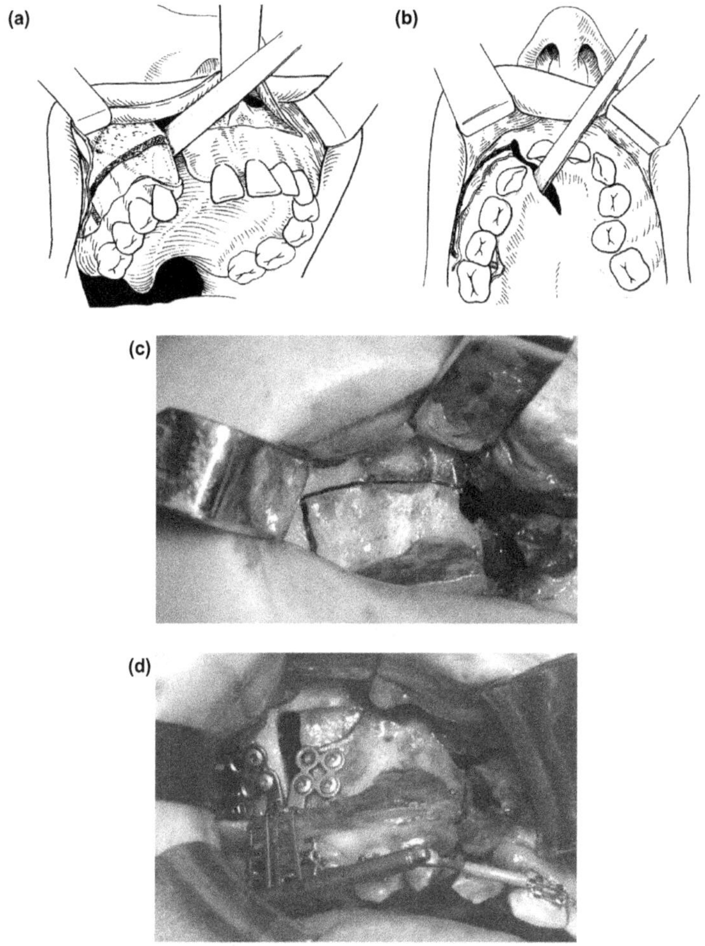

Figure 12.12 Segmental alveolar distraction. The completion of segmental alveolar distraction.

ensure the fragment moves easily and the 3-dimensional vectors are correct (Figure 12.12d).

4. The wound is sutured without the need for relieving incisions. Postoperative care is as stated above.
5. The distractor is activated after 5 days to achieve 0.5–1.0 mm a day guided by the rigid arch wire within tubes attached to each tooth on the segment to ensure controlled forward movement.

(e)

(f)

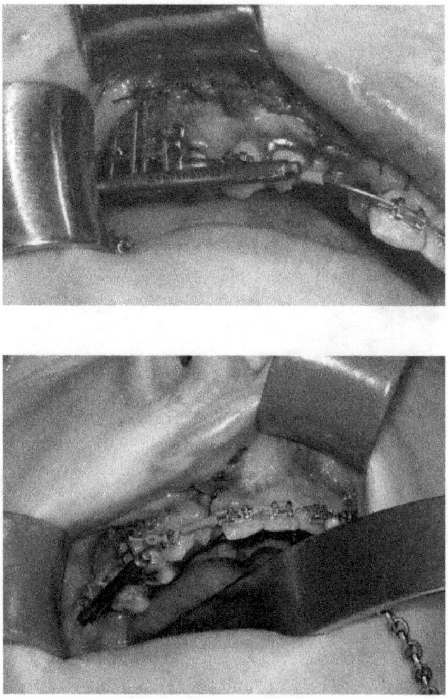

Figure 12.12 (*Continued*)

On completion of the distraction, as seen in Figures 12.12d–12.12f, a consolidation phase of 4–6 weeks is required to ensure maturation of the callus.

6. The distractor is then removed under an general anaesthetic and a gingivoperiosteoplasty is performed as for an alveolar bone graft to complete the closure. Bone grafting is rarely required as the alveolar cleft has been closed as a function of the osteodistraction.

Residual Fistulae

Small Fistulae

A double-layered closure is the most reliable technique, as is described in the alveolar bone grafting section. Figures 12.13a and 12.13b show

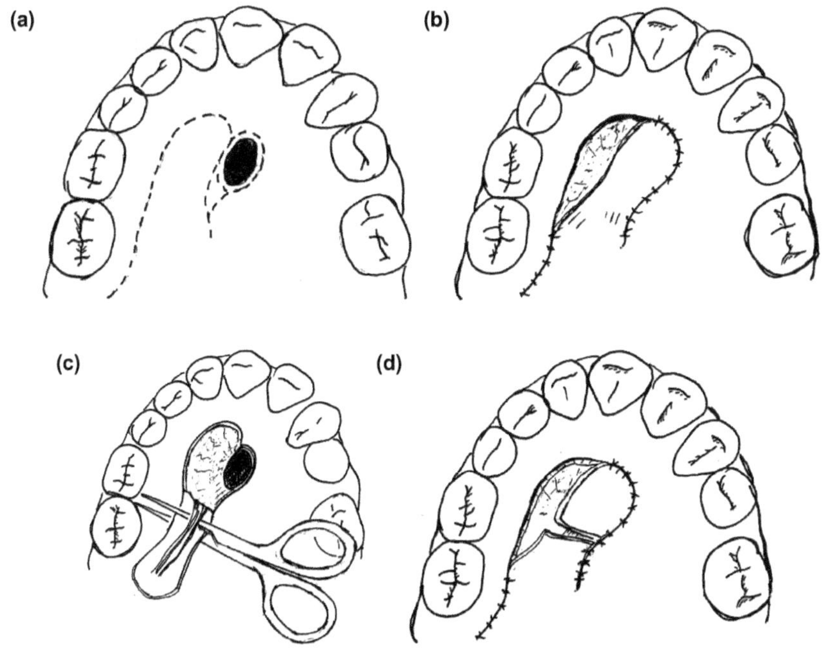

Figure 12.13 Closure of a small residual palatal fistula.

a rotation flap based on the posterior palatal vessels, which must be patent. Reflection of the flap and skeletalising the exposed vessels gives a more manoeuvrable island flap.

The Surgical Treatment (Figures 12.13a to 12.13d)

1. Outline the fistula with a pen and the adjacent contralateral pedicled flap.
2. Infiltrate with a local anaesthetic containing vasoconstrictor.
3. Incise the margin of the fistula and undermine and elevate the inner fistula margin tissue into the nose sufficiently to close with a purse string suture using a small J shaped needle. This will ensure a double layered closure.
4. Incise the outline of the pedicled flap down to bone and elevate back to the posterior palatine foramen.

(a) (b) (c)

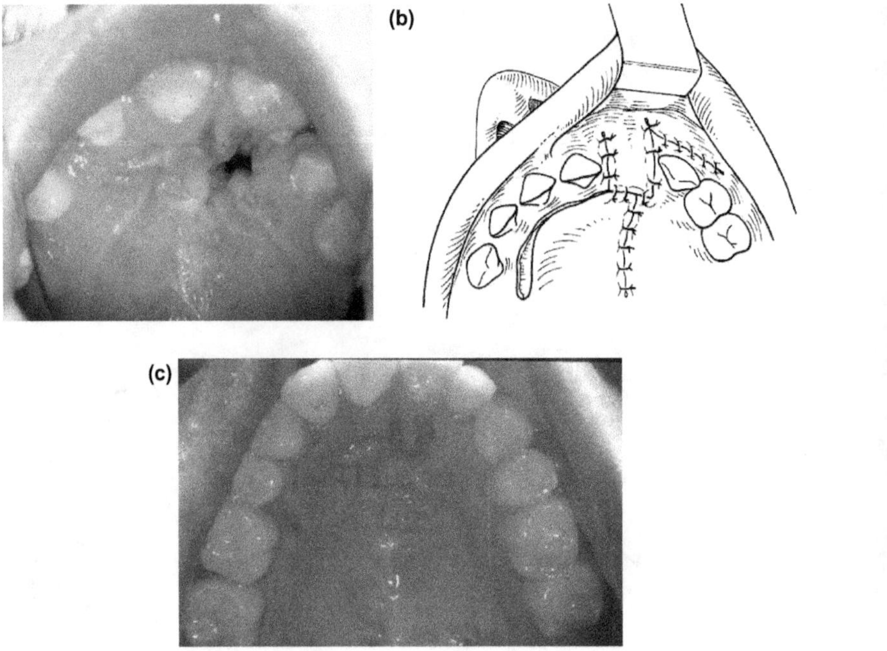

Figure 12.14 Large palatal fistula closure.

5. Separate the vessels visible on the under surface from the overlying submucosa with fine scissors, carefully and widely. This may be difficult due to scarring from previous surgery. If they have been thrombosed due to previous surgery go to point 8.
6. Cut the thick mucosal pedicle leaving the island flap attached by its palatine vessels.
7. Rotate the island flap over the lined fistula and suture with interrupted 4/0 vicryl sutures. The bare area should be covered with a Surgicel R pack sutured around the margins and oversewn for stability.
8. If the vessels are not readily separable, rotate the broad based pedicled flap (Figure 12.13b) suture and pack the bare area.

A pedicled sliding flap is shown in Figures 12.14.

Closure of Large Fistulae in Cases Presenting Late

The Problem

Large defects of the anterior hard palate require a different strategy. They result from the expansion and advancement of grossly collapsed maxillary dental arches. Large fistulae also exist in some older patients due to the pattern of surgery practised 40 years ago or more. Such large oronasal communications become a major problem when full dentures are worn.

The Surgical Treatment

1. Unilateral or bilateral segmental alveolar distraction slowly closes the dental and alveolar gap and will generate bone in the alveolar region (see above) but if not available a flap will be required.
2. Tongue flaps.
    - The tongue has an extremely good blood supply and has been extensively used for reconstruction of large palatal fistulae.
    - Reconstruction is performed in two stages. The second stage to divide the pedicle and inset the flap may be 10–14 days from the initial procedure.
    - The use of lingual mucosa over the alveolus is an unfavourable environment for tooth eruption and long term maintenance of periodontal health.

Lateral tongue flaps are reliable axial flaps and tend to be well tolerated and stable, despite tongue movements during the transfer stage.

Anterior-based dorsal tongue flaps are random flaps and are less well tolerated during the period of transfer as they are distorted by movements of the tongue. This may occasionally prejudice the blood supply. However, they provide an ideally shaped tissue transfer and leave little or no deformity of the tongue. The width is made slightly greater than the defect with two to three millimetres of muscle included with the mucosa to ensure the blood supply.

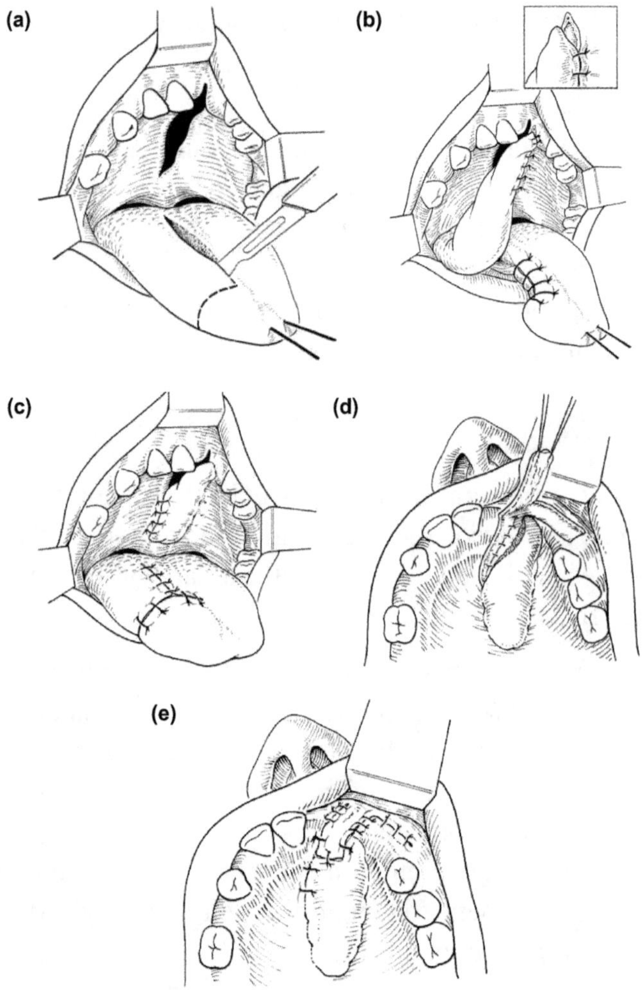

Figure 12.15 The lateral tongue flap used to close a palatal fitula.

The Surgical Treatment

The Lateral Tongue Flap

1. The tongue margin is injected with 1:200,000 adrenaline in 0.25% laevobupivacaine. Hypotensive anaesthesia is used if

available. A 2/0 black silk mattress stay suture through the tip facilitates access.

2. The flap is incised comprising the lateral one-third of the tongue based posteriorly, but excluding the tip (Figure 12.15a).
3. A marginal flap of palatal mucosa is raised from the recipient site area to facilitate suturing and to increase the area of contact (Figure 12.15b). The free tip of the tongue flap is then sutured with 5/0 vicryl to the anterolateral lip of the fistula. The margin of the flap is firmly sutured to the adjacent palatal mucosa. It is better to close a left-sided fistula with a right-hand tongue flap, and *vice versa*, as it is found in practice that the flap lies more naturally when so arranged.
4. The tongue flap remains with its dual attachment for 14 days, at which point a further anaesthetic is administered. An inexperienced anaesthetist may find difficulty in intubating a patient with a tongue flap attached to the anterior palate because of the obvious problems associated with the insertion of a laryngoscope. To avoid this problem, the base of the flap can be severed under local anaesthetic prior to the induction of general anaesthesia but in practice this is rarely necessary.
5. After division, the tongue flap free edges are sutured to palatal mucosa round as much of the fistula as possible (Figure 12.15c). The flap will be used as a split tube but it is usually impractical to form a sutured nasal layer at this stage. As long as the transferred flap can be attached completely to one side of the fistula, the nasal surface can be left until later. The flap remnant attached to the tongue is fashioned to fit back into the side of the tongue. Tongue shape can usually be restored almost to normal.
6. As it is rarely possible to complete the closure of a large oronasal fistula when the tongue flap is first separated, 2–3 further weeks later the remaining free edge of the fistula is separated into the oral and nasal layers. The tongue flap is split along its free margin and its nasal surface used to complete the nasal

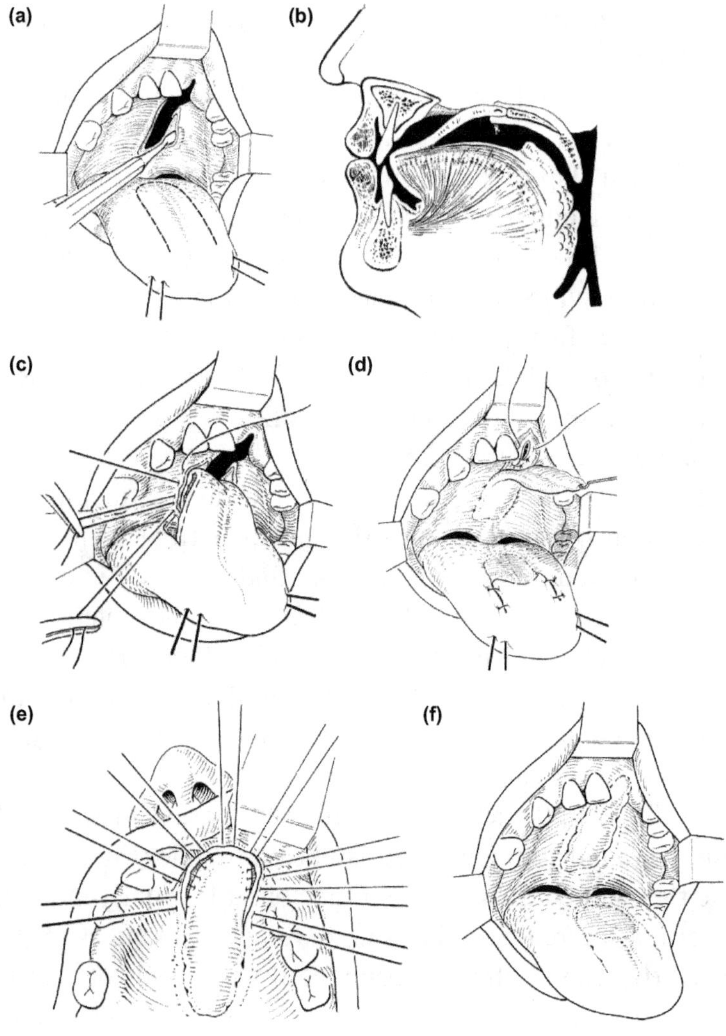

Figure 12.16 The anteriorly based dorsal tongue — stage 1 (**a–c**) and stage 2 (**d–f**).

layer. The oral mucosal defect is closed, partly by the oral surface of the tongue flap and partly by a vestibular flap, as shown in Figures 12.15d and 12.15e. Separation of an oral and nasal layer means that a bone graft can be inserted at this stage if necessary.

7. The completed flap tends to be somewhat bulky, however carefully it has been trimmed. If it is intended to be used as a denture-bearing area, it may be thinned later.

The Anterior Based Dorsal Tongue Flap

1. The tongue is held forward with two lateral 2/0 black silk stay sutures. The flap is marked with ink and the site injected with local anasesthetic and a vasoconstrictor (Figure 12.16a).

   As the mucosa and submucosal muscle is profusely supplied with a rich vascular plexus, especially at the tip of the tongue, the base of the flap does not have to overly the proximal blood supply. The anterior base provides a flap that is easy to insert but restricts the tongue's movements during the transfer stage.
2. The posterior and lateral margins of the fistula are incised with a No. 11 blade and raised with Mitchell's trimmer to provide a shelf-like flap. This stage helps to estimate the width and length of the flap. A base of 3 cm allows a flap of 5 or 6 cm in length.

   The tongue flap is incised to a depth of 4 mm to include an undersurface of submucosal muscle, and is then carefully dissected free. Bleeding points on the donor site are sealed with bipolar diathermy to ensure only localised coagulation.
3. The tongue flap is set into the palatal mucosa shelf margins, with the raw submucosal surfaces in contact and the papillated lingual mucosa facing upward towards the nose (Figure 12.16b). This is done with a series of 5/0 vicryl mattress sutures. These are left untied and clamped with mosquito forceps to allow freedom of access until the maximum number of sutures is inserted (Figure 12.16c). They are now carefully tied with a triple knot and cut short. There is no need to close the nasal layer at this stage.
4. The flap may be rested by inserting loose intermaxillary tie wires through eyelets around the teeth in upper and lower dental arches.

5. Three weeks later the base is divided and the flap (with its raw surface now re-epithelialised) trimmed and set in anteriorly in the same way as was the tip (Figure 12.16d). If the anaesthetist anticipates difficulty in intubation, the flap can be incised under local anaesthetic just prior to the intubation procedure. Ideally this should be done in the operating theatre. Excess flap is sutured back on to the de-epithelialised donor site, which heals spontaneously with minimal defect (Figures 12.16e and 12.16f).
6. If a cancellous bone graft is inserted, the nasal mucosal layer is raised and closed with 4/0 vicryl (Ethicon Ltd, Edinburgh, UK).

Note: This technique, which provides an easy and reliable means of inserting the flap margin, is possible because of the rapid epithelialisation of the raw muscle on the undersurface of the flap. Furthermore, it takes on the normal mucosal character instead of remaining a patch of tongue on the palate.

Extraoral Flaps

If intraoral tissue is not sufficient for the largest fistulae a microvascular transfer of a free radial skin flap or free radial fascial flap can be combined with local mucosal turn-over flaps to close the nasal layer together with bone to fill any bony defects of the alveolus and hard palate.

Residual Oronasal Fistulas in the Soft Palate

Oronasal fistulas in the soft palate require correction if there is a loss of oral pressure during speech. The best approach in the presence of poor speech is a complete re-repair of the soft palate. This improves the function of the velopharyngeal mechanism and speech improves as a consequence.

Residual Nasolabial Fistulae

If left until alveolar bone grafting there will be less overall scarring. Presurgical orthodontic expansion gives good access to the whole cleft. The fistula is excised and good nasal layer should be reconstructed as described above in the alveolar bone graft section. The interpositional bone graft improves the success of the closure.

Orthodontic Considerations

The objectives of presurgical orthodontic treatment for the cleft patient are not the same as non-cleft patients. The most obvious differences are;

i) Management of the dental gap in the cleft region.

In the unilateral case with a full dentition on the non-cleft side, closure of the space in the cleft gap may not be aesthetic, whereas in the bilateral case where both maxillary lateral incisors are missing, a satisfactory aesthetic result can be achieved by bilaterally closing the space. However, closure of the spaces will change tooth contacts and may make intercuspation difficult to achieve.

Orthodontic alignment following the alveolar bone graft will optimise the bone support for the teeth. It also aligns the tooth roots to produce the best possible incisor and canine crown angulation thereby facilitating a range of restorative options for replacing the missing lateral incisor. Adequate alveolar bone will enable the insertion of a dental implant.

ii) Transverse dento-alveolar collapse.

Achieving sufficient maxillary expansion and transverse stability is a great challenge. Orthodontic expansion of the dental arch must be within a reasonable expectation of stability. Dental relapse disturbs the surgical result in both the antero-posterior and lateral dimensions. Permanent transverse retention may be needed to overcome rigid palatal scarring.

With significant transverse deficiency surgical widening at the time of the maxillary advance may be considered but a posterior cross-bite is preferable to the creation of a fistula or losing segments due to ischaemic necrosis.

Orthognathic Surgery

Orthognathic correction should be delayed until facial skeletal growth is complete.

Specific Problems in Cleft Patients

- The Class III skeletal problem affects the paranasal, nasal, infraorbital, and zygomatic regions in the anteroposterior and lateral planes, and may even cause exorbitism with poor eyelid support.
- The associated malocclusion frequently includes anterior open bites and posterior cross bites which impair eating, speech and the long-term health of the teeth and their supporting bone.
- The deformity also impairs nasal breathing and drainage, olfaction and hearing.
- Dental development may also be delayed in both arches but is most evident in the cleft segment and may compromise the presurgical orthodontics.
- The repaired alveolar cleft is a potential site for fracture at the time of the down-fracture.
- If the maxillary alveolus has not been reconstructed, alignment of the alveolus can be incorporated into the orthognathic procedure. However it complicates the planning of the surgery and increases the potential morbidity. Segmental osteotomies are less stable than one-piece maxillary osteotomies.

- Previous surgery produces scarring of the labial and buccal vestibule, the palate and behind the maxillary tuberosities. This presents problems with the surgical incisions, mobilisation and postoperative closure of the surgical wound.
- A pharyngeal flap may make advancement of the maxilla difficult and will need to be divided. The patient has to be informed well in advance.
- Earlier distraction osteogenesis is an option for management of the maxilla if the patient has gross skeletal deformity (see later).

Preparation of the Patient for Surgery

Other congenital defects such as cardiac abnormalities will require consideration. The preparation of the patient and parents starts earlier than in the non-cleft population. Families with cleft lip and palate children get considerable support from self-help organisations. Despite this these deformities have profound psychological effects and the support of a clinical psychologist is often helpful.

Dental Care and Preparation

Oral hygiene instruction, dietary advice, periodontal and restorative treatment should be initiated before pre-surgical orthodontic preparation. The early loss of teeth has catastrophic consequences for any future orthodontic, orthognathic and restorative dental treatment.

Treatment Planning

The basic facial and orthognathic evaluation is the same as the non-cleft case with important refinements.

a) Lip-incisor relationship.

   As in the non-cleft case, the lip to maxillary incisor relationship is extremely important. The major surgical moves are predominantly in the maxilla and with a tight, previously scarred upper lip, small skeletal moves have a pronounced effect on the incisor exposure. Surgical and orthodontic changes in incisor angulation will have a similar effect.

b) Asymmetries.

Both dental and skeletal asymmetries are dominant features, often with compensatory asymmetries in the mandible. Where possible, preoperative orthodontic management will make the surgical correction technically easier. If dental asymmetries are to be corrected after surgery, space will need to be maintained.

c) Preoperative speech assessment and counselling.

Ideally all cleft patients should have a full preoperative speech assessment with nasoendoscopy and videofluoroscopy. The patient with adequate velopharyngeal function preoperatively generally maintains function, unless the maxillary advance is large. Patients with borderline velopharyngeal function are at risk of developing hypernasality postoperatively. These patients need to be identified and followed up for evaluation and corrective treatment.

The Choice of Osteotomy Operation

Maxillary Hypoplasia

- The LeFort I osteotomy will give acceptable results at the occlusal level with antero-posterior advancement and vertical lengthening.
- Transverse maxillary widening can be accomplished by a paramedian osteotomy of the hard palate on the non-cleft side within the constraints discussed above.
- Patients with severe hypoplasia of the infraorbital and malar regions can be improved by the high LeFort I level osteotomy. Graft augmentation either at the same time or as a secondary procedure combined with a rhinoplasty may be necessary.

- The modified LeFort II or Kufner LeFort III osteotomy, do not give accurate control of movement in asymmetrical cases.
- Nasal airway obstruction may arise from a deviated nasal septum narrowing of the nares, hypertrophied turbinates, nasal polyps and posterior choanal constriction from sub-periosteal bone and asymmetrical vomer flaps.
- Pharyngeal obstruction can be caused by hypertrophied adenoidal tissue or pharyngeal flaps.
- The management of these problems is an essential part of the orthognathic procedure. Paradoxically the adenoid mass may contribute to velopharyngeal function and its removal may precipitate velopharyngeal inadequacy.

Implications for the Mandible and/or Chin

- Although many cleft patients may also have a latent mandibular hypoplasia, there is invariably a relative mandibular prognathism. Functional, aesthetic and surgical considerations may need a mandibular setback. The maxillary surgical limitations are severe palatal scarring, borderline velopharyngeal insufficiency or a tight inferiorly based pharyngoplasty flap.
- During maxillary advancement and inferior positioning, the anterior maxilla is differentially positioned more inferiorly. This will produce a posterior open bite deformity unless a mandibular ramus procedure is undertaken simultaneously. Differential down grafting of the anterior maxilla also results in a counter clockwise rotation of the mandible which may make the chin retrogenic. This can be corrected by a simultaneous augmentation genioplasty.

Maxillary Advancement in the Previously Bone Grafted Maxilla

At the time of orthognathic surgery all oro-nasal fistulae should have been closed and the dentoalveolar arcade should be intact. Presurgical orthodontics will have aligned and coordinated the dental arches. In these ideal circumstances the osteotomy technique is similar to a non-cleft patient undergoing maxillary surgery. However, infection, bone and soft tissue necrosis, delayed healing, loss of teeth and relapse all occur with greater frequency.

Special Considerations — The Osteotomy Cuts and the Down-Fracture

- In most cases a standard vestibular incision taken higher in the labial sulcus gives good access posteriorly and ensures a good vascular supply buccally. Care must be taken to preserve the parotid duct.
- Subperiosteal dissection is carried out with elevation of the soft tissues to the infraorbital nerves superiorly and to the pterygomaxillary fissures on both sides. The nasal mucosa is elevated bilaterally from the nasal floor.
- In bilateral cases, where the blood supply to the premaxillary region is compromised due to gross scarring from previous surgery, a full labial incision and down fracture may be unwise and a tunnelling approach is preferable from a small vertical incision in the mid line to give access to the premaxillary bone to enable full mobilisation of the maxilla.

Ancillary Surgical Manoeuvres

Segmental Maxillary Surgery

- If vertical steps are present in the maxillary arch, orthodontic segmental levelling is undertaken and the maxilla expanded prior to surgery. However with severe displacement and gross arch collapse this may not be achievable. Segmental distraction osteogenesis may be an appropriate alternative.
- Although surgically moving segments vertically avoids intrusive and extrusive orthodontic mechanics and may be more stable long term it is the most difficult of the three options.

- Surgical expansion, segmental alignment and levelling require interdental osteotomy cuts for which a minimum of a 3 mm of interdental space needs to opened by the orthodontist by tipping the roots away from the osteotomy site or bodily opening up a gap prior to surgery. Endodontic and periodontal complications will follow without careful presurgical planning.
- The palatal and interdental cuts are performed from above, following the down-fracture. A limited vertical tunnelling approach laterally facilitates access to the buccal cortical plate which is divided with a fine bur but the interdental cut is completed with a narrow 5 mm Osteotome. Ideally orthodontic bands rather than bonded brackets should be placed on the teeth adjacent to the interdental osteotomy site as bonded appliances do not withstand the forces needed to mobilise the maxilla in segmental cleft surgery.
- A large rectangular arch wire with surgical hooks should be wired to the orthodontic bands to aid fixation. A heavy supplemental arch wire fitted into distal tubes is required to help locate and stabilise the occlusal relations of the segments, with the help of a wafer in addition to the bone plate osteosynthesis. This can be a high impact acrylic intermediate wafer. The wafer can be left *in situ* for two weeks post-operatively to supplement the fixation.

Airway Considerations

- Whilst the maxilla is down fractured contouring of the inner aspects of the nose can be achieved easily and time should be taken to bur out any bony excesses in the nostril on the cleft side.
- Asymmetries in the piriform region can be corrected which may interfere with the repositioning of the maxilla or distort the nose. The mucosa of the nostril floor can also be repaired at this stage.
- With a unilateral cleft the septum is usually deviated towards the non-cleft side inferiorly with a bowing towards the cleft side.

A septoplasty may be necessary to correct the aesthetic and functional problems. The subnasal approach after the down-fracture provides excellent access to the cartilaginous septum, the vomer and the perpendicular plate of the ethmoids.

- Partial or complete inferior turbinectomies may be indicated if they are enlarged and cause nasal obstruction. Submucosal turbinectomies can be performed under direct vision through an incision in the nasal mucoperiosteum.
- Antral and nasal polyps can be removed at the time of down fracture.
- Pharyngeal flaps raise additional concerns for the anaesthetist and surgeon. The pharyngeal flap that has a broad base or small portals may make intubation difficult and restrict the nasal airway postoperatively. The flap will need to be divided several weeks preoperatively and the patient's speech and language reassessed postoperatively. Inferiorly based flaps may restrict maxillary advancement but at the time of down fracture access to the flap is relatively good and the flap may be lengthened. Superiorly based flaps are less restrictive on maxillary advancement and can also be lengthened at the time of maxillary advancement. Soft palate re-repair or a repeat pharyngeal flap should be considered carefully as they may further impair the maxillary vascular supply.
- Bone grafting — cortico-cancellous bone grafts should be used to fill the voids created by any inferior positioning of the maxilla as this will improve the stability of the osteotomy postoperatively. Bone grafts should also be shaped and placed to address any specific cosmetic deficiencies and asymmetries. These bone grafts can be tailored to meet the individual requirements of the patient and rigidly fixed to the surface of the maxilla and zygomas with mini screws or wire.
- Mucosal asymmetries of the lip may be corrected by using asymmetric V to Y closures of the labial mucosa. Final lip correction should be left until postsurgical orthodontic refinement

of the occlusion including any minor changes in the incisor position, or cosmetic dental treatment have been completed.

Postoperative Manoeuvres

Intermaxillary elastics to orthodontic archwires may be used to assist in providing proprioceptive input in guiding the jaws into occlusion but should not be used in an attempt to recover a situation where the skeletal elements are incorrectly related. The prolonged use of elastic traction should be avoided as there is a risk of a bony non-union of the maxilla.

As a prophylactic measure, extraoral elastic traction using a face mask can be used in patients who are considered particularly at risk of relapse either due to scarring or who have had large surgical moves anteriorly and inferiorly. The value of this is uncertain (Figures 12.17a and 12.17b).

Effects on Speech

Maxillary advancement increases the velopharyngeal distance so that postoperatively, patients are at risk of developing velopharyngeal

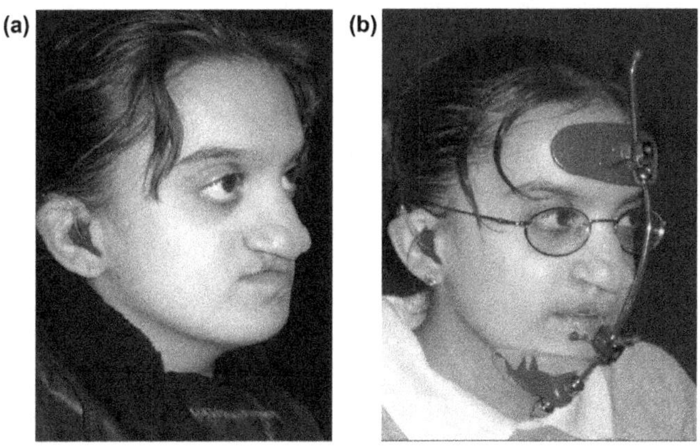

Figures 12.17 After maxillary surgical advancement, extraoral elastic traction support may be useful in a patient at risk of relapse.

incompetence. The soft palate mechanism in non-cleft patients has considerable reserve capacity and can adapt to an increase in length. The repaired cleft soft palate does not have this capacity to adapt especially after major advances. The patient with borderline velopharyngeal incompetence preoperatively is likely to develop worsening of their speech postoperatively.

Lip and Nose Changes with Maxillary Surgery (See also Chapter 14 "Rhinoplasty Surgery")

- Mismanagement of the soft tissues during closure of the labial vestibular incision may cause shortening and thinning of the upper lip.

  The V to Y closure of a maxillary vestibule incision may increase the vermilion show in patients with a thin upper lip.
- Maxillary advancement widens the alar base, increases the projection and elevation of the nasal tip and the width of the nares.

  Various surgical manoeuvres can be used to prevent these unwelcome side effects. These include an alar base cinch suture, recontouring the bony piriform aperture either by trimming and/or asymmetric bone grafting and alar base resections.

Achieving Stability

Stability after orthognathic surgery is unpredictable due to scarring. The factors that increase stability include:

- Meticulous orthodontic preparation and quality of the occlusion achieved.
- Avoiding segmental procedures and unfavourable surgical moves.
- Surgical overcorrection where possible. The cleft maxilla usually requires a least a 9 mm advancement.

- Ensuring that all adhesions are divided so that the maxilla can be advanced passively into the planned position. If this is not possible then a compromise position must be planned and if necessary incorporate a mandibular setback.
- Alveolar bone grafting.
- Bone grafting for inferior repositioning of the maxilla.
- Internal rigid fixation for all moves.

Skeletal Relapse

Most relapse occurs within the first few months. Where the relapse is significant, the options depend upon the occlusal relationship. If the occlusion has compensated for the skeletal relapse, then masking procedures such as onlay bone grafts may be an option.

If the occlusion cannot be recovered through postoperative orthodontics, then further skeletal surgery must be considered but with no guarantee that the osteotomy will not relapse again. Maxillary distraction may be a reasonable option in the management of relapse.

Dentoalveolar Relapse

Transverse dentoalveolar relapse is a problem following large orthodontic or surgical palatal expansions. Such patients may require permanent palatal retention. However it is better to accept a planned posterior cross bite than put the maxilla in an unstable position, as relapse at one site may undermine the stability of the whole maxilla.

Mid Face Distraction Osteogenesis

Indications

For the majority of patients, conventional orthognathic surgery gives excellent results that are stable and aesthetically pleasing. However there are some situations when distraction should be considered:

Severe Maxillary Deficiency and Complex Three-Dimensional Deficiency

- With gross maxillary hypoplasia and a severe degree of scarring, the degree of advancement may be beyond the expected limits of stability of a conventional osteotomy. Distraction of the maxilla is preferable to a surgical compromise such as a mandibular setback.
- If the deformity is complex particularly in the upper mid face then a higher level osteotomy with distraction often gives a better result than a modified LeFort I with masking onlay bone grafts or modified LeFort II and LeFort III osteotomies that are difficult to perform and can give unsightly steps particularly over the radix of the nose.
- Slow expansion of the maxilla may produce a more stable increase in the width of the maxilla and face than surgical repositioning or presurgical orthodontics.
- Relapse surgery for distraction is less than a repeat osteotomy and full mobilisation with down fracture is not needed. One is less likely to run into poor vasculature problems in the re-operation site. By slowly advancing the maxilla the resistant forces may be overcome more easily.

Stability and Effects on Speech

Some claim that distraction produces less disturbance of speech with reduced incidence of velopharyngeal incompetence. The potential advantage of an increase in soft tissue following distraction also is helpful for the closure of large fistulae.

Disadvantages

- The procedure takes longer than conventional surgery and involves at least two stages.
- The control of the movement vectors in maxillary distraction is difficult and less precise than an osteotomy.

- Simultaneous mandibular procedures may be necessary and must be coordinated with the maxillary distraction to overcome a prolonged period without a functioning occlusion.

Method and Choice of Distraction Device

- The surgery is similar to conventional orthognathic surgery but instead of the maxilla being placed into the surgical wafer at the end of the procedure and fixed with plates, a distractor is applied.
- The choice of distractor is determined by the desired direction and distance the maxilla needs to be moved.

Internal Distractors

Are partially buried and give excellent control over vectors, but require

- adequate bone on both sides of the osteotomy cuts to fix them,
- extensive sub-periosteal stripping that may impair new bone formation, and
- a patient with good manual dexterity to turn the appliance either inside the mouth or externally in the temple region.

Extra-Oral Distractors

Are easier to activate, but

- give less control over the vectors of distraction,
- do not control the posterior maxilla well, and
- require a frame that is a disadvantage particularly if in place for the duration of the stabilisation phase.

LeFort I Distraction (Figures 12.18a to 12.18e)

LeFort I distraction is performed by carrying out a standard or modified higher level LeFort I osteotomy cuts. If any of the

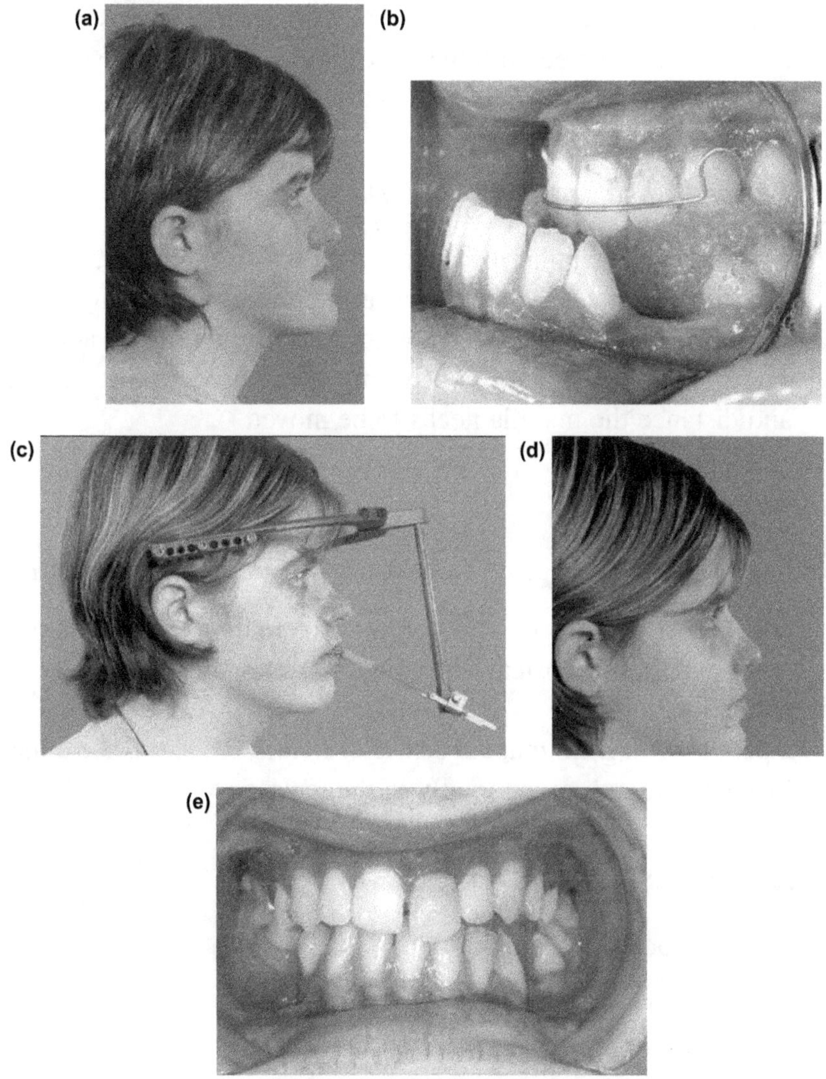

Figure 12.18 An external distraction frame used for maxillary advancement.

previously described ancillary manoeuvres are needed then a maxillary down-fracture is incorporated into the procedure before the distractor is applied. External distractors are connected to the maxilla either with cap splints, or pre-formed arch bars, or directly to plates fixed to the bone or both. This depends on the desired moves and the need to control vectors during the distraction procedure. Controlling the vector can be difficult as often the distractor position is determined by the lip and nose and a compromise may have to be made.

LeFort II Distraction (Figures 12.19a to 12.19g)

For patients with severe maxillary hypoplasia a higher level of distraction is needed to improve the mid face aesthetics. This may need to be performed in combination with a mandibular sagittal split osteotomy to improve the mandibular plane angle and to allow for the elongation of the maxilla in the vertical dimension. Further wires are attached to the hypoplastic malar bones to guide their distraction forwards. Slow distraction at this level seems to give a better shape to the nose than a standard LeFort II advancement that would normally require bone grafting and which can lead to steps and irregularities.

LeFort III (Kufner) Distraction

If there is significant orbital rim hypoplasia then distraction at the LeFort III level may be useful, particularly as bone grafts in this area are difficult to contour and produce disappointing results in the short term and are notoriously unstable in the long term. The location of the scar needs to be considered. Stretching skin that would normally hide beneath underwear over the iliac crest can lead to the normscar being invisible when dressed. This scar can be stretched by the weight of the skin and poor support from the fascia underneath. A scar directly over the iliac crest eminence can be visible but heals much better. To avoid a stretched scar.

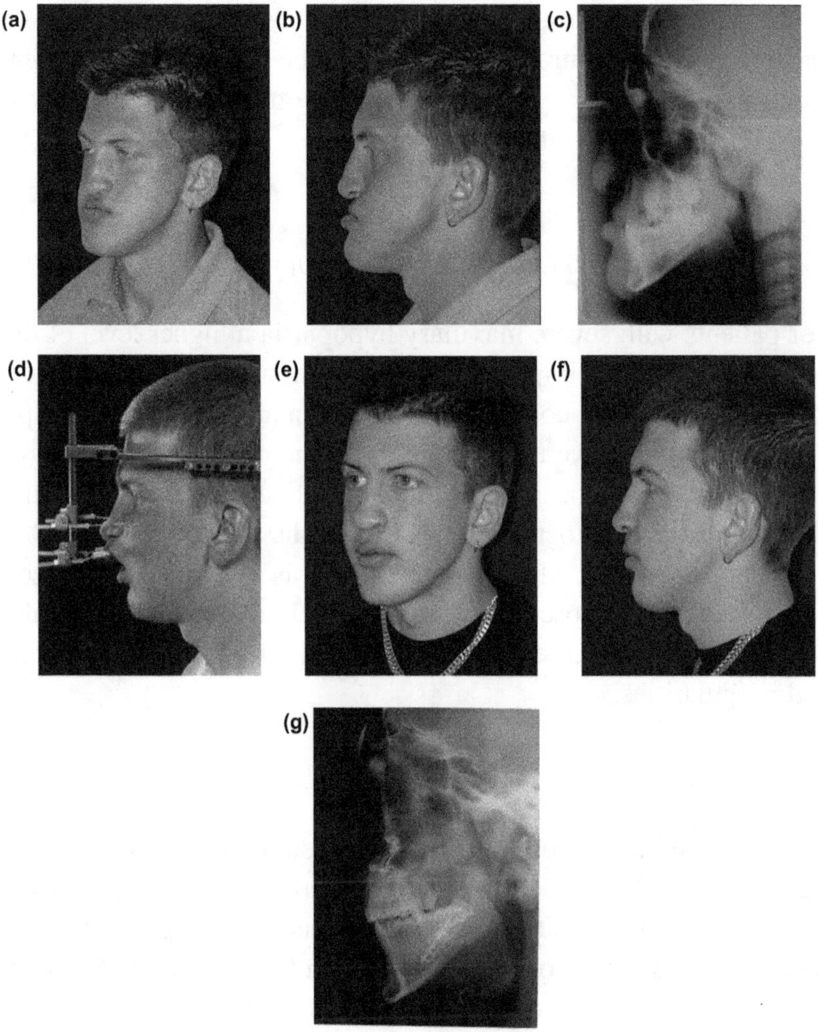

Figure 12.19 Simultaneous differential distraction of the maxilla at two or more levels may produce a better balanced facial contour.

Chapter 13

Ankylosis of the Temporomandibular Joint

Malcolm Harris

Introduction

There are many causes of limited mouth opening (trismus) which may be classified as follows.

Intra-articular trismus (intracapsular)

- Closed lock due anterior displacement of the meniscus without reduction.
- Osseous or fibro-osseous ankylosis, secondary to trauma, infection or osteoarthritis.
- Fibrodysplasia ossificans progressiva (formerly myositis ossificans).
- Ankylosing spondylitis, juvenile rheumatoid arthritis.

Extra-articular (extracapsular)

- Trismus.
- Disuse muscle atrophy, contractures secondary to intra-articular ankylosis or psychogenic trismus.

- Post-radiotherapy and thermal scarring.
- Post-traumatic scarring.
- Oral submucous fibrosis.
- Post-cancrum oris scarring.
- Fibrodysplasia ossificans progressiva (formerly myositis ossificans).

Only the management of intra-articular ankylosis with its marked disturbance in facial skeletal growth will be considered here.

Aetiology

Although most causes of extra-articular ankylosis are self-evident the aetiology of intra-articular ankylosis is obscure. It is uncommon in the West and the prevalence seems to be higher in tropical and sub-tropical countries although there is no reliable epidemiology.

Certain factors are significant; extra- and intracapsular joint trauma are common in children and adults but ankylosis is very rare (Figures 13.1a–13.1e). Experimental ankylosis is very difficult to produce in animals without inserting a bone graft.

Removal of the meniscus produces a condylar overgrowth similar to the ankylosis deformity but without fusion (Figures 13.2a–13.2c).

However the rare fibrodysplasia ossificans progressiva which has an unexplained short first toe (Figure 13.3) and widespread heterotopic bone formation, is associated with an excess of the bone morphogenetic protein 4 (BMP 4) gene which may be due to a deficiency of the BMP inhibitor genes, curiously named gremlin (DRM) and noggin. Also the progressive ankylosis gene ank produces intra-articular and peri-articular joint fusion in man and mice.

The outcome of such a localised abnormal genotype could be a deficiency of RANKL (receptor activator of nuclear kappa ligand) a key messenger responsible for osteoclastogenesis, when the affected structures are challenged by trauma or infection.

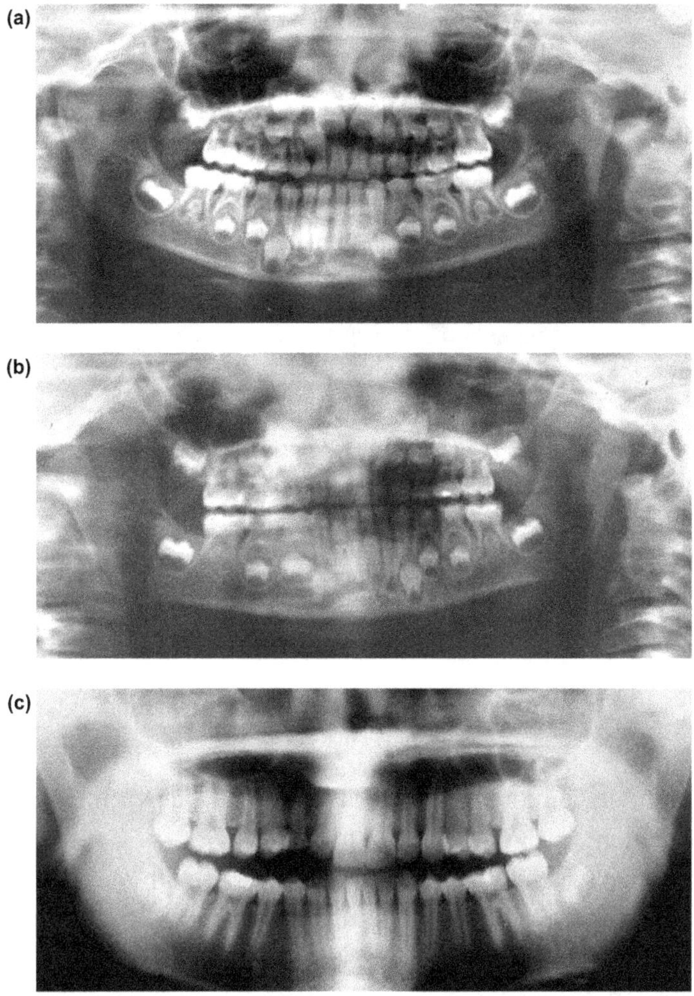

Figure 13.1 (**a**) Radiograph showing bilateral intracapsular fractures at 6 years. (**b**) Condylar remodelling 6 months later. (**c**), (**d**) and (**e**) Normal growth without ankylosis at 14 years.

The natural history is usually infantile and pre-adolescent loss of the meniscus due to:

- birth trauma with displacement of the meniscus;
- juvenile joint infection — middle ear, mastoid or haematogenous; and

(d) (e)

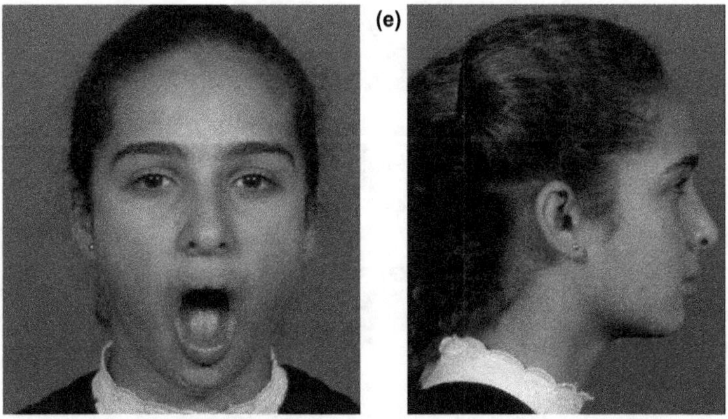

Figure 13.1 (*Continued*)

- juvenile rheumatoid arthritis (Stills disease), plus the unexplained tendency for local ectopic bone formation (see BMP 4, noggin, gremlin and ank above).

The idiopathic intracapsular bony fusion appears to arise through the following sequence of events.

i) Condylar damage and loss of meniscus due to traumatic displacement, inflammmation or infection.
ii) Irregular reparative condylar overgrowth with varying degrees of mechanical, fibrous and bony ankylosis with ossification of the joint capsule.
iii) Extra-articular ankylosis due to masticatory muscle contracture.

The same pattern is less frequently seen in adults following trauma, ankylosing spondylitis or osteoarthritis.

Presentation

Ankylosis in children produces impaired mandibular growth with bilateral deformity in all dimensions. This deformity is asymmetrical in unilateral cases with a straight small hemimandible on the

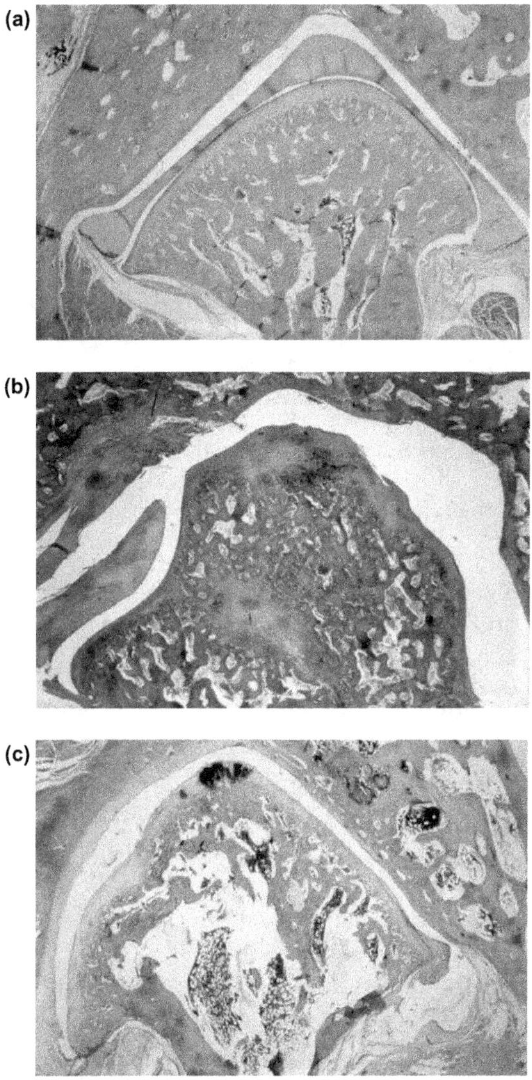

Figure 13.2 (**a**) Normal rabbit condyle and meniscus. (**b**) Hemi-condylar overgrowth following partial meniscectomy. (**c**) Total meniscectomy showing condylar overgrowth with mechanical but not bony ankylosis, illustrating a modelling role of the meniscus on condylar growth (loaned by Dr. Rudolph Sprintz).

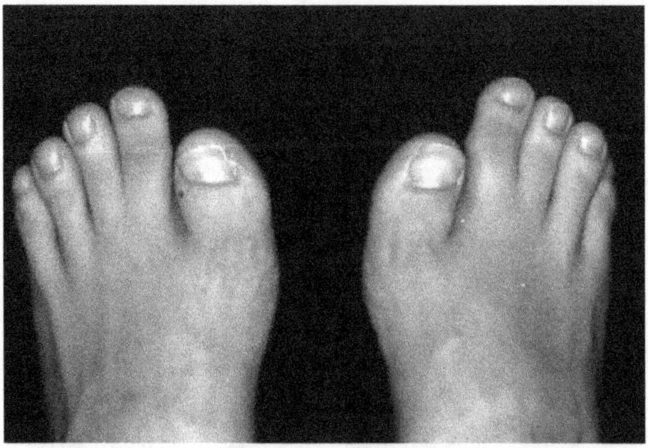

Figure 13.3 Short great toe characteristic of fibrodysplasia ossificans progressiva.

ankylosed side, and a marked contralateral bowing deformity. Retrognathia and retrogenia (Figures 13.4a–13.4c) become more apparent with age. This produces an occlusal cant down to the normal side. In rare bilateral cases the mandible is short but symmetrical. In all cases the inter-incisal opening can be up to 10 mm even with total bony fusion reflecting the bone elasticity within the masticatory system. There appear to be two causes of the impaired growth pattern.

i) The loss of the condylar fibrocartilage.

   Although the condylar growth cartilage is not considered to be the primary growth centre for the entire mandible, it makes a significant contribution to the height of the condylar head, neck and the ascending ramus including the angle of the mandible. This can be seen very clearly after perinatal ankylosis following birth trauma when the dental lamina has to extend backwards into the ascending ramus due to the lack of local alveolar bone at the angle (Figure 13.4f). The contralateral intact condylar growth centre continues to grow down and forwards towards the affected side producing the characteristic bowing deformity.

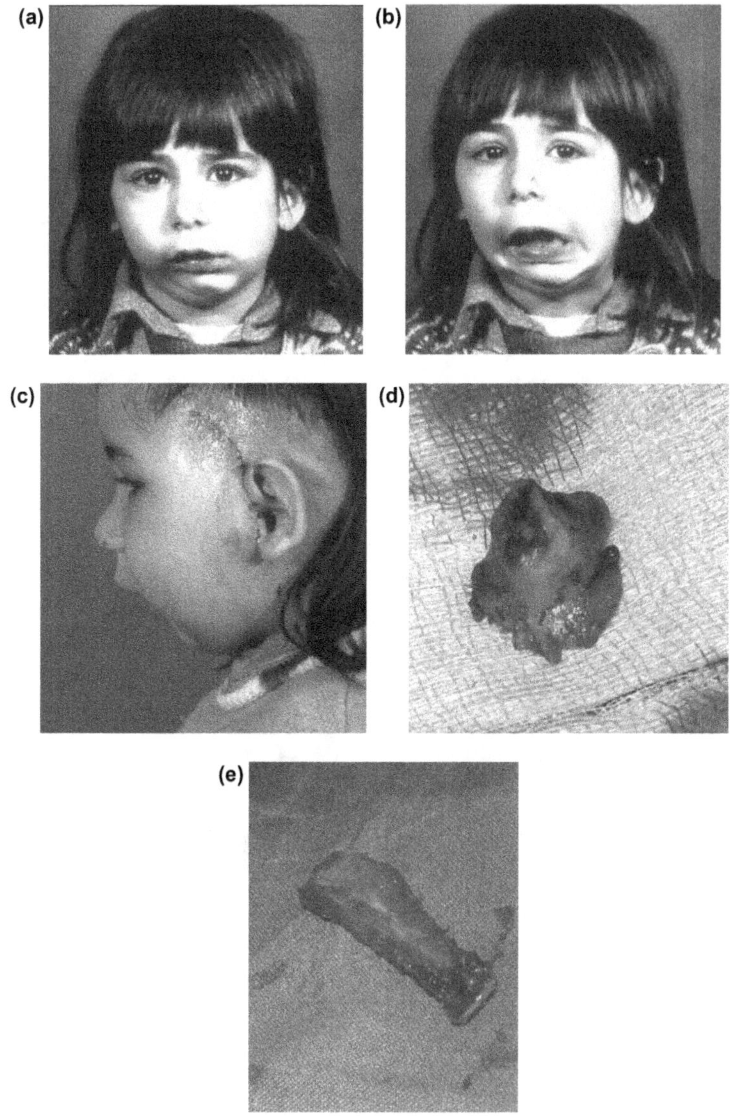

Figure 13.4 Left TMJ ankylosis following birth trauma showing characteristic facial deformity at 4 years (**a**), (**b**) and (**c**). Excised ankylosed condyle showing the wide adherent margin (**d**). Costochondral graft (**e**). The radiograph shows inverted mushroom ankylosis and extension of the dental lamina into the shortened ascending ramus.

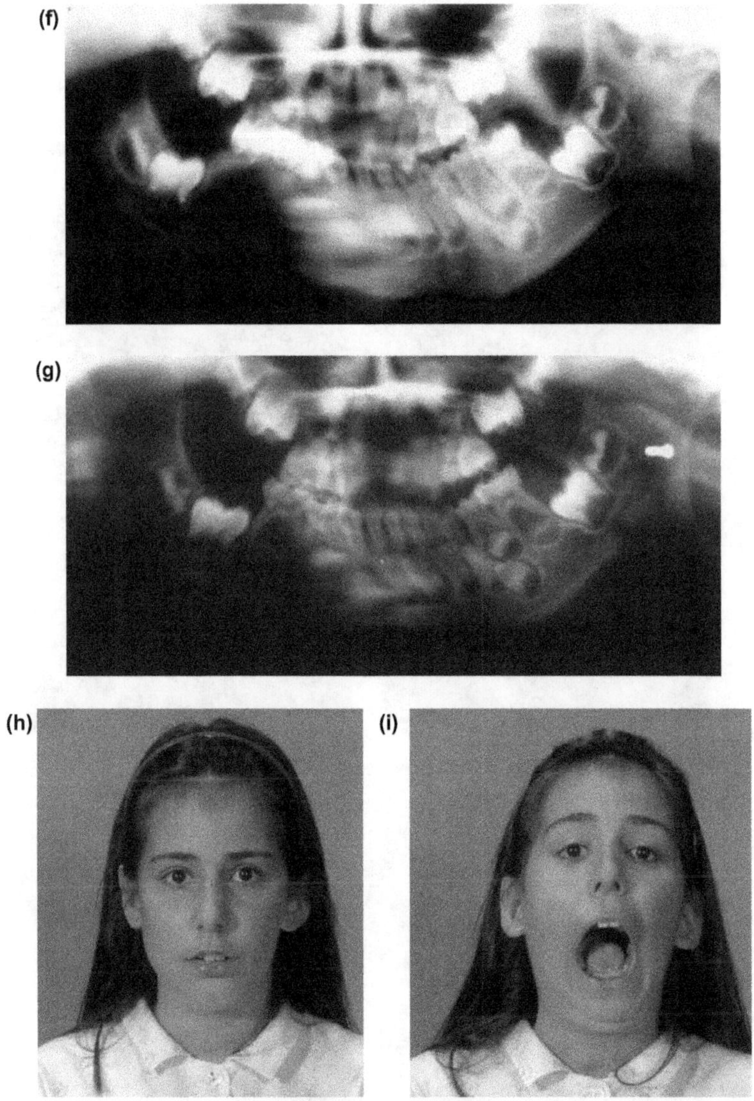

Figure 13.4 (*Continued*) **(f)** and **(g)** Following division of the ankylosis, ipsilateral coronoidectomy and costochondral graft. Early pre-adolescent arthroplasty allows catch-up growth and remodelling at 13 years **(h)** and **(i)**, 19 years **(j)** and **(k)** and at 27 years. **(l)**, **(m)**, **(n)**, **(o)** Inadequate growth of the costochondral graft is seen as deviation of the chin at rest and on opening, with a secondary limitation of the ipsilateral maxilla producing inclination of the occlusal plane. The ankylosis defect or surgery has also produced winging of the left ear.

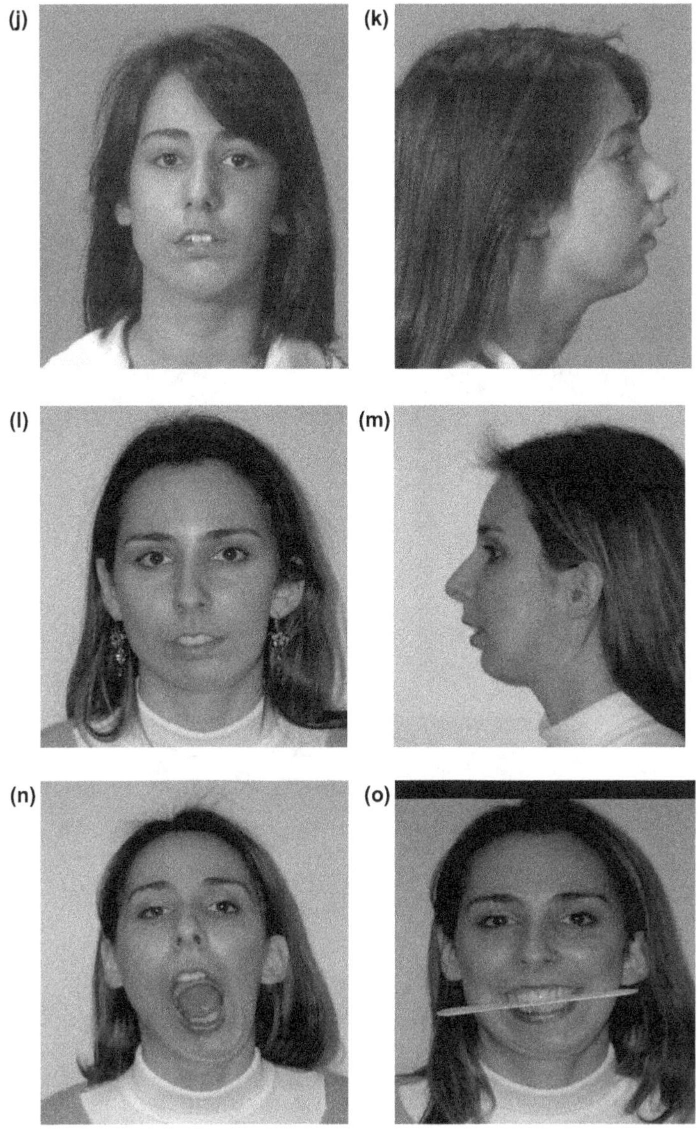

Figure 13.4 (*Continued*)

ii) The loss of function.

Persistent impaired function of any bone inhibits its linear and cross-sectional growth as can be seen in the ankylosed mandible in Figures 13.5a–13.5d. However this is avoided when the

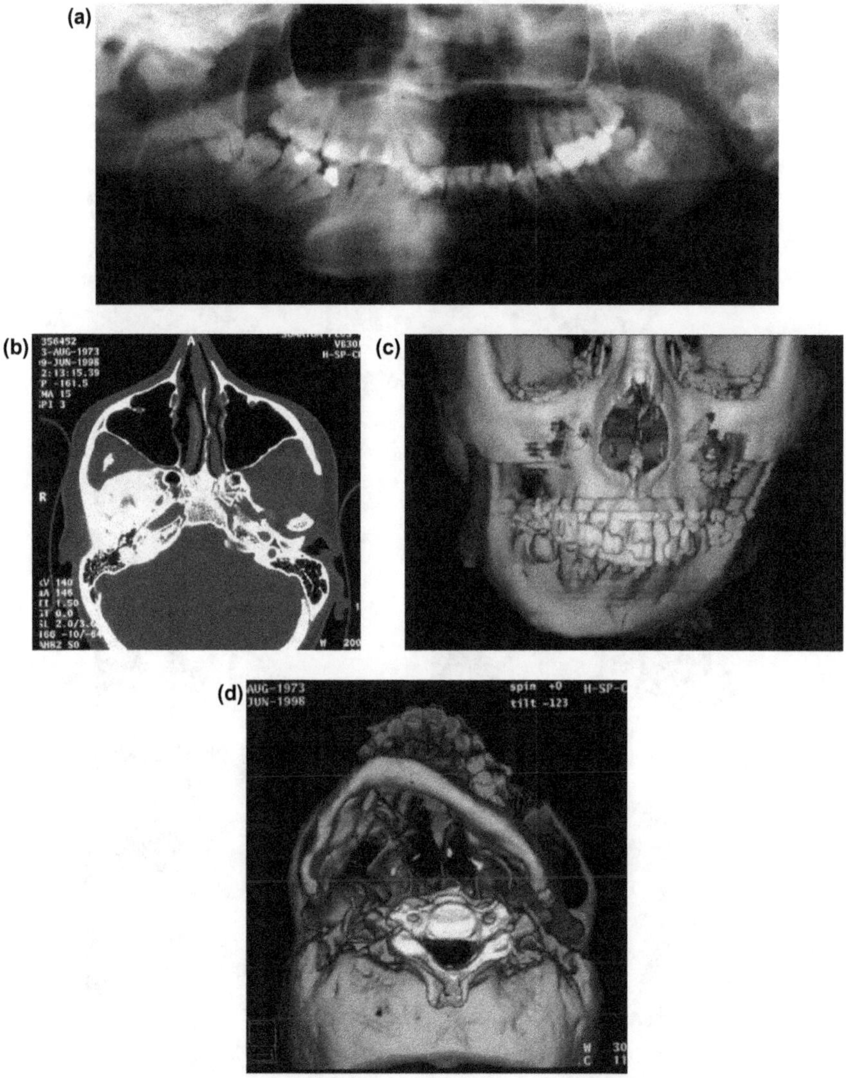

Figure 13.5 Imaging showing (**a**) apparent fibrosseous ankylosis of right TMJ but (**b**) shows complete fusion with base of skull. (**c**) 3D CT shows straight ankylosis side with deformed growing contralateral side with occlussal cant and (**d**) lower border of mandible shows impaired growth in all dimensions (case of Kieren Coghlin).

mandibular body is freed early before the adolescent growth spurt and function is restored. Figure 13.4 shows the natural history of a childhood ankylosis treated with a costochondral graft from the age of 4 through to 27 years.

However it is interesting to compare this with the outcome of a simple gap arthroplasty where the mandible can develop normally even without a condylar growth cartilage replacement (Figure 13.6).

It has been estimated that from 3–16 years the ascending ramus grows approximately 2 cm in height and the body of the mandible 2.5 cm in length. The aims of treatment are to:

- restore the ramus height and its growth potential as early as possible,
- release the functional growth of the mandibular body, and
- prevent secondary deformity.

Treatment Principles

- Excise the bony fusion as early as possible.
- Reconstruct.
- Prevent recurrent ankylosis.
- Restore function.
- Correct the secondary deformity.
- Correct the occlusion.

There are many treatment strategies depending on the age of the patient the duration of the deformity and degree of secondary deformity, but in all cases, success depends on preventing recurrence of the localised idiopathic fibrodysplasia ossificans.

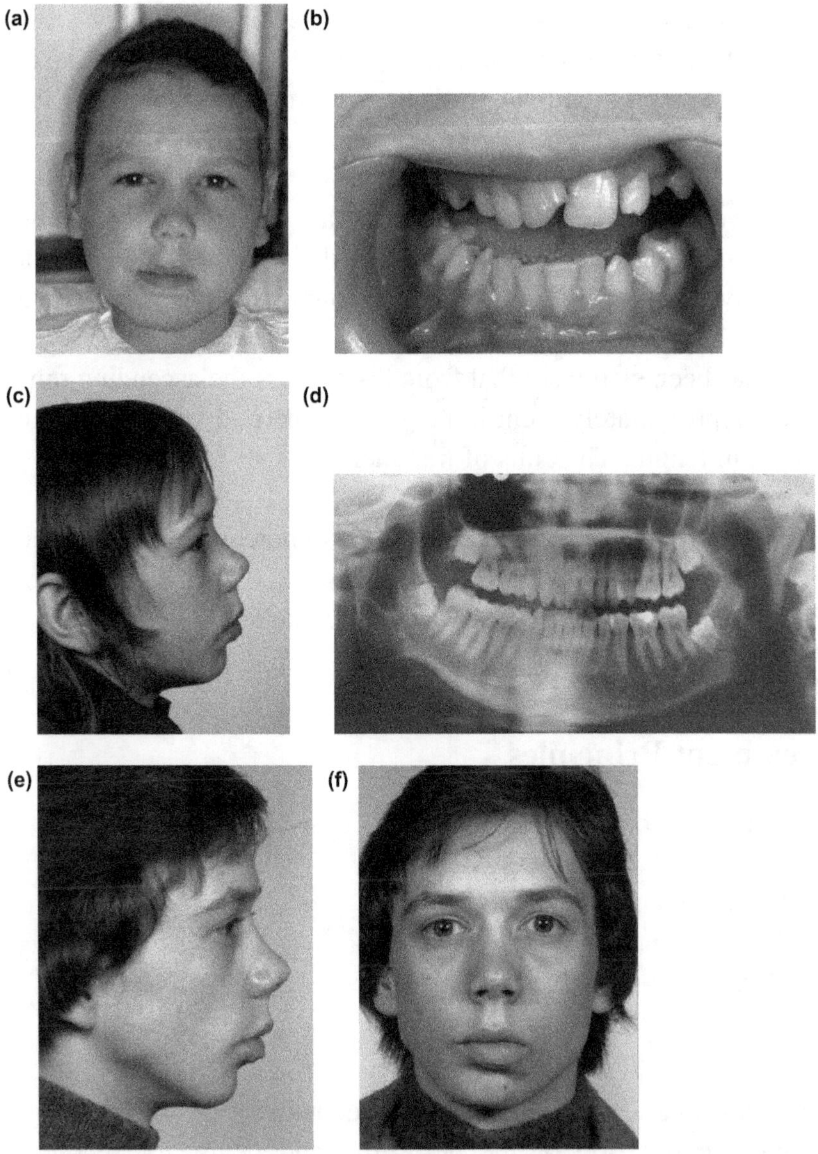

Figure 13.6 Post-traumatic right TMJ ankylosis at 10 years (**a**) and (**b**) treated with only a wide gap arthroplasty. (**c**) and (**d**) Facial growth and a functional pseudarthrosis. Normal growth and function at 19 (**e**) and (**f**) and 26 years with excellent opening but asymmetry limited to the loss of the condylar head and neck height (**g**)–(**i**).

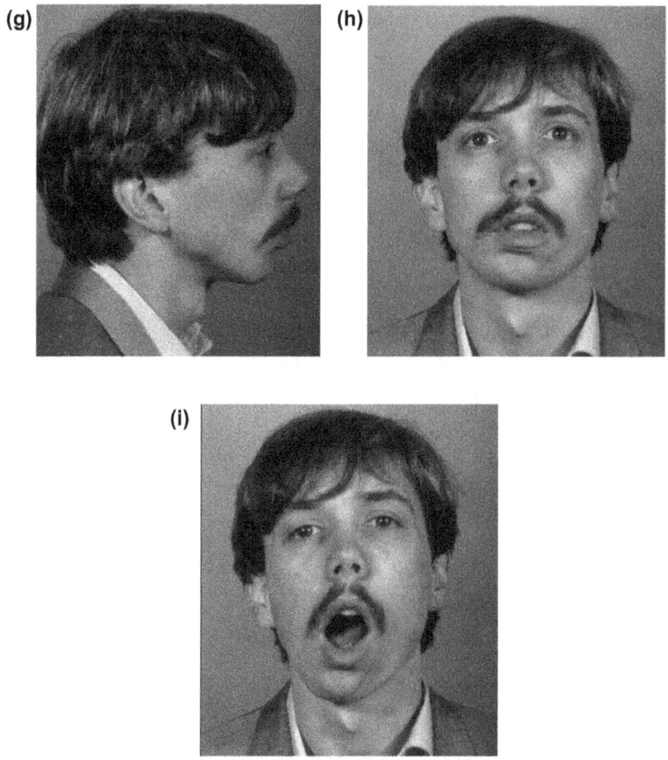

Figure 13.6 (*Continued*)

Treatment Choices

1. Pre-adolescent ankylosis presenting in childhood.

    a) Excision with the insertion of an interpositional temporalis myofascial peninsular flap and reconstruction with a costochondral growth centre to restore function and ramus growth.
    b) Bilateral coronoidectomies (coronoidotomies).
    c) Or excision of the ankylosis creating a simple gap arthroplasty with an interpositional temporalis myofascial peninsular flap followed by distraction osteogenesis (see below and Chapter 10).

The anteroposterior deficiency and asymmetry in childhood is usually self-corrected with catch-up growth.

2. The pre-adolescent ankylosis presenting during or post-adolescence.

    a) Excision with the insertion of an interpositional temporalis myofascial peninsular flap or a sialastic “membrane” and reconstruction with a costochondral graft to restore function and ramus growth if early enough.
    b) Bilateral coronoidectomies (coronoidotomies): the earlier the restoration of function the more spontaneous growth and remodelling will be achieved in adolescence.
    c) Or as the alternative to the excision of the ankylosis, simply creating a gap arthroplasty with an interpositional temporalis myofascial peninsular flap and the addition of distraction osteogenesis (see point 5 below and Chapter 10).

3. Pre-adolescent ankylosis presenting after the completion of facial growth.

    a) As 2 above, with a rotational advancement genioplasty.
    b) Marked retrognathia will require a sagittal split or inverted L osteotomy.

4. Late ankylosis in adults with no interference with facial growth.

    a) Division of the ankylosis conserving ramus height, sculpting the condylar head with the interposition of an articular membrane such as a temporalis myofascial peninsular flap, a 2 mm sialastic membrane or the retrieved meniscus (Figures 13.7a–13.7d).
    b) Bilateral coronoidectomies (coronoidotomies).

In all cases the tendency for localised fibrodysplasia ossificans to produce a recurrent fusion must be inhibited by a 7-day pre- and 2-month postoperative course of bisphosphonate, which is currently alendronic acid 10 mg a day in the morning.

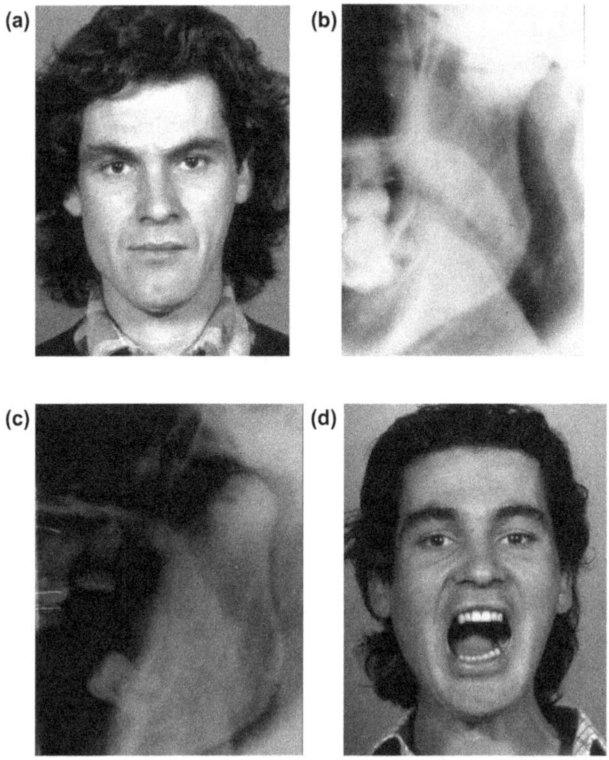

Figure 13.7 (**a**) Left TMJ ankylosis following adult trauma does not impair facial growth. (**b**) Linear radiolucency within the fused "golfball exostosis" is site of failed division of bony mass. (**c**) Separation at skull base, with insertion of sialastic membrane and coronoidectomy, provides function. (**d**) Without loss of ramus height.

5. Distraction osteogenesis (see Chapter 10).

There is now evidence that

- division of the ankylosis,
- bilateral coronoidectomies (otomies) to free temporalis contractures,
- a myofascial interpositional arthroplasty, and
- distraction osteogenesis

restore movement and function and simultaneously elongates the deformed mandible. As bisphosphonates delay bone formation their role in distraction osteogenesis is as yet unpredictable.

Preoperative Imaging (Figure 13.5)

- OPG.
- True lateral skull.
- CT scan with 3D reconstruction.
- Standard orthognathic photographic series.

Timing

Resection of the ankylosis should be carried out as early as possible to enable normal growth and avoid secondary deformity. The exception is any extra-articular jaw osteotomy which should be deferred until facial growth has ceased.

Surgical Approach

The preoperative preparation differs from the standard orthognathic workup in several respects.

1. The anaesthetist must be skilled in the intubation of patients who are unable to open their mouths. This has been been made easier by the use of fibreoptic intubation but still represents a challenge especially in cases with marked retrognathia. The facilities for a tracheostomy should always be available.
2. The temporal area must be shaved and cleaned before the patient is taken into theatre. This facilitates the incision and prevents hair straying into the operative field.
3. The face and mouth are cleaned with aqueous povidone iodine and draped, exposing both ears for access and orientation.

A small piece of sterile petroleum jelly gauze (tulle grasse) is inserted into the depths of the external auditory meatus. A large piece will work its way out within minutes of starting the operation.

4. The incision is marked with a surgical pen, from the temporal area (2 cm above and 2 cm anterior to the tip of the pinna) diagonally downwards and backwards to the attachment of the ear, and then following the junctional contour to the upper end of the tragal cartilage. It then follows the crest of the cartilage down to the lobe and then skirts behind it (Figure 13.8a).
5. The whole length is infiltrated with bupivocaine and adrenaline to achieve local vasoconstriction.
6. Incise the skin with a No. 15 blade from above downwards, retraction with skin hooks will reveal the superficial veins which are coagulated with bipolar diathermy and divided. The incision along the crest of the tragus will reveal but preserve the cartilage. With fine tooth forceps the skin is dissected forwards off the cartilage and then the attachment of the lobe can be divided from front to back. The length and depth of this incision are crucial for comfortable exposure of the deeper structures (Figure 13.8b). This "parotid" incision gives excellent access to the acending ramus, eliminates the need for an additional submandibular approach and leaves a totally discrete scar.
7. By keeping the temporal incision well back, the orbito-frontal branches of the facial nerve will be safe in the upper anterior flap. The main trunk of the VII nerve emerges from the stylomastoid foramen one and a half fingers breadths below the tragal cartilage (the external auditory meatus) and passes forward 1–2 cm beneath the skin surface deep to the superficial lobe of the parotid gland, and so remains safely enclosed in the depths of the lower anterior flap. The auricular temporal vessels will be encountered but should be readily controlled with bipolar diathermy and 3/0 vicryl ties.

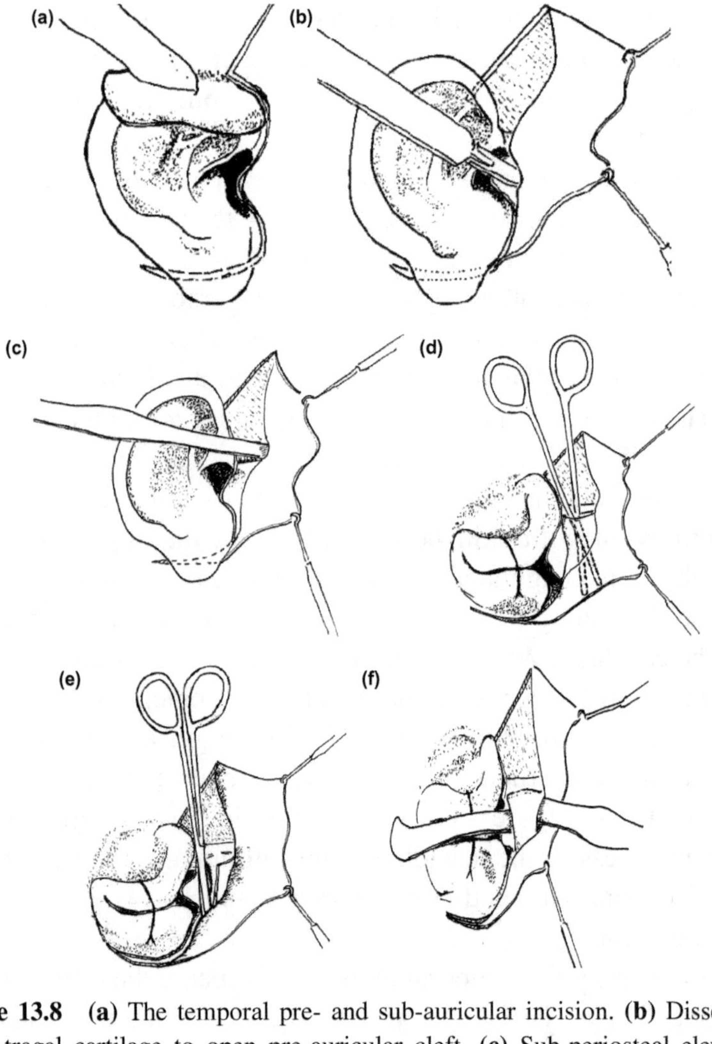

Figure 13.8 (**a**) The temporal pre- and sub-auricular incision. (**b**) Dissection along tragal cartilage to open pre-auricular cleft. (**c**) Sub-periosteal elevation along zygomatic arch. (**d**) Creation of vertical pocket in the plane of the root of zygoma and the ankylosis. (**e**) Dividing the posterior partition of the pocket to expose the ankylosis. (**f**) Isolating the ankylosis with retractors. (**g**) The bony fusion has been separated with a bur and fine osteotome, the condylar neck has been divided together with a coronoidectomy. The ramus decortication is for the costochondral graft. (**h**) Division of the ankylosis with preservation of ramus height in an adult without facial deformity. (**i**) A sialastic interpositional membrane suspended from the glenoid fossa.

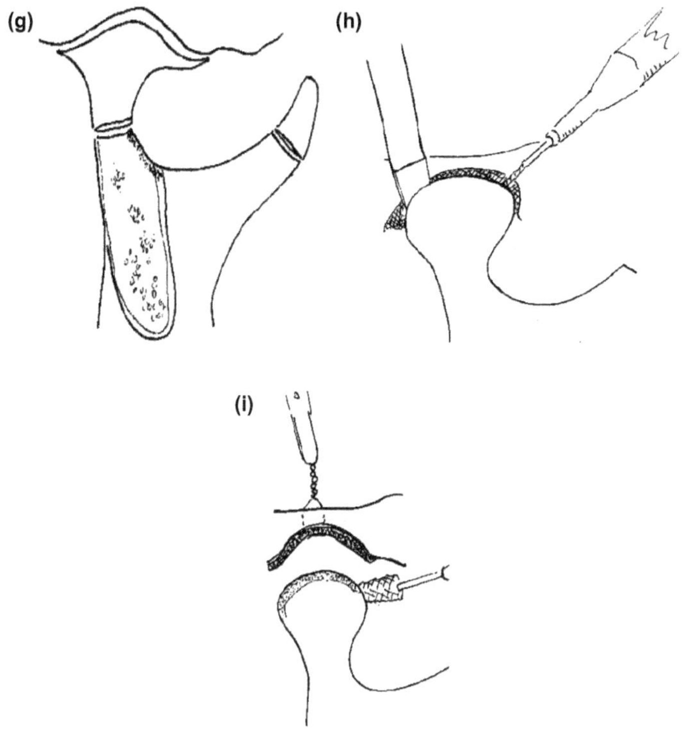

Figure 13.8 (*Continued*)

8. After arresting all bleeding points, the incision is deepened through the temporalis fascia down to muscle and down to bone at the root of the zygomatic arch. A small vessel at this point must be coagulated. Below the arch there is a natural vertical cleft in the deeper tissues that can be opened with the blade along the anterior surface of the cartilaginous external auditory meatus and then with Macindoe scissors (Figure 13.8b).
9. Confirm the periosteal incision on the root of the zygomatic arch is down to bone with the rasp end of a Howarth periosteal elevator, reverse it and insert the elevator firmly forward along the surface of the arch. This will raise a tent of fascia both above and below the arch which must be released with scissors

at both ends of the incision (Figure 13.8c). Posteriorly it is convenient to fold the ear and suture the lobe to the pinna with 2/0 vicryl.

10. The operative plane below the arch is now developed obliquely downwards and forwards with a periosteal elevator and then Macindoe scissors from the surface of the root of the zygoma onto the surface of the ankylosis (Figure 13.8d). This creates a pocket overlying the ankylosis with a posterior partition separating it from the vertical pre-auricular cleft. This partition must be divided with scissors to create a free peri-articular area to work in (Figure 13.8e).
11. It is now possible to expose the arch as far forward as the zygomatic bone itself. Where the flap can be held with a small Langenbeck retractor.
12. In all cases the joint capsule has been ossified and has disappeared so that sub-periosteal exploration down from the arch will immediately expose the lateral aspects of the ankylosis.
13. Carefully but firmly push the elevator distally around the condylar neck and leave it or a malleable strip against the deeper aspect of the bone as a retractor. Repeat this on the anterior surface of the condylar neck area. With marked loss of ramus height, the space below the arch may be tight admitting only a narrow instrument such as a Frear elevator as a retractor (Figure 13.8f).
14. The child's ankylosis differs morphologically from the fusion occurring in an adult. In the child the fusion resembles an upturned mushroom (Figure 13.8g) whereas adult cases tend to be a proliferative golf ball. The line of fusion should be visible or estimated and is explored by firmly tapping a 5 mm osteotome progressively deeper into its depth at three or four points. It should now be possible to lever the bony mass away from the skull base. The mass is separated by a bur cut at the base of the condylar neck (Figure 13.8g).

Sub-periosteal dissection forward to the anterior border of the ramus can usually enable the coronoidectomy (otomy) to be done through the pre-auricular incision.

15. There are two forms of adult ankylosis:

    (i) simple bony fusion following osteoarthritis or ankylosing spondilitis and
    (ii) those following trauma with an exostotic mass continuous with the zygomatic arch and skull base.

    Both have no loss of ramus height, and simply require a line of cleavage. The former is usually apparent and can be separated with a narrow osteotome. The exostotic form has to be estimated and cut deeply with a tungsten carbide fissure bur. A sturdy 1 cm osteotome is then necessary to lever this bony mass from the overlying skull base preserving it to be sculpted into a new condyle with an acrylic bur (Figure 13.8h).
16. In the adolescent and adult the temporalis and its tendon and to a lesser extent the other elevator muscles have undergone a degree of contracture which must be released with a bilateral coronoidectomy or otomy. This can be done on the ankylosis side by extending the sub-periosteal exposure forward over the ascending ramus and retaining access with an Obwegeser channel retractor passed around the anterior border. The lower bur cut instead of just sectioning the neck can be extended simultaneously forward just below the sigmoid notch to the anterior border of the ramus to include the coronoid process (Figure 13.9a).
17. At this point it is essential to inspect the specimen and also explore the depths of the wound on the ankylosis side as the fusion of a fractured condylar neck to skull base can be wrongly assumed to be the complete ankylosis, whereas the medially displaced condyle is often fused with the skull base above and to the medial aspect of the ascending ramus

(a)

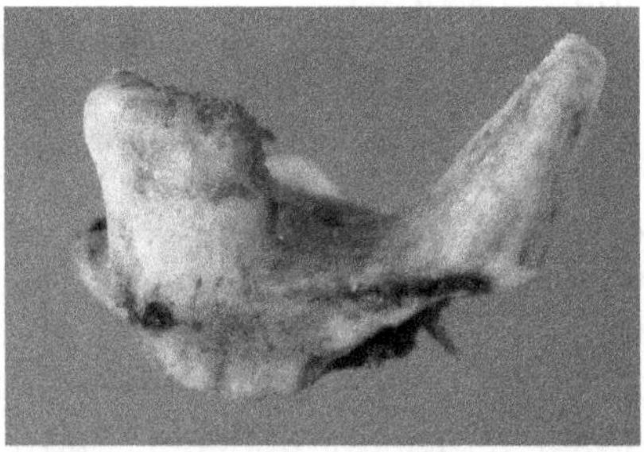

(b)

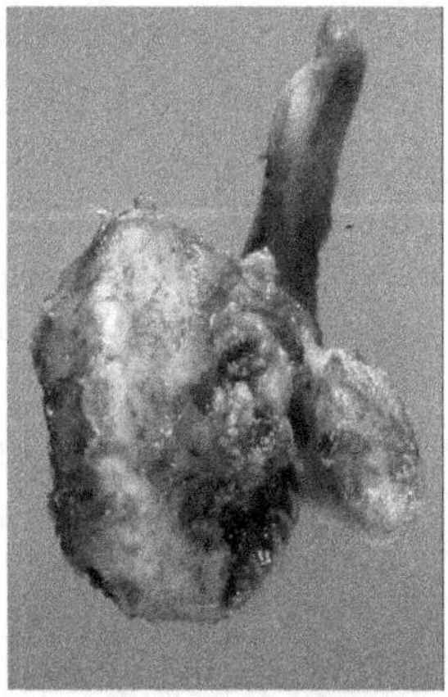

Figure 13.9 (**a**) and (**b**) Combined excision of ankylosis and coronoid showing the major restraint to opening was the concealed medially displaced condylar head which was fused to both the skull base and ascending ramus.

below. If this is the case the aberrant condyle must also be separated and removed (Figure 13.9b). In post-traumatic cases the exploration should also attempt to locate and retrieve the meniscus.

18. A contralateral coronoidectomy or otomy is essential to give maximum opening. This is done intraorally after stretching the mouth open with a Featherstone or similar self-retaining gag. Two blade (Lacs) retractors are required and are pressed, one on each side of the anterior border of the ascending ramus. Incise downwards between them through the mucosa and muscle to the bone. Elevate the periosteum and muscle layer on both sides of the ascending ramus and insert the blade retractor (Lacs) in each pocket, then using the forked Langenbeck retractor, the coronoid is exposed and grasped with curved Kocher forceps and divided obliquely at its base with a bur. The last remaining bony bridge which is the anterior rim of the sigmoid notch is fractured with an osteotome

(a)

(b) (c)

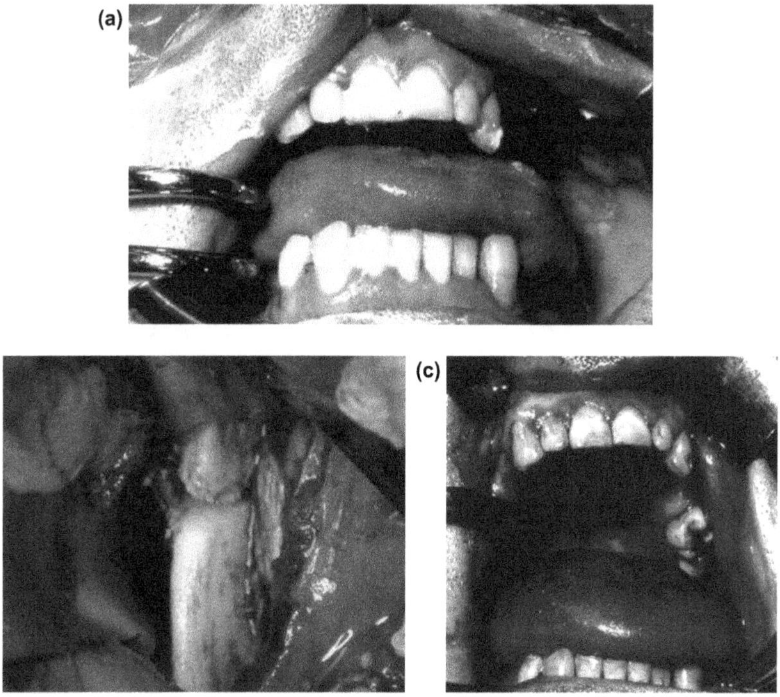

Figure 13.10 (**a**) Opening after resection of fused condylar head and coronoidectomy. (**b**) Intraoral contralateral coronoidotomy and (**c**) significant increase in mouth opening.

inserted in the bur cut and twisted. As the coronoid process is elongated its removal can be difficult and is probably unnecessary. The stretched opening of the mouth can now with effort be doubled (Figures 13.10a to 13.10c).

19. Reconstruction using the costochondral graft.

    - Where growth or ramus height are required a costochondral graft is harvested and trimmed to provide a suitable articular surface (Figure 13.11).
    - A groove is prepared on the lateral surface of the ramus by superficial decortication with a bur and an osteotome.

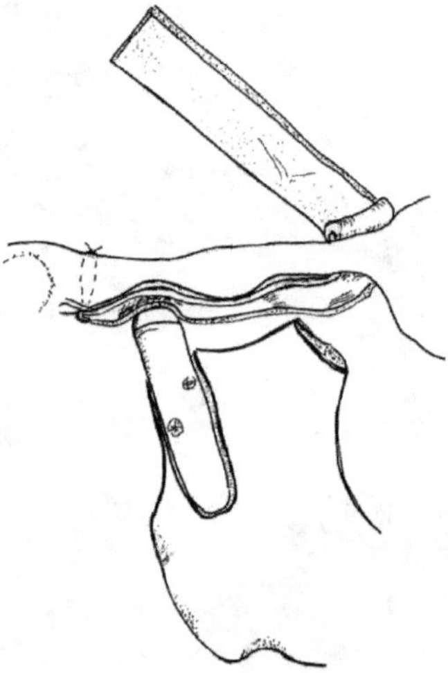

Figure 13.11 Costochondral graft with temporalis myofascial peninsular flap rotated downwards through the zygomatic arch and backwards to act as a meniscus.

- The bite is propped open 10 mm in the ipsilateral molar area with a folded tonsil swab side and the rib placed on the groove with the costal cartilage extending up against the glenoid fossa and 2 screws inserted to fix it.
- The meniscus is replaced if it can be localised from a medial fracture displacement. Otherwise the choice is a temporalis myofascial peninsula flap or a 2 mm sialastic membrane.
- The 2 cm broad myofascial flap is outlined postero-superiorly as shown with its base at the origin of the arch. It is incised down to the calvarium, elevated and firmly pulled (and pushed) down and under the zygomatic arch with a heavy suture passed through its mobile distal end. This suture can be passed down through the arch with a wire "pull" loop, a pair of curved Kochers or Adsons right angled forceps. It is then pulled backwards into the

condylar fossa and anchored with a heavy suture passed upwards through a drill hole, done from above through the most disto-medial point of the roof of the glenoid fossa (Figure 13.11). This procedure is much easier with the condyle subluxed from the fossa by maximally stretching the mouth open and then reduced to sit beneath the flap.

- Of the many autogenous and alloplast materials used as alternative interpositional membranes, 2 mm sialastic has proved to be ideal for this role suspended by 0.5 wire from the glenoid fossa. The margins must be carefully trimmed to avoid overextension (Figure 13.8i).

20. Reconstruction preserving the condyle.

    This is useful in late onset ankylosis where there is a proliferative fusion and no loss of ramus height. The bone is sculpted into a neocondyle and the fossa trimmed to accommodate it with an acrylic bur. In these cases a myofascial flap or 2 mm sialastic sheet are used as an interpositional membrane as described above (Figures 13.8h and 13.8i).
21. Reconstruction with a prosthetic joint. With the many autogenous alternatives, prosthetic total joint replacement is rarely required but may be essential in the older osteoporotic or rheumatoid patient. The principles are the same as the costochondral graft with the exception that the occlusion has to be carefully defined. Alloplastic joints do not remodel and have to be accurately placed to avoid morphoincompatibility where function will erode the tense overlying tissues leading to exposure and infection.
22. Post-adolescent cases require an augmentation and rotation genioplasty (Figures 13.12a to 13.12c). In a bilateral case, if an advancement osteotomy (or distraction osteogenesis) is required, ideally this follows preparatory orthodontics.

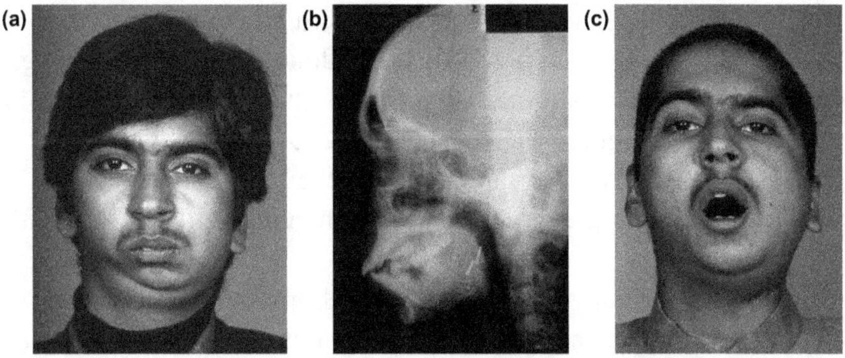

Figure 13.12 (**a**) Characteristic adult asymmetrical retrognathia from left TMJ ankylosis in childhood. (**b**) and (**c**) After costochondral graft arthroplasty and rotation advancement genioplasty.

The osteotomy is not usually necessary when the ankylosis is treated before adolescence especially with a costochondral graft or with distraction osteogenesis.

23. Vacuum drains are inserted, and the wounds closed with subcutaneous 3/0 vicryl and 5/O prolene for the skin. A firm turban pressure dressing is applied, ensuring that gauze or wool is placed behind the pinna of the ear to avoid compression ischaemia.
24. Postoperative care. Analgesics and antibiotics are prescribed as usual with the addition of daily alendronic acid 10 mg in the morning for 2 months. This is taken 30 minutes before breakfast when upright to avoid oesophagitis. A fluid and soft diet is essential to achieve a compromise between rest and function to be followed by stretching exercises with a modified laboratory chemistry clamp (Figure 13.13) at least 3 times a day for 6 months.
25. The closure of the maxillary cant can be facilitated by taking impressions and a squash bite as soon as possible (intraoperatively is inappropriately messy) and the models mounted to

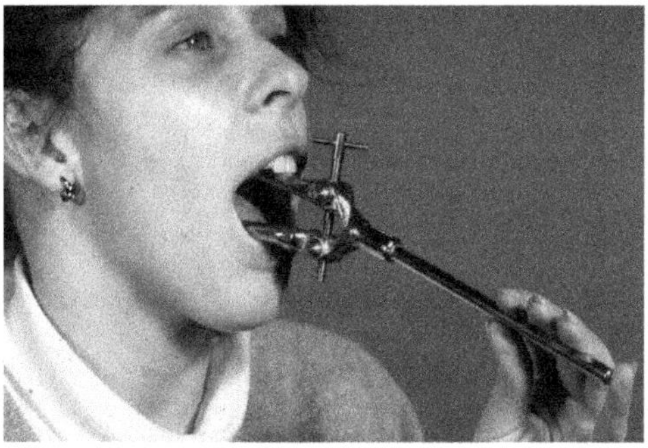

Figure 13.13 Modified laboratory retort (chemistry) clamp with plastic tubing to protect teeth, provides well controlled stretching exercises.

enable a maxillary plate with a lateral bite wedge to keep open the ipsilateral buccal occlusion until an orthodontic assessment and the insertion of a functional appliance to level the occlusion (Figures 13.14a to 13.14c).

Complications

- Damage to the orbital and frontal branches of the facial nerve is to be avoided by careful flap design.
- Limited opening due to inadequate bone removal especially on the medial aspect of the condylar neck — will be revealed by a CT scan and requires a repeat arthroplasty.
- Persistent limited opening due to a failure to do a bilateral coronoidectomies or otomies. These may be done intraorally but must be supplemented by stretching exercises and bisphosphonates.
- Postoperative fibrodysplasia ossificans in the medial pterygoid and masseter can occur and will also require bisphosphonates and stretching exercises for 2–3 months (Figures 13.15a and 13.15b).

(a)

(b)

(c)

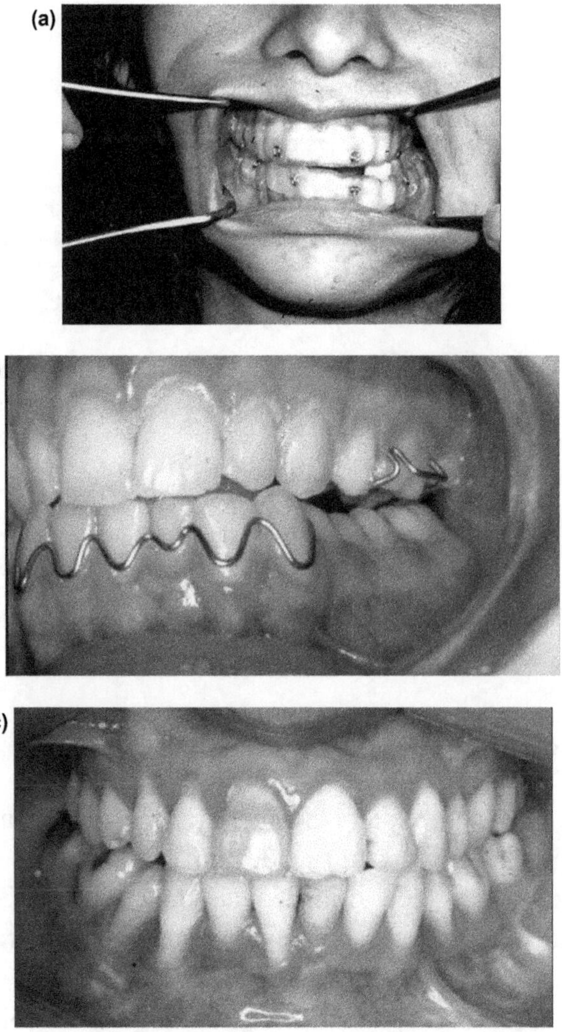

Figure 13.14 (**a**) Acrylic wedge to maintain postoperative lateral open bite and ramus height. Another patient to show (**b**) functional appliance to facilitate closure of postoperative lateral open bite (**c**) closure achieved.

- Marked malocclusion will require orthodontics and an osteotomy.
- Failure of the costochondral graft to grow. With function this acts as an interpositional arthroplasty enabling mandibular

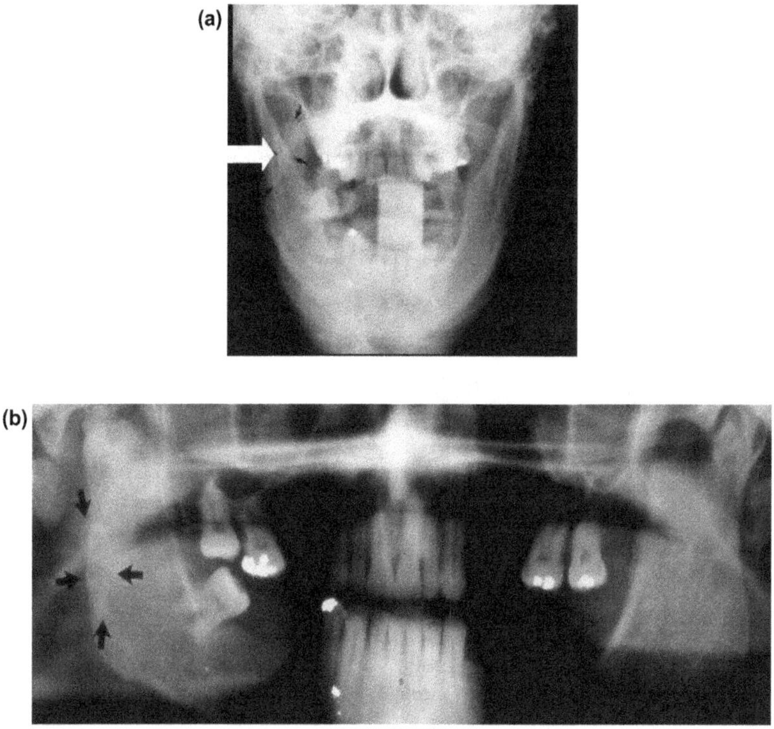

Figure 13.15 (**a**) and (**b**) Gradual postoperative onset of impaired opening due to fibrodysplasia ossificans of the medial pterygoid muscle. Treated with 3 months bisphosphonate and stretching.

growth. Asymmetry is rarely great can be corrected by an osteotomy or distraction osteogenesis when mandibular growth has completed.

- Fusion of the graft with re-ankylosis requires a repeat arthroplasty and bisphosphanates or distraction osteogenesis.
- Excess growth of the graft with a pseudohemimandibular elongation can be corrected by trimming the articular end of the graft and levelling the occlusal plane orthodontically (Figures 13.16a–13.16f).
- Pneumothorax (see Complications and Emergencies section).

(a) (b) (c) (d) (e) (f)

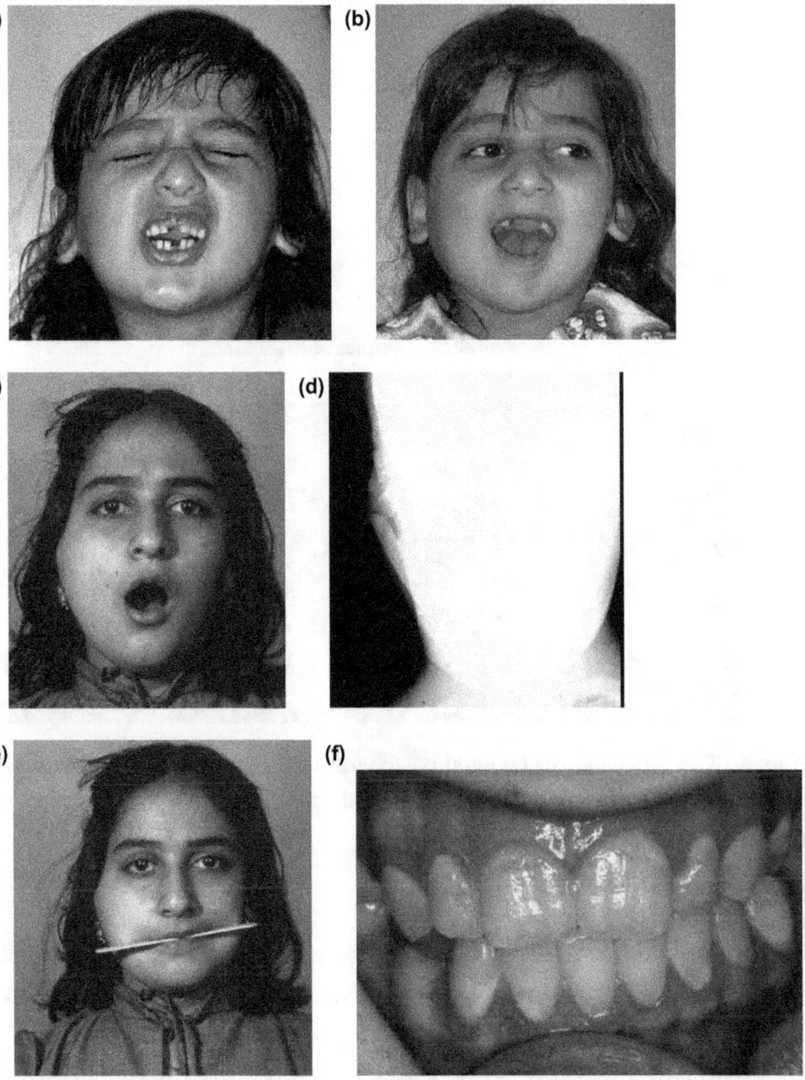

Figure 13.16 (**a**) Ankylosis in a 5-year-old. (**b**) Postoperative opening. (**c**) and (**d**) Pseudohemimandibular hyperplasia due to costchondral overgrowth at 12 years with lateral displacement of overgrown graft. (**e**) and (**f**) Occlussal cant.

Summary

The excision of the ankylosis, joint reconstruction with a costochondral graft and bilateral temporalis myotomies remain the most common management. However there is evidence that restoration of growth and function may also be achieved with an interpositional arthroplasty as described for the adult case, and distraction osteogenesis as an alternative to a costochondral graft (see Chapter 9).

Chapter 14

Rhinoplasty Surgery

Santdeep H. Paun

Introduction

Rhinoplasty surgery forms a vital part of the functional and aesthetic management of congenital or traumatic deformities of the facial skeleton. This chapter will cover important aspects of

- nasal anatomy,
- assessment of the deformity,
- surgical planning, and
- operative procedures.

It is essential that the reader refers to a comprehensive or specialist texts for detailed aspects of the surgery.

The nose is a complex structure cantilevered on the mid face. Its complex role embraces the senses of smell and taste, respiration, aesthetics and sex and so rhinoplasty surgery requires careful consideration. All mid face orthognathic surgery will affect the nose to a degree. LeFort I operation impactions broaden the alar width, and with inadequate trimming of the nasal septum they will lead to septal buckling and obstruction or deviation of the nasal tip. Advancements will raise the nasal tip and straighten out profile curvatures. For these reasons it is undesirable to do a rhinoplasty before, during or within 6 months of a mid face osteotomy.

Nasal Anatomy

It is important to understand the complex nasal anatomy which is made difficult by the nomenclature. The upper border of many structures is designated cephalic (headwise) and the lower border caudal (tailwise). The anterior surface of the nose is dorsal and posterior structures are posterior. Unfotunately some terms have been introduced in relation to the supine anaesthetised patient, so that what might be considered as anterior and posterior nasal sites are described as "high" and "low".

Figures 14.1 and 14.2 show the anatomical subunits of the nose, which is conveniently divided in thirds. The upper third consists of the bony pyramid, made up of the nasal bones with their articulation to the frontal processes of the maxilla and the bony septum. The

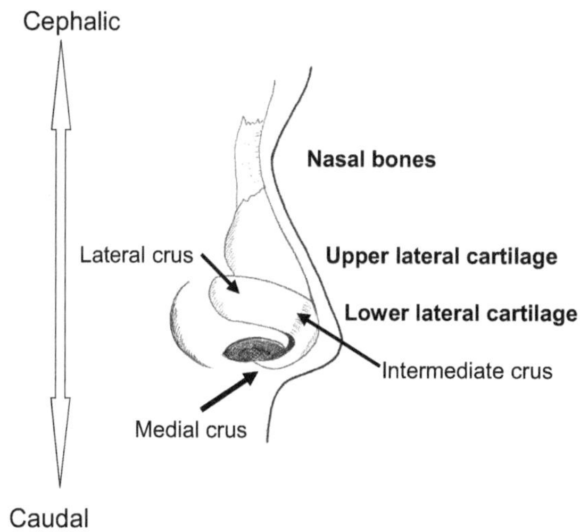

Figure 14.1 External anatomy of nose (lateral view).

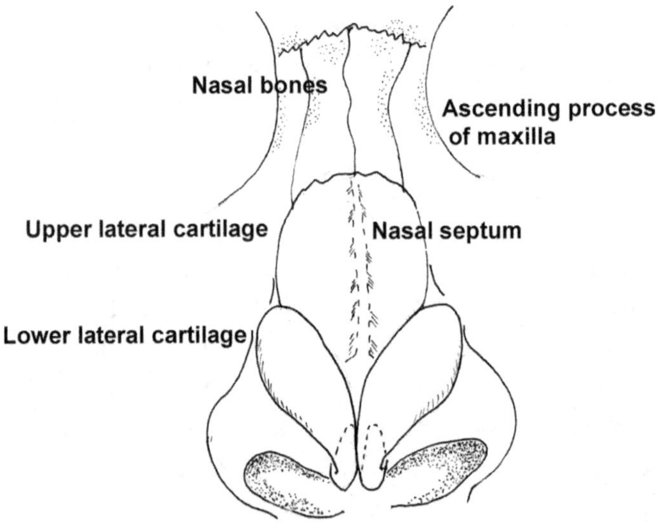

Figure 14.2 External anatomy of nose (frontal view).

paired upper lateral cartilages insert just under the caudal (lower) end of the nasal bones and their fusion with the midline cartilaginous septum in a "T" type configuration forms the middle third ("vault") (Figure 14.2). The attachment of the caudal aspect of the upper lateral cartilage to the cephalic (upper) aspect of lower lateral cartilages forms the boundary to the lower third of the nose and is referred to as the scroll attachment. The paired lower laterals, sometimes called the alar cartilages, form the a prominent part of the lateral surface of many noses and the nasal tip, They are divided into the lateral, intermediate and medial crurae — or processes (Figures 14.3a and 14.3b). The intermediate crurae form the "domes" and are the tip defining points of the nose.

The medial crura curve medially and backwards and their terminal processes, the so-called footplates abut against the border of the caudal aspect of the nasal septum and form the cartilaginous columella.

The columella with its cartilage and skin provide the external (caudal) border of the septum from the tip to the nasolabial angle.

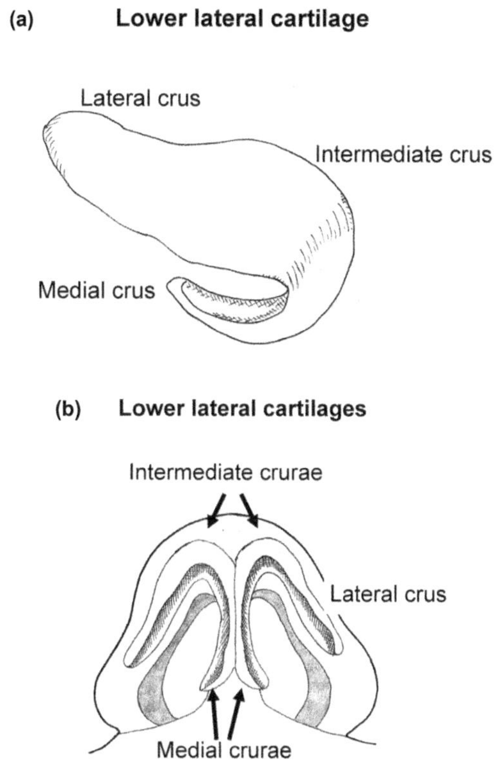

Figure 14.3 (**a**) and (**b**) Lower lateral cartilage anatomy.

The outer margin of the nares are the soft tissue alar lobules that are devoid of cartilage.

The overlying superficial musculoaponeurotic system (SMAS) of the nose is a complex layer which provides a rich vascular supply covering to the underlying skeleton and is derived from the superior labial and facial arteries and corresponding venous and lymphatic vessels accompanying these. Its intrinsic aponeurotic muscles have elevator, depressor, compressor and dilator functions which contribute to olfaction and facial expression.

The external anatomy of the nose is readily studied in any crowded place.

Assessment

History

A detailed history covering the functional and aesthetic aspects of the nose is mandatory.

To assess function, the patient is asked specifically regarding the presence and duration of nasal obstruction, sinus disease and allergic type symptoms. It is important to document prior medical and surgical treatments and their efficacy in treating any functional or aesthetic complaints.

A detailed history of traumatic injuries to the nose and surrounding facial skeleton is essential especially if operated on, and an indication of the pretraumatic appearance of the nose is helpful. It is particularly important to gauge the patient's specific concerns about the appearance of each subsection of the nose with direct questioning. A generalised vague reference to a dislike of the overall look of the nose or any suggestion that the surgeon should decide where the problems lie is to be discouraged and may be suggestive of a dysmorphic disorder (see Chapter 16). The patient's thoughts about the overall improvement desired are sought and realistic expectations estimated. A general medical history should screen the patient for bleeding disorders, cardiovascular and respiratory disease and importantly a psychiatric history.

Examination

A detailed examination of the internal and external aspects of the nose is performed. Anterior rhinoscopy to detail mucosal, caudal septal and turbinate deformities is supplemented with an endoscopic evaluation of the posterior nasal cavity and middle meatal areas to exclude infective or obstructive sinonasal disease. The internal nasal valve area which is bounded by the upper lateral cartilage, inferior turbinate, nasal septum and nasal floor is specifically examined and any high septal deformity noted. This is the narrowest

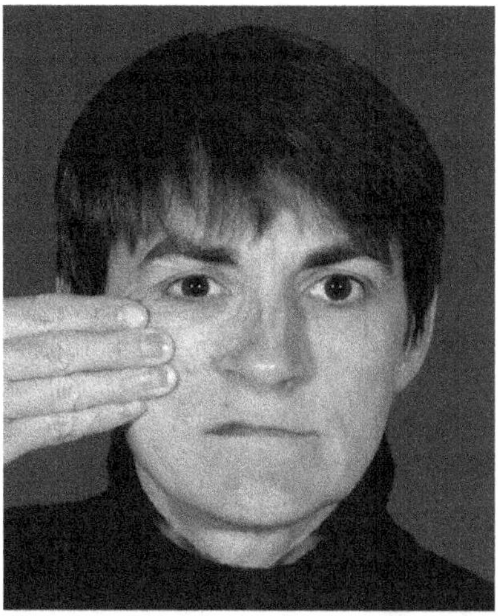

Figure 14.4 Demonstration of Cottle's test.

part of the nasal airway and significant internal nasal valve collapse can be demonstrated by Cottle's test (Figure 14.4) in which the airway improves when the cheek adjacent to the mid third of the nose, i.e. the upper lateral cartilage is pulled laterally.

The importance of the balance of the nose to other aspects of the face is important. Assessment of this relationship should form the initial part of the external examination process. The patient's ethnic characteristics must also be considered. Facial and nasal asymmetries are documented and detailed to the patient.

The skin-soft tissue envelope is important and is critical in predicting postoperative changes. Thinner skin may show minor postoperative irregularities whilst very thick skin can hide any corrections made.

An initial evaluation of the underlying skeletal aspects of the nose considers three fundamental parameters: length (nasion to tip), projection of the dorsum and rotation of the nasal tip. Detailed examination should then document deformities in relation to these factors.

External deformity is most easily assessed and documented in nasal thirds. The frontal (b), lateral (a and c), oblique (d and e) and basal views (Figures 14.5a to 14.5g) are all separately visualised.

- The upper bony pyramid is examined for deviation, irregularity and the extent of any dorsal hump. The width of the base of the dorsal pyramid is determined and the dorsum palpated to ensure there is no "open roof" type deformity.

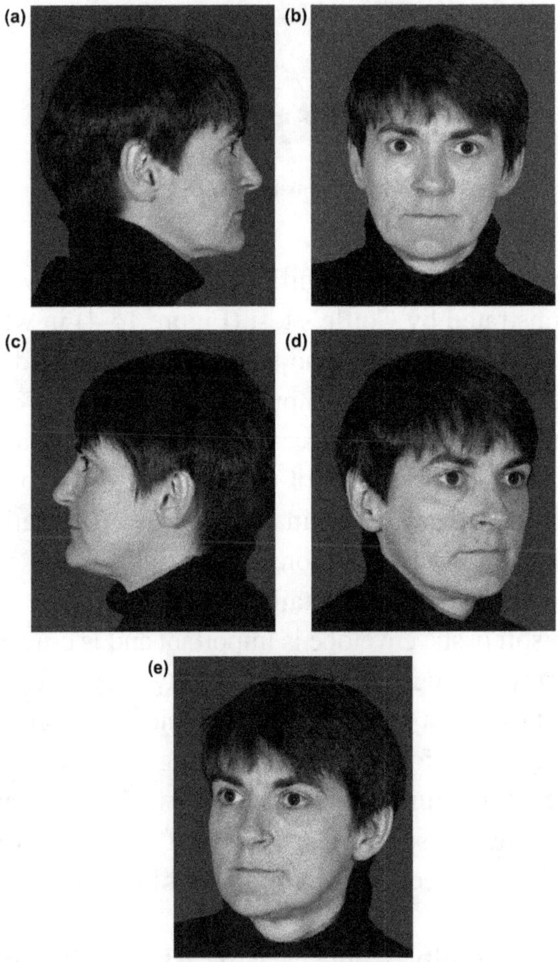

Figure 14.5 (**a–e**) Standard photography views.

(f)

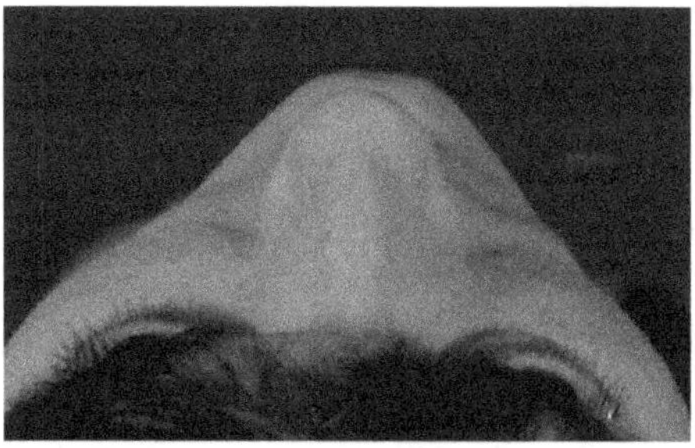

(g)

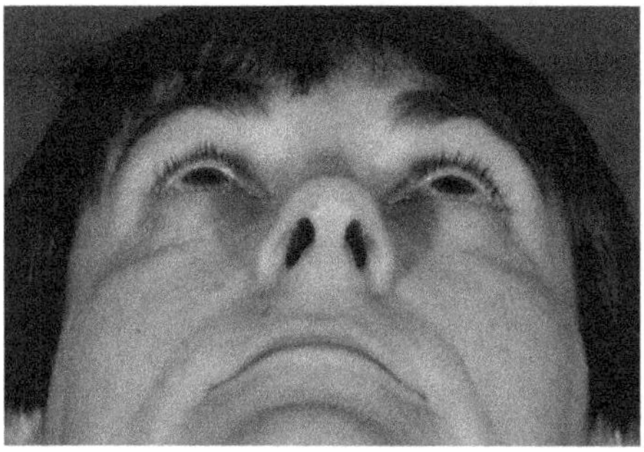

Figure 14.5 **(f)** and **(g)** (*Continued*)

- Similar deformities are sought in the mid third of the nose which is cartilaginous. In this area, an assessment of any externally visible collapse in the nasal valve area is made by inspection and Cottle's test.
- The lower third nasal tip region, which is made up of the lower lateral cartilages is assessed for asymmetry, bulbosity, projection and rotation. A judgement regarding the width of the alar base in relation to the facial proportions is made. The alar width should match the normal intercanthal distance.

Documentation

Documentation of all aspects of the examination is critical for clinical and medicolegal purposes. A rhinoplasty assessment form can be very useful in this regard. It ensures all the areas of the evaluation are considered methodically and can be used for standardising the assessment for all patients.

The patient's expectations and all discussion points are clearly noted. A surgical plan is formulated to correct the specific deformities. It is essential to ensure the patient is given realistic expectations for the outcome of intended surgery, and limitations together with potential complications are discussed. It is very important to ensure that improvement is indeed likely and a risk benefit profile needs to be detailed to the patient prior to obtaining consent and carefully noted.

The surgical approach, be it endonasal or external, should be discussed with the patient and incisions outlined and documented.

Photography and Computer Imaging

Preoperative photography is an absolute requirement for analysis and medicolegal purposes. Standard view photographs form a useful way of communicating deformities and potential changes to the patient. They assist in operative planning and are invaluable for reference during surgery. In combination with postoperative images, they allow self- and peer-reviewed assessment of results.

Standardisation is critical both from the views taken and lighting and background conditions. Digital SLR photography lends itself well to computer archiving and digital imaging. A standard neutral background such as pale grey, green or blue is used. The camera should be two metres from the subject and an appropriate zoom used to compose the image using the portrait outline. An overhead lamp, a "kicker" above the patients head can help eliminate unwanted shadows (Figure 14.6).

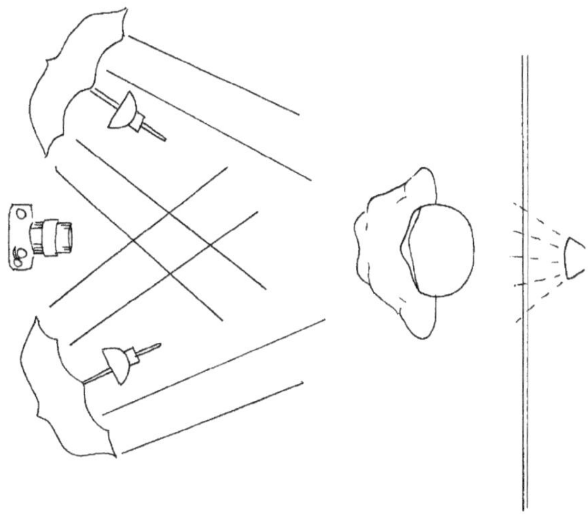

Figure 14.6 Photography setup.

The standard views are as follows (Figures 14.5a to 14.5g):

1. Straight frontal view. The patient looks directly into the camera with the eyeline in a horizontal plane.
2. Lateral view. The patients Frankfort plane should be horizontal. This view assesses dorsal profile and is critical in assessing the three basic parameters of length, projection and rotation of the nose. The nose-chin relationship is also clearly demonstrated. A separate lateral view with the patient smiling may outline dynamic movement in the nasal tip.
3. Oblique views. These views are at taken at 45 degrees to the frontal views and can outline asymmetries and contours.
4. Basal view. This view is taken looking up the nose and focuses on the nasal tip detailing asymmetry and deformity.
5. "Birds eye" view. This view is taken from the top of the patient looking down the nose. It can be useful in showing the subtleties of deviation of the nose.

With digital imaging simple morphing is possible with photo-imaging software. With rhinoplasty surgery, they can be very useful in showing patients potential changes and postoperative outcomes. This is most useful in detailing profile changes in the lateral view but with some experience frontal views can be morphed to show potential width reduction and refinement in the nasal tip. Dedicated programmes have measurement abilities and so can be extremely helpful in operative planning. It is important not to convey unrealistic changes to the patient — this will be a source of dissatisfaction afterwards. As a rule a slight underestimation of the postoperative result is generally favourable. Most surgeons choose not to give printed images to the patient of the predicted changes but if you do so, a printed waiver should make clear that the image is only an indication of the likely result.

Surgical Approaches

As a general rule, it is best to limit surgical tissue dissection to a minimum to reduce the risk of vascular compromise of the skin-soft tissue envelope. In this way, additional scarring is prevented and healing is more predictable. Limited dissection also makes it easier to judge the underlying structural components and position of placed underlying grafts.

There are two basic approaches to the nasal skeleton:

i) the endonasal or closed approach and
ii) the external or open approach.

The advantages and disadvantages of each are much debated and many authors advocate one method to the exclusion of the other. Each offers benefits in specific situations and should be within the repertoire of a rhinoplasty surgeon.

The least traumatic method of dissection to achieve the specific goal should be used and as such the endonasal approach is favoured for all simple cases unless a better result using the open technique.

Endonasal Approach

The endonasal approach only requires incisions within the nose with no visible external scars (Figures 14.8 to 14.10). Minimal soft tissue dissection is needed, making this method favourable for less marked deformities and is ideal for correcting bony dorsal irregularities. Its benefits lie in the limited soft tissue disruption allowing early and predictable healing due to the comparatively reduced scar tissue formation. Its main limitations are the restricted exposure of the underlying nasal skeletal elements. The endonasal approach can further be divided into delivery and non-delivery approaches dependent on whether the lower lateral cartilages are fully delivered. With delivery the cartilage is exposed and withdrawn from its overlying subcutaneous layer. The incisions required for these are detailed later.

External Approach

The external approach requires a mid-columellar skin incision which is joined to bilateral marginal incisions (Figure 14.11). More soft tissue dissection is required but provides an unparalleled view of the nasal structures, facilitating diagnosis and correction by bimanual tissue handling. Other benefits include binocular vision for the surgeon, control of bleeding with diathermy, precise placement and suturing of struts, battens, shield and spreader grafts. This approach also offers a definite teaching advantage although this should not be thought of as an indication for its use. The external approach is favoured for most major reconstructive rhinoplasty and revision surgery, particularly where the nasal tip needs addressing. Recent incision refinements and surgical technique have overcome some of the earlier criticisms of a columellar scar, delay in resolution of the supratip skin oedema, loss of tip projection and extra operating time. However with this approach, it may be difficult to assess the supra-tip area and the desired tip projection due to the lack of traction of the soft tissue prior to closure of the columella incision. Specific indications for the external approach in rhinoplasty include:

- congenital deformities such as the "cleft lip nose",
- extensive revision surgery,
- severe nasal trauma,
- the markedly deviated nose,
- marked tip deformities, and
- situations where assessment of the exact pathology is difficult.

Extended applications of the external approach enable greater exploration of the nasal skeleton and the advantages this affords. It has been advocated for nasoseptal perforation repair, access to the nasal dorsum for treatment of nasal dermoids and even as an approach to hypophysectomy.

Operative Techniques

Anaesthesia

Rhinoplasty surgery is usually performed under general anaesthesia although local anaesthetic and sedation are also possible. The face is prepared with an aqueous detergent and draped to reveal the eyes, the corneas are simply protected with lacrilube ointment. The intranasal mucosal cavity is prepared preoperatively with a (10%) cocaine vasoconstrictor solution. Local anaesthesia with a vasoconstrictor is then injected to further minimise intraoperative bleeding. A dental syringe and needle are used with a 2% lidocaine and 1:80,000 adrenaline cartridge. The injection sites are as follows (Figures 14.7a to 14.7d):

a) along lateral wall of nose through intercartilaginous area,
b) base of the columella and collumellar region if the external approach is used,

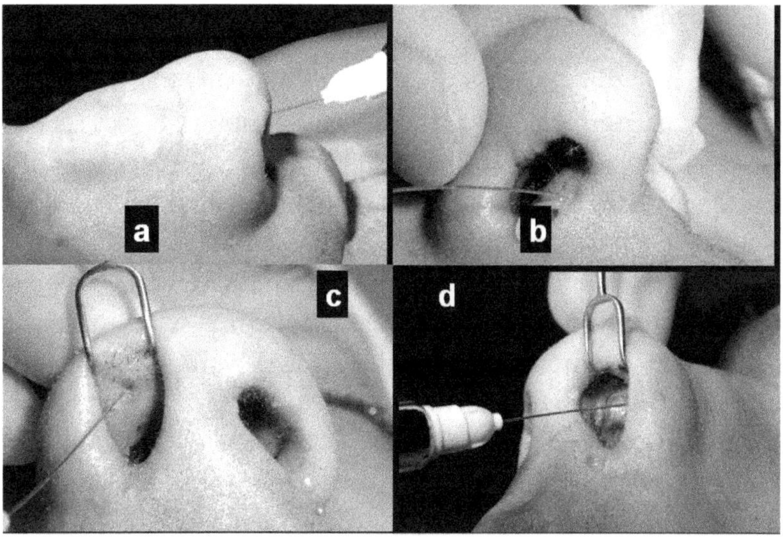

Figure 14.7 **(a)–(d)** Local infiltration technique for rhinoplasty.

c) vestibular and non-vestibular aspects of the lower lateral cartilages (the alar cartilages),
d) caudal septal cartilage area, and
e) alar bases if reduction is planned (*not shown*).

Injection over the immediate dorsum is best avoided as the resultant swelling can make assessment of this area difficult. Lateral nose depot injections can be massaged upwards into the dorsal area to reduce bleeding when the skin-soft tissue envelope is being elevated. Leaving adequate time for the anaesthesia to take effect is essential to its haemostatic advantage.

Incisions

Elevation of the skin and soft tissue envelope is facilitated by various incisions.

1. *Intercartilaginous*

The intercartilaginous incision (Figures 14.8a to 14.8c) is the most commonly used in endonasal rhinoplasty. It allows direct access to the mid and upper thirds of the nose but affords no exposure of the tip cartilages. It is often used in combination with other incisions if tip surgery needs to be performed.

The incision is made in the area separating the upper and lower lateral cartilages. A small linear hollow is seen intranasally demarcating the area between the caudal border of the upper lateral and the cephalic border of the lower lateral cartilages. It is usually seen and easily palpable when the alar margin is retracted upwards and everted using a two-pronged skin hook (Figure 14.8a).

- An incision is made into this hollow laterally (Figure 14.8b) and the blade is then turned forwards and medially along the intercartilaginous junction and onto the caudal septum to make a transfixion incision below the caudal cartilaginous septum, i.e. the incision passes through the membranous septum between the medial crura and the caudal septum.
- It is important to ensure this transfixion incision does not extend more than half way along the columella as further extension risks dividing the medial crural attachment to the caudal septum. This is one of the major tip support mechanisms, and division may result in postoperative tip ptosis. Conversely, an extended full transfixion incision can be utilised as a manoeuvre for deprojection of the tip if required.
- With retraction of the lower lateral cartilage, the overlying skin-soft tissue envelope can be gently elevated off the cartilaginous dorsum of the upper lateral cartilages by sharp dissection upwards using a sawing motion with a No. 15 blade in a supra-perichondral plane (Figure 14.8c).

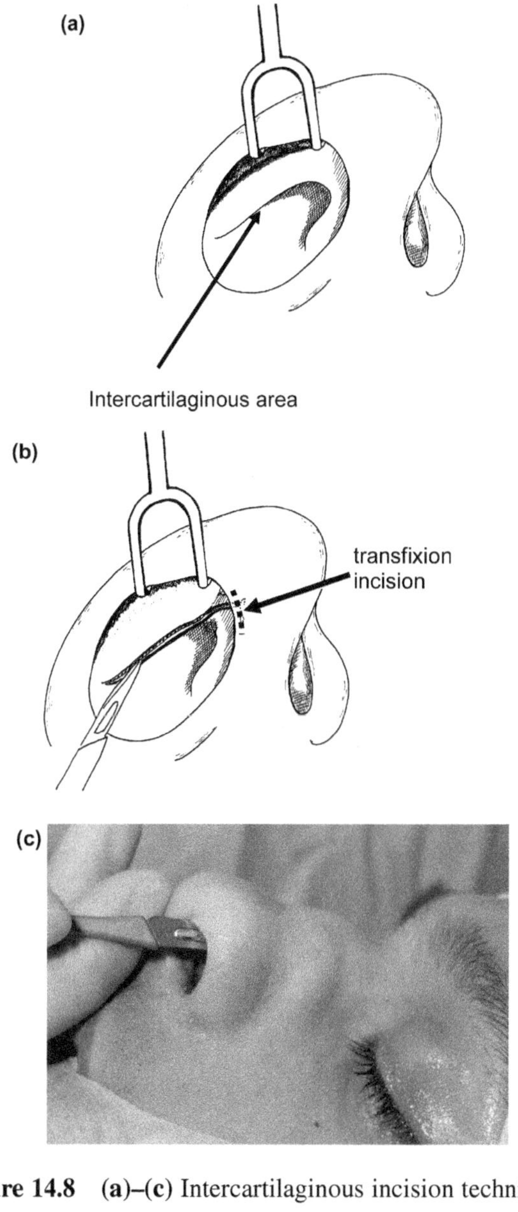

Figure 14.8 **(a)–(c)** Intercartilaginous incision technique.

- After the cartilaginous vault is freed of overlying tissue, an incision is made into the caudal end of the periosteum of the nasal bony pyramid.
- The periosteum and its overlying procerus muscle can then be elevated using the side of a Joseph elevator. Such elevation needs extend only far enough laterally to gain access to a dorsal hump.
- The intercartilaginous incision approach does not expose the lower lateral cartilages although retrograde exposure of the cephalic border may allow volume reduction of this area.

Whilst these incisions are mucosal and as such should heal very well, it is the author's preference to close these with fast absorbing sutures (4.0 Vicryl Rapide — Ethicon).

2. *Cartilage Splitting (Intracartilaginous, Transcartilaginous)*

The cartilage splitting incision facilitates volume reduction of the cephalic border of the lower lateral cartilages. It is frequently performed in addition to reduction of the dorsum.

- The cephalic border of the lower lateral cartilage is identified in the vestibular region and a length of at least 8 mm of cartilage is marked to be left as an intact strip.
- An incision is then made through the vestibular skin which is then freed from the lower lateral cartilage (Figure 14.9a).
- The cephalic edge of the cartilage requiring excision is exposed and incised at the appropriate level as determined by the amount of cartilage to be removed.
- The incised cephalic part of the cartilage can then be freed from the overlying soft tissue and skin and removed ensuring symmetrical amounts are taken.

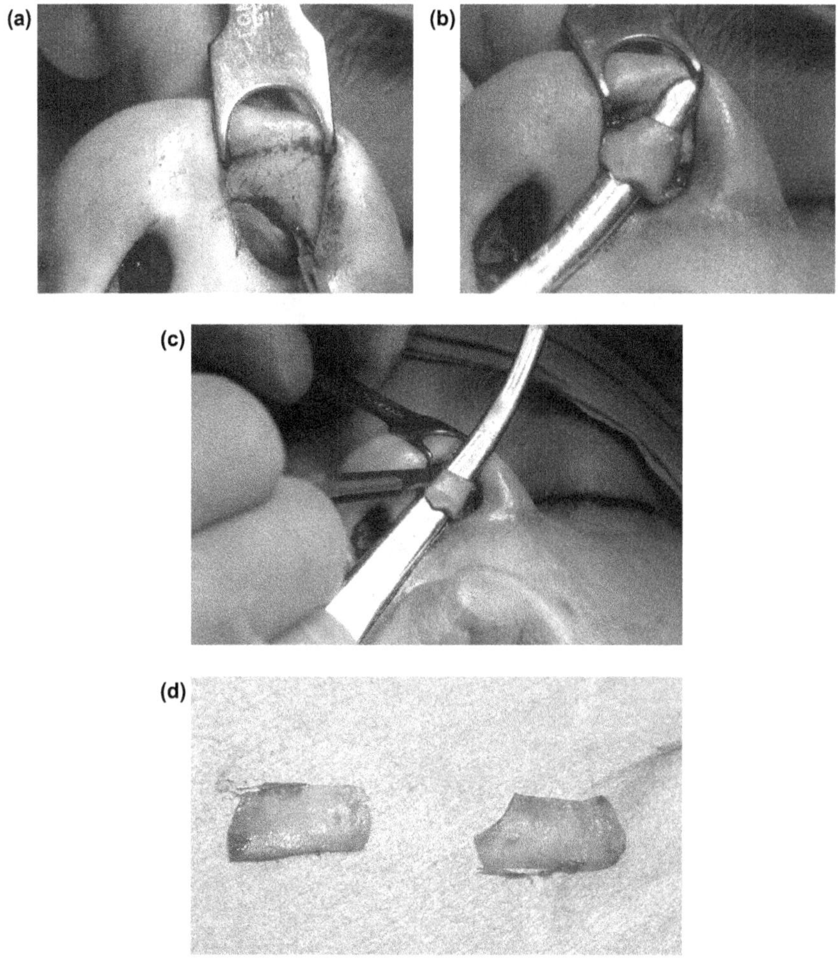

Figure 14.9 (**a**)–(**d**) Cephalic resection of the lower lateral cartilages via the cartilage splitting incision. (**b**) The entire cartilage mobilised from which a strip (**c**) from the cephalic border is incised leaving continuity, and then excised (**d**).

- Exposure of the nasal dorsum can then proceed as before.
- An alternative way of removing the cephalic border can be done when performing both the intercartilaginous and cartilage splitting incisions. A bipedicled chondrocutaneous

flap is delivered and can be "bucket handled" into the nasal cavity allowing accurate resection of the cephalic cartilage (Figures 14.9b to 14.9d).

The cartilage splitting incision does not allow full exposure of the lower lateral cartilages and is deemed a "non-delivery" approach. As such this incision will not allow adequate correction of a major tip deformity where significant manipulation of the lower lateral cartilages is required.

3. *Marginal Incision*

The marginal incision follows the caudal margin of the lower lateral cartilages allowing the whole cartilage to be delivered and is the choice in dealing with more complex tip abnormalities using an endonasal approach. This margin is often, but not always, at the junction of the hair bearing and non-hair bearing skin in the vestibular area.

- Exposure is enhanced by retraction of the alar margin with a wide double-pronged skin hook and pressure with the middle finger on the upper margin of the alar lobule allowing eversion of the vestibular surface of the nostril. An impression of the caudal edge is then seen and palpated (Figure 14.10a) and an incision is then made through vestibular skin.
- Dissection proceeds using sharp Iris scissors in the supraperichondrial plane on the non vestibular side (Figure 14.10b). The dissection extends to the cephalic border of the cartilage and when combined with an intercartilaginous incision allows full exposure of the whole alar cartilage (Figure 14.10c).
- The cartilages can now be inspected and modified in any required way. Marginal incisions are closed with multiple fine absorbable sutures.

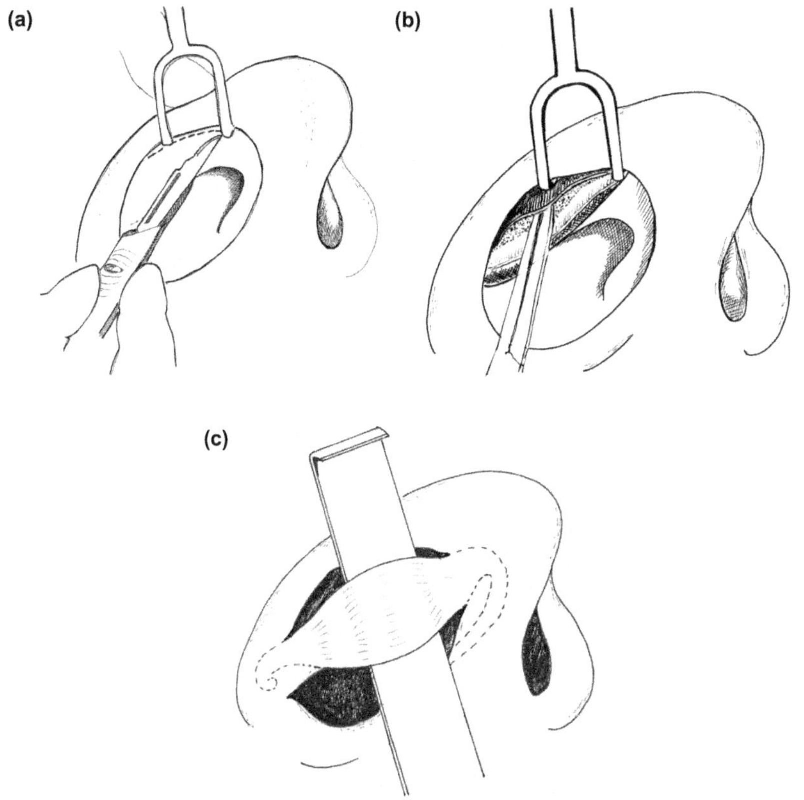

Figure 14.10 **(a)–(c)** Marginal incision to fully expose and deliver lower lateral cartilages.

4. *External Approach*

Whilst many variations of the columella incision have been advocated, the broken transcolumellar inverted V incision is most commonly used and the author's preferred configuration.

- The incision is made in the mid columella region overlying the medial crural footplates to ensure adequate support on closure thus preventing a depressed scar (see Figure 14.11a).

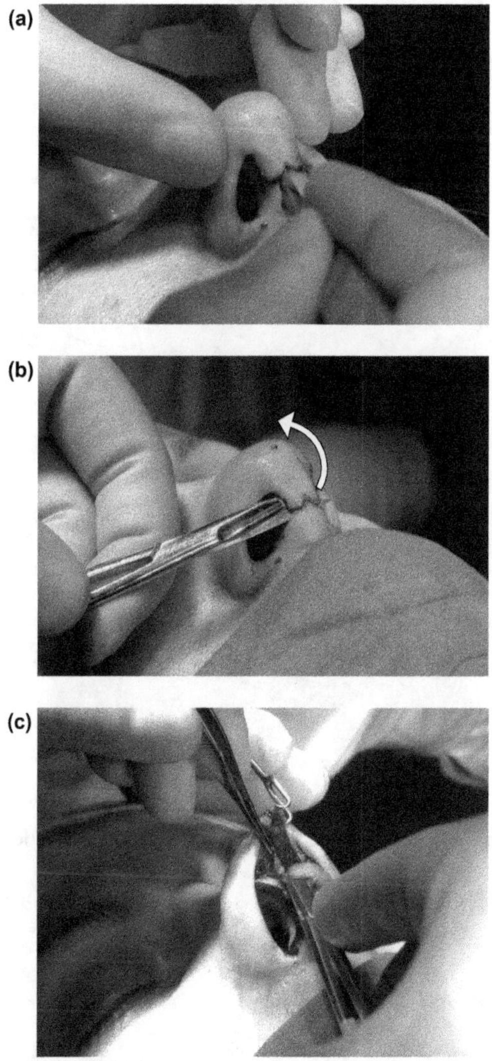

Figure 14.11 (**a**)–(**c**) External approach technique.

- It is essential to protect the integrity of the caudal end of the medial crura just beneath the incision to prevent postoperative notching in this area. This may be done by initially making only relatively superficial incisions inside the columellar margin which extend laterally to enable reflection to expose the tip.

- These marginal vestibular extensions of the transcollumella incisions are placed 2 mm inside the vestibule and joined by careful undermining of the columella skin with sharp Iris scissors. The scissors can then be used as a guard upon which the transcolumella incision is completed (Figure 14.11b).
- It is relatively easy to identify the caudal end of each of the medial crura and use this as a guide in extending the marginal incision more laterally using angled Converse/Walter scissors with a spreading movement (Figure 14.11c). These hug the caudal surface of the cartilage and cut the overlying soft tissue.
- To obtain adequate exposure of the nasal skeleton, the marginal incision should be extended laterally at least halfway along the lateral crus. Although the major tip support mechanisms are respected in the external approach, the disruption of the skin-soft tissue envelope overlying the lower lateral cartilages and the division of the medial intercrural ligamentous fibrous tissue leads to loss of some of the minor tip support mechanisms. Some ptosis of the nasal tip should therefore be anticipated in all cases.
- The columella incision is closed with five separate 6.0 nylon simple sutures. Eversion of the skin edges ensures favourable healing and vertical mattress sutures may be needed to ensure this. The initial closure of the incision is in the midline at the apex of the inverted V. If there is any risk of tension, a subcutaneous PDS suture is used in addition to the skin sutures. The marginal incisions are closed with fine rapidly absorbing sutures.

The Operative Sequence

The sequence of surgical correction in septorhinoplasty is widely debated. Some advocate correcting any nasal tip abnormality first, prior to addressing the dorsal deformity. The advantage stated is that trying to achieve dorsal correction to match the form of the nasal tip is easier than *vice versa*. Further, as the external nasal splint is applied shortly after corrective osteotomies, this reduces the ecchymosis and swelling that inevitably follows. Conversely it can be argued that the more aggressive methods of dorsal reduction and osteotomies are better performed prior to the fine nasal tip work. Whichever sequence used, it is generally accepted that septal correction should precede any correction of external deformity and that alar base corrections are performed as the final part of the operation.

1. ***Septal Surgery (Figure 14.12a)***

Septoplasty surgery is not detailed in this chapter but forms an essential and difficult part of the correction of the traumatic and functionally impaired nose. Whilst bony restoration of the dorsum may improve the upper third aesthetics, septal surgery (essentially the quadrilateral septal cartilage) is important in allowing the cartilaginous dorsum to be re-aligned.

- Caudal septal deformities can displace the leading edge of the septum from behind the columella into the nasal airway, giving rise to nasal obstruction in this area (Figure 14.12b).
- The caudal septum also provides a firm support for the columella and trauma or surgical overresection of the caudal septum may lead to columellar retraction.
- Traumatic injuries may cause fractures within the quadrilateral cartilage of the septum leading to functional problems as well as loss of support in the supratip area — the “saddle” nose. A similar appearance may occur after a traumatic septal haematoma and abscess where there is necrosis of the cartilage.
- Over-resection of cartilage during septoplasty itself may also predispose to this deformity.

(a)

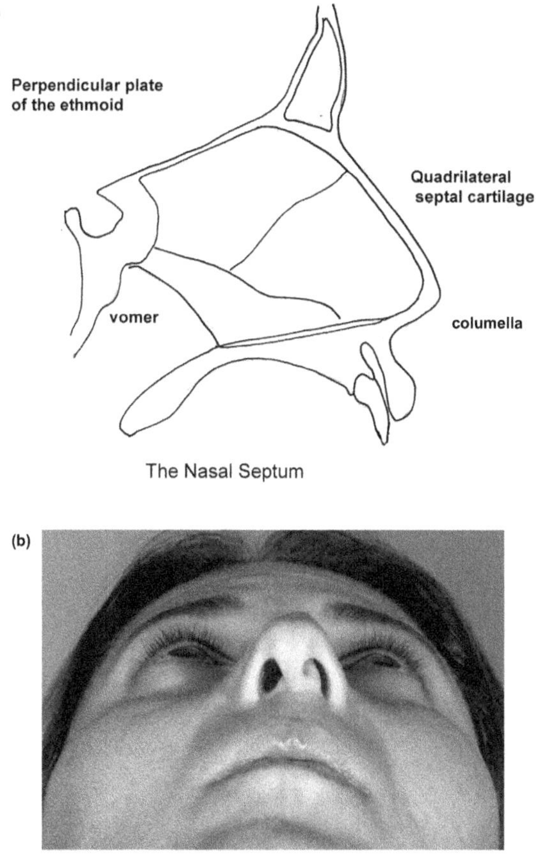

Figure 14.12 (**a**) Anatomy of the nasal septum. (**b**) Dislocated nasal septum leading to functional and cosmetic deformity.

- Harvesting of the quadrilateral cartilage is often required for grafting purposes. However it is important to leave substantial support for the dorsum in the form of an L shaped dorsal and caudal septal butress at least 10 mm wide.
- The rhinoplasty surgeon is required to be able to perform standard septoplasty techniques to achieve predictable functional and aesthetically pleasing results.

Correction of the Osseocartilaginous Dorsum

1. *Hump Reduction*

It is important to judge the extent of resection required from the dorsum prior to local infiltration and elevation of the skin-soft tissue envelope. Attention should be given to the difference in thickness of this envelope at various aspects of the dorsum, it being thinnest at the rhinion, the lowest and most prominent point of the internasal suture. The dorsal hump consists of a bony and cartilaginous component. Endonasal approaches give more restricted views of this area but exposure is maximised by placing an Aufricht retractor along the dorsum under the skin and soft tissues (Figure 14.13).

External rhinoplasty exposure of the upper third of the nose may allow more accurate diagnosis and precise correction, although lack of traction of the tissues makes judgement more difficult.

- The initial incision occurs through the cartilaginous dorsum at the decided level by cutting through the cartilage from cephalically at the osteocartilaginous junction downwards caudally (Figure 14.14a).

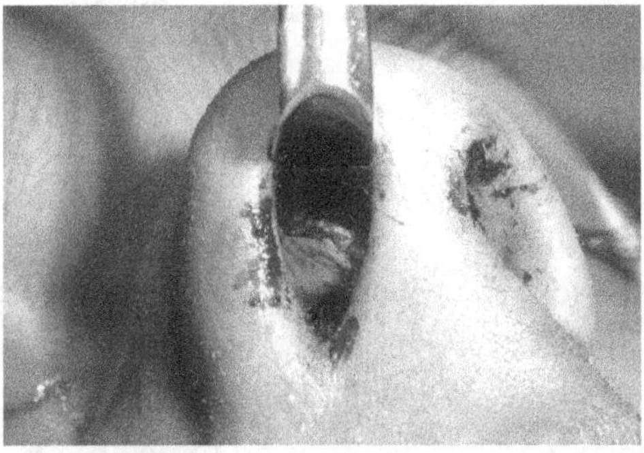

Figure 14.13 Aufricht retractor placed along dorsum of nose in endonasal approach.

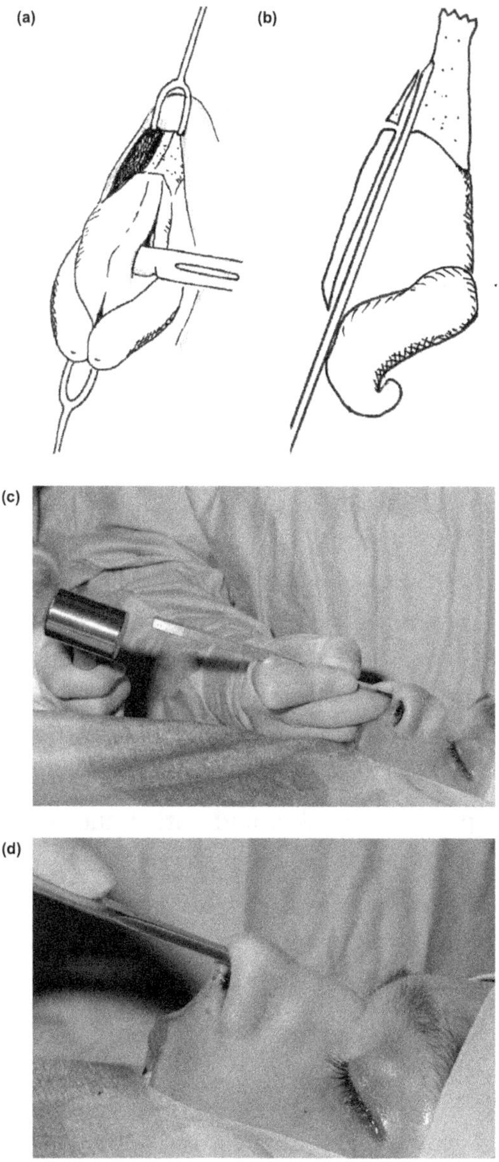

Figure 14.14 **(a)–(d)** Removal of dorsal hump.

- An osteotome can now be placed under the resected cartilage fragment with its edge facing the bone cephalic to this (Figure 14.14b). It is important at this stage to ensure the osteotome is held in a perfectly horizontal plane to ensure symmetrical bony removal (Figure 14.14c). The exception to this is when excising a bony hump in the presence of a bony pyramid deviation with nasal bones of unequal height. In this case the plane of the osteotome must be altered. An assistant performs a series of double taps with a mallet onto the osteotome to initially engage and then cut through the bone. If the soft tissues have been adequately mobilised, an en-bloc osteocartilaginous hump can be removed. This resected fragment is boat shaped and should consist of part of the nasal bones and the upper laterals/cartilaginous septum complex.
- Symmetry of resection of these structures is checked on the removed fragment. Coarse tungsten-carbide rasps can now be used to "fine tune" the dorsal resection to remove any significant excess bone and finer diamond rasps used to smooth any irregularities in the resected bone (Figure 14.14d).
- An important final step here is to turn the rasp upwards and gently sweep under the skin and soft tissue for removal of any small residual fragments which may otherwise be palpable or visible as postoperative irregularities.
- Rasping of the dorsum alone without using the osteotome is advocated by some surgeons. Due care is advised using this method as repeated use of a rasp may inadvertently traumatise the overlying skin, especially when thin, which can cause some persistent erythema. Bony reduction with powered instrumentation is a new and elegant alternative to the osteotome.

A common mistake is resection of the bony hump without appropriate reduction of the cartilaginous vault. This risks leaving a "pollybeak" deformity which can also occur secondary to soft

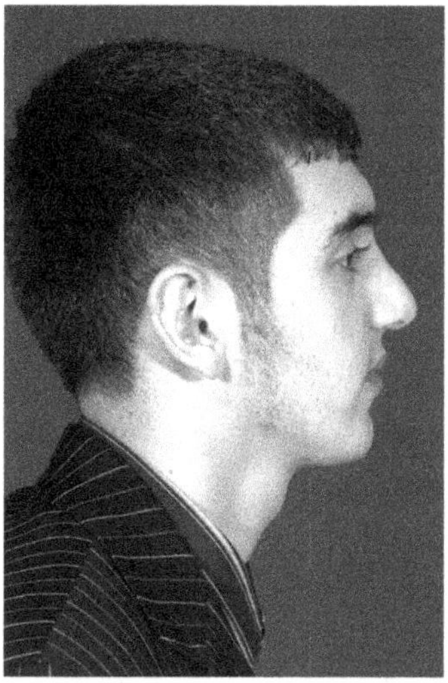

Figure 14.15 Pollybeak deformity in a revision rhinoplasty patient.

tissue scarring when the plane of dissection in this area is incorrect (Figure 14.15).

2. *Osteotomies*

Mobilisation of the bony vault is achieved by osteotomy. The bony pyramid may need

- re-alignment if deviated,
- narrowing at the base, or
- closure of the "open roof" that is an inevitable consequence of hump reduction.

Many aspects of the technique have been refined to produce predictable results with minimal ecchymosis and oedema.

- Local infiltration of the tissues lateral and medial to the bony vault with lidocaine and adrenaline is helpful in reducing bleeding. Microosteotomes are used and should be sharp and small (approximately 2–3 mm).

Medial osteotomy

The medial osteotomy extends from the caudal bony vault upwards in a slightly oblique fashion (Figure 14.16a).

- The osteotome is introduced intranasally and engaged into and advanced along the medial aspect of the nasal bone. A distinct note change is usually heard if the thicker frontal bone is reached. This medial fracture controls the site where a lateral bony back fracture occurs.

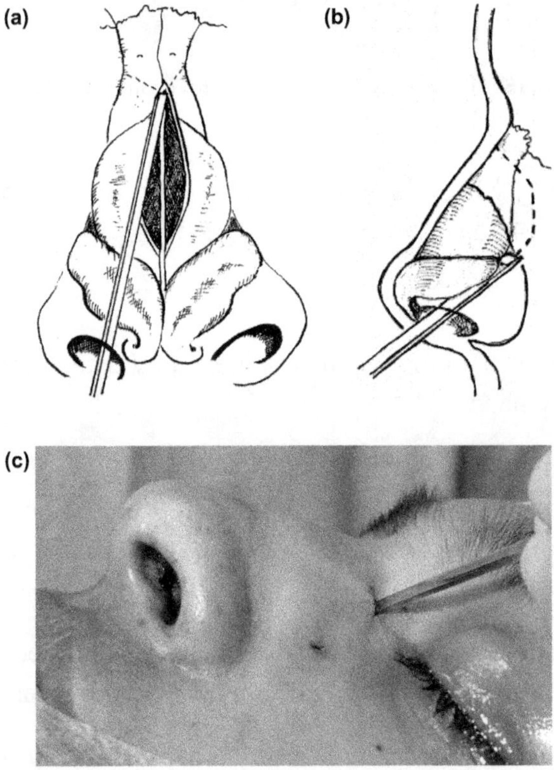

Figure 14.16 (**a**) Medial osteotomy. (**b**) Lateral endonasal "high-low-high" osteotomy. (**c**) Lateral percutaneous osteotomy.

Lateral osteotomy

The lateral osteotomy may be performed endonasally or percutaneously.

Endonasally;

- A stab incision is made intranasally in the mucosa overlying the pyriform aperture just above the attachment of the inferior turbinate to the lateral nasal wall.
- A thin guarded microosteotome is used, designed to preserve the medial periosteum and a laterally positioned guard allows palpation of the edge of the osteotome at all times. The so called high–low osteotomy refers to the supine patient where the upper nasal bone area is "high" and the lower bone is "low".
- The "high-low-high" osteotomy proceeds as follows: initially the osteotome is introduced *high* on the lateral wall of the pyriform aperture (Figure 14.16b). The osteotomy is extended down to and then *low* along the nasofacial groove. As it is extended upwards it is slowly curved from lateral to medially and ends *high* at the level of the medial canthus. This leaves a small triangle of bone at the base of the pyriform aperture which, if infractured, may lead to nasal blockage.

Extension of the lateral osteotomy beyond this level into the thicker nasofrontal bone risks a "rocker deformity" where infracture of the nasal bone causes protrusion at the superior fracture site. If a medial osteotomy has been performed, a controlled back fracture is achieved by twisting the osteotome medially.

The lateral osteotomy may also be performed percutaneously.

- Stab incisions are made through the skin at two points; midway between the medial canthus and the edge of the pyriform aperture low in the nasofacial groove and superiorly between the medial canthus and the top of the dorsum (Figure 14.16c).

- A sharp 2 mm microosteotome is introduced and a series of perforations are made low along the lateral nasal wall and a superior osteotomy is fashioned with perforations at the level of the medial canthus.
- Each perforation is made to go through the bone but not the medial periosteum. As the bone is perforated a distinct change in tone (fall in pitch) is heard with the tapping sounds.
- Studies have shown that the small stab incisions are entirely invisible postoperatively. The percutaneous lateral osteotomy is simple to learn and execute and allows precise, predictable fractures to be made.

Intermediate Osteotomy

The intermediate osteotomy is used to correct an extreme deviation of the nasal pyramid where one nasal sidewall is far longer than the other. Medial and lateral osteotomies alone in this case could not create bones of equal height and residual postoperative deviation is the norm. The intermediate osteotomy effectively shortens the longer side allowing the nasal bones to be repositioned into the mid line. When performed bilaterally it can be used to narrow a very wide nasal dorsum. The osteotomy is placed along the mid aspect of the lateral nasal wall and it is important to perform it prior to the lower lateral osteotomy as it cannot be done if the lateral wall is mobile.

Nasal Tip Surgery

Surgery of the nasal tip is by far the most complex aspect of rhinoplasty surgery and requires a sound appreciation of the anatomy and aesthetic facial parameters. Preoperative assessment should define what specific anomalies are present and the objectives for correction.

The problems encountered may be thought of as being due to

- volume excess,
- under- or overrotation,
- under- or overprojection,
- width problems, or
- intrinsic tip deformities.

It is beyond the scope of this chapter to describe each aspect of complex tip correction in detail. The basic concepts can be divided into

- volume reduction,
- tip remodelling procedures,
- placement of (usually) cartilaginous grafts.

Projection and rotation of the tip are intricately related and manoeuvres to correct one may well affect the other.

The tripod concept of the nasal tip is a very useful model to predict changes in these parameters with modifications of the alar cartilages, and is detailed later.

Volume Reduction

Where there is isolated volume excess of the nasal tip giving rise to bulbosity, cephalic resection of the lower lateral cartilage may be adequate to increase definition and cause mild narrowing (see Figures 14.9a to 14.9d). Access to the cephalic border of this cartilage as previously described may be via a cartilage splitting incision or by retrograde dissection from an intercartilaginous incision. The external approach is not required for isolated cephalic reduction but precise and symmetrical resection is optimal using this technique.

Judgement is critical in ensuring enough cartilage is removed to give a noticeable change in the definition but leaving as much cartilage behind as possible. Overzealous cephalic strip resection can lead to a "visoring" effect due to alar retraction caused by contraction as healing occurs. An absolute minimum of 8 mm width of residual cartilage continuity is recommended but in the presence of an anatomically narrow alar cartilage this may need to be reconsidered. If vestibular mucosa is not preserved, this too can contribute to contracture and promote further retraction.

When employing an endonasal approach, marking in the vestibular area is useful to ensure the incision is made in the correct position — an instrument can be used to make an imprint in the vestibular skin or a needle placed percutaneously in the appropriate place. Symmetrical reduction is essential — both resected cartilages are compared to ensure this is the case.

Following reduction, a small void is created in cephalic region of the lower lateral cartilages. Healing and contracture may cause some upward rotation of the tip to fill the void. Overall this is often a favourable change although care should be exercised in an already overrotated tip. This method cannot be relied upon as a powerful or indeed completely predictable method of causing significant tip rotation.

Rotation Deformities (Figure 14.17a)

Correction of the underrotated tip can be done with various manoeuvres based on the tripod concept. This concept proposes that the conjoint medial crura are one limb of the tripod with each lateral crus representing a separate lateral limb (Figure 14.17b). Manipulation of any part of the tripod can be used to predict changes in the projection and rotation of the nasal tip. The LeFort I maxillary advancement will correct an underrotated tip by advancing the conjoint medial crura and caudal septum. Most rhinoplasty

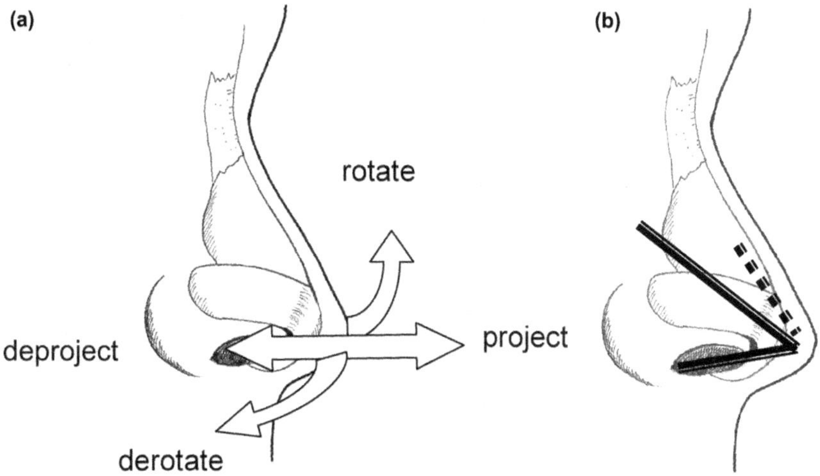

Figure 14.17 (**a**) Surgical anatomy terminology. (**b**) Tripod model of lower lateral cartilage dynamics. The tripod limbs represent the two lateral crurae and the conjoined medial crurae as the third limb.

techniques for rotation problems rely on the tripod manoeuvres of the nasal tip.

- Thus division and overlay of the lateral crura will produce a marked tip rotation upwards, but will also cause some tip deprojection (Figure 14.18a).
- Lateral crural steal techniques which recruit the lateral crura medially using domal suturing can enhance rotation and also be usefully employed for increased projection (see also projection deformities below) (Figures 14.19a and 14.19b).

An over rotated nasal tip is an unaesthetic "piggy nose". Options for correction are more limited with this situation.

- A graft in the tip/infratip area will give an illusion of counter-rotation and increased length of the nose.
- A caudal septal extension graft also gives a similar effect.

- In order to accomplish counter-rotation in extreme cases, a skin-cartilage composite graft may be needed in space created between the upper and lower lateral cartilages.
- Division and overlap of the medial crurae is another option, although this also deprojects the tip.

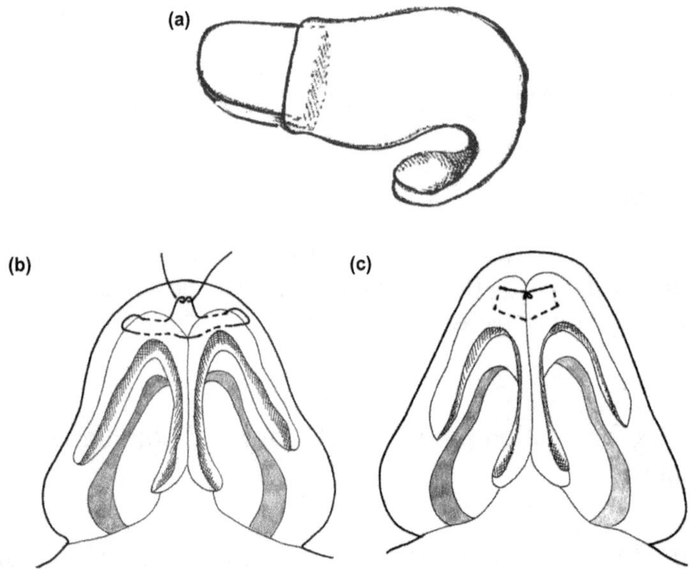

Figure 14.18 (**a**) Division and overlay of lateral crura to cause tip rotation. (**b**) and (**c**) Dome suturing technique.

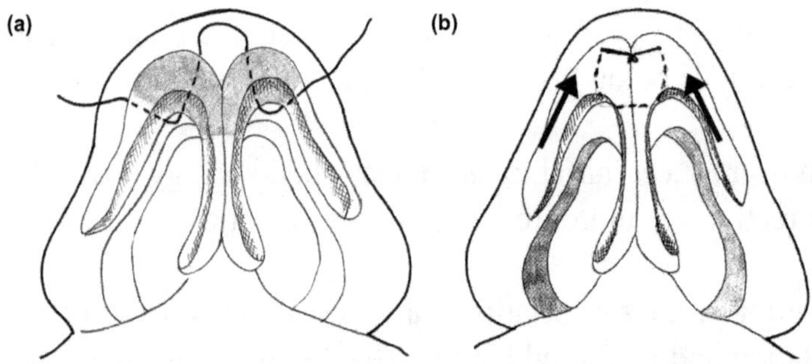

Figure 14.19 (**a**) and (**b**) Lateral crural steal technique to increase tip projection.

Projection Deformities

Increasing the projection of the nasal tip is often desirable in rhinoplasty surgery. As with rotation problems, this can be achieved by reorientation of the alar cartilages or by addition of cartilaginous struts or grafts. Variations of basic techniques are widely described. Commonly performed procedures include the following:

1. *Domal Sutures*

Suture modification of the nasal domal area can refine the shape of the nasal tip into a more aesthetic configuration.

- Domal sutures can convert a "boxy" or trapezoidal configuration of a nasal tip into a more aesthetic triangular configuration (Figures 14.18b and 14.18c). Sutures are placed within an individual dome (intradomal or a single dome unit) and the two domes can then be approximated (interdomal or a double dome unit).
- Mild projection of the nasal tip can also be achieved by transdomal suturing using 6.0 nylon, that causes the domes to be elevated.
- To increase the projection even further, the lateral crus of the lower lateral cartilage is mobilised fully from the vestibular skin. This lateral crus can then be recruited towards the domal area and a new dome created and sutured in a newly projected position — the so-called "lateral crural steal" (Figures 14.19a and 14.19c). This procedure also causes a degree of tip rotation.
- Vertical dome division with resuturing — The Goldman technique is the original and perhaps most well described method of dome division. The many modifications of this technique all describe vertical division of the lower lateral cartilage usually 2–3 mm lateral to the existing dome. The medial cut ends of cartilage are then sutured back to back thereby increasing

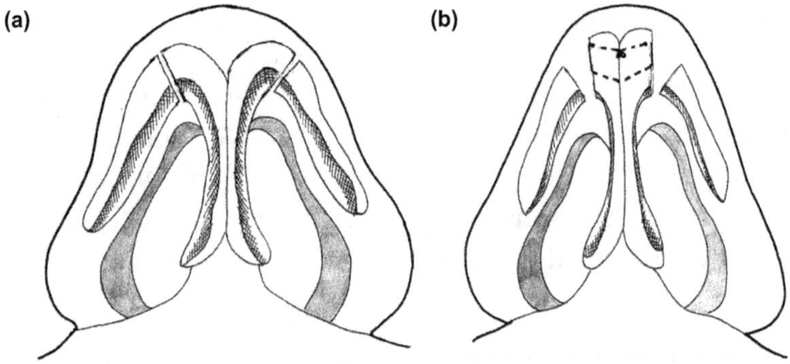

Figure 14.20 (**a**) and (**b**) Goldman technique of dome division.

projection of the tip and can be trimmed to the exact height required and if required, can be shortened to deproject the tip (Figures 14.20a and 14.20b). The residual lateral cartilages are left and generally prolapse medially. Vestibular skin may be preserved intact although the original description of this technique suggested incision through this. Current management of the nasal tip has veered away from this technique towards suture modification. Criticisms of its use have included its relative irreversibility and the creation of a very sharply defined, "tent pole"-like appearance to the tip particularly in the presence of thin skin.

These techniques are, however, still very useful and with appropriate selection of patients give excellent form to the tip.

2. *Grafts and Struts*

Autogenous grafting material is always a preferred source of tissue. Grafts are usually harvested from the quadrilateral cartilage of the septum or auricular conchal bowl (Figure 14.21). Placement on the nasal tip region can cause projection changes. Dependent on the area required for projection, various cartilage grafts have been

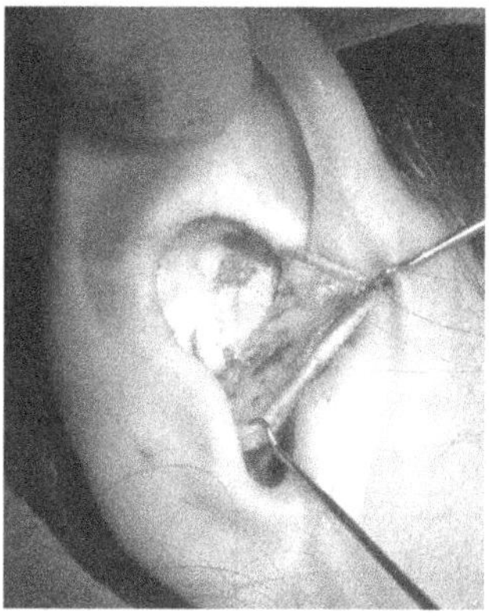

Figure 14.21 Harvest of auricular cartilage via an anterior approach.

described. Grafts are sutured into place using fine non-absorbable sutures when performing an external approach, or by specific placement in precise pockets if approached endonasally.

The columellar strut is extremely useful in maintaining and to some extent increasing tip projection. With the inevitable loss of tip support with any of the described approaches, ptosis may be anticipated in the postoperative period and placement of a cartilaginous strut between the medial crurae can help prevent this (Figure 14.22).

Placement of grafts in the premaxillary region can be sometimes used to give an illusion of tip rotation and projection.

Deprojection of the tip is less often required and can necessitate a number of manoeuvres based on the tripod concept.

- Division of the medial crural footplate attachment to the caudal septum with an extended full transfixion incision will lose one of the major tip support mechanisms and should cause some deprojection and counter-rotation.
- Vertical division of the alar (lower lateral) cartilages with overlay and suturing of the edges should also decrease projection. Such an overlay can be fashioned in the lateral crurae to give increased rotation and decreased projection.

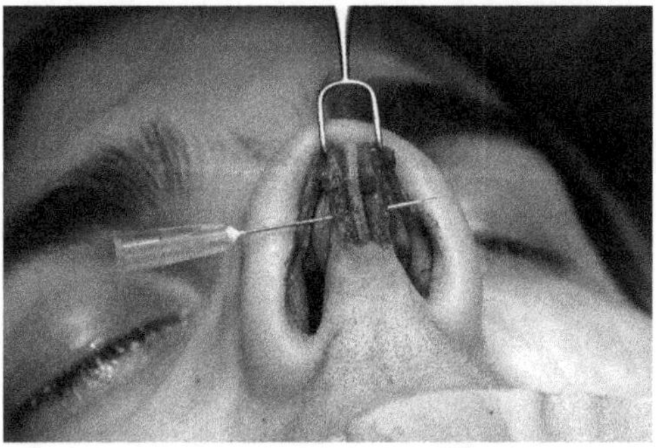

Figure 14.22 Insertion of cartilaginous columellar strut.

Other techniques include:

- Reduction of the nasal spine.
- The previously described vertical dome division with excision of the excess medial crurae and reconstruction with sutures.
- The "tongue-in-groove" technique of septocollumellar suturing remains a further option and is a useful way of establishing both projection and rotation of the nasal tip. A disadvantage of this method is the rigidity and lack of mobility such a procedure imparts to the tip in some patients.

Alar Base Reduction

Assessment of the alar base is made preoperatively and reduction planned if required. Change in tip dynamics may influence the alar base width perioperatively such as in marked deprojection of the overprojected "tension" nose. In this case, the alar base is generally flared as a result of the other corrective procedures and the patient should be told of the possibility of needing reduction.

Alar base reduction is generally divided into correction relating to excess alar flare, excess nostril size or a combination of these. It is universally agreed that alar base reduction is performed as a final step in the operation after all other deformities have been corrected. Conservative reduction is important to avoid the complications of asymmetry and over-reduction which are both difficult to correct.

Nostril Size

Excision of a wedge of skin and soft tissue from the nostril floor alone will reduce the internal dimension of the medial border of the nostril (Figure 14.23a). Subtle alteration of the alar curve can be effected too, but this manoeuvre will not affect the width of the alar bases.

Alar Flare

More marked changes in alar flare are achieved by extension of an incision within the nostril into the alar facial junction.

- The incision is not made within, but rather 1–2 mm above the alar facial crease as this minimises postoperative scarring and visibility. A wedge is removed from this area allowing reduction in the bulkiness of the ala and the width of the base can be narrowed as well (Figure 14.23b).
- If significant alar flare reduction is needed a larger wedge is excised and a small back cut onto the lateral edge of the nostril facilitates adequate medialisation of the alar bases (Figure 14.23c).

Combination

The combination of alar flare and excess nostril size is corrected with a rectangular shaped resection of alar tissue. Symmetrical marking of the excision is critical to diminish the postoperative dissatisfaction of asymmetry (Figure 14.23d).

Eversion of the skin edges with fine non-absorbable sutures (6.0 nylon) are used to ensure an accurate closure.

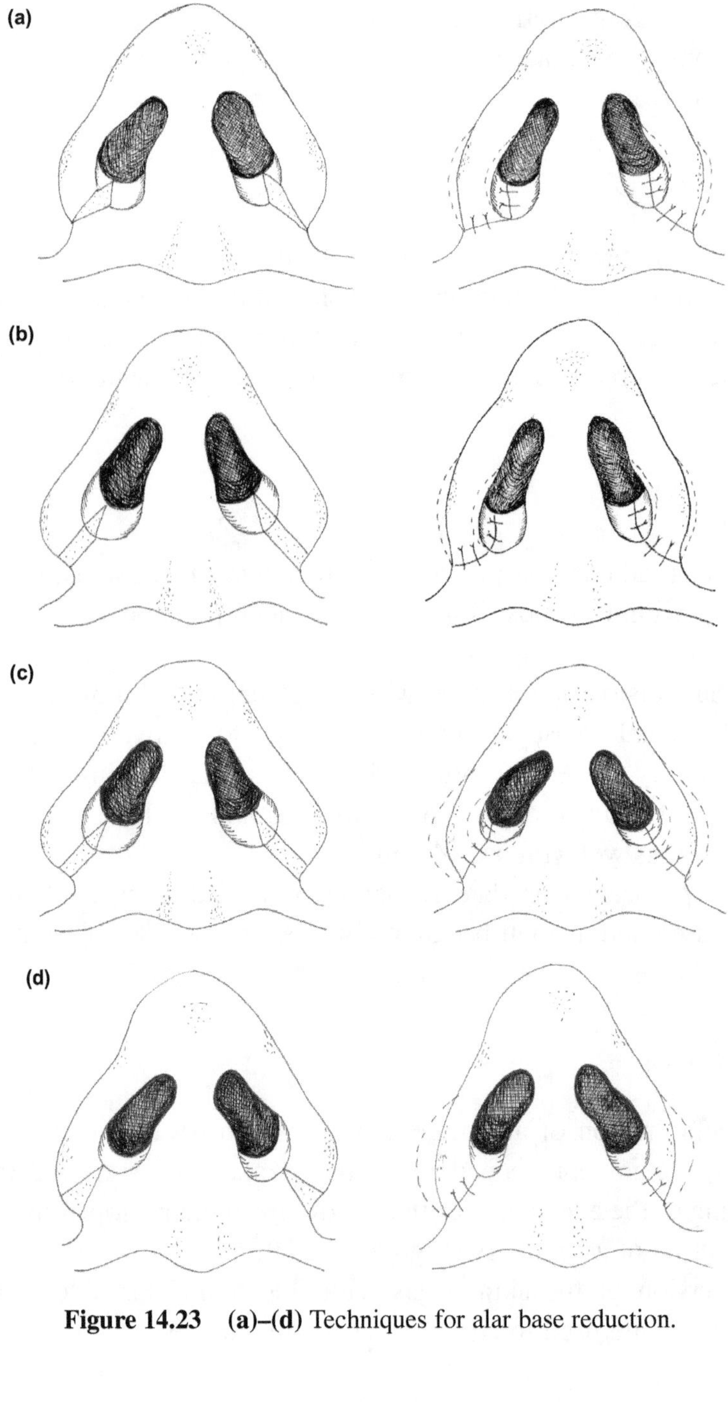

Figure 14.23 **(a)–(d)** Techniques for alar base reduction.

Sequential lowering of the cartilaginous dorsum

Although the en-bloc resection of the bony and cartilaginous dorsum has been the preferred option of many surgeons, the risk of collapse of the mid third of the nose caused by over-resection of the upper later cartilages has led to the means to strengthen the mid vault area. An alternative to the traditional method is deconstruction of the cartilaginous dorsum with sequential lowering. The upper lateral cartilages can be divided from the quadrilateral septal cartilage extramucosally initially and the midline septal cartilage resected alone to the desired level. The upper laterals are thus left intact at this point. The bony hump is then lowered, either by rasping alone or by using an osteotome with subsequent rasping as already described. The upper lateral cartilages will now remain proud and can be infolded to form autospreader grafts thus protecting against long term collapse in this area. This method of dorsal reduction is particularly helpful whenthere is a large cartilaginous hump and where there is insufficient septal cartilage available to fashion traditional spreader grafts.

Postoperative Care

Generally, meticulous technique and closure can avoid the need for postoperative nasal packing altogether and this is preferable as the presence and removal of such packs can be extremely uncomfortable. Packing materials, if required, include nasal tampons, ribbon guaze packing that may be impregnated by Bismuth Iodoform Paraffin Paste (BIPP) or non-stick dressings such as Telfa or Melonin. Packing is generally removed a few hours after surgery although can be left overnight.

Intranasal silastic splints are generally not required but are used in patients in whom postoperative synaechiae between the lateral wall of the nose and septum are a risk. Such patients include those with preoperative nasal adhesions from prior trauma or surgery or those who have significant perioperative septal mucoperichondrial tears. Splints are also used routinely after septal perforation closure. Silastic splints are available preformed or may be custom-made from sheets and are sutured to the nasal septum anteriorly. The splints are removed two weeks postoperatively in the outpatient setting.

A dorsal dressing is applied at the end of surgery to stabilise the nasal bones following osteotomies. Initially, steristrips are placed firmly along the dorsum to help re-approximate the dorsal skin and soft tissue envelope to the underlying skeleton. It is important to place one strip across the nasal tip area moulding and holding the tip into a desired position whilst the healing process occurs. Many options for the splint are available including preformed thermoplastic and metallic splints and the author's favoured custom tailored Plaster of Paris. A 5-layer 5 cm × 5 cm triangle of plaster is used. The sharp squared edges are rounded off into gentle curves in particular to ensure the cephalic edge of the plaster does not impinge upon the medial canthus of the eye. The plaster is soaked in warm water and is applied over the steristrips and held firmly whilst it sets and fixes the bony dorsum in the desired position. This creates a small but adequately protective splint that is further secured by taping over the plaster onto the face thereby ensuring it remains in position. Brown coloured micropore is used to act as an effective camouflage of the plaster itself (see Figure 14.24). The dorsal plaster splint is removed a week postoperatively as are any external sutures.

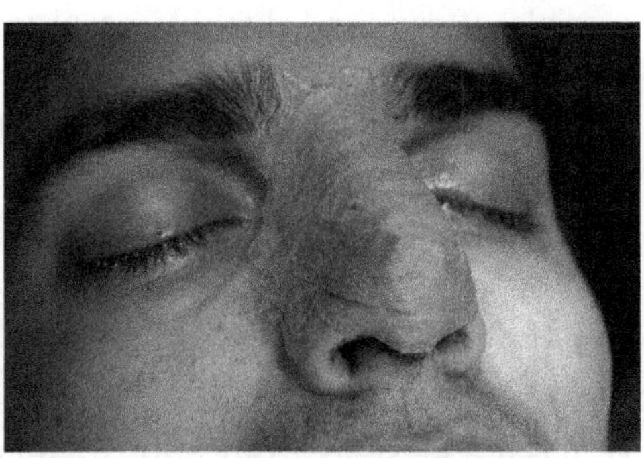

Figure 14.24 Nasal splint.

Revision Surgery

Revision corrective procedures remain one the most challenging aspects of rhinoplasty surgery. As techniques evolve, the rhinoplasty surgeon is ever seeking an ultimate postoperative result that will please both the discriminative patient and surgeon alike. New computer-aided preoperative techniques aimed at predicting eventual improvement in cosmesis coupled with the unprecedented number of media articles on cosmetic surgery appear to be increasing patient expectations. The inadequately informed patient is likely to be more critical of postoperative results. Increasing rates of revision surgery may be predicted in Europe, reflecting trends in North America.

The need for revision rhinoplasty may arise from either inadequate or overzealous primary surgery, most often the result of poor judgement by an inexperienced surgeon. Furthermore, postoperative scarring can turn a shorter-term good cosmetic result into a suboptimal one with time. In both cases, the resultant localised loss of contour or deficiency of the support mechanisms may in turn be associated with functional problems.

The revision rhinoplasty patient may further present with psychological issues including the body dysmorphobic disorder, relating to the original surgery and these must be both recognised and addressed during any preliminary consultation. In doing so, the important distinction between a patient-perceived or truly inadequate postoperative result can be made. In the former case it is particularly important not to convey false expectations regarding a revision procedure to the expectant patient. A doctor/patient rapport must be built laying the foundations for extended counselling in order to convey a realistic outcome for any revision surgery. Where a personality disorder is apparent, referral to a clinical psychologist or liaison psychiatrist may be essential.

Retrospective analyses have identified lower-third deformities followed by middle-third deformities as the most commonly encountered problems requiring secondary surgery.

Most authors would agree that revision surgery should not be planned for at least one year following the last operation. This time allows maturing of scar tissue, diminishing the risk of further deformity due to poor tissue healing following subsequent surgery. Whilst this remains a good general guideline, early correction of minor deformities such as an inadequate osteotomy may allay patient anxieties without compromising overall results. Other deformities that may be similarly rectified at an early stage include alar base widening that may be evident following the original surgery, alar retraction and minimal bony dorsal deformities requiring little soft tissue dissection. The majority of revisions, however, are best deferred and a clear explanation regarding the reasoning will usually temper patient pressure. The advantage of soft mature scar tissue during the revision operation facilitates easier dissection. "Shrink-wrapping" of the skin over the structural components is also well established by a year and will identify any irregularities at this stage, although the overall process continues further for some years. However, nasal tip revision surgery may need to be deferred somewhat longer than 12 months as adequate healing and shrink-wrapping may not be complete.

A particular challenge in revision rhinoplasty surgery is the unpredictability of the findings during surgery. Soft tissue contractures and scarring may mimic underlying structural deformity, and even with meticulous planning, the surgeon must remain able to adapt or even change the planned techniques to suit the discovered anomaly. Camouflage grafts are not always predicted for use but should be considered as being required to help correct such unforeseen deformities when formulating the preoperative plan. Experience in a variety of techniques is naturally a prerequisite to undertaking this sort of procedure due the very nature of this unpredictability.

Case Reports

Three cases are presented as examples of the complexity of the rhinoplasty challenge (see Figures 14.25 to 14.27).

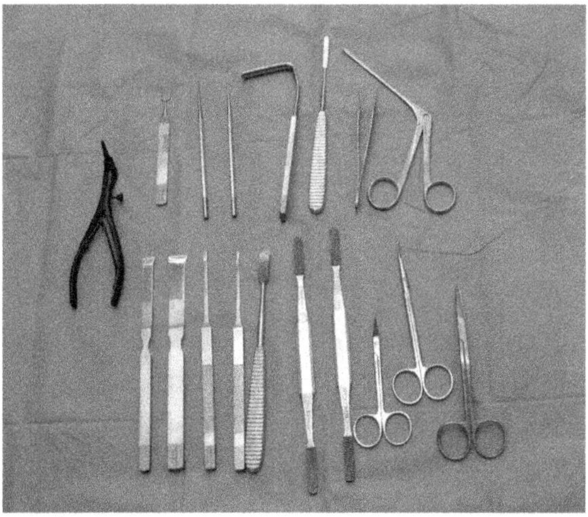

Figure 14.25 Basic rhinoplasty instruments. Instrument list (from left to right), Top row: Cottle's speculum, double pronged wide hook, single/double pronged micro hook, Aufricht retractor, Joseph periosteal elevator, Brown-Adson toothed forceps, Blakesley-Wilde forceps. Bottom row: Osteotomes — 14 mm/10 mm/ guarded 2.2 mm/2 mm, tungsten carbide glabella rasp, tungsten carbide dorsal rasps, Walter scissors, Kilner scissors, Foman scissors.

Patient Examples

Patient 1 — Dorsal Hump and Tip Ptosis (Figure 14.25)

Problems: Dorsal hump, slight deviation of bony dorsum, low take off point of nose from face, ptosis of nasal tip, excess columellar show. Retrognathia — patient not seeking correction of this.

Important Considerations: Large dorsal hump reduction may be the initial intervention for an inexperienced rhinoplasty surgeon. This would lead to a overlong, ptotic looking nose which would be more unaesthetic than the initial presentation. Projection and rotation of the tip here is the key to

(a) (b) (c) (d) (e) (f)

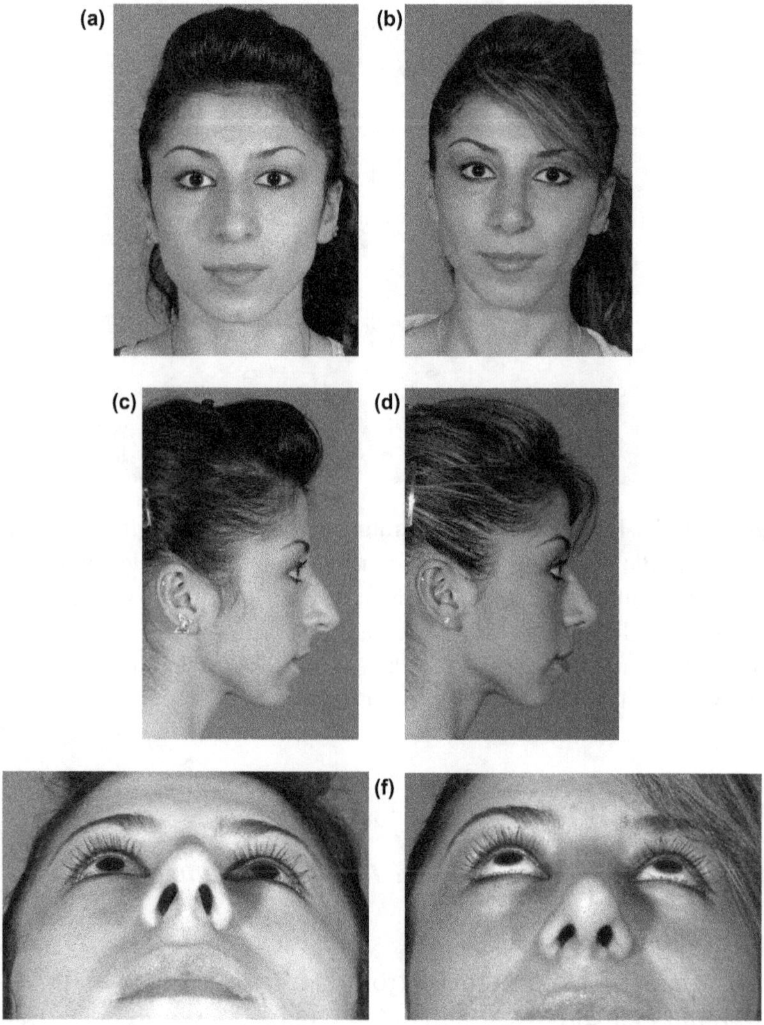

Figure 14.26 Dorsal hump and tip ptosis.

improving the nasal balance. The "take off point" of the nose is also very low on the face with a shallow nasion — an ideal being approximately at the level of where the upper eyelashes point to on the lateral view. Augmentation of the radix area together with the tip changes mean a much smaller dorsal hump reduction is required.

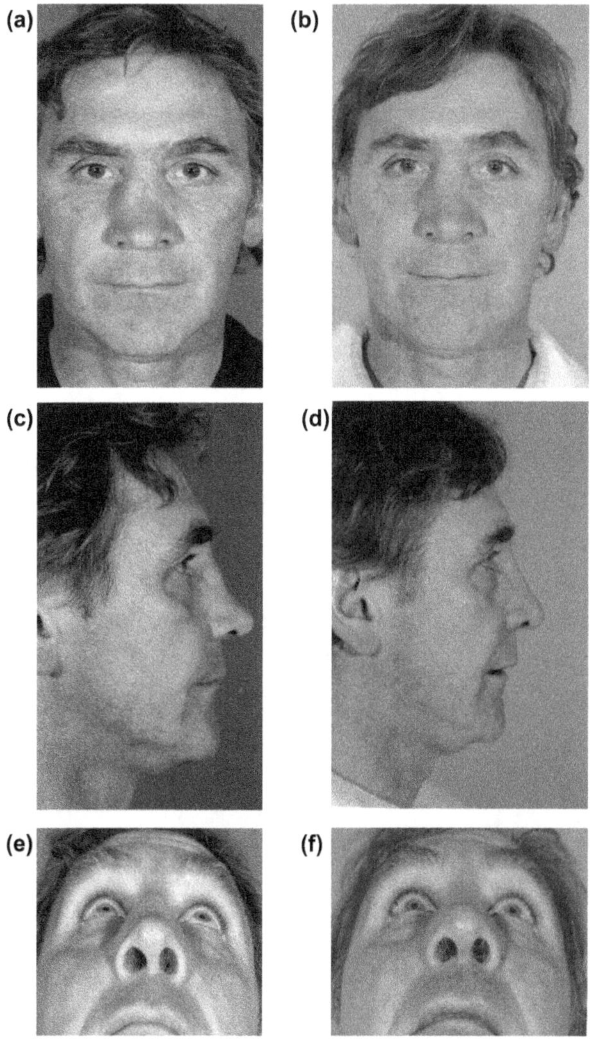

Figure 14.27 Post-traumatic saddle deformity.

Surgical Plan: External approach septorhinoplasty; lateral crural steal and suturing to rotate and project tip, minor cephalic volume reduction of lateral crurae, columellar strut harvested from septal cartilage for support, reduction of caudal and membranous septum, dorsal bony and cartilaginous dehump (minor), medial and lateral endonasal osteotomies, crushed radix graft harvested from septal cartilage to augment nasion.

Patient 2 — Post-Traumatic Saddle Deformity (*Figure 14.27*)

Problems: Post-traumatic saddle deformity, scar overlying dorsum, bony deviation to right, columellar retraction, broad nasal tip (patient unconcerned regarding this). Nasal obstruction with internal nasal valve collapse.

Important Considerations: Given the extent of the saddle deformity, septal cartilage harvest would be impossible and alternative sources are required. Scar revision, if required, should be deferred.

Surgical Plan: External approach rhinoplasty; auricular cartilage harvest for augmentation of dorsum with 2-layer graft, columellar strut and spreader grafts, tip refinement with dome suturing, medial and lateral percutaneous osteotomies.

Patient 3 — Shallow Dorsal Hump and Boxy Tip (*Figure 14.28*)

Problems: Dorsal hump, wide, "boxy" configuration to nasal tip with excess cephalic volume of lower lateral cartilages. Nasal obstruction with septal deviation and idiopathic perforation.

Important Considerations: Subtle improvements are only required here for restoration of cosmesis and improvement of brow-tip aesthetic lines.

Surgical Plan: Septorhinoplasty with closure of septal perforation; minor dorsal bony and cartilaginous dehump, medial and

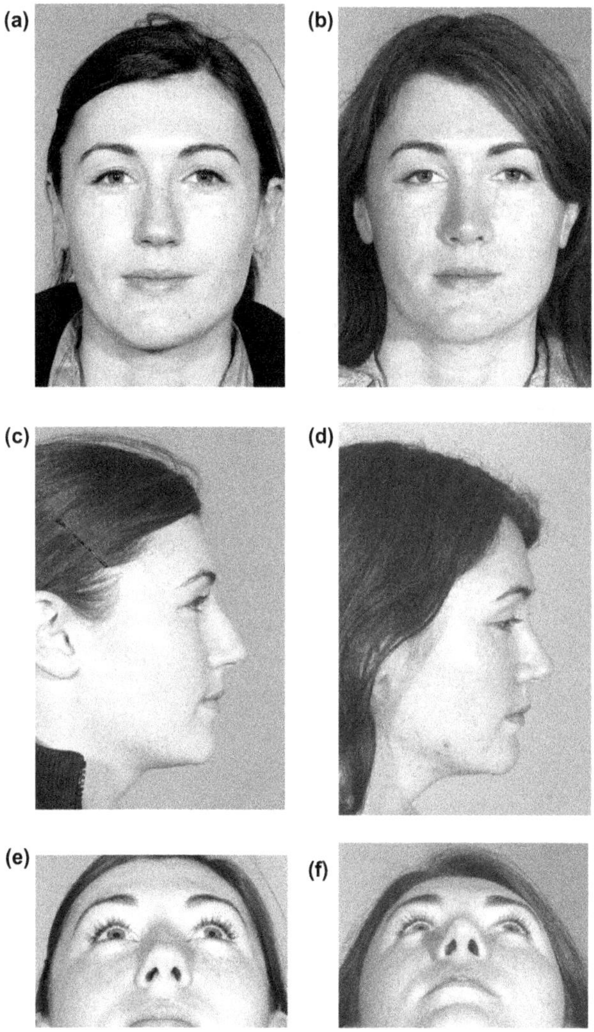

Figure 14.28 Shallow dorsal hump and boxy tip.

lateral endonasal osteotomies, dome suturing of lower lateral cartilages and volume reduction of cephalic margins. Septal perforation closure with bipedicled mucoperichondrial flaps and interpositional graft.

Conclusions

Rhinoplasty surgery is a complex aspect of aesthetic and reconstructive surgery of the face. Its important relationship to other orthognathic procedures is clear and the principles outlined in this chapter should provide a sound understanding of the basic concepts of this type of surgery.

The wide array of operative techniques involved in rhinoplasty necessitates a thorough understanding of the anatomy of the osseocartilaginous vault and septum, surgical principles and healing processes associated with these operations.

Chapter 15

Emergencies and Complications

Dan Harris and Malcolm Harris

Introduction

Problems will vary from the orthognathic to those of a more general nature, which can be life threatening. Although orthognathic surgery is usually carried out on young fit adults, life-threatening complications may arise. Careful technique, and expertise in the management of serious emergencies are essential. This includes the understanding the mysteries of medical monitoring.

Medical Monitoring (Figure 15.1)

ECG: a basic knowledge of abnormal PQRST complexes and arrhythmias is essential for interpreting the ECG. "Three-lead" monitoring gives an interpretable rhythm-strip but is no replacement for a full "12-lead" ECG assessment when acute cardiac problems are suspected.

Heart rate (HR): derived from the ECG and the monitor can be set to detect bradycardia and tachycardia.

Arterial blood pressure (ABP): is measured by direct cannulation of the radial, brachial, dorsalis pedis or femoral arteries. The

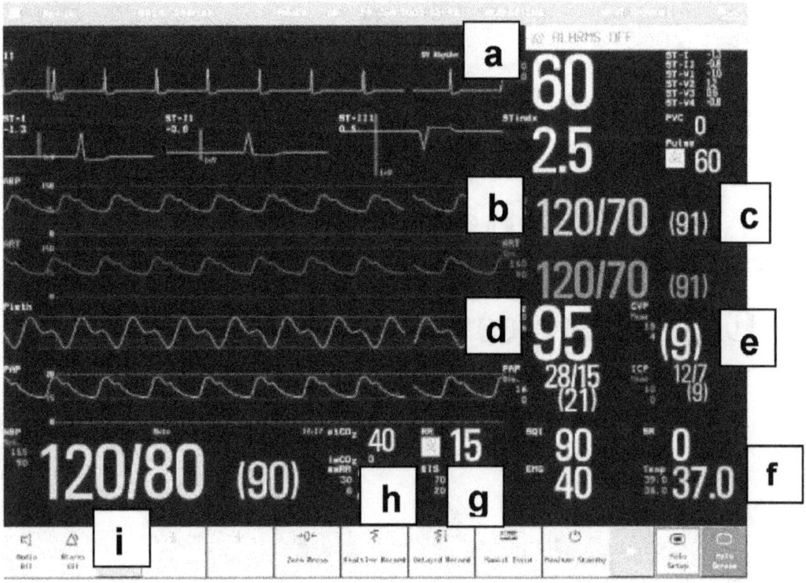

Figure 15.1 Intensive Care Monitor (by courtesy of Panasonic). **(a)** Heart rate. **(b)** Continuous invasive blood pressure (BP). **(c)** Current mean arterial pressure. **(d)** Oxygen saturation. **(e)** Central venous pressure. **(f)** Temperature. **(g)** Respiratory rate. **(h)** End tidal CO_2. **(i)** Non-invasive cuff BP.

mean arterial pressure (MAP) is denoted in brackets. Non-invasive monitoring (NBP) is done with an appropriately-sized pneumatic cuff placed either around the upper arm or lower leg.

Central venous pressure (CVP): is useful as an indication of right ventricular preload. Serial readings (i.e. the trend of CVP measurements) are far more useful than single readings. The normal value is 2–6 mmHg. Respiration (RESP): is normally 14–20 a minute.

Oxygen saturation of arterial blood (SpO_2): is usually measured by a digital pulse oximeter based on the light absorptive properties of oxygenated and deoxygenated Hb. Oxygen saturation monitoring, which assesses oxygenation, not ventilation, is no substitute for arterial blood gas assessment as there are both extrinsic and intrinsic reasons why the reading may be inaccurate.

Carbon dioxide: is expressed in a graphic form by the capnograph. Capnography is an indirect monitor that not only helps in the differential diagnosis of hypoxia, but also provides information about CO_2 production, alveolar ventilation and respiratory patterns.

Temperature: can be monitored by mouth, axilla, tympanic membrane, oesophagus and rectum. Rectal and oesophageal measures are the most accurate.

Complications

1. *Oedema and Infection*

Oedema is reducible with pre- and postoperative dexamethasone and antibiotic cover as described earlier. Contrary to some popular practice vacuum drains can dramatically reduce the swelling arising from mandibular osteotomies, and the minivacuum drain is equally valuable for infraorbital haematomas following dissection through a subciliary incision. The same applies to the iliac crest donor site. Where possible leave drains for at least 24 hours after they cease to function.

Where there is gross postoperative swelling and pain, the presence of a haematoma is more likely than oedema alone. Treatment should be the release of the haematoma, especially if expanding, as it may be the presenting feature of a persistent arterial bleed, which needs to be identified and arrested.

There is some dispute as to whether clean operations require more than one pre- and postoperative antibiotic bolus. However prospective trials have shown that a five-day course produces less postoperative infection at the sagittal split site.

2. *Bleeding Problems*

a) *Minor Haemorrhage*

Even with healthy patients not receiving any medication which would predispose to excess bleeding, intraoperative blood loss is significantly reduced by the administration of an antifibrinolytic agent such as tranexamic acid 25 mg/kg orally or 0.5–1 g by slow intravenous injection pre- and postoperatively.

Tearing the periosteum on the medial aspect of the ascending ramus exposing it for a sagittal split may produce a troublesome bleed, which can be controlled with a hot wet tonsil swab and pressure for 3 minutes. Damage to the facial vessels through the base of the subperiosteal pouch prepared for the mandibular buccal cortex cut responds to the same pressure and patience. Rarely the maxillary, tonsillar or lingual arteries may be damaged, giving rise to prolonged serous haemorrhage. Again, packing firstly with a swab, and secondly with a large piece of oxidised cellulose (Surgicel) should be sufficient, assisted by 0.5–1 g t.d.s. tranexamic acid (Cyclokapron, Kabi) given intravenously or orally. If vigorous bleeding persists the external carotid may need to be tied off, as described below.

b) *Persistent Haemorrhage*

Failure to control bleeding despite efficient conservative measures may be due to:

i) A patent damaged artery, either the maxillary or tonsillar that require identification and ligation. Do not delay ligation of the external carotid if significant bleeding persists despite local ligation, packing and antifibrinolytic therapy for more than 30 minutes. This should allow time for essential investigation.
ii) A latent coagulation defect or defibrination. In both cases there is an evident lack of clot formation on the drapes and the wound oozes "watery blood".

c) *Investigations and Management*

Ensure early that adequate blood is available for replacement; if not, send venous samples for full blood count, cross-matching and a clotting screen which must include the thrombin time, prothrombin time (PT or INR), thromboplastin generation test, fibrin degradation products and a platelet count. The following are found in rare cases of acute defibrination: prolonged prothrombin time (PT), activated partial thromboplastin time (APPT) and thrombin time (TT), with increased fibrin degradation products and reduced platelets. The increased fibrin degradation products have an anticoagulant effect.

Maintain the circulation with crystalloid solution until packed cells or fully cross-matched blood are available. Remember the circulating blood volume in an average adult is around 5 litres (75 ml/kg), and transfusion is required after a 20%–30% loss. In a child the circulating blood volume is equal to the weight in kilogrammes × 80 ml, and therefore a relatively small volume will equal a 20% loss.

Any patient when given a large volume of blood replacement (1–1.5 times the circulating volume within 24 hours) will require fresh frozen plasma (FFP) the highly concentrated, cryoprecipitate and platelets. At this stage a clinical haematologist should guide all blood product prescribing. If no lab results are available give 1,000 mls of FFP for each 6 units of red cells. If lab results are available and show the PT ratio to be >1.5 the prescribed volume of FFP should be 15–20 ml/kg.

Two "pools" of cryoprecipitate should also be given if lab results are not yet available and bleeding is ongoing, or if results are available and fibrinogen levels are <1.5 g/L.

d) *Ligation of the External Carotid Artery*

Clean the neck with detergent and iodine. Resist the temptation to use an aesthetic skin crease incision, as this will limit access if the neck is distended with blood. Always incise obliquely along the anterior border of the sternomastoid muscle (Figure 15.2a). Remember the carotid bifurcation is just below the level of the hyoid bone. Therefore incise obliquely downwards from two fingers' breadth below the angle of the mandible to the level of the prominence of the thyroid cartilage along a line drawn from the mastoid process to the sternal notch. Deepen the wound through fat,

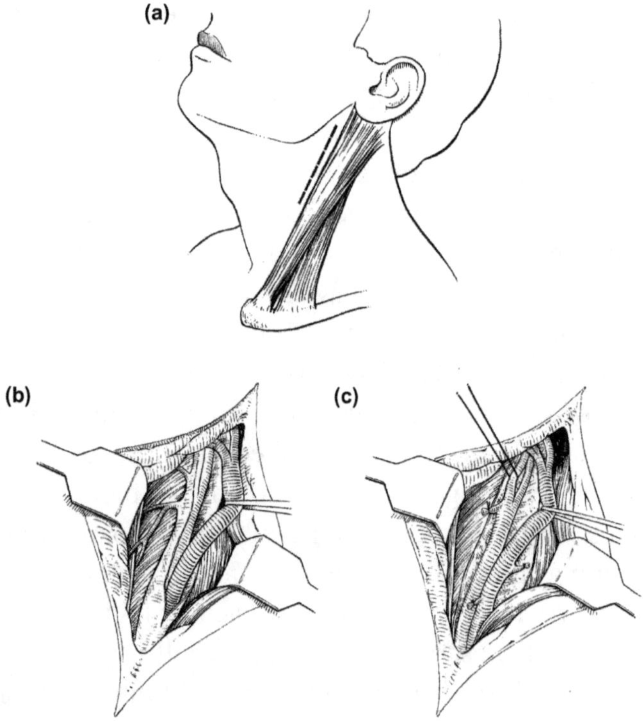

Figure 15.2 (**a**) Skin incision at the upper anterior border of sternomastoid. (**b**) Opening of carotid sheath with retraction of internal jugular vein to reveal the carotid artery. (**c**) Ligation of external carotid artery.

platysma and fascia using a No. 10 or 20 blade until the anterior border of sternomastoid muscle can be felt and seen.

The sternomastoid must be retracted firmly with a broad Langenbeck. The carotid triangle contains fine filamentous fascia, unless it has become infiltrated with oedema due to prolonged bleeding into the neck.

The carotid sheath fascia overlying the internal jugular vein is picked up with toothed forceps and incised along the vessel with McIndoe scissors. A nylon tape is passed around the internal jugular, once revealed, and attached to artery forceps; the vein is retracted distally with the sternomastoid muscle (Figure 15.2b).

The carotid will now be palpable and partially visible; again, fascia will need to be divided to expose the bifurcation. This may be obscured by one or more small veins, which must be tied with 3/0 polyglycollate or linen and divided. The external carotid is anteromedial to the internal carotid and can be identified by its branches. The superior thyroid artery often arises at the bifurcation and has to be ligated with a black silk or linen and divided to gain access to the main trunk. Ligatures are more easily passed around the vessel with small Adson's artery forceps as they have a more pronounced right angle curve. Rather than search for a specific vessel it is better to tie the external carotid at its base. There is no need to divide it (Figure 15.2c).

A vacuum drain is inserted and sutured to the skin with 3/0 black silk and the wound closed in three layers using 3.0 polyglycollate for the platysma and subcutaneous layers and 5/0 interrupted Prolene sutures for the skin.

An absorbent non-adhesive dressing is then secured with adhesive tape.

e) *Coagulation Defects*

Persistent bleeding despite local and carotid ligation indicates either a factor deficiency (the most common unsuspected defect being von Willebrand's disease) or disseminated intravascular coagulation (DIC). By now the laboratory results should be available. A prolonged thromboplastin generation test suggests a missing clotting factor. The prothrombin time (INR) will not be of value unless this is an anticoagulant or advanced liver disease problem, which is unlikely in an osteotomy patient. If however, there are also raised fibrin degradation products and deficient platelets, DIC should be assumed to be the problem. DIC management should be as follows.

i) Maintain tissue perfusion and oxygenation with intravenous fluid support and supplemental oxygen.

ii) Fresh frozen plasma (FFP), which contains clotting factors as well as the natural anticoagulants antithrombin III and protein C, is given as follows:

If no lab results are available. 1 litre of FFP for each 6 units of red cells.
Or 15–20 ml/g if lab results show the PT ratio to be >1.5. If lab results are not yet available and bleeding is ongoing "2 pools" of cryoprecipitate are given as they also are if results are available and fibrinogen levels are <1.5 g/L.

iii) Platelet transfusion, 1 Adult Therapeutic Dose (ATD) of platelets should be given in bleeding cases where no results are available or if the platelet count is known to be below 75×10^9/L.

iv) Antifibrinolytic agent (tranexamic acid 0.5–1 g IV) must be administered 1g as a bolus over 10 minutes followed by second gram as an infusion over 8 hours. However once this process has been recognised it is essential to consult a clinical haematologist for advice.

v) Any patient receiving a large volume of blood replacement (1–1.5% of the circulating volume within 24 hours) will require FFP, cryoprecipitate and platelets. At this stage a clinical haematologist should guide all blood product prescribing. Recombinant activated Factor VII (rFVIIa, NovoSeven™) is now not recommended in the majority of haemorrhage protocols.

vi) The patient has by now been infused with 5–10 litres of fluid, much of which will be distending the bladder. This will require an indwelling catheter (see below), not only to decompress the bladder but also to help calculate the state of fluid balance and renal perfusion.

vii) Continued bleeding into the tissues may fill the soft palate, the lateral wall of the pharynx and the neck, constituting a serious threat to the airway postoperatively. Blood will also have passed the throat pack into the larynx and almost certainly into the stomach. The airway can be managed by prolonged endotracheal intubation but this will be dependent on skilled postoperative intensive care. If support is not available, an early decision should be made to carry out a tracheostomy, which not only guarantees the airway but also prevents aspiration into the lungs of blood or gastric contents and allows aspiration of accumulated secretions from the bronchi.

viii) Remember to administer metoclopromide 10 mg. Metoclopromide is a dopamine antagonist, which stimulates gastric emptying, and small intestinal transit whilst also enhancing the strength of oesophageal sphincter contraction.

ix) Before the patient leaves the theatre a Ryles nasogastric tube should be passed to aspirate the blood and bile reflux from the stomach. Gastric acid reduction as a prophylaxis against aspiration may also be achieved by giving a proton pump inhibitor such as omeprazole 40 mg by slow intravenous injection. Under normal conditions the effects of proton pump inhibitors are enhanced if the drug is given the evening before surgery and again 2 hours prior to surgery commencing. However this is not possible in cases of surgical emergency.

f) *Secondary Haemorrhage*

The patient may suddenly bleed profusely postoperatively in the ward, or even at home. The common causes are a partially divided large vein or untied artery in the depths of a mandibular osteotomy wound. Occasionally an undetected coagulopathy such as von Willebrand's is the underlying problem, especially when the bleeding is repeated.

The management must commence with pressure applied to the bleeding site with swabs, and rapid transfer to theatre for exploration and haemostasis, as described.

As with all severe haemorrhage up to 10 mg intravenous morphine should be given immediately by slow intravenous injection as a sedative analgesic, together with tranexamic acid 1 gram intravenously over 10 minutes to help conserve clotting factors and clot in favour of haemostasis.

g) *Gastric Haemorrhage*

The chance of stress-induced gastric erosion is small, even after prolonged orthognathic surgery. However, the combination of a patient with a history of peptic ulceration, a stressful surgical procedure, anti-inflammatory steroids and analgesics can produce a gastric bleed. Abdominal discomfort, tachycardia, true melaena and/or haematemesis and a fall in haemoglobin (a late sign) should alert one to this possibility. Initial treatment should include intravenous fluid support and administration of a proton-pump inhibitor (omeprazole), first as an intravenous bolus dose (40 mg), then as an intravenous infusion for 72 hours. Early endoscopy should be considered after consultation with a gastroenterologist so that the bleeding point can be injected or banded.

The aim of drug treatment is to raise gastric pH to above 4, thereby stabilising any clots that may have formed at the bleeding site. This is the reasoning behind the use of proton pump inhibitors over H2 receptor blockers such as ranitidine, which have a lesser effect on pH.

With vulnerable patients a regular prophylactic proton pump inhibitor, such as omeprazole or lansoprazole, should be administered as well as eliminating both steroids and non-steroidal anti-inflammatory analgesic drugs from the intraoperative and postoperative regimen.

3) *The Airway*

After an uneventful operation, the airway should be maintained with a nasopharyngeal tube, which is sucked out throughout the postoperative 12–18 hours at 30-minute intervals. Unless the nurse ensures that the fine suction catheter passes beyond the end of the nasopharyngeal airway tube, the end will gradually become blocked with blood clot and will become an efficient airway obstruction (Figure 15.3a) the same can occur with a tracheostomy tube (Figure 15.3b). Some anaesthetists leave an endotracheal tube *in situ* which with modern closed suction units can be kept unobstructed with minimum effort and nursing intervention.

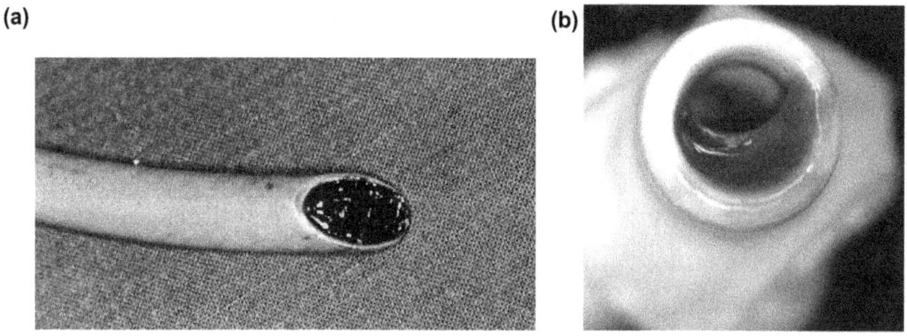

Figure 15.3 Clot obstructing (**a**) endotracheal tube and (**b**) tracheostomy tube.

A facemask with 40% oxygen at a flow rate of approximately 5 litres/min ensures adequate tissue perfusion. In intensive care or high dependency units an intra-arterial line may have been inserted to monitor blood gases and invasive blood pressure is displayed on the cardiac monitor as a continuous arterial pressure trace. But this is not an alternative to the provision of a good airway by careful suction and good nursing. Continuous monitoring via a peripheral oxygen saturation probe will give early warnings of evolving airway obstruction and hypoxia.

Nasal obstruction with blood clot and mucous crusting can be prevented by steam inhalations containing Friar's Balsam or some similar aromatic vapour.

Occasionally an asthmatic patient develops acute bronchospasm and airway obstruction despite the dexamethasone cover. This may be resolved by a salbutamol nebuliser; 2.5–5 mg of salbutamol in a pre-prepared solution via a nebuliser mask on 8 litres oxygen per minute repeated as required, with 500 mcg of ipratropium bromide (an antimuscarinic bronchodilator) added 6-hourly. In addition intravenous magnesium (2 g in 100 ml normal saline) over 30 minutes is now an accepted part of The British Thoracic Society Guideline for severe acute asthma management. Magnesium induces relaxation of bronchial smooth muscle in acute asthma by interfering with calcium transport mechanisms and intracellular phosphorylation.

With these basic conservative measures, emergency tracheostomies are rarely needed.

h) *Emergency Airway Procedures*

Acute upper airway obstruction is more likely to follow trauma then operative procedures. In the non-intubated patient, obstruction secondary to haemorrhage into the neck tissues may prevent the clinician from inserting an endotracheal tube through the cords to establish airway patency. In such cases needle cricothryroidotomy and surgical cricothyroidotomy may be used to maintain ventilation and oxygenation whilst formal endotracheal intubation is attempted.

i) Needle cricothyroidotomy and jet insufflation can provide supplemental oxygenation for around 20–30 minutes, the time constraint being carbon dioxide retention, as only minimal expiration is possible through the obstructed airway via this method. This relatively simple technique buys time to perform more definitive airway procedures by a clinician skilled in difficult and emergency situations.

Technique

Attach a 12–14 gauge cannula to a 10 ml syringe.

With the patient in a supine position extend (neutral in acute trauma) the patient's neck whilst controlling the head.

Palpate the cricothyroid membrane and then stabilise the trachea between thumb and forefinger of the nondominant hand to prevent lateral movement.

Puncture the skin in the midline with the cannula needle directly over the membrane, directing the needle at a 45° angle caudally.

Insert the needle through the lower half of the membrane, aspirating as the needle is inserted.

Aspiration of air indicates entry into the tracheal lumen, at which point the catheter can be carefully advanced into the lumen whilst withdrawing the needle.

Oxygen tubing attached to a Y-connector or with a hole cut into the side is attached to the hub of the catheter.

Intermittent insufflation can be achieved by occluding the open limb of the Y-connector or the hole in the tubing with a finger for 1 second and releasing for 4 seconds, during which oxygenation and then some passive expiration can occur. Expiration is limited as it occurs through the partially obstructed airway and not through the lumen of the inserted catheter.

Oxygen flow is commenced at 10 litres per minute and increased in increments of 1 litre until chest wall movement is observed during the period of hole occlusion.

As well as allowing oxygenation via jet insufflation, needle cricothyroidotomy can be used to carry out a retrograde intubation. After initial insertion of the needle through the membrane has been confirmed by aspiration of air, a guide wire is passed through the needle cephalad. This wire should pass upwards into the pharynx and then grasped with forceps to be brought out through the mouth. An endotracheal tube can then be passed over the wire into the larynx. The wire is removed once the tube reaches the level of the membrane and the tube is then passed further into the trachea.

ii) Surgical cricothyroidotomy involves the insertion of a small endotracheal tube or tracheostomy tube through the cricothyroid membrane. Using this method the patient can be successfully oxygenated and ventilated with a bag valve system with supplemental oxygen until intubation or retrograde intubation is achieved. This technique is not recommended for children under 12 years of age in whom damage to the cricoid ring is likely.

Technique

Place the patient in the supine position with the neck in a neutral position.

Prepare the skin and anaesthetise the area if the patient is conscious.

Identify the cricothyroid membrane between the thyroid and cricoid cartilages.

Stabilise the thyroid cartilage with the non-dominant hand to prevent lateral movement.

Carefully make a transverse skin incision over the membrane and then incise through the lower half of the membrane.

Open the airway by using either a haemostat, a tracheal spreader, or by inserting the scalpel handle through the incised membrane and rotating it through 90°.

Insert the endotracheal or tracheostomy tube through the incised and opened membrane, directing it distally into the trachea.

Inflate the cuff and secure the airway using either sutures or ribbon ties.

Attach a bag valve system that is connected to a high flow oxygen source to the tube and ventilate the patient, observing for chest wall movement to indicate lung inflation.

iii) Tracheostomy: The need for elective tracheostomy has diminished with improved anaesthetic techniques and emergency care. However, the emergency tracheostomy, especially where there has been marked uncontrolled blood loss into the tissues, is still essential for untroubled postoperative care if prolonged endotracheal intubation cannot be adequately supervised. It provides an assured airway with reduced dead space, easy access for the aspiration of secretions from the bronchi below and prevents aspiration into the bronchi from above.

Technique

Place a sandbag between the shoulders and maximally extend the head on the neck to elevate the trachea (Figure 15.4a).

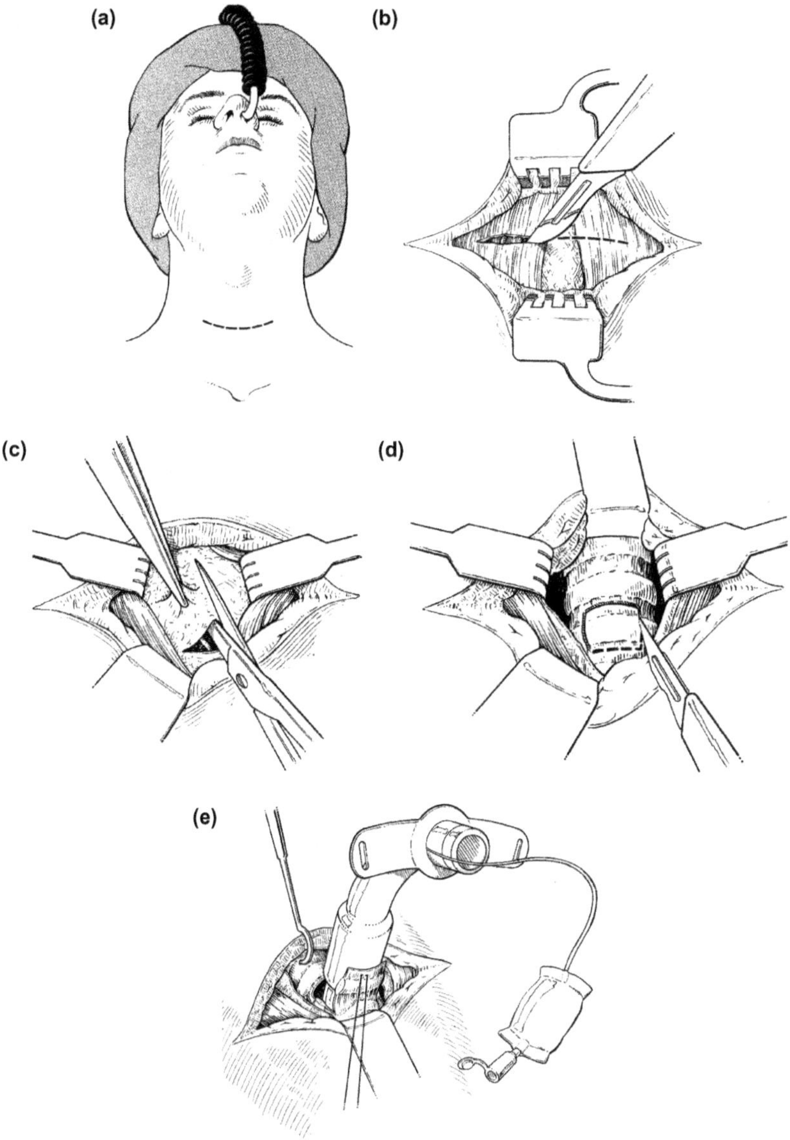

Figure 15.4 Tracheostomy technique, details on pages 480 and 480.

Prepare the skin from the lower border of the mandible to below the clavicles with povidone-iodine. If there is no hurry, mark the incision and infiltrate it with a vasoconstrictor solution.

A horizontal 5 cm incision is made halfway between the prominence of the thyroid cartilage and the sternal notch with a No. 10 blade. Incise through the fatty superficial fascia and platysma down to the muscle layer, revealing the anterior jugular veins on both sides. These may be divided and tied, or undisturbed and ignored if there is any urgency. Retract the flaps with cat's paws or a self-retaining retractor (Figure 15.4b).

Incise vertically in the midline with a knife or scissors, separating the intramuscular fascia and revealing the pretracheal fascia.

Retract the strap muscles laterally.

Lift up the pretracheal fascia with toothed forceps and incise upwards with scissors to reveal the isthmus of the thyroid, and then downward, avoiding if possible the centrally placed inferior thyroid vein (Figure 15.4c). If the thyroid isthmus is large it may be retracted upwards with a broad Langenbeck. Occasionally it may be necessary to clamp the isthmus with long curved haemostats and divide it. To prevent bleeding, the margins should be carefully tied with 2/0 polyglycollate before releasing the clamps.

Re-position the retractors inside the pretracheal fascia on either side of the trachea. If time allows, or if using local analgesia, infiltrate between the second and third tracheal ring with 1 ml 2% lignocaine containing 1:80,000 adrenaline for haemostasis, then inject another 1–2 ml into the lumen. This anaesthetises the mucous membrane and helps to suppress the violent cough reflex when inserting the tube.

Make a horizontal slit between the second and third tracheal ring with a No. 15 blade and extend it downwards bilaterally. The trachea may be steadied by passing a tracheal or skin hook beneath the upper ring and gently elevating. The simplest technique is now to remove a circular disc of trachea and then pass a 1/0 black silk stay suture around the lower ring and clip it outside the lower wound margin (Figure 15.4d).

Some surgeons prefer a Bjork flap, which is an inverted U hinged inferiorly (Figure 15.4e). The upper margin of the flap is sutured to the skin surface. This enables re-intubation if the tracheostomy tube is displaced or removed. However, the tracheal defect tends to be larger and there may be a greater incidence of post-tracheostomy stenosis.

Choose a suitable size of tracheostomy tube, 33 to 39 for small to large individuals, and test the cuff by inflating with air.

Insert the tracheostomy tube gently as the anaesthetist withdraws the endotracheal tube, carefully sucking all blood from the area. Inflate the cuff with a 20 ml syringe, noting whether it is self-sealing or requires clamping and sealing with its own spigot (Figure 15.4e).

The endotracheal tube is now completely removed and the anaesthetic hose connected to the tracheostomy tube.

Suture the skin margins beneath retaining flanges with interrupted 3/0 Prolene or silk as far medially as possible. Cover the wound margins with an acriflavine-impregnated gauze swab or Telfa pad which has been prepared with a T-shaped cut to fit around the tube.

Tie the tube flanges behind the neck with tapes to prevent displacement.

Postoperative Care

Secretions must be sucked out regularly every half hour, and more frequently if necessary, with a fine catheter and using an aseptic technique

The tracheostomy oxygen must be warmed and humidified.

High volume, low-pressure cuffs no longer need to be released at intervals to prevent ischaemia of the tracheal mucosa but the cuff pressure should be checked.

A chest radiograph must be taken postoperatively to exclude pleural damage and pneumothorax. Note: surgical emphysema of the neck may be dramatic but is of no consequence.

Daily physiotherapy is essential, with gently catheter suction and warm saline to loosen the secretions.

Once the oral and cervical swelling has receded and the chest radiograph is clear, the tracheostomy should be removed. The skin is cleaned with detergent (Savlon) and the tube is sucked out with the patient upright and is then withdrawn. Steri-strips may be used to close the margins of the wound, which is then covered with a dry gauze adhesive dressing and is left unchanged, and sealed for 10 days. Complete spontaneous closure usually takes place in a week. If there is any delay, swabs taken from the wound will show gross antibiotic resistant contaminants. Avoid the temptation to use exotic antibiotics when local cleansing with 0.05% hibitane or povidone-iodine dressings is all that is required.

As osteotomy cases do not require a prolonged tracheostomy, replacement of the tube does not arise.

4. *Drainage of a Pneumothorax*

Occasionally, despite every care on removing a rib graft, there is a breach in the pleura and the patient develops a pneumothorax. The presenting signs are breathlessness and tachypnoea with absent breath-sounds over the area. The typical radiographic appearance where the visceral pleura is breached is a demarcated peripheral area devoid of lung markings — here seen on the left side (Figure 15.5a). However Figure 15.5b shows a mottled oval opacity of surgical emphysema in the right lung field overlying a pneumothorax where both visceral and parietal pleura have been breached following costochondral graft removal.

The most convenient, comfortable and cosmetically pleasing site for drainage is in the fourth or fifth intercostal space just anterior to the mid-axillary line. To achieve this, the patient must be comfortably positioned, either reclining on the bed with the ipsilateral arm behind the head to expose the axilla, or leaning forward, with folded arms resting on a pillow on the bed-table. The surgeon should scrub,

(a) (b)

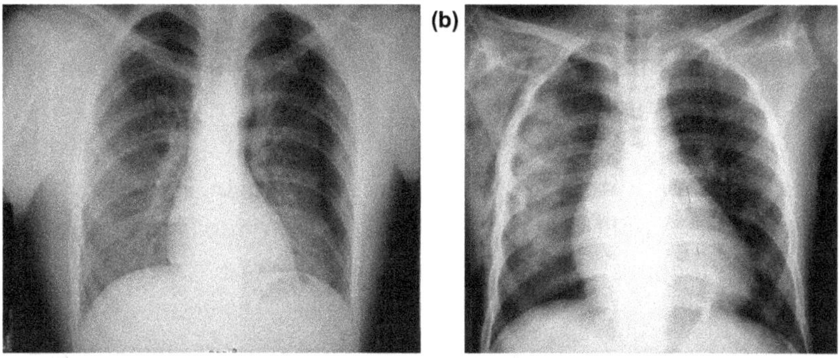

Figure 15.5 (**a**) Left pneumothorax due to breach of visceral pleura producing a demarcated peripheral area devoid of lung markings. (**b**) Oval mottled opacity of surgical emphysema overlying right pneumothorax due to breach in parietal and visceral pleura.

gown and put on gloves. The skin is prepared with povidone-iodine and, with sterile towels to isolate the area, is infiltrated with 1% or 2% lignocaine. Then with a 21-gauge needle (green hub) the chest wall is infiltrated to the pleura (up to 3 mg/kg), at which level air can be aspirated. Always keep to the upper rib border to avoid the intercostal neurovascular bundle that runs along the inferior border of the rib. A small skin incision is made and then blunt dissection used through the superficial fascia and intercostal muscles to the pleural space.

Small calibre chest drain sets (8–14 F) come with a Seldinger technique insertion kit. The method involves passing dilators of increasing size into the pleural space over a guide wire that has initially been introduced through a hollow needle. This creates an almost bloodless and atraumatic tract into the space required, through which the chest drain can be passed prior to connecting it up to an underwater drainage system. The use of the rigid trochar is contraindicated for all sizes of drain due to the risk of intrathoracic injury.

Two sutures are routinely inserted, the first to assist closure of the wound after drain removal, usually a mattress suture, and the second, a stay suture to secure the drain. "Purse-string" sutures are no longer recommended due to the less pleasing scar and increased pain whilst *in situ*.

The catheter position and pneumothorax are then checked with an anteroposterior chest radiograph. The catheter may be removed 24 hours after radiographic evidence that the lung is fully inflated. The drain should be removed whilst the patient performs either Valsalva's manoeuvre or during expiration. Provided aseptic techniques have been used, there is no role for prophylactic antibiotic administration for chest drain insertion.

Vomiting

Postoperative vomiting in patients with intermaxillary fixation was a well-recognised problem. Predisposing factors are blood escaping intraoperatively and postoperatively into the stomach, where partial digestion together with bile reflux creates an irritant stagnant mixture. An additional factor is the emetic effect of opiate analgesics.

Prevention

i) Avoid intermaxillary fixation by using internal rigid fixation.
ii) A 12–16 FG nasogastric tube passed at the time of the anaesthetic induction enables postoperative aspiration of gastric contents. The tube is attached to a bile bag to create a closed collecting system for any spontaneous reflux. As the patient is monitored throughout the postoperative night the stomach should be aspirated hourly and the fluid loss noted. Initially flushing the tube with 20 ml water before aspiration prevents the end becoming clogged with clot.

The administration of an antiemetic, e.g. metoclopromide 10 mg intravenously at the end of the operation, and with any required opiate analgesics, reduces drug-induced emesis (up to a maximum of 30 mg/24 hours). Metoclopromide 10 mg intravenously should also be given at any other time if vomiting is anticipated. 5HT antagonists such as ondansetron block the action of 5HT in the intestine and CNS, which also has an antiemetic effect. This is introduced after the administration of metochlopramide. With a fully conscious patient it is often the nasopharyngeal airway that provokes the problem.

Management

The patient who is being nursed in a 45° sitting position should be sucked out immediately through both sides of the nose with a broad-core catheter. The buccal sulci will also require clearing.

Contrary to popular belief, cutting intermaxillary fixation — if used, is neither essential nor the most efficient way of managing the vomiting patient.

Paradoxically, nasal suction is more efficient than opening the mouth and attempting to clear the oropharynx of vomitus in a conscious patient.

5. *Iliac Crest Problems*

The removal of bone from the iliac crest for orthognathic purposes is becoming less popular. However, the inverted L osteotomy may require a substantial amount of corticocancellous bone to correct a very small mandible.

Postoperative pain is the most frequent complication and can be reduced by drainage and analgesics. Some surgeons leave a fine cannula for infusion of a long acting local analgesic such as bupivacaine (Marcain). It is difficult to be certain if this is of significant value.

If a large graft has been removed near the anterior superior iliac spine, this may fracture with sudden movement once the patient is mobilised (Figure 15.6). No treatment is required apart from reassurance, rest, analgesics and physiotherapy.

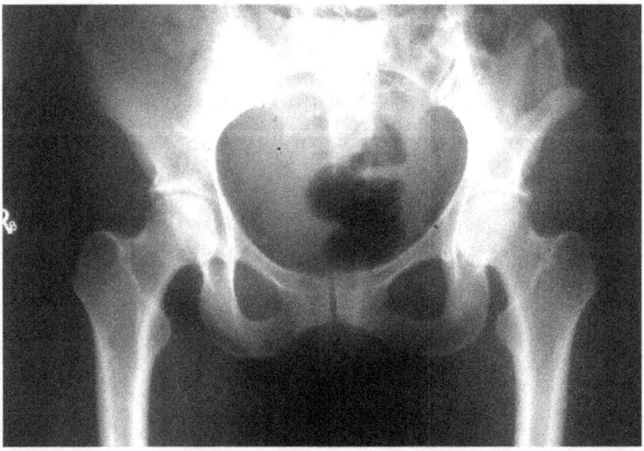

Figure 15.6 Fracture at the base of the anterior superior iliac spine with collapse of the preserved iliac crest lid.

6. *Catheterisation*

Catheterisation is necessary for prolonged surgical procedures, especially where large quantities of fluid have been infused. This is uncommon with orthognathic cases except where there has been unexpected major blood loss. Another occasional indication is the patient, usually male, who has postoperative urinary retention. This may be due to opioid-induced sphincter spasm, diffidence in using a urinal, or a combination of both, leading to gross distension. Any associated agitation will resolve with catheter insertion and bladder drainage and does not need to be controlled with intravenous benzodiazepines.

Technique

As with all separate aseptic procedures, each area must be freshly prepared and the surgeon re-gloved and gowned.

Clean the external genitalia carefully with sterile saline and towel the area. Place a receiver between the abducted thighs. A No. 14 or

16 Foley catheter is the optimum choice; its retaining balloon can be tested by inflating with air. Note: if there is obstruction, try a smaller gauge (10–12 FG) or a firmer, curved Coudé catheter.

With males the penis is held vertically in sterile gauze. Sterile lubricating gel with lignocaine is instilled into the urethra. After giving the lignocaine a minute to work the catheter is then passed vertically downwards to the lower border of the pubic symphysis. With continued pressure on the catheter the penis is rotated downwards (caudally) so that the catheter may traverse the angle at the penoscrotal junction in the bladder. In cases of prostatic enlargement or stricture this may be difficult and will require expert help.

With females it is important to part the vaginal labia to reveal the external urethral orifice within the vestibule. The inexperienced attack the base of the clitoris, which is above the urethral orifice, with the catheter tip.

Once the catheter is in the bladder, urine will pass into the receiver. Gentle aspiration may be required initially to clear obstructing gel from the tip of the catheter. Push the catheter in maximally and fill the balloon with 10 ml sterile water (always check the balloon volume first); a gentle pull should indicate its retention. Attach the catheter to a collection bag to complete a closed drainage system; monitor urinary outflow, which should exceed 30 ml/h. Remember to change the bag every 24 hours if it is retained. Remove the catheter as soon as possible.

7. *Deep Vein Thrombosis*

This is a rare event in orthognathic patients, usually occurring unexpectedly in young women. As a precaution, all women should cease taking oestrogen containing contraceptive pills 4 weeks prior to surgery. If this has been overlooked, subcutaneous low molecular weight heparin prophylaxis should be considered, i.e. Dalteparin Sodium 5000 units preoperatively followed by a daily injection for 5–7 days. Both high and low risk patients benefit from elasticated thromboembolic-deterrent stockings being worn during the operation. Any complaint of postoperative calf tenderness must be taken seriously, especially when there is an increase in circumferential measurement and/or local erythema. Lower limb Doppler ultrasonography should be carried out and if this is positive (or not possible) the patient is anticoagulated to prevent extension of the thrombus and embolism.

An oral anticoagulant such as warfarin should also be started at 10 mg/day for the first 3 days, or as guided by your local anticoagulation clinic. A baseline prothrombin time is recommended prior to anticoagulation if any liver disease is suspected. Subsequent prothrombin times (INR) should be 2–2.5 times normal and taken on the second and third days of treatment and then weekly to confirm a stable ratio. Follow up in the anticoagulation clinic should be organised prior to discharge from hospital. The usual maintenance dose of 3–9 mg is taken at the same time each day for 3–6 months. Novel Oral Anticoagulant drugs (NOACs) are now available such as Rivaroxaban which is a direct inhibitor of activated factor X (factor Xa) and with daily dosing does not require monitoring of the INR.

8. *Fixation Problems*

These are infinitely varied but fortunately become uncommon with experience.

i) Infection may occur around screws and plates. Miniature plates are an essential part of the osteotomy and surprisingly in the maxilla rarely get infected. If drainage and a course of antibiotics do not suppress the infection, the plate and screws have to be removed. Similarly, uninfected bone plates may become palpable subcutaneously or submucosally and also require removal.
ii) Incorrectly placed screws and plates may displace the bony parts. This occurs more commonly in the third molar area with

the sagittal split operation, but is also with Le Fort I procedures where maxillary displacement can distort the nasal septum. Less commonly plates break. Whenever displacement or loss of control takes place, the patient should be taken back to theatre for correction. Pious hopes that the problem will go away or will be correctable by postsurgical orthodontics always prove to be futile.

iii) The use of screws or buccal plates for rigid fixation of the mandible can create occlusal discrepancies if it is not appreciated that the osteotomy is carried out with the patient anaesthetised and supine. If the condyle is pushed to the back of the fossa when temporary intermaxillary fixation is put on to facilitate the insertion of the bicortical screws or buccal plate, on its release, with the patient conscious and upright, the condyles will tend to recoil downwards and forwards. This is favourable for the Class 2 Division I mandibular advancement but gives a postoperative prognathous malocclusion with the Class 3 set-back. To avoid these artefacts (a) the model surgery should be based on a conscious supine centric relation squash bite and (b) the ascending ramus proximal fragment should be displaced backwards for Class 2 advancements but pulled forwards prior to fixation with the Class 3 mandibular setback.

Such problems were less likely to happen with a loose interosseous wire loop at the osteotomy site and prolonged intermaxillary fixation for 6 weeks. This enabled the ascending ramus proximal fragment to achieve an optimum condyle-meniscus-fossa relationship by functional adjustment brought about by swallowing and speech.

iv) Disturbed muscular proprioception and intracapsular oedema may also give a transient deranged postoperative occlusion when using rigid fixation. In these cases, light elastics for 7 days will help to restore the occlusion to the planned relationship. The final occlussal wafer is often left *in situ* even where there is no occlussal problem. This is very uncomfortable for the patient and there is no evidence that it helps. However, if after this elastic "proprioceptive regimen" there still appears to be marked displacement and malocclusion — re-operate.

9. *Relapse*

Relapse is any postoperative change in the planned or achieved dental or skeletal relationships. Most arise from inadequate planning or inappropriate surgical technique. The latter may be roughly divided into two overlapping groups: those arising from (1) operative structural causes and (2) postoperative functional causes.

a) *Operative Structural Causes of Relapse*

Inadequate bone, cartilage or periosteal separation. Osteotomy cuts and soft tissue dissection must provide absolute freedom of movement of the parts and allow effortless repositioning. Tight bone plates will not correct reluctant anatomical components but will cause some malalignment elsewhere. Common sites are as follows.

i) Inadequate separation of the proximal mandibular bone and the medial pterygoid muscle from the buccal plate when doing a sagittal split. A finger firmly inserted to the depth of the split is used to remove the restraining periosteum and muscle fibres, which hold the two cortices together at the lower border.
ii) Inadequate bone removal from the posterior wall of the antrum or separation of the pterygoid plates in a Le Fort I impaction can also create problems.
iii) The untrimmed nasal septum will create a buckling effect and either displace the maxilla and disturb the occlusion, or displace the nose and produce an asymmetric tip deformity, and obstruct the airway. Late correction will require a rhinoplasty.
iv) Where a mandibular osteotomy has been done with the pious hope of eradicating temporomandibular joint pain in a patient

with a meniscus displacement, the osteotomy may not only give rise to more pain initially but may create intracapsular adhesions and limited opening postoperatively.

v) Occasionally lower lip sag may follow a bone graft procedure to increase the chin depth by augmentation, or a mandibular forward movement with a genioplasty. It is difficult to be sure whether it is due to inadequate freeing of the periosteal pouch and overlying soft tissues, or failure to re-attach the mentalis high enough on the anterior mandibular surface, or abnormal muscle activity. The last cause would be inadequate orbicularis tone or decreased mentalis elevated activity.

   The lip sag should be avoided by the creation of a large loose periosteal pouch to accommodate the enlarged chin, carefully suturing the divided mentalis to the deep muscle fibres on the alveolar surface, and the application of a firm pressure dressing overlying the labiomantal groove. Once formed it can be eliminated in some cases by vigorous exercising of the lower lip, i.e. the lip is actively stretched upwards over the incisor edges. If this fails, it will be necessary to deglove and reposition the soft tissues upwards using heavy polyglycollate (Vicryl) sutures to elevate the soft tissues of the chin.

vi) Tooth damage may occur with the bone cuts of segmental osteotomies, either apically or laterally. Avoid the former by marking the estimated apical site with a shallow bur hole prior to the section. Lateral root damage arises when burs are used interdentally. Only the buccal and lingual (palatal) bone should be cut with a bur and the actual division should be made with a fine osteotome or saw.

Although root damage often appears to be self-limiting and most teeth survive, occasionally the exposed dentine undergoes progressive resorption. An attempt may be made to preserve the tooth by root canal therapy with calcium hydroxide. However, should root loss progress, extraction and an implant or bridge will be required to salvage the situation.

Segmental cuts in the older patient with incipient periodontal disease may also create intractable bony pockets unless anticipated. The cuts must be done carefully with a fine osteotome after prior periodontal therapy followed by postoperative oral hygiene instruction.

b) *Postoperative Functional Causes of Relapse*

i) The most notorious is the recurrent anterior open bite following attempted correction with a mandibular osteotomy. This will occur in patients with a high mandibular-maxillary plane angle where the low posterior facial height reflects a short pterygo-masseteric sling. This is stretched as the mandible is rotated around the fulcrum created by the occluding molar crowns when the anterior teeth are brought into occlusion to close the gap. The inelastic ligaments and the return of postoperative muscular tone may even produce a relapse despite internal fixation. This is avoided by a posterior maxillary impaction equivalent to the anterior open bite to be corrected.

ii) Postoperative tooth movement can be favourable, especially with the spontaneous or assisted closure of lateral open bites. However, unfavourable tooth movements may arise.

- Repositioned lower incisors are proclined by a large or "anteriorly postured" tongue.
- Upper incisors are proclined by the lower lip after a maxillary segmental pushback procedures is carried out on a marked Class II, Division 1 patient without a mandibular forward correction to an edge to edge relationship.
- Continued eruption (occlusal drift) of the lower incisors will follow an anterior segmental setdown unless they are placed in a stabilising contact with the cingula or incisive edges of the opposing teeth.

- Expansion of the maxillary premolar and molar segments may tilt those teeth buccally. Subsequent palatal drift will produce intercuspal contact on closure with the creation of an anterior open bite. Major expansion of the palate should be done surgically with a midline osteotomy to avoid dental relapse.
- Idiopathic periapical and internal resorption may occur in teeth adjacent to an osteotomy cut, even without untoward bur contact. The cause is unknown but may be due to a vascular response to the adjacent surgery.
- Orthodontic depression of lower incisors in adults, before surgery, may cause proclination with alveolar dehiscence and gingival recession. Furthermore, the proclined incisors may then upright spontaneously once fixation is removed.

If, after a considerable input of time and energy if both surgeon and patient, are agreed something has gone seriously wrong with the operative correction — start again!

c) *Nerve Damage*

i) It is important to warn the patient preoperatively of impaired sensation that may arise in the mental or mylohyoid nerve distribution of the lower lip and chin following a sagittal split or anterior segmental operation, and in the infraorbital area following a maxillary osteotomy. The former usually recovers in 2–6 months, although some patients have a permanent deficit, which is less noticeable if the operation is otherwise successful.

   When the inferior dental nerve is exposed and torn during the sagittal split, it may be possible to hold the separated ends together with a 6/0 Prolene suture prior to fixation.

ii) Facial nerve damage with weakness can be localised following external incisions for a subsigmoid (subcondylar) osteotomy but will involve a wider distribution of the facial nerve if it is damaged near its main trunk. This can occur with a sagittal split pushback or an intraoral subsigmoid (subcondylar) operation. The cause is probably traumatic instrumentation. They prognosis is usually very good, with gradual recovery over 6–8 weeks.

iii) The lingual nerve is rarely damaged during an osteotomy. However, persistent impaired lingual sensation after 6 weeks requires open exploration and repair. This is most easily done by removing the overlying sublingual salivary gland.

iv) A rare disturbance is nasal vasomotor hyperfunction, which may occur after a Le Fort I osteotomy. The patient develops continuous rhinorrhoea, which simulates a cerebrospinal fluid leak. The cause is uncertain and may be either loss of sympathetic vasomotor control or damage to the sphenopalatine ganglion with enhanced stimulation. There is no satisfactory treatment.

10. *Emotional and Psychiatric Problems — see also the Psychopathology of Facial Deformity; Chapter 16.*

These vary from postoperative depression, often manifested as a refusal to take food or medication by mouth, to more dramatic states. Many patients would be spared a reactionary depressive state if they had been carefully warned of postoperative problems on admission. Good nursing care and attentive surgical staff are the treatment of choice.

Agitation can arise both from intolerance of intermaxillary fixation (which is now uncommon) or nasal airway obstruction. Both can now be avoided. However, not only is it essential to clear the nose by inhalations and suction, but always seek an underlying structural obstruction, such as a displaced nasal septum.

Unanticipated anxiety of an alien environment, especially the intensive care unit, may precipitate postoperative psychotic behaviour. This can be controlled by intravenous antipsychotic drugs such as haloperidol, which can later be given orally.

Emotionally unstable individuals, especially those who have a history of body dysmorphic disorder, may also become aggressive and difficult to control. Again, an antipsychotic drug regimen is essential, together with preoperative and postoperative psychiatric advice. Unfortunately some patients get legal aid to express their illogical complaints through a solicitor. It is wise to report the problem to risk management in an NHS hospital who can if necessary provide legal support. With private patients the surgeon will need to seek the advice of their medical defence society.

Dissatisfaction can be avoided by repeated preoperative discussion about the operative procedure, the immediate and late complications and, most important of all, the patient's aesthetic expectations. All these should be recorded.

Finally an explanatory handout of the operation covering common complications is essential.

Chapter 16

The Psychosocial Aspects of Facial Deformity

Susan J. Cunningham

Introduction

The face has the principal receptors for sight, sound, taste and smell, Overt sexual significance, and the means of expressing non-verbal emotion. Facial attractiveness is one of our most important social characteristics and the psychopathology of facial deformity is a spectrum which extends from common emotional problems in the normal to manifestations of personality disorders, neurosis, depression and psychosis.

1. Social Aspects of Facial Deformity

Perceptions of facial attractiveness vary from person to person and also amongst different racial groups. However it appears that those who display an attractive face are perceived as being more friendly, sensitive and successful than those who are unattractive. This unfair social advantage does not take into account compensatory factors such as intellect, personality and motivation. Certain facial stereotypes are inappropriately portrayed as being associated with particular characteristics, for example a Class III malocclusion may be perceived as aggressive or a marked Class II as weak or less intelligent. Other facial features, for example bat ears or large noses, are a source of teasing in childhood, creating a hypersensitive awareness, which undermines self-confidence. There is also evidence that less attractive individuals are discriminated against in a wide range of situations from early life through to adulthood.

We now appreciate that dentofacial deformity may be a severe handicap in many situations. This supports the view that many individuals who request orthognathic surgery have suffered the effects of discrimination or imagine discrimination in order to make them seek treatment which has inherent discomfort and risks. Therefore a psychological assessment of all orthognathic patients is a vital part of the planning procedure. It is vital to identify problems before inappropriate planning decisions have been made and ideally a liaison psychiatrist or clinical psychologist would undertake this role. However where constraints are placed on the provision of an optimum service, the orthodontist or surgeon must be responsible for the initial screening and refer those patients of particular concern.

2. The Psychological Assessment

The social acceptance of aesthetic orthognathic surgery has increased the demand for treatment. Hence the treatment plan should be based not only on aesthetics and function, but also on the patient's perception of what they wish to obtain from treatment. Patients perceive their facial appearance and in particular their profile, differently from clinicians. This emphasises the need for good communication from the outset when planning surgery. This process is critical and may take several visits to identify the patients' subjective problems and the changes they are seeking. The clinician must then decide whether these expectations can be met. The following approach is essential to avoid overlooking problem areas and should be done on a one-to-one basis and not in a large multidisciplinary clinic, where patients are reluctant to disclose personal details. A number of patients will require referral to a liaison psychiatrist or clinical psychologist for a more thorough assessment before proceeding further.

Patients should be considered for referral prior to agreeing to undertake treatment where there is:

i. intuitive concern for motivation
ii. a history of previous cosmetic surgery
iii. minimal facial deformity or no evident problem
iv. expectations which exceed surgical feasibility
v. an obsessional concern for certain features.

There are a number of key questions which may necessitate further psychological assessment:

- *What is the main complaint?*
  This establishes how the patient perceives their problem. Accuracy is not important, for example the patient may feel they have a prognathic mandible when actually they have a retrognathic maxilla. However, they should be able to recognise a problem. Those who offer vague non-specific complaints such as "I don't like my face" tend to make poor surgical patients compared with those who are clear about their complaint — "I think my chin sticks out and is not symmetrical".

- *What does the patient expect from treatment?*
  This is important and the way this question is phrased can influence the response. It is helpful to ask "How do you think this treatment will affect your life?" Those patients who want to look better and feel more self-confident are classified as expecting primary gain from treatment and tend to be good

surgical patients. Patients who require psychological assessment include those who:

(i) are concerned with secondary gain such as promotion, a better job or new partner
(ii) do not have any idea what they expect from treatment
(iii) are not able to verbalise their answers to these questions.

- *How long has he/she been concerned about their face and why seek treatment now?*

  Patients should always be asked how long they have had these concerns. Those who have become concerned only recently should be assessed by a psychologist/psychiatrist as their worries may have been triggered by a recent adverse life event such as redundancy, divorce, or bereavement. It is then appropriate to delay treatment until the patient has reached a more stable state before any intervention.

- *How does their dentofacial deformity interfere with their life?*
  A patient who can function at work, socialise with friends and has an acceptable body image despite the facial deformity is more likely to be satisfied following treatment. Those who have become reclusive as a feature of their concerns must be investigated further, especially where the discrepancy clearly does not justify this abnormal behaviour pattern.

- *What is the main source of motivation?*
  The internally motivated patient usually has long standing feelings about their appearance, which impair their enjoyment of life, whereas the externally motivated patient may be seeking treatment to please someone else such as a parent, partner or employer. Externally motivated patients may require a change in their environment rather than surgery. They require careful psychological assessment and counselling prior to consideration for

treatment. Patients who are internally motivated usually make better patients for orthognathic intervention.

- *Does the patient have family support?*
  This important issue is frequently overlooked. Patients should not be refused treatment if they have little family or social support. However, in this situation, the orthognathic team may need to offer more support than usual, particularly in the immediate pre- and postoperative periods when patients are at their most vulnerable. This is where a liaison orthognathic nurse or social worker can play an extremely important role.

- *Has the patient previously sought treatment elsewhere?*
  Patients who embark upon numerous consultations, "doctor shopping" often do so because they are dissatisfied with a previous rejection or a treatment plan which does not meet their unrealistic expectations. Others may already have undergone previous dentofacial operations or cosmetic procedures. Such a history should be investigated fully, prior to agreeing to further intervention (see the section on Body Dysmorphic Disorder, BDD).

- *Has the patient received any medical treatment that may be of importance?*
  Has the patient undergone any previous psychiatric treatment? The diagnosis of psychiatric disorders is difficult for those with little or no training but a medication history can be an invaluable clue. Some clinicians find it useful to utilise screening questionnaires such as the Hospital Anxiety and Depression (HAD) scale or the Orthognathic Quality of Life Questionnaire, although such questionnaires are relatively limited in what they can tell you about the patient. The general medical history may include conditions that make orthognathic treatment inappropriate or impossible, such as haemophilia, severe thallasaemia, acromegaly or bone dysplasias.

If any of these questions raise doubts treatment must be delayed pending specialist assessment, followedby an interdisciplinary case conference. This delay will also help determine how motivated the patient is to proceed with surgery.

3. Satisfaction and Dissatisfaction with Treatment

The majority of patients are satisfied with the outcome of orthognathic surgery even where there are minor discrepancies in the result. Careful management appears to be the key factor. Patients who experience less pain and numbness than expected, tend to be more satisfied and enjoy higher self-esteem. This reinforces the need to inform patients of all possible problems they may encounter and give strong personal support if complications arise.

Many problems are due to poor clinician/patient communication, rather than deficient technical skills or poor surgical outcome. Occasionally there is no obvious justification and the adverse reaction is the result of a psychiatric problem triggered by the surgery. This may include litigation, obsessional behaviour, seeking additional surgical procedures, depression, frank psychosis and physical assault of the surgeon or staff.

Most forms of post-surgical dissatisfaction can be avoided by careful prior assessment and realistic explanations of the procedure in terms of pain, swelling, difficulties eating or speaking, and the amount of time which will be required away from work or college. It is now mandatory to include, in the process of informed consent, the possibility of all complications, which may be overlooked. Not only should the information be given verbally but also reinforced with detailed information leaflets or other aids as most patients remember only a small or selective part of what they are told in a clinic, especially when nervous. The nursing staff should also be trained to inform and counsel all orthognathic patients pre- and post-operatively, and advice must be provided for the immediate family. (*See the Eastman Consent Process at the end.*)

It is important that the surgeon is vigilant in the postoperative phase and does not delegate aftercare to inexperienced junior staff. Many clinicians take postoperative morbidity for granted and ignore the psychological upheaval arising from a long anticipated change. Patients may also experience strong negative feelings when facing postoperative orthodontic treatment which should be kept to a minimum. If overt postoperative depression is diagnosed it must be treated medically rather by ineffectual reassurance. A course of anti-depressants and psychiatric care will produce a marked improvement. Frank psychosis is extremely rare but requires immediate attention from a psychiatrist.

Subjective Disorders of Appearance

Body Dysmorphic Disorder (*BDD*)

Body dysmorphic disorder describes the patient with a persistent subjective feeling of ugliness or a physical defect which is minor or not obvious. This condition was formerly known as dysmorphophobia but is now termed Body Dysmorphic Disorder (BDD) and can involve any part of the body. The aetiology is obscure, although the prevalence is 4 times higher in first-degree relatives of BDD patients and is related to other disorders concerned with body image such as the eating disorders anorexia and bulimia. In order to make this diagnosis, the following criteria must be fulfilled:

- There is a preoccupation with a defect in the appearance. The defect is either imagined, or if a minor defect, the individual's concern is inappropriately excessive.
- This preoccupation causes significant distress to the patient and dominates all aspects of their life. Suicidal ideation is common and suicidal attempts have been identified in a significant percentage of patients.

Presenting Features

The area of concern may remain the same over a long period or change with time. It frequently affects the face, therefore orthodontists maxillofacial, ear nose and throat and plastic surgeons should be fully aware of the presenting features.

It usually begins during adolescence although there is often a delay in seeking treatment hence symptoms persist over a number of years. Those suffering from BDD may spend hours thinking about their "defect", studying it in the mirror or attempting to camouflage the area. A high proportion of patients avoid social relations and may become housebound and suffer impairment of their academic or work performance. BDD patients require early identification and careful assessment at their initial appointment. It is important not to risk making matters worse by drawing the patient's attention to other potential "defects". Referral letters may be misleading if the practitioner has uncritically accepted the patient's complaint. However, a history of numerous referrals, with or without intervention, is pathognomonic of the condition. Some patients will avoid disclosing visits to other clinicians or will demand constant reassurance about the supposed defect and attend appointments with photographs or diagrams to show idealistic faces that they wish to emulate. Such patients have frequently researched the management of facial disfigurement on the internet, use medical terminology and "lead" the initial assessment so that the unwary clinician feels forced into undertaking treatment. It is vital that clinicians are aware of the inevitable poor outcome in carrying out unnecessary treatment for such persuasive patients.

The Body Dysmorphic Disorder Examination (BDDE) and the Body Dysmorphic Disorder Modification of the Yale-Brown Obsessive Compulsive Scale (BDD-YBOCS) may prove useful where a tentative diagnosis has been made. However the analysis and management from this point, requires a psychiatrist familiar with the condition.

Treatment Options

Surgery and BDD

BDD patients may constantly pursue surgical treatment for their "problem" and consult numerous surgeons in the hope of finding someone who is willing to operate on them. However, surgery rarely improves the situation and should only be considered when there is a detectable and remediable defect and the patient complies with psychiatric care. Unfortunately inappropriate surgery makes the condition worse with the patient frequently finding a new problem. The unsuspecting clinician may then be faced with an extremely distressed and dissatisfied patient.

Medication management

Medical management is empirical although selective serotonin re-uptake inhibitors are currently the first line pharmacological treatment option. However, the lack of controlled clinical trials has made the assessment of outcome uncertain.

Counselling and psychological therapy

A number of different psychological treatment options are available including cognitive behavioural therapy and systematic desensitisation. BDD symptoms seem to be significantly reduced in subjects who have undergone this form of therapy and studies have shown that the disorder appears to have been eliminated in up to 82% of cases immediately post-treatment and 77% at follow-up.

Racial/Ethnic Dysphoria

Dentofacial aesthetic norms vary between racial groups and when planning surgical changes consideration should be given as to whether they are racially appropriate. Some non-Caucasian patients,

(a) (b)

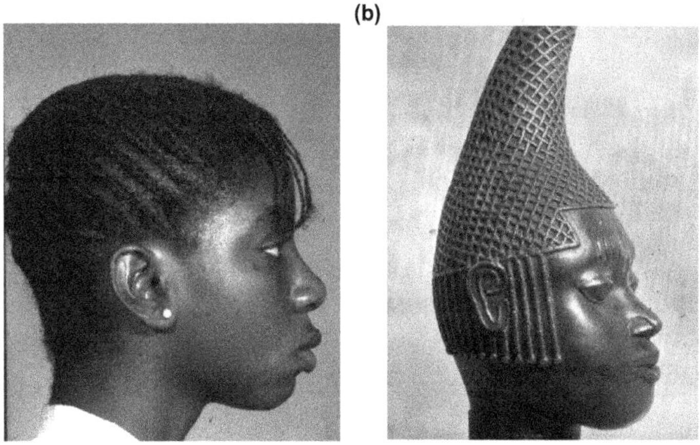

Figure 16.1 (**a**) and (**b**) British girl of Nigerian origin who wanted to look like her European school friends, compared with the ideal beauty of the Benin bronze.

influenced by popular Caucasian features, may demand changes which are either unsuitable or unattainable. An example of this would be an African girl seeking a European profile (Figure 16.1a and 16.1b). Her bimaxillary protrusion reproduces exactly the natural beauty of her tribal origin, seen in the classic sculpture of a Benin bronze. This could be altered with upper and lower segmental surgery but might not produce the aesthetic satisfaction this adolescent patient anticipated. She responded well to orthodontics and counselling. The merits of surgical change in such cases must be carefully discussed between patient, orthodontist, surgeon and psychologist.

Gender Dysphoria or Gender Reassignment Surgery

The need for gender reassignment was considered an uncommon BDD variant in which the patient wishes to change gender. However this is now recognised as a medically necessity for many whose lives are profoundly influenced by this complex bio-psycholo-endocrine disorder where the individual seeks to acquire the sexual appearance and function of their self-identified gender.

Treatment for transgender patients includes endocrine manipulation, reconstructive surgery to the face, breasts and genitalia and specialised psychological support, especially as these patients experience serious mental distress and social hostility. Forty percent attempt suicide if untreated.

The demand for a less prominent mandible or more prominent malar bones facial epilation (depilation) in an otherwise satisfactory face can be difficult to understand unless seen as part of this overall problem. Measures of successful management are probably unreliable and persistent regret can occur after sex reassignment surgery. This may be due to unresolved gender dysphoria, described as a fluctuating sense of identity, which may even lead to suicide.

Conclusions

Patients who seek orthognathic surgery for dentofacial deformity may harbour emotional concerns and all require careful psychological assessment, sound informative discussion and comprehensive information. This is summarised below.

It is essential to detect those with or without facial deformity who have latent psychopathology which requires specialist treatment. Also important is that some clinicians are unaware that the Bolam principle no longer exists to protect those who claim to be no more negligent than their colleagues.

The Eastman Consent Process*

This is designed to provide all potential orthognathic surgery patients with the information as to the risks and benefits of all aspects of the treatment that a large body of patients undergoing such treatment would expect to be given.

---

* Based on the decision in Montgomery vs. Lanarkshire Health Board by the UK Supreme Court on the 11 March 2015 by courtesy of Nigel Hunt.

It is achieved in a variety of ways which include:

i. Patients attend a group information clinic where 5 or 6 patients together with their parents, or partners or close relatives are given a presentation by an orthodontist, a surgeon, liaison psychiatrist and hygienist as well as meeting and questioning a patient who has been through the experience.
ii. They also receive a copy of a DVD produced by the British Orthodontic Society as well as hard copy patient information leaflets.
iii. The specific risks and benefits expected in each of their particular cases are then reiterated subsequently at an individual meeting with the multidisciplinary team.
iv. See also the "The Information Sheet for Patients Undergoing Orthognathic Surgery".

Chapter 17

Non Surgical Facial Aesthetics — Part 1 Clinical Anatomy and the Aging Face

Rui Ming Ho and Fooi Chin Ng

Introduction

The Greek word *aisthētikós* — aesthetics, is used to describe the principles and philosophy that define the concept of beauty. Non Surgical Facial Aesthetics (NSFA), is the means of achieving this without surgical intervention. However this practice should be Non Surgical Facial Cosmetics as the process of creating beauty is cosmesis, *kosmētikos*.

As the clinical assessment of beauty is a subjective judgement by the patient and clinician, satisfactory NSFA success can only be realized if both share achievable aims.

The demand for cosmetic procedures to improve facial aesthetics are many and varied. The available facial cosmetic procedures include restorative dentistry, orthodontics, orthognathic surgery and facial-plastic surgery. These invasive procedures aim to improve facial form and function and their criteria of need are mostly dento-skeletal and the means of correction are dealt with in earlier chapters.

NSFA is applicable to a wide range of problems but the most common clinical problem which may benefit from NSFA is the "aging face" although an increasing number of adolescents and younger adults seek change driven by subjective dissatisfaction. Where this need is obsessional and inappropriate the condition is identified as the body dysmorphic disorder in which the dissatisfaction is obsessional and may persist despite repeated interventions. This is discussed in Chapter 16.

Hence assessment and treatment must be based on correctable disorders of the facial drape involving the skin, muscles and connective tissue.

The Structure of the Skin

The skin is the largest organ in the body whose components are the epidermis, dermis and its associated connective tissues.

The main cell in the epidermis is the keratinocyte which forms a barrier to retain moisture and resist insult from the external environment. Other cells include, melanocytes Langerhans cells and Merkel cells.

Melanocytes produce the pigment melanin. The number of melanocytes does not differ significantly between individuals and their race. It is the type of melanin and the size of the melanosome that causes variation in the skin type and colour. The melanosome, an organelle in the melanocyte, synthesises the melanin which gives the skin colour and photo-protection.

Langerhans cells are antigen-presenting immune cells of the skin and mucosa. They are present mainly in the stratum spinosum. They provide protection against infection by transporting antigenic materials to the lymph nodes. Merkel cells are mechanical sensory cells. They are involved in "touch" and neuro-endocrine functions.

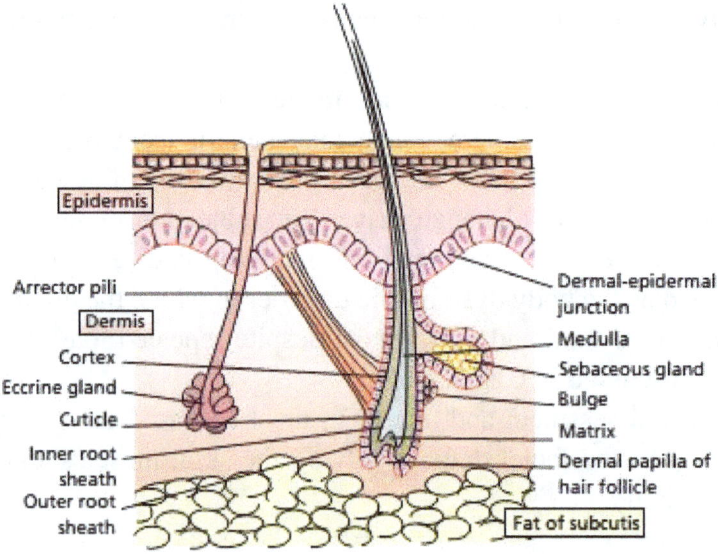

Figure 17.1 The structure of the skin.
Source: Burns T *et al. Rook's Textbook of Dermatology, 4 Volume Set, 8th Ed.*, Wiley (2013).

The bulk of the dermis is collagen, elastic fibres and hyaluronic acid, which are produced by fibroblasts and smooth muscle cells. Collagen provides the tensile strength of the dermis and is vital for the cutaneous scaffold. The two main types of collagen are collagen type I and type III, which coexist within the same fibril and make up more than 80% of the collagen in the dermis. The elastic tissue is bundles of elastin proteins, and gives the skin its elasticity. With age this elastic function is lost which contributes to a sagging skin.

Hyaluronic acid (hyaluronan) is a large glycosaminoglycan molecule. It has many functions including a lubricating role in muscular connective tissues that enhances the invaluable sliding function between adjacent tissue layers. Without this sliding function, there will be impedance and stiffness in muscular and connective tissue movement that may affect facial expression. It is also vital to maintain the moisture of the skin due to its ability to bind to water molecules.

The Aging Process and the Skin

Cutaneous aging is the result of two biological processes, the intrinsic (genetic) and extrinsic due to solaraging, smoking and atmospheric pollution. Both processes affect the epidermis and the underlying dermis. When skin is exposed to excessive ultra violet B rays (UVB), it causes sunburn and photochemical damage of DNA, with inflammation, premature aging, premalignant and malignant changes. The damaged dermis cells produce less hyaluronan and its accumulated degradation products initiate inflammation. Removal of these molecules is important for the resolution of the repair process.

The combined effects of degenerative changes vary considerably with the individual. Some will not respond to NSFA therapy and intervention may do more harm than good, whilst many older faces continue to retain their aesthetic quality despite the passing years. In general, aging will lead to the following skin changes:

- thinning of the skin,
- loss of hydration producing a dry skin,
- skin laxity,
- rhytides (wrinkle) formation,
- uneven skin tone or marked dyspigmentation,
- fat pad migration and localised obesity.

Racial Aging Differences

The most obvious difference between individuals of different races is that of skin colour and type. Darker skin types with an increased melanin content are better protected against the harmful effects of ultraviolet (UV) radiation and are not as susceptible to photo-aging as lighter skin.

Dyspigmentation and uneven skin tone are more common with darker skin types. Vitiligo is a distinctive patchy total loss of

Table 17.1 Summary of skin aging effects.

Component	Effect from aging	Consequence
Keratinocytes (Epidermis)	Decreased production renders the skin barrier less able to retain moisture and resist external damage	Dry skin
Melanocytes (Epidermis)	Decrease number of active melanocytes	Dyspigmentation and uneven skin tone
Collagen (Dermis)	Breakdown of collagen with decreased synthesis	Skin laxity and wrinkle formation
Elastic tissue (Dermis)	Degradation and decreased synthesis	Skin laxity and wrinkle formation

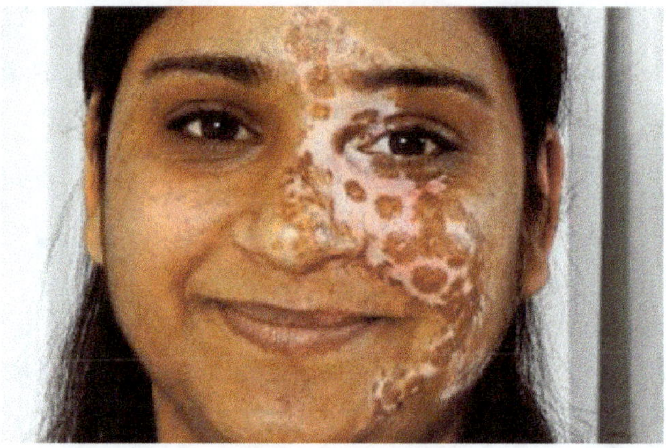

Figure 17.2 Segmental vitiligo (NHS choices).

pigmentation which is not age related and is probably an autoimmune condition currently camouflaged with cosmetics.

Beside the difference in melanin, the dermis in Caucasian skin is generally thinner and less compact as compared to Asian and

Table 17.2 Summary of racial aging differences.

Caucasians	Asians	Africans
Earlier onset of wrinkle formation and sagging as compared to darker ethnic skin types. Sagging due to skin laxity.	Dyspigmentation more prevalent than Caucasian.	Dyspigmentation more prevalent compared to Caucasian counterparts.
More susceptible to UVB photoaging.	Less susceptible to photoaging compared to Caucasian counterparts.	Less susceptible to photoaging as compared to Caucasian and Asian counterparts. Has a natural sun protective factor of approximately 13.
		Mid face aging is more prominent compared to the upper face. Brow ptosis is not as significant as the Caucasian counterpart. Sagging due more to heaviness of the tissues than skin laxity.

Black skin which makes it more susceptible to rhytid formation at an earlier age.

Facial Aging and the Integument (Figures 17.3 and 17.4)

The youthful face is maintained by a network of facial ligaments especially the zygomatic, masseteric and mandibular ligaments that arise from the deep fascia to penetrate the overlying envelope of the Superficial Muscular Aponeurotic System (SMAS) and

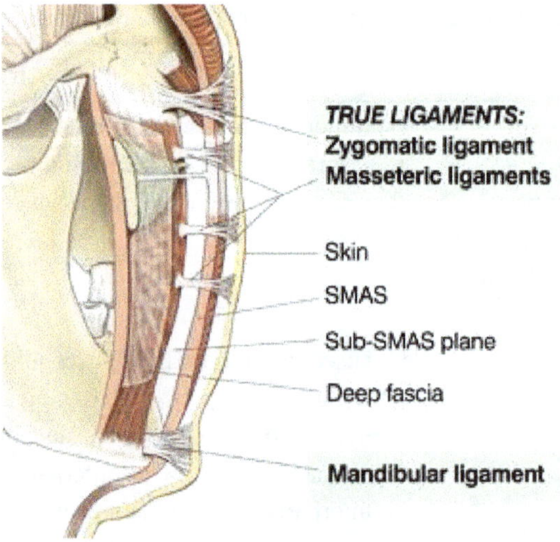

Figure 17.3 The layers of the facial integument (the tissues of the skin), whic are penetrated by the facial ligaments from the deep fascia through the SMAS to the subcutaneous layer.

gain attachment to the subcutaneous layer to create a scaffold which retains the contour of the compartmental fat pads. Thus the SMAS is a flat layer of tendinous connective tissue which envelopes the muscles of facial expression and extends upwards from the fascia over the pectoralis major and deltoid to the superficial temporalis fascia. It is the degeneration of the compartmental septa, ligaments and the muscles of facial expression together with gravity that permit the migration of fat in the plane between the superficial and deep fascia. This is the dominant aging feature and the most conspicuous results are the malar fat pad which migrates downwards and forward from beneath the malar bone to accentuate the naso-labial crease and the descent of the buccal and submental fat to the lower border of the mandible.

There is also the loss of skeletal support due to dental attrition and tooth loss, and osteoporotic jaw remodelling which contribute

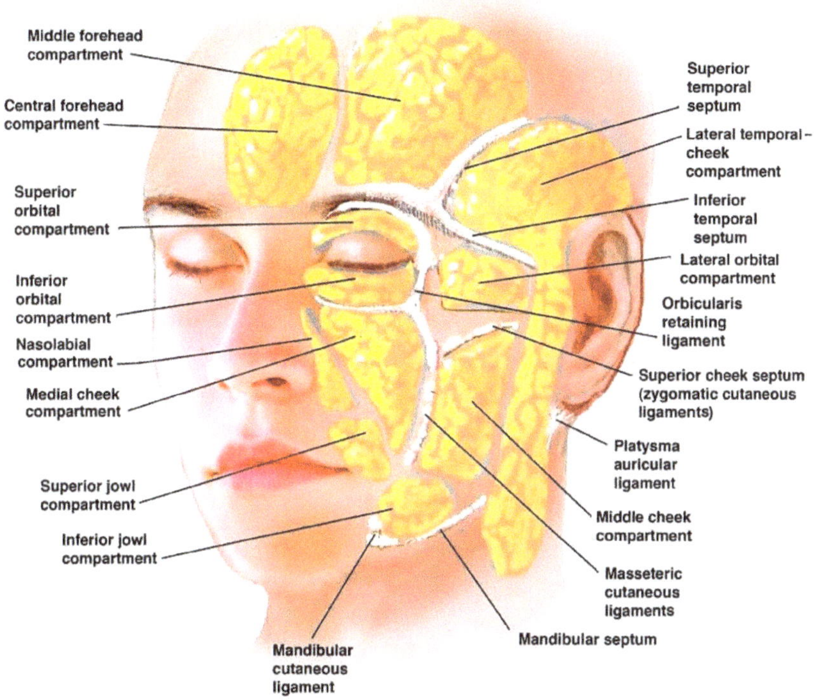

Figure 17.4 This illustrates the complex of superficial fat compartments divided by the zygomatic, masseteric and mandibular septa and ligaments. These connective tissue compartments and their fat content provide the contours of the youthful face which is animated by the muscles of facial expression which are attached to the overlying elastic dermis.

Source: Alghoul M, Codner MA, Retaining ligaments of the face: review of anatomy and clinical applications, *Aesthet. Surg. J.* **33**(6): 769–782 (2013).

to the aging facial contour and loss of facial volume. Unless masked by obesity the face becomes narrower and irregular with hollowing of the temporal, periorbital and buccal areas, and a scalloped mandibular jaw line. The lips also lose their cupid's bow fullness.

The Muscles of Facial Expression

The muscles of facial expression are unique in structure and function. They are situated within the SMAS and arise from the facial bones to be inserted into the superficial fascia and dermis of the skin. They are innervated by the facial cranial nerve VII and oculomotor nerve III(levator palpebrae superioris) which harmoniously activate contraction or relaxation to express both negative and positive facial emotional responses. The orchestration of these muscles can display emotions which vary from anger and grief to humour and happiness. A remarkable form of non-verbal communication (Figure 17.5).

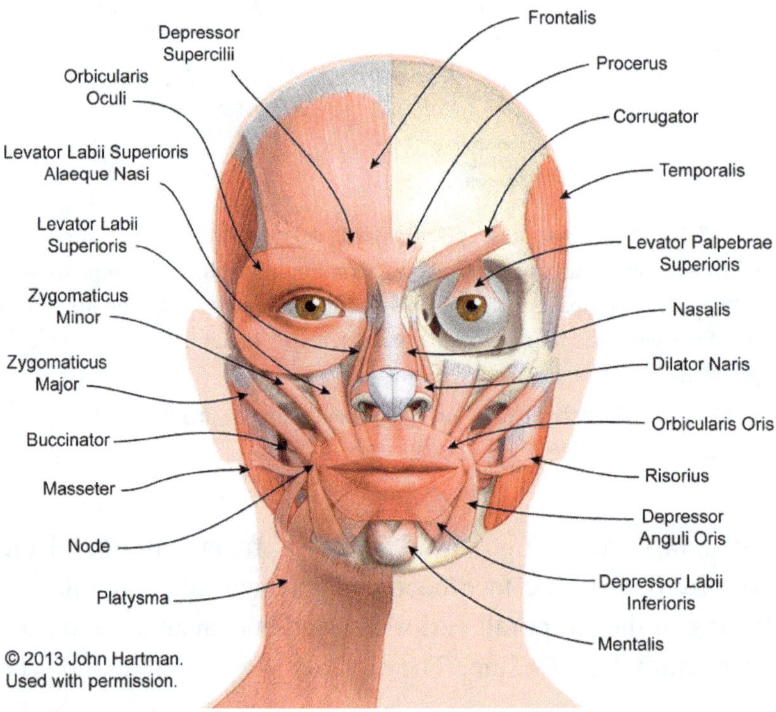

Figure 17.5 This diagram of the muscles of facial expression clarifies their structure and function as described below.

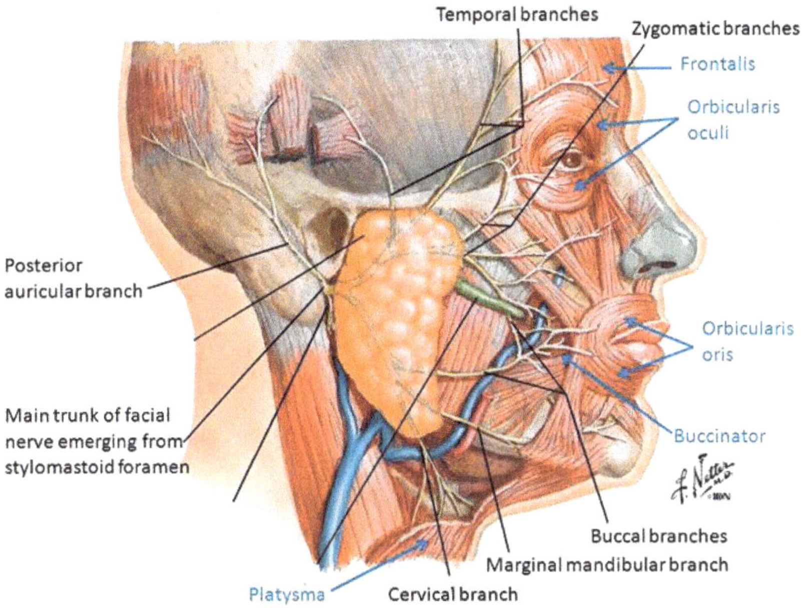

Figure 17.6 The muscles of facial expression are innervated by the facial nerve (VII) apart from the levator palpebrae superioris in the upper eyelid, which is innervated by the oculomotor nerve III (not shown).

Source: Netter FH, *Atlas of Human Anatomy*, *5th Ed.*, Saunders (2010).

The Origin and Function of the Muscles of Facial Expression (Figures 17.5 and 17.6)

(i) Frontalis

Origin: The skin over the brows. Insertion: The galea aponeurotica.

The occipito-frontalis is a broad musculo-fibrous layer overlying each side of the calvarium of the skull, from the occiput to the eyebrow. The occipitalis is connected to the frontalis, by a tendinous aponeurosis, the galea aponeurotica. The frontalis is the only elevator of the upper face and raises the eye brows and creates forehead wrinkles. In treating the frontalis muscle, the glabellar complex (the corrugators and procerus) are often treated together so as to balance the upward and downward traction forces.

(ii) Levator Labii Superioris Alaeque Nasi (LLSAN)
Origin: Frontal process of maxilla.
Insertion: Alar of nose and upper lip.
The levator labii superioris alaeque nasi elevates the upper lip and the nostrils.

(iii) Levator Labii Superioris
Origin: Infra-orbital margin of maxilla.
Insertion: Lateral half of the upper lip.
This muscle elevates the upper lip and contributes to the formation of the naso-labial fold on animation.

(iv) Risorius
Origin: Fascia of the masseter muscle.
Insertion: Corner of mouth.
The risorius pulls the corners of the mouth laterally and backwards. Injection of this muscle with BTX-A can cause an asymmetrical smile.

(v) Corrugator Supercilii
Origin: Deep to the orbicularis oculi muscle. It arises from the deep medial end of the superciliary arch of the orbital margin.
Insertion: Superficially into the skin laterally at the middle of the brow.
The corrugator pulls the eyebrows medially and inferiorly. It causes vertical wrinkles above the nose and around the medial eyebrow region.

(vi) Procerus
Origin: The nasal bones.
Insertion: Skin between the brows.
The procerus draws the eyebrows inferiorly and causes horizontal wrinkles over the bridge of the nose.

(vii) Orbicularis Oculi
Has an orbital component and palperbral, i.e. eyelid component.
Origin: The orbital part arises from the medial palpebral ligament, the adjacent the adjacent frontal process of the maxilla and nasal aspect of the frontal bone.

Insertion: It forms a continuous circular ring around the orbit and is inserted into lateral palpebral ligament.

The orbicularis oculi enables blinking, squinting and forceful closing of eyelid.

The central palpebral part closes the eyelids gently whilst the circumferential peripheral orbital part closes the eyelids forcefully. It is the lateral orbital part that contributes to Crow's Feet.

In some individuals, the inferior palpebral part of the orbicularis oculi is thick and is prominent especially on smiling and/or squinting the eyes. In such cases, BTX-A can be administered in this region to relax the muscle and make the eyes appear larger.

(viii) The levator palpebrae superioris

Origin: From the lesser wing of the sphenoid bone, above its optic foramen.

Insertion: Inserts under the skin of the upper eyelid, and its superior plate. The superior tarsal muscle, a smooth muscle, is attached to the levator palpebrae superioris, and inserts on the superior tarsal plate as well.

It broadens and decreases in thickness and becomes the levator aponeurosis.

Innervation: The oculomotor nerve.

(ix) Masseter

Origin: Zygomatic arch and maxillary process of zygomatic bone.

Insertion: Angle of mandible and lateral surface of the ramus of mandible.

The masseter is a powerful muscle of mastication and elevates the mandible during chewing. Masseteric idiopathic "hypertrophy" is a hyperplasia that creates a thick muscle producing a broad square face. BTX-A injected into this muscle will reduce the bulk and aesthetically enhance appearance.

(x) Mentalis

Origin: The mentalis originates from the anterior recess of the mandible below the incisors.

Insertion: Inserts into the skin overlying the chin in a V-like pattern. It protrudes the lower lip and causes wrinkling and a "cobbled-stone" appearance to the chin when contracted.

With BTX-A, an active mentalis can be relaxed to improve this "cobble-stone" wrinkling of the chin.

(xi) Orbicularis Oris

Origin: The maxilla and mandible in the midline.

Insertion: Is a continuous band of muscle around the mouth inserted into skin and the mucous membrane of the lips.

The orbicularis oris "purses" the lips and causes wrinkling around the lips. These wrinkles are sometimes referred to as "smoker's lines" due to repeated contraction of the orbicularis oris during smoking. Infiltrating this muscle with BTX-A can improve the appearance of these wrinkles around the lips.

(xii) Depressor Anguli Oris

Origin: The mandible below the canine, premolar and 1st molar.

Insertion: Inserted into the skin at angle of the mouth.

The depressor anguli oris (DAO) causes the downturn of the corners of the mouth during frowning. In certain individuals, an overactive or strong depressor anguli oris (DAO) can give a sad appearance but with BTX-A, this can be improved by relaxing the muscle.

(xiii) Depressor labii inferioris

Origin: Oblique line of the mandible.

Insertion: Lower lip medially.

The depressor labii inferioris (DLI) is not routinely treated in facial aesthetics. Its function is to pull the lower lip downwards and laterally. It arises from the mandible deep to the depressor anguli oris, and inserts superiorly and medially into the lower lip.

A complication resulting from involvement of the depressor labii inferioris is a crooked smile which can occur following injection of the depressor anguli inferioris or mentalis due to wrong placement of BTX-A or because of the spread of BTX-A to the DLI.

N.B: The relationship of the labial group of muscles from deep to superficial is: Mentalis > Depressor Labii Inferioris > Depressor Anguli Oris.

(xiv) Platysma

The platysma is a thin broad muscle of facial expression and has three parts: It arises from the superficial fascia on the upper part of the pectoralis major and deltoid muscles.

Insertion: The anterior fibres run across the clavicle and up the neck to insert onto the lower border of the mandible, forming the pars mandibularis. More lateral intermediate fibres, the pars labialis continue across the lower part of the face, deep to the depressor anguli oris muscle to insert into the lateral half of the lower lip (Figure 17.5), and the superficial musculo-aponeurotic system (SMAS) of the face. The lateral fibres travel over the mandibular attachment of the masseter, deep to risorius, where they insert onto the modiolar musculature, and the skin around the angle and lower part of the mouth, this is the pars modiolaris part.

Platysma expresses surprise and wrinkles the skin of the neck in an oblique direction (Figure 17.7). It also draws down the lower lip and angle of the mouth and on contraction it tenses the skin of the neck and produces palpable vertical rippling.

Spasmodic contractions of platysma occur in nervous tics and belly dancers use the muscle to elevate the breasts.

Treating platysma with BTX-A prevents this contraction and improves the appearance of the platysmal bands and gives more definition to the jawline.

But with age laxity of the skin and the SMAS, the vertical bands become prominent even *without* contraction. This is the platysma dewlap or "Turkey Neck". In such cases, surgical options such as a platysmaplasty should be considered as the use of BTX-A will not be useful.

(xv) Zygomaticus Minor

Origin: Anterior aspect of lateral surface of the zygomatic bone.
Insertion: Skin of upper lip just medial to the corner of the mouth.

The zygomaticus minor assists with the elevation of the upper lip. This muscle is not routinely injected with BTX-A because it can cause an asymmetrical smile that is unsightly.

(xvi) Zygomaticus Major

Origin: Posterior aspect of lateral surface of the zygomatic bone.
Insertion: Corner of the mouth.

The zygomaticus major pulls the angle of the mouth superiorly and laterally. Likewise, this muscle is not routinely injected with BTX-A as it can result in an asymmetrical smile and unbalanced facial expression.

The Muscular Control of Emotional Facial Expression

Facial expression is a complex means of non-verbal emotional communication and was exploited by the classical Greek and Japanese theatre. More recently Darwin was criticised for his observation that facial emotional expression was universal for both humans and nonhuman primates. However 20th century research confirmed Darwin's observations and at least the six emotional expressions for anger, disgust, fear, happiness, sadness, and surprise are seen within and across cultures (Figure 17.7). They are a worldwide human response to common stimuli which are not influenced by literacy.

These six universal facial expressions of emotion are a small part of a range of 44 possible independent movements of the human facial musculature called Action Units (AUs) (Figure 17.7). Non-surgical facial aesthetics requires an understanding of this neuro-anatomical complexity. For example the lateral part of the frontalis (pars lateralis) can move independently of the medial frontalis (the pars medialis) and as each requires separate innervation for the separate functions, frontalis is anatomically two muscles.

Another example of the composite action unit is the emotional reaction that brings the brows down and together which is a combination of three anatomical separate muscles that do not usually act independently in humans: the corrugator supercilli, depressor supercilli and procerus.

Although the basic expression of facial emotional response is universal it is possible to learn masking strategies to conceal a spontaneous response. This can vary from a totally concealed impassive facial response to an exaggerated reaction.

These "emotional faces" (Figure 17.7) are associated with widespread magnetic resonance imaging (MRI) activation in the

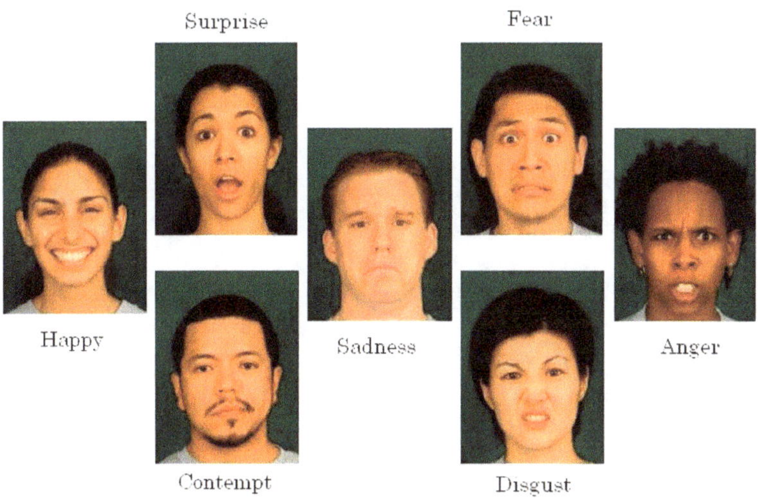

Figure 17.7 The seven universal facial expressions of emotion.

Source: Matsumoto D, Hwang HS, Reading facial expressions of emotion, *Psychol. Sci. Agenda*, American Psychological Association (May 2011).

visual, limbic, temporoparietal and prefrontal areas, and the putamen and cerebellum.

Clinical Segmental Aging Changes *(See also the treatment sections in Chapter 18)*

1. **Aging of the upper third of the face**
   a. The loss of forehead subcutaneous support reveals the underlying bony margin of the anterior temporal fossa and often the temporal artery and veins (not shown here).
   b. With the loss of subcutaneous collagen and elastin recoil, the frontalis, procerus and corrugator muscles which overly the glabellar, produce fixed wrinkles (Figure 17.8).
   c. The lack of subcutaneous support at the superior and lateral orbital margin creates skin flaccidity between the eyelid and eyebrow with varying degrees of ptosis so that the cutaneous eyebrow descends below the orbital rim and produce a lateral fold which may encroach on the lateral

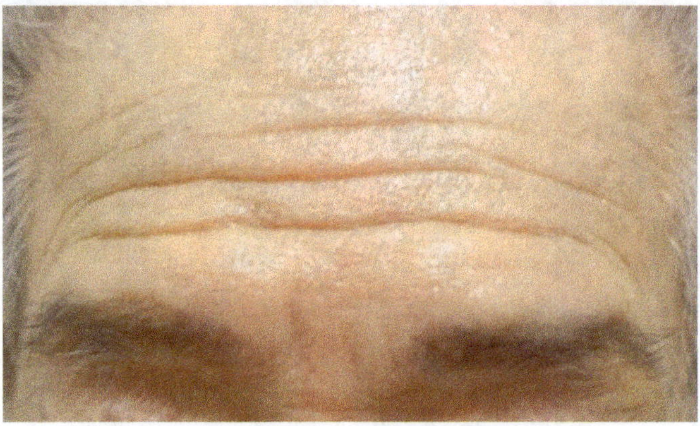

Figure 17.8 Fixed upper face wrinkles.

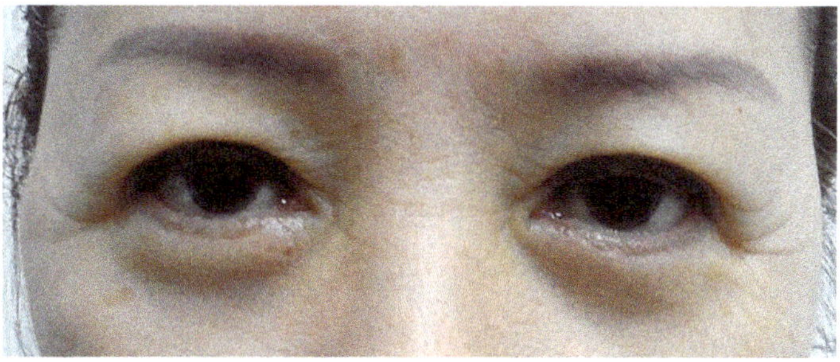

Figure 17.9 Ptosis of upper lids.

visual field. These stigmata are usually symmetrical (Figure 17.9).

2. **Aging of the midface**

   a. The principal midface change is the loss of the infraorbital connective tissue scaffold which allows the inferior migration of the

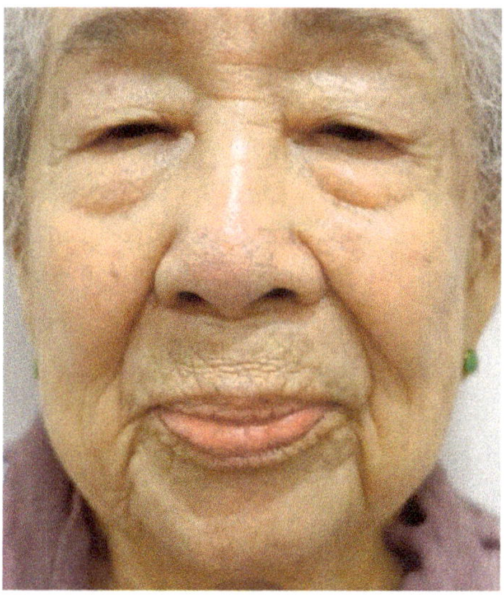

Figure 17.10 The elderly scalloped midface contour with 1. bulging of the infra-orbital fat pads (fat bags) 2. descent of the buccal fat (chubby cheeks) which are continuous with the deep temporal fat above 3. the nasolabial folds medially and 4. the rhytides below.

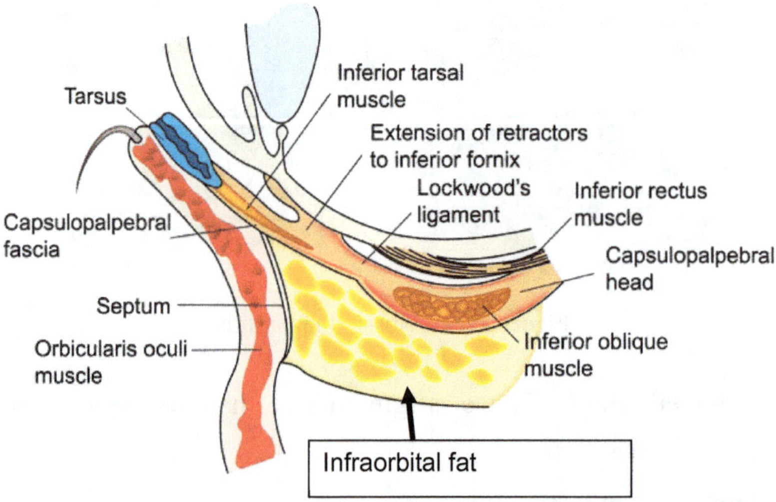

Figure 17.11 **(a)** Sagittal section of the lower lid showing the relations of the infraorbital fat below Lockwoods ligament and posterior to the orbital septum. The fat can herniate over Lockwards ligament or herniate outwards through a weakened septum.

buccal fat pads to produce a sagging appearance of the malar prominence and cheeks and a deep naso-labial fold below (Figure 17.10).

Medially the loss of infraorbital subcutaneous connective tissue also expose the infraorbital fat pads the "palpebral bags" which create the tear-trough depression. This overlies the osteocutaneous tear trough ligament. This ligament runs obliquely downwards and laterally from the medial canthus to the mid-papillary line where it joins the palpebro-malar groove, the groove between the lower eyelid and the malar bone. With age, deepening of the tear trough produces dark infra-orbital hollows.

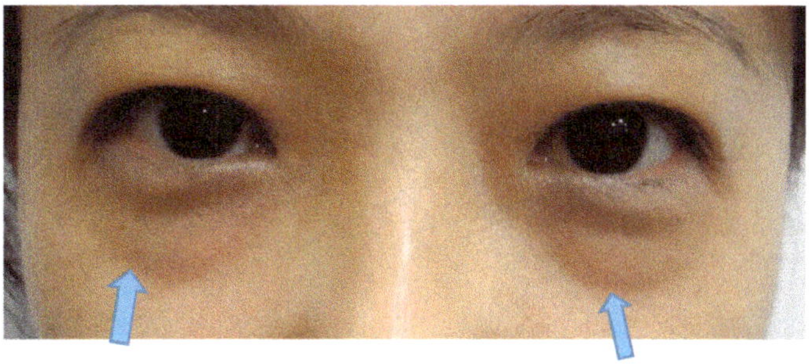

Figure 17.11 (**b**) A moderate tear trough depression deformity which joins the lateral palpebro-malar groove in the mid-papillary line with infra-orbital darkening.

b. Intraorbital fat may herniate anteriorly due to laxity of Lockwood's ligament which is the hammock-like ligament of the globe. This causes descent of the globe and a weakened orbital septum (Figures 17.10 and 17.11a to 17.11c).

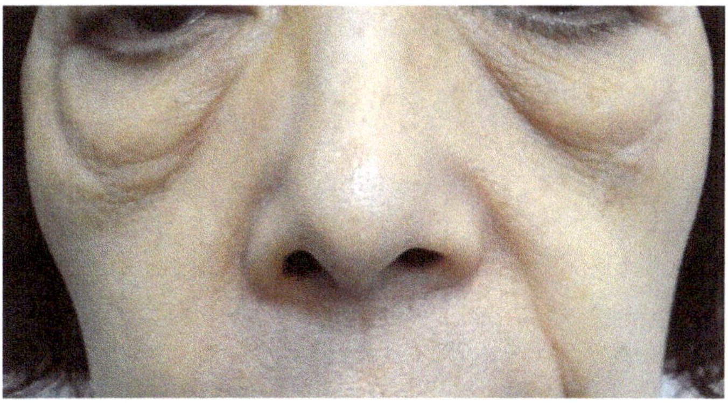

Figure 17.11 (**c**) Advanced aging of the mid face with descent of the infraorbital fat pads to produce "large palpebral bags" and marked tear troughs. See also the correction with fillers Chapter 18

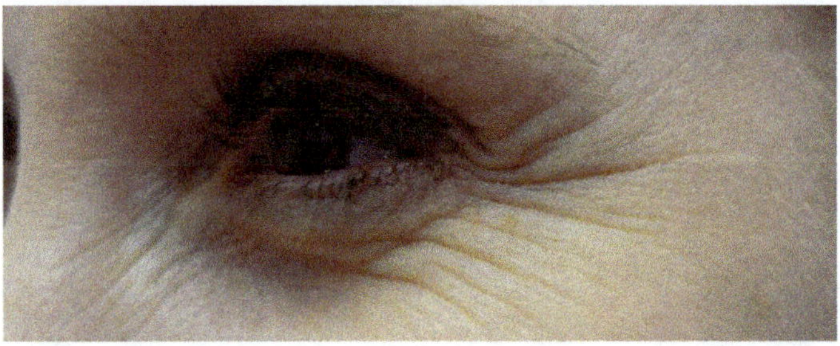

Figure 17.12 "Crow's feet" (rhytides).

c. The periorbital loss of subcutaneous elastin allows the orbicularis oculi muscle and its peripheral muscular insertions to create lateral canthal lines ("crow's feet" rhytides) (Figure 17.12).

The Nose and Ears

There is often enlargement of the nose and ears especially the lobes but the explanation of these changes has been attributed to:

i) Continuous chondrocyte driven cartilage growth enlarging the nose and pinna of the ear.
ii) The effect of gravity producing ptosis of the nasal tip due to reduced support by degenerate collagen and subcutaneous elastin which allows separation of the the upper and lower lateral nasal cartilages. A gravitational explanation is more obvious for the ear lobe (Figure 17.14a).
iii) In some patients the enlargement of the nose is partially due to the relative loss of surrounding facial volume.

3. Aging of the lower face

i. The descent of the compartmental facial fat towards the lower margin of the mandible will create changes from mid to lower

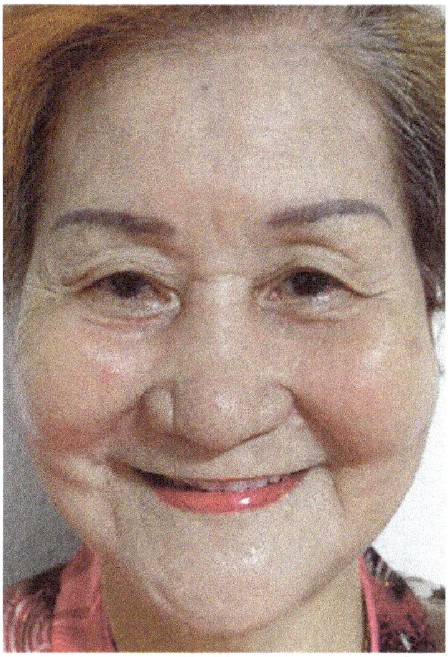

Figure 17.13 The aging nose.

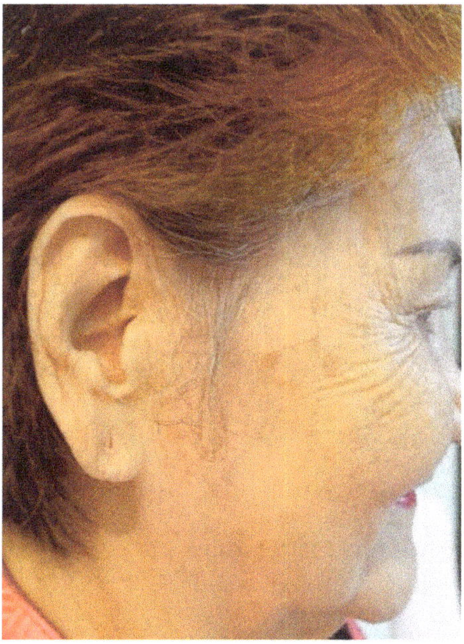

Figure 17.14 (**a**) The aging ear and periorbital "crow's feet" rhytides.

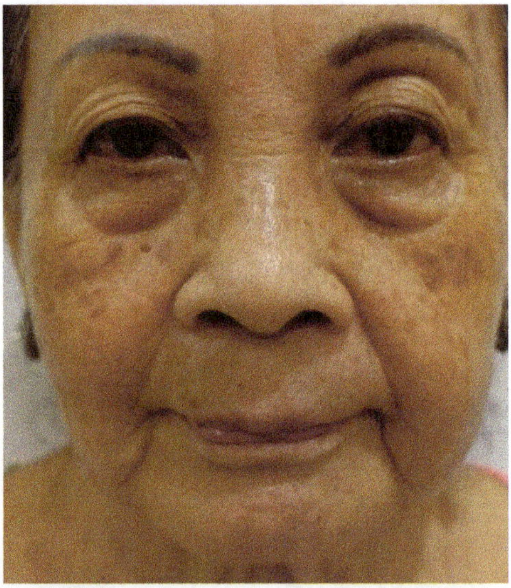

Figure 17.14 **(b)** Jowls overlying the mandibular border which extend distally from the marionette lines. Note also the eye bags, the naso labial rhytides and dyspigmentation.

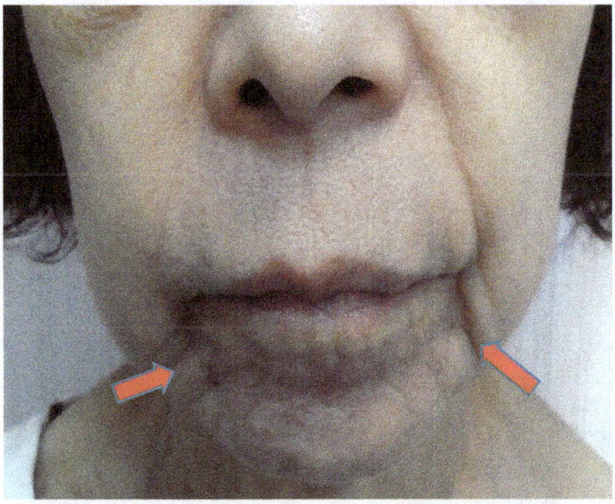

Figure 17.15 The loss of mid face volume with marked nasolabial fold which is continuous below with the arrowed marionette lines.

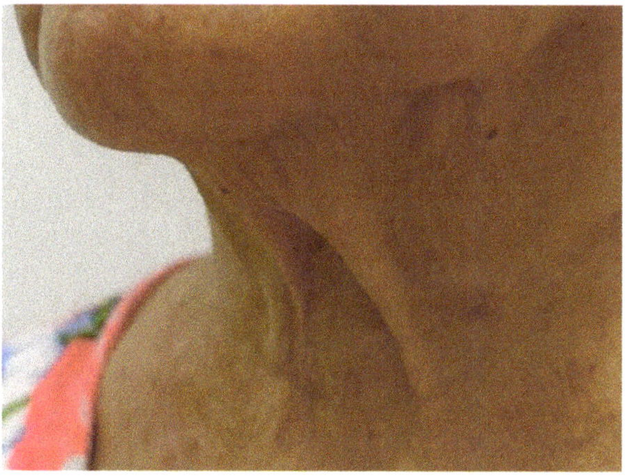

Figure 17.16 Dewlap skin folds give the "Turkey" neck appearance.

facial volume. Figures 17.13 to 17.16 show the varied contours from the midface down to the scalloped mandibular margin and to the platysma area of the neck. With the laxity of the overlying perioral skin there is also deepening of the nasolabial fold which extends down to the marionette rhytides which arise from the oral commissure (Figure 17.15).

ii. The loss of submental elasticity and facial ligament retention, also contribute to the sagging of the skin over the borders of the platysma muscle. This combined laxity of the skin, platysma and SMAS give rise to the vertical dewlap bands of the neck (Figure 17.16).

iii. Blunting of the cervico-mental angle (Figure 17.17) can be attributed to a combination of:

- excess submental adipose tissue

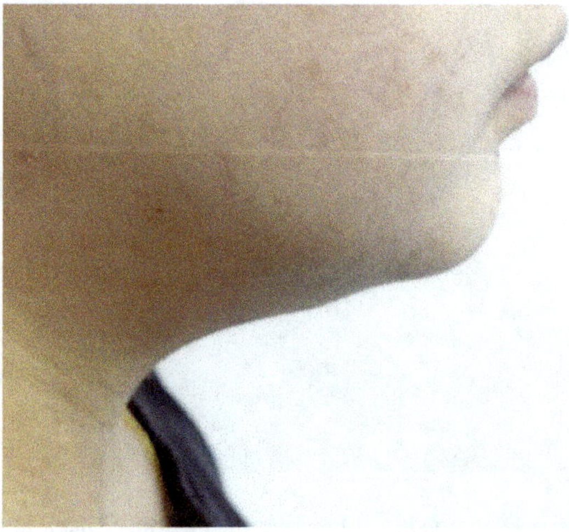

Figure 17.17 Blunting of cervico-mental angle in a young adult due to an excess of submental adipose tissue which may be a genetically determined feature.

- skin laxity
- drooping of the medial border of the platysma muscle and the SMAS
- hypertrophy of a submandibular gland

In the case of Figure 17.17, if blunting of the cervico-mental angle is primarily due to excess adipose tissue, then liposuction may be a more definitive treatment.

(Note: Lipolytic agents are not approved in some countries during the time of writing this chapter.)

Chapter 18

Non Surgical Facial Aesthetics — Part 2 Injectable Neuromodulators and Fillers

Rui Ming Ho and Fooi Chin Ng

Introduction

Facial Rejuvenation with Injectable Neuromodulators

Botulinum Toxin (BTX) is a neurotoxin produced by the anaerobe bacterium, *Clostridium botulinum*. Although it has seven serotypes, only types BTX-A and BTX-B are used in facial aesthetics of which type A makes up the majority of the current usage and will be the serotype discussed. It causes degrees of flaccid rather than rigid or tetanic paralysis by blocking acetylcholine which activates muscle contraction on release at the motor nerve terminal.

The three main products of BTX-A and their applications are:

1) Onabotulinumtoxin A (Botox®, Botox Cosmetic®)
   I. Botox — Cervical dystonia, severe primary axillary hyperhidrosis, strabismus, and blepharospasm
   II. Botox Cosmetic — Moderate to severe glabellar lines

2) Abobotulinumtoxin A (Dysport®) — Cervical dystonia, moderate to severe glabellar lines
3) IncobotulinumtoxinA (Xeomin®) — Cervical dystonia, blepharospasm

The relative doses of the three different products are as follows:

1 U Botox® is equivalent to 2.5 U Dysport®
1 U Botox® is equivalent to 1 U Xeomin®

Usually syringes with 30 G needles can be used to administer 0.5 cc or 1 cc of BTX-A.

Mechanism of Action

In facial aesthetics, BTX-A is excellent for eliminating lines of skin movement and wrinkles and it targets the neuromuscular junction at the specific site where it is injected, inhibiting muscle contracture for up to 4–6 months.

There are generally two different types of wrinkles (rhytides):

1) **Dynamic wrinkles**
   These are wrinkles that are seen with muscle contraction and on facial animation. BTX-A is highly effective to treat these muscle contractions.

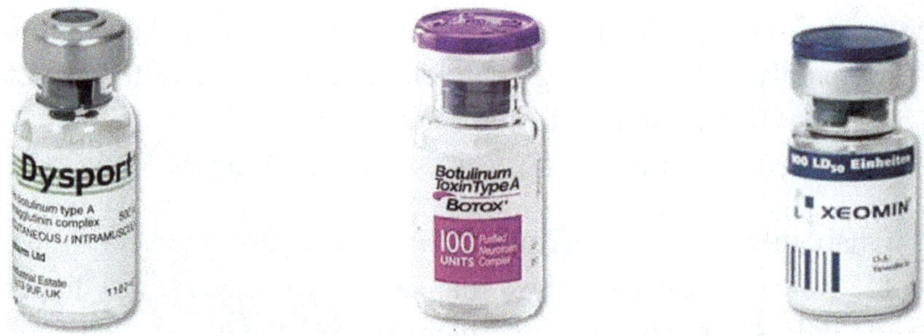

Figure 18.1 The different brands of BTX-A.

2) **Static wrinkles**
   These are wrinkles that are seen at rest. With repeated contraction, dynamic wrinkles will progress to static wrinkles. BTX-A may not be sufficient to smooth static wrinkles but is used to prevent further deepening of the wrinkle. Other aesthetic modalities such as dermal fillers p 553 and laser skin resurfacing are used in combination with BTX-A to achieve better results.

Neuromuscular Physiology

In normal muscle contraction, the terminal end of a neuron contains acetylcholine vesicles. Acetylcholine forms a Synaptic Fusion Complex with 3 SNARE proteins which are *Synaptobrevin, Syntaxin and SNAP-25,* which on neuronal stimulation facilitate the acetyl choline release into the synaptic cleft space between the neuron and muscle fibre.

The released acetylcholine binds to the acetylcholine receptors on the muscle fibre and generates the action potential that produces muscle contraction.

When BTX-A is introduced into the neuro-muscular junction, it prevents the release of acetylcholine as follows:

a) BTX-A has a heavy chain which facilitates its entry into the neuron.
b) Once inside the neuron, the light chain of BTX-A cleaves the SNAP-25 protein that is one of the SNARE proteins.
c) This prevents the formation of the Synaptic Fusion Complex.
d) Without the Synaptic Fusion Complex, the vesicles are unable to release acetylcholine into the synaptic cleft.
e) The result is the loss of muscle contraction.

Excess paralysis of the muscle from too much BTX-A can be treated by injection in the opposing muscle or waiting for the effect to wear off which may take up to 4–6 months.

The dilution of BTX-A Botulinum toxin is administered by diluting the powder in 2.5 mls of normal saline and injecting it directly into neuromuscular tissue. It can take 24–72 hours to take effect, but may take as long as 7–14 days for the full effect.

Neutralising antibodies to BTX-A rarely occur and are manifested by a lack of response to the neurotoxin injection. It is possible that high dose BTX-A administered at short time intervals may increase the possibility of antibodies to BTX-A. To minimise this occurrence, always start with the lowest possible effective dose and repeat at the longest time interval possible.

Case Studies

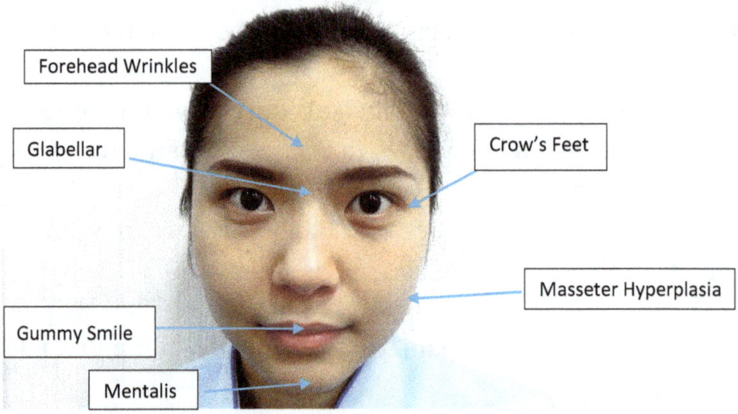

Figure 18.2 Facial areas commonly treated with BTX-A.

1) **Forehead wrinkles (Figure 18.3)**
   The Frontalis muscle is targeted as marked with 1 U BTX-A at each point.

Possible complications:

a) Brow and eyelid ptosis
   The injector must assess the patient carefully and avoid administering too high a dose of BTX-A as this can result in an

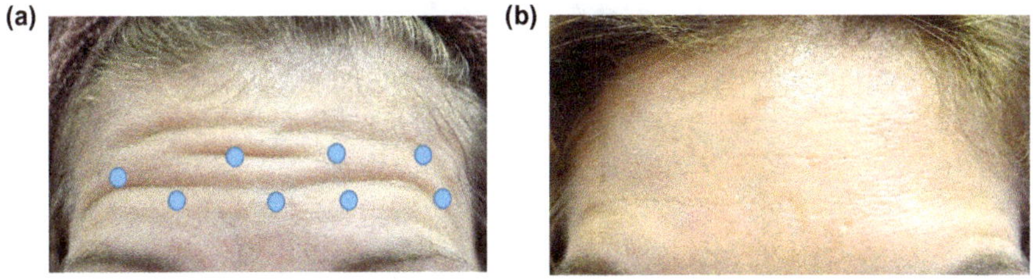

Figures 18.3 (**a**) Before injection. (**b**) One week after 8 U BTX-A.

unnatural "frozen" look. The amount of BTX-A to be used will depend on the clinical condition. Keep the injections at least 1.5 cm above the brow so as to decrease the risk of brow ptosis and eyelid ptosis. Eyelid ptosis occurs due to the spread of BTX-A into the upper eyelids.

The patient should remain upright for 4 hours post injection and avoid massaging the points of injection to prevent the spread of BTX-A to adjacent muscles.

The management of brow and eyelid ptosis:

i) Explanation and reassurance. As the effects of BTX-A are not permanent, the undesirable effects will resolve over time.
ii) For eyelid ptosis, apply the alpha-2 adrenergic agonist, brimonidine eye drops with a dosage of 1 drop per affected eye three times a day. This is used to stimulate Muller's muscle (the superior tarsal muscle) to elevate the affected eye lid by 1–3 mm. This smooth muscle is on the underside of the levator palpebrae superioris, which is the principal elevator of the the upper eyelid.

b) The "Spock-look" (Figure 18.4a)

If the lateral frontalis is not paralysed adequately, the lateral fibres of the frontalis will still contract and pull more strongly upwards. This will cause the eyebrows to be raised and give the "Spock-look". It is essential to treat the frontalis muscle for forehead wrinkles, with BTX-A evenly distributed across the entire muscle so as to prevent this "Spock-look" surprised appearance.

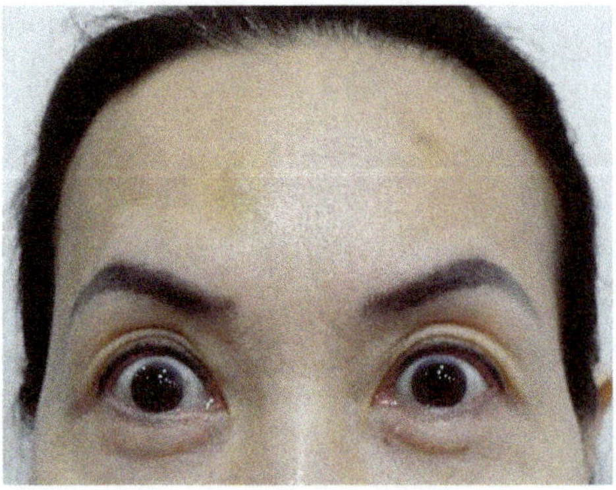

Figure 18.4 (**a**) The surprised "Spock" look.

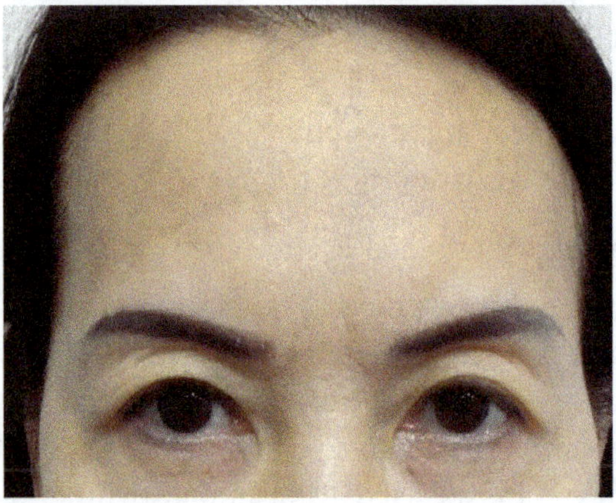

Figure 18.4 (**b**) After correction of the "Spock" look.

Management: Remedied by treating the lateral frontalis with a small dose of BTX-A (1–2 U) each side.

2) **Frown lines Figure 18.6a**
Muscles targeted: Corrugator Supercillii and Procerus.

Possible complications:

a) Brow ptosis — If BTX-A is placed incorrectly and into the frontalis muscle instead of Procerus and Corrugator a brow ptosis may occur.

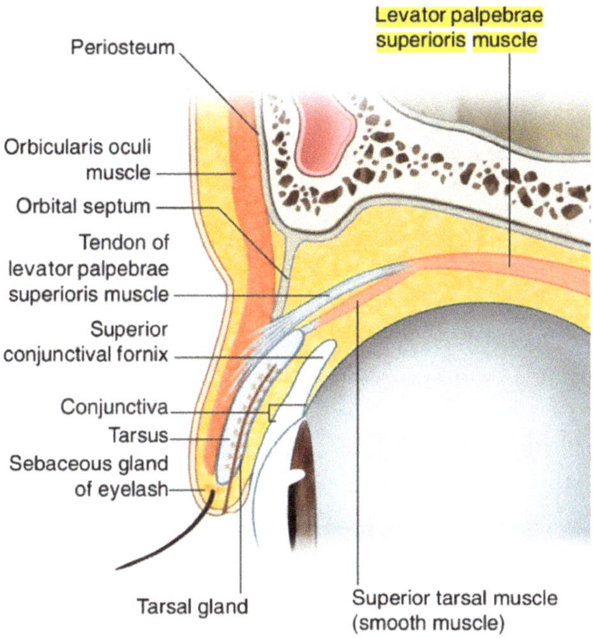

Figure 18.5 Anatomy of the upper lid showing the Superior tarsal muscle — Mullers muscle deep to the Levator palpabraesuperioris (LPS) muscle. This smooth muscle can be stimulated to enhance lid elevation when LPS is paralyzed by excess Botox.

Source: Netter FH, *Atlas of Human Anatomy*, *5th Ed.*, Saunders (2010).

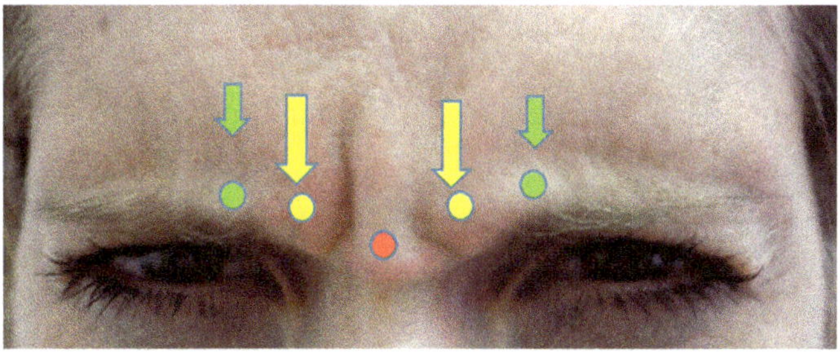

Figure 18.6 (**a**) 4 U BTX-A is injected into Procerus (red middle circle) and 2 U BTX-A into each point of Corrugator. The yellow medial aspects of the corrugators are injected deep while the green lateral aspects more superficially.

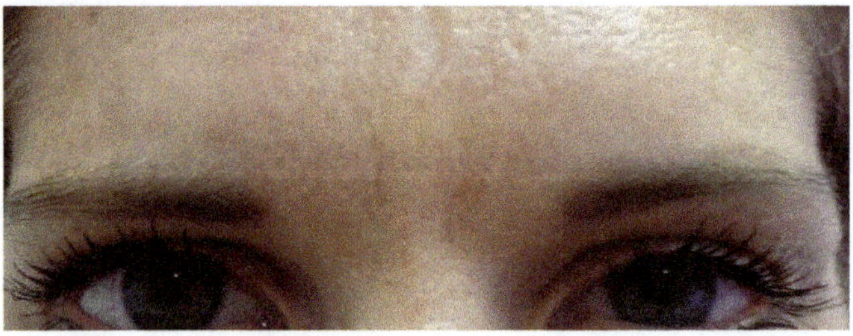

Figure 18.6 (**b**) One week after the total of 12 U BTX-A administered to the glabellar complex.

Management of complications

i) Explanation and reassurance. As the effects of BTX-A are not permanent, the undesirable effects will resolve over time.

3) **Crow's feet (Figures 18.7a and 18.7b)**
   Muscles targeted: Orbicularis Oculi.

Possible complications:

Cheek ptosis and a crooked smile may occur if BTX-A is administered into the zygomatic muscles below. As a guide, keep BTX-A injections above the zygomatic bone to minimise the risk of injecting into the zygomatic muscles.

Management of complications: Explanation and reassurance.

4) **Bilateral masseteric hyperplasia (hypertrophy)— The square jaw**
   Muscle targeted: Masseter (Figure 18.8a).

- Superiorly: A line drawn from the ear lobe to the corner of the mouth
- Inferiorly: The inferior border of the mandible
- Anteriorly: The anterior border of the masseter
- Posteriorly: The posterior border of the masseter

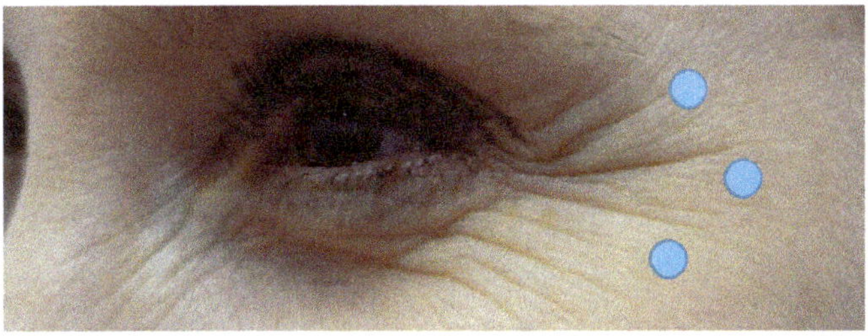

Figure 18.7 (**a**) 4 U BTX-A are injected into each point seen before injection.

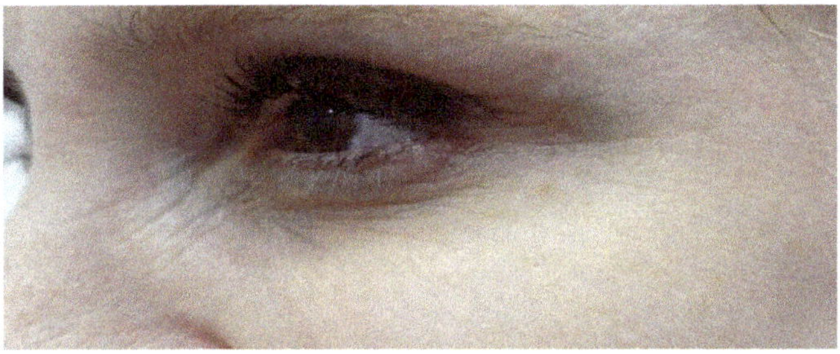

Figure 18.7 (**b**) One week after treatment with 12 U BTX-A.

The main structures to be aware of during the injection of the masseter are the parotid, its duct and the facial nerve. The surface anatomy of the parotid duct is the red line drawn from the tragus of the ear towards a point mid way between the alar of the nose and angle of the mouth. This safety zone minimises the risk of injuring the parotid duct (Figures 18.8a and 18.8b).

The facial nerve courses superficial to the masseter. Injections into the masseter should be deep so as to avoid the buccal branch of the facial nerve which supplies the orbicularis oris, buccinator and zygomaticus. Involvement of the facial nerve will result in an assymetrical smile.

Deep injections ensure that the deep head of the masseter is targeted as well. If the deep head of the masseter is missed, uneven muscle movement or muscle bulging can be seen during contraction of the masseter.

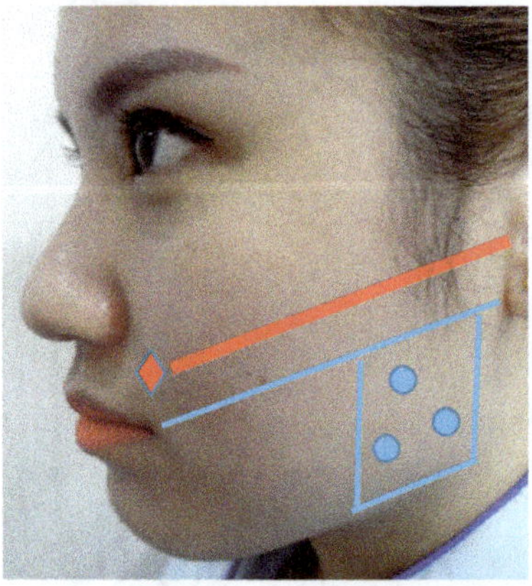

Figure 18.8 (**a**) The safety zone for injection of the masseter is demarcated by the blue rhomboid margins.

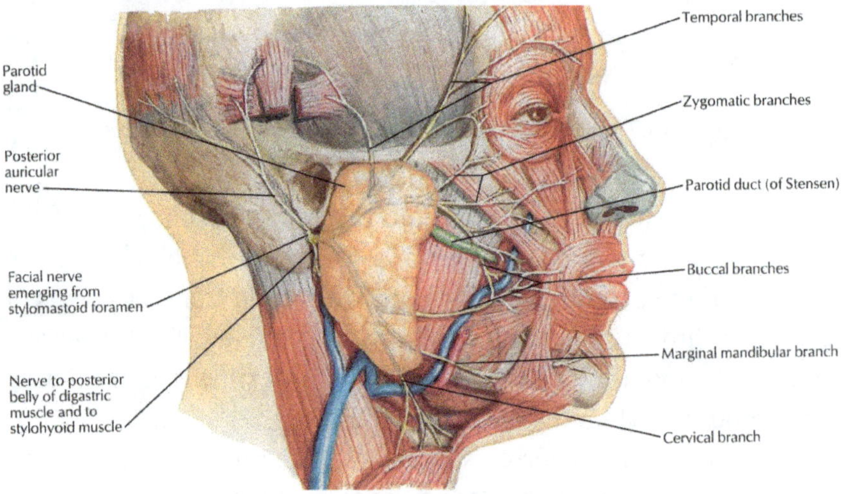

Figure 18.8 (**b**) The masseteric injection safety zone in relation to the parotid salivary gland and duct.

Source: Netter FH, *Atlas of Human Anatomy*, *5th Ed.*, Saunders (2010).

Injections should also be kept 0.5 cm to 1.0 cm above the inferior border of the mandible so as to avoid the marginal mandibular branch of the facial nerve (Figure 18.8b).

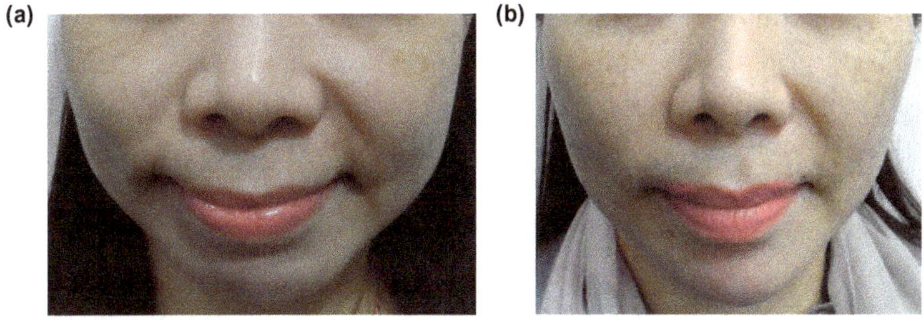

Figure 18.9 (**a**) Masseteric hyperplasia before BTX-A. (**b**) Five months after 10 U BTX-A at each of 3 blue points within the safety zone (Figure 18.8b).

Additionally, injections should not be administered too anteriorly as the risorius can be affected and also give rise to an asymmetrical smile.

Figures 18.8a and 18.8b are diagrams depicting the safety zone for masseteric BTX-A injections, illustrated by the blue points within the rhomboid areas.

Possible complications:

a) Always use the markings (above) as a guide to minimise the risk of parotid duct perforation.

   Prescribe analgesia and antibiotics if parotid swelling indicates evidence of an ascending parotid infection.

b) Crooked asymmetrical smile
   This occurs when BTX-A is injected too anteriorly and superficially and has spread or been injected into the risorius muscle. The affected side will not be able to retract the corner of the mouth distally.

   Management: Explanation and reassurance.

c) Uneven muscle movements and bulging if the BTX-A acts on different parts of the muscle with differing concentrations. This may occur in patients with large masseters and inaccurate injection points and depth.

Management:

i) Additional BTX-A injections to the area that bulges.
ii) Explanation and reassurance.

5) The "gummy smile"

A smile that shows too much gingivae can be distracting and unsightly. With BTX-A, the exposure on smiling can be reduced. The targeted muscles are Levator Labii Superioris Aleque Nasi (Figure 18.10).

Possible complications:

a) Elongation of the philtrum due to increased distance between columella and vermillion border.
b) "Frozen" upper lip and difficulty in smiling.
c) Difficulty in pursing lips.

Management: Explanation and reassurance.

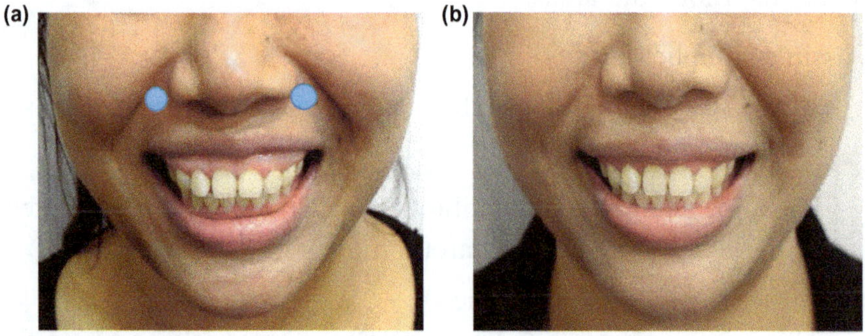

Figure 18.10 (**a**) Before 2 U BTX-A to each point in the alar groove. (**b**) One week after 2 U BTX-A to each Levator Labii Superioris Aleque Nasi.

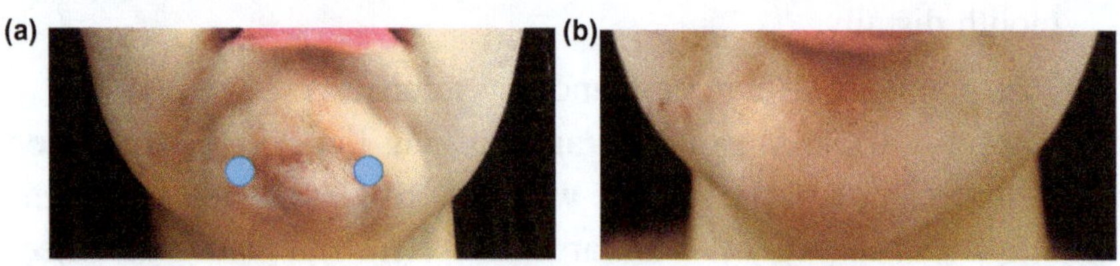

Figure 18.11 Cobble stone wrinkles of the chin. (**a**) Before 10 U BTX-A. (**b**) One week after 10 U BTX-A into each point of mentalis.

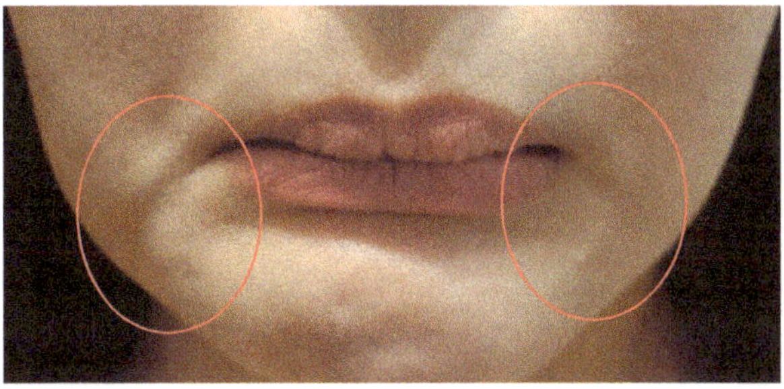

Figure 18.12 (**a**) Contraction of the DAO.

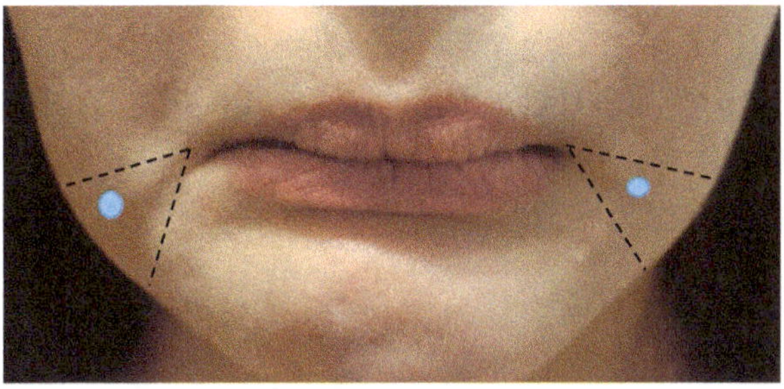

Figure 18.12 (**b**) Points of injection to target the DAO.

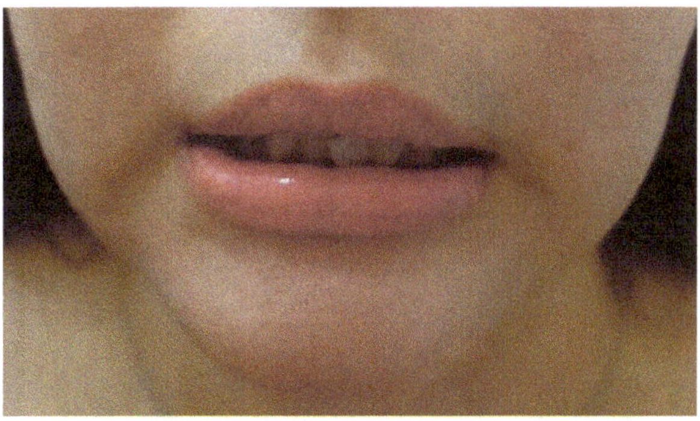

Figure 18.12 (**c**) Elimination of drooping of the commisures after BTX-A injection.

6) **"Cobble stone" wrinkles of the chin**
   Muscle targeted: 10 U BTX into each mentalis muscles (Figures 18.11a and 18.11b).

Possible complications:

a) A crooked smile which occurs when BTX-A has inadvertently been injected into the Depressor Labii Inferioris.

   Management: Explanation and reassurance.

7) **Drooping of the mouth corners (Figures 18.12a to 18.12c)**
   An overactive Depressor Anguli Oris pulls the corners of the mouth downwards and gives a "sad" appearance. BTX-A can be injected into the muscles to relax the tension on the oral commissures.
   The muscle targeted is the Depressor Anguli Oris.
   Dose: Can start with 2 U BTX-A for each Depressor Anguli Oris.

Possible complications:

Crooked smile: This can occur if the levator anguli oris muscle is affected. Always locate the muscle by facial animation and inject laterally instead of medially.

Management: Explanation and reassurance.

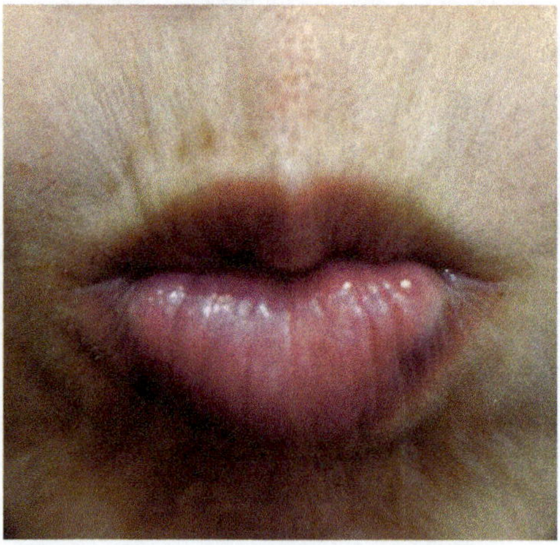

Figure 18.13 (**a**) Bar code peri-oral wrinkles on animation.

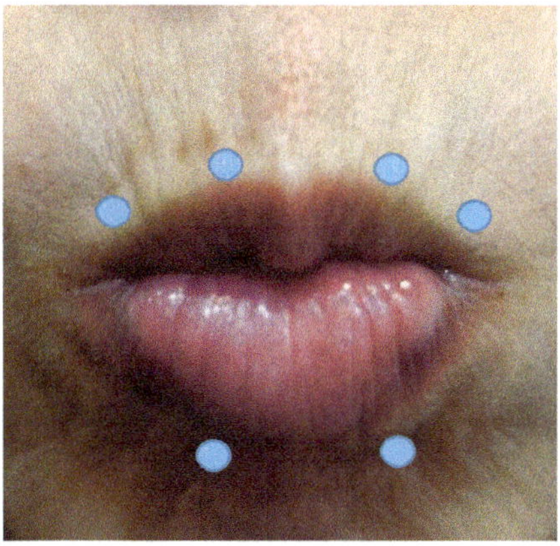

Figure 18.13 (**b**) 1 U BTX-A is injected at each point.

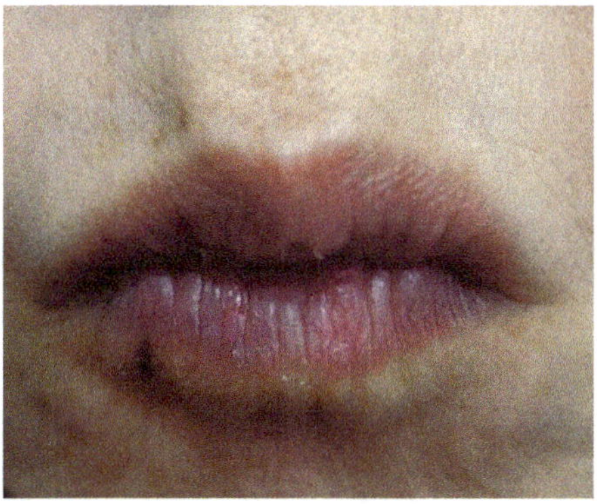

Figure 18.13 (**c**) Peri-oral region 2 weeks after BTX-A injection. Note the softening of the peri-oral wrinkles between Figures 18.13b and 18.13c.

8) Peri-oral wrinkles

Peri-oral wrinkles or "bar code" lines around the lips are unsightly and give a stern and aging look. This appearance can be improved by the administration of BTX-A into the orbicularis oris muscle to relieve the tone which condenses the labial connective tissue to cause the rhytides.

Muscle targeted: Orbicularis oris.

Dose: A total of 4 U BTX-A into the upper peri-oral region and 2 U BTX-A into lower peri-oral region.

Possible complications:

a) A crooked smile

This can occur if the Depressor Labii Inferioris is affected when the lower peri-oral wrinkles are treated. To avoid this, the lower peri-oral wrinkles are not treated or treated with low doses of BTX-A i.e. 4 U for the upper lip and 2 U for the lower lip perioral wrinkles.

Management: Explanation and reassurance.

9) Cervical dystonia

Dystonia is characterized by involuntary sustained muscle contractions of opposing muscles resulting in twisting and repetitive movements. It is incompletely understood but relief of the dystonic grimacing and associated discomfort is improved markedly with botulinum toxin with apparent effects 3 days to 2 weeks following treatments. After 3 months, the effects of the botulinum toxin will diminish.

Possible complications:

A ceiling dose of 100 U of BTX-A to the sternocleidomastoid muscle with no more than 50 U at each site given no less than 12 weeks apart, is recommended. Adverse effects are uncommon although a flu-like syndrome has been reported, but it is generally short-lived. Other adverse effects include muscle soreness, headaches, light-headedness, hypertension, weakness, diarrhoea, and abdominal pain. Patients, should be informed of the potential weakness in the injected area or in nearby muscles.

10) Opening the palpebral fissure

Injection of 1–3 U of BTX-A into a hypertrophic inferior orbicularis oculi muscle can "open the eye". Avoid this in older Caucasian females as it can accentuate laxity in the infraorbital skin (Figures 18.14a and 18.14b).

11) Platysma

Plastysma injections have been advocated to improve the definition of the jaw line by decreasing the downward contraction

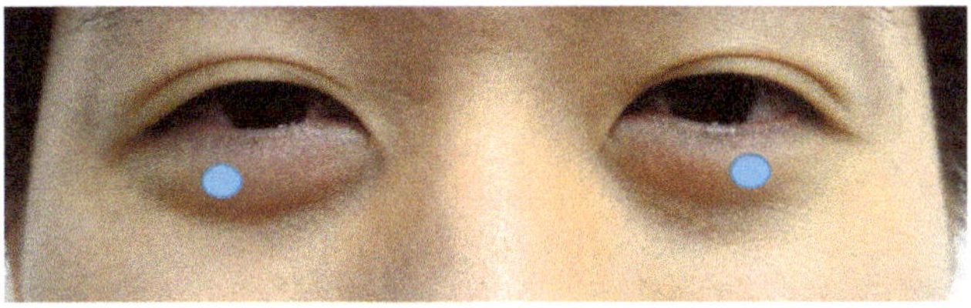

Figure 18.14 (**a**) 1–3 U of BTX-A at each point.

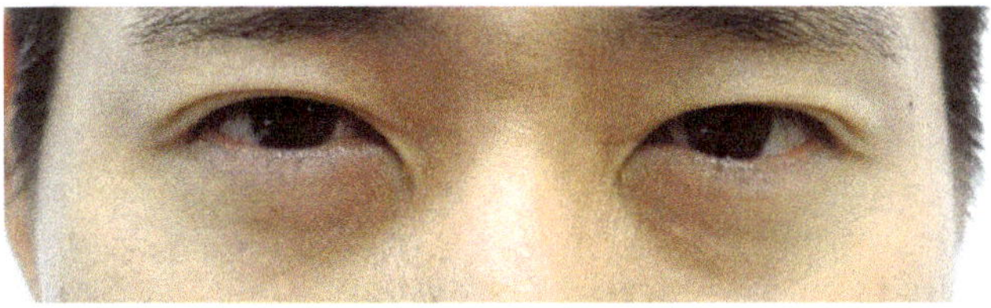

Figure 18.14 (**b**) Two weeks after BTX-A injection. Note the reduction in size and prominence of the inferior orbicularis oculi.

of the muscle. This is intended to eliminate the vertical platysma banding that is associated with the contraction. However such use of a neuromodulator should be reserved for:

i. younger patients who are not in need of surgical intervention,
ii. some cases of post-surgery residual banding, and
iii. those patients who have undergone treatment to reduce submental chin fat.

In cases where sagging is apparent with prominent vertical bands *without* contraction due to sagging of the unsupported skin, surgical options such as a platysma-plasty should be considered for this "Turkey Neck" platysma dewlap (Figure 18.15).

12) Intra-dermal BTX-A

Botulinum toxins have known inhibitory effects on both acetylcholine and vasoactive intestinal polypeptide. These mechanisms of action have prompted clinicians to use hyper-diluted

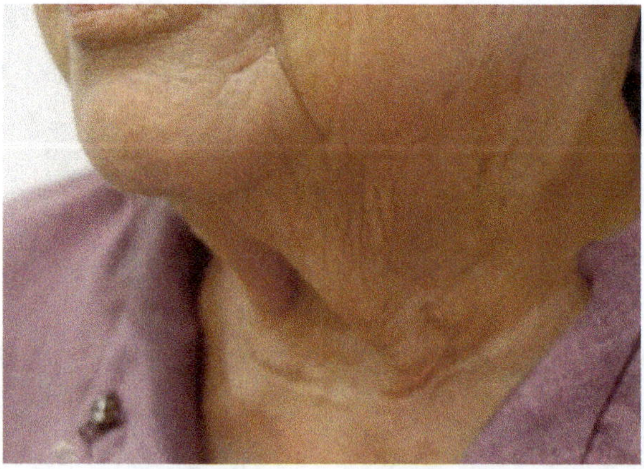

Figure 18.15 The "Turkey Neck" Platysma dewlap.

botox delivered into the dermal plane to improve the appearance of pores, acne, rosacea, and flushing. Such applications, lack evidence-based studies and require more conclusive investigation. A potential side effect of injections that are too deep may interfere with the muscles of facial expression.

13) Botox and the treatment of idiopathic myofascial pains including the Temporo-Mandibular Joint Pain Dysfunction Syndrome (TMJPDS/Facial Arthromyalgia FAM)

The temporo-mandibular joint pain dysfunction syndrome (FAM) presents as pain in the temporo-mandibular joint and associated musculature aggravated by mastication. It is intermittent and lasts from weeks to months and belongs to a wide group of idiopathic pains, which include atypical (idiopathic) facial pain which is non-joint and non-muscular, atypical (idiopathic) odontalgia, headache, neck, back, and pelvic pain and irritable bowel. Two or more may occur in the same patient simultaneously or sequentially.

FAM has been attributed to a variety of dysfunctions including bruxism and malocclusion without evidence and treated symptomatically with bite guards, occlusal equilibration, ultrasound and other modalities.

The analgesic action of botulinum toxin is unlikely apart from a placebo effect and has been attributed to toxin action on nociceptive neurons. There is no therapeutic confirmation supported by controlled trials.

The essential diagnosis and management of an idiopathic pain is facilitated by recognising that such patients have a bio-psycho-social disorder where the "bio" appears to be impaired central analgesic function involving serotonin and noradrenaline. The "psycho" is an inherent predisposition to somatisation which is probably a manifestation of "central pain sensitization where the patient is is overly concerned with the pain symptoms. The social component represents the effect of adverse life events which may be chronic ill health in the family,unemployment, academic adversity and even the problems of moving house.

Hence the treatment can include evidence based explanation and reassurance, Cognitive Behavioural therapy by a "pain trained" psychologist, a serotonin or noradrenaline reuptake inhibitor such as venlafaxine or a tricyclic antidepressant (nortriptyline) administered to provide central pain control but not for depression.

Conclusion

Neuromodulator injections are a very important component of non-surgical rejuvenation. Knowledge of the neurophysiology of the injected product and the anatomy of the face are vital factors in the final result. The most important variables are the skill, experience and the artistic eye of the clinician.

Dermal Fillers

Introduction

The origin of dermal fillers can be traced back to 1893 when Gustav Adolf Neuber, (1850–1932) described the first transplantation of arm adipose tissue to the lower margin of the orbit to correct adherent scars due to osteomyelitis. The first dermal filler approved by the United States Food and Drug Administration (FDA) was zyderm, made of bovine collagen. In 2003, the FDA approved the first hyaluronic acid (HA) filler, restylane. Since then numerous types of filler have been introduced for "volumization" to enhance tissue thickness and help overcome the following:-

1) skin laxity and wrinkles,
2) muscle and facial ligament atrophy,
3) loss of the dermis facial fat pad volume.

These changes result in a shrunken or sagging appearance with a loss of facial projection. Dermal fillers are designed to replace volume without the need for surgical structural support.

Fat Compartments and Ligaments of the Face

The concept of the facial fat compartment anatomy has helped non-surgical facial aesthetic management by the addition of volume to the age depleted soft-tissue compartments (see Chapter 17 Figures 17.3 and 17.4). The optimum strategy is to start the compartmental correction from the skeletal framework. A neglected cosmetic foundation is to correct restorative dental problems such as missing teeth and restorations, periodontitis and occlusal support before embarking on the overlying neuro muscular or filler procedures.

The results from fillers are immediate, except for Sculptra® where the effects are gradual and appreciated from the third month onwards. The longevity of the filler material depends on the type of fillers used (see Table 18.1). For instance neocollagenesis is collagen rejuvenation in the dermis layer where collagen loss has produced aging wrinkles.

As the effects from fillers wear off, additional filler material can be administered to revolumise the area.

Table 18.1 Main types of dermal fillers.

Type of filler	Composition	Mechanism of action
1) Hyaluronic acid E.g. Juvederm® Restylane® Teosyal® Revanesse® *(Lasts from 6 –24 mths)*	Hyaluronic acid gel +/– lidocaine	• Direct volumisation • Integration into dermal tissues • Draws water molecules more than 1000×
2) Calcium hydroxyapatite E.g. Radiesse® *(Lasts 12 mths+)*	Calcium hydroxyapatite microspheres in a gel carrier composed of sterile water, glycerine and sodium carboxymethylcellulose +/– lidocaine	• Direct volumisation • Neocollagenesis
3) Poly-L-lactic acid E.g. Sculptra® *(Lasts 24 mths+)*	Poly-L-lactic acid polymer particles from the alpha-hydroxy-acid family; has to be reconstituted with sterile water	• Neocollagenesis • Volumisation over time
4) Polymethylmethacrylate (PMMA) E.g. Bellafill® *(Lasts 12 mths for acne scars and 5 yrs for nasolabial folds)*	PMMA microspheres in water based gel composed of bovine collagen and lidocaine	• Direct volumisation • Creates matrix that supports collagen production • Long lasting (up to 5 years or more)

The Nerves and Arteries of the face

Knowledge of the facial nerve supply is essential to inject fillers without direct damage or compression of a sensory or motor nerve. Both can produce transient anaesthesia, permanent neuropathic pain or muscle weakness. The vascular anatomy must also be carefully respected to avoid complications such as tissue haemorrhage or thrombosis.

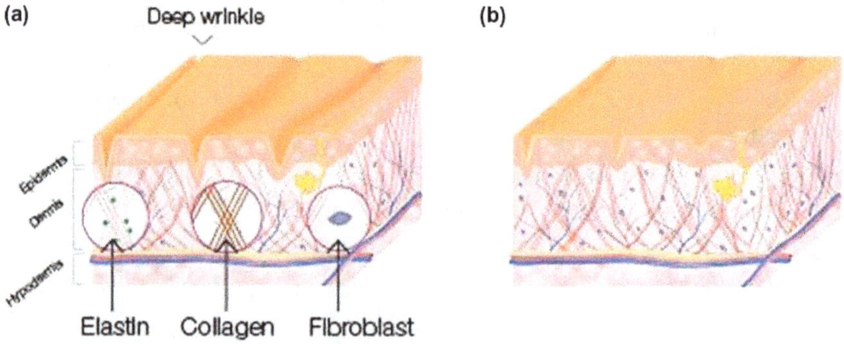

Figure 18.16 **(a)** Illustrating dermal loss. **(b)** The dermis after filler has replaced elastin, collage and fibroblasts.

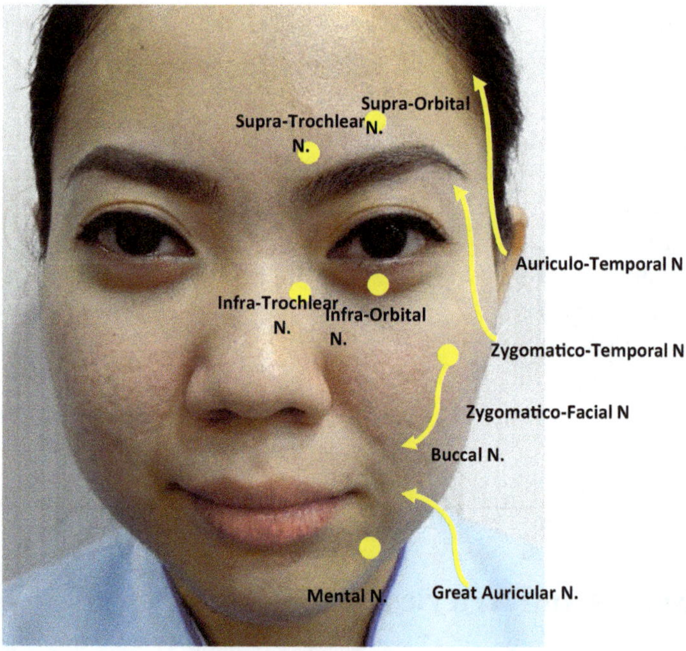

Figure 18.17 The cutaneous sensory distribution of the terminal branches of the trigeminal nerve (V). It is important to visualise that in clinical practice there is substantial anatomical overlap of these terminal branches.

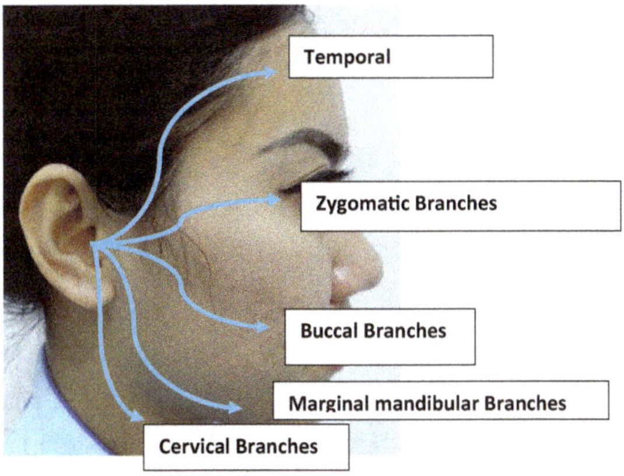

Figure 18.18 The motor branches of the facial nerve (VII).

Arteries of the Face

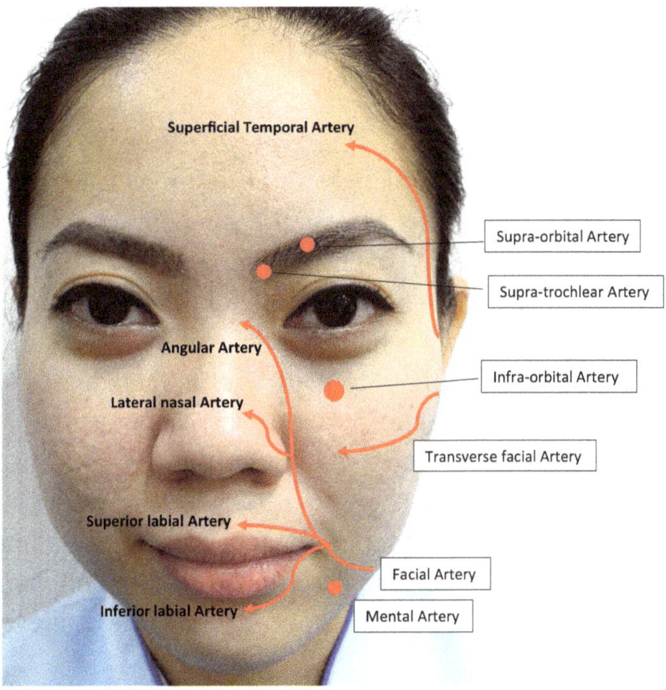

Figure 18.19 The main arteries of the face to be aware of during injection which is avoided by prior aspiration.

The Clinical Applications of Dermal Fillers

1) Wrinkles

When dynamic wrinkles progresses to static wrinkles, BTX-A alone may not be sufficient to treat these lines. A combination of BTX-A and a filler may be employed to achieve a better outcome

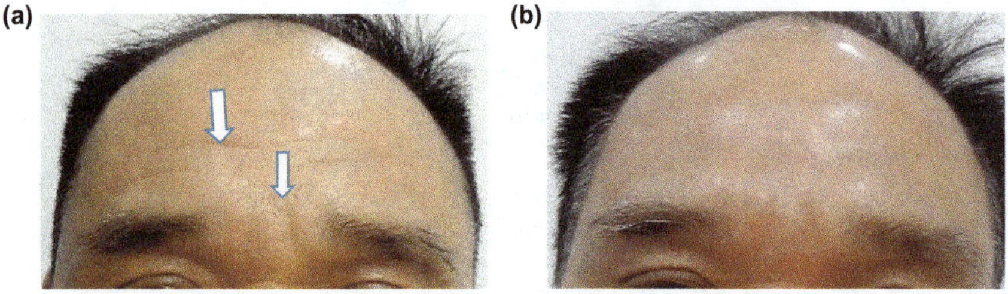

Figure 18.20 (**a**) Before. (**b**) Two weeks after a combination of BTX-A and 1 cc Juvederm® Volbella fillers applied directly beneath the forehead and glabellar wrinkles. The fillers were used because BTX-A alone was not enough to smooth the forehead.

2) Eyebrow fillers

The administration of fillers to the brow region is intended to improve the shape of the palpebral fissures by lifting the brows and eyelids. The apex of the natural brow is usually at the junction of the medial two-thirds and lateral third (see blue arrows) but this is not always a reliable guide especially in males.

The injection of fillers to the brows is intended to improve the shape of the palpebral fissures. The shape of the palpebral fissure of the eyes is improved with a more prominent arch at the superior border and shows more of the pupil and iris. Figure 18,21 shows that this change produced by filler volumisation may be confined to the palpebral fissure width and considered inadequate. A more positive brow lift may be achieved with Botox or surgery.

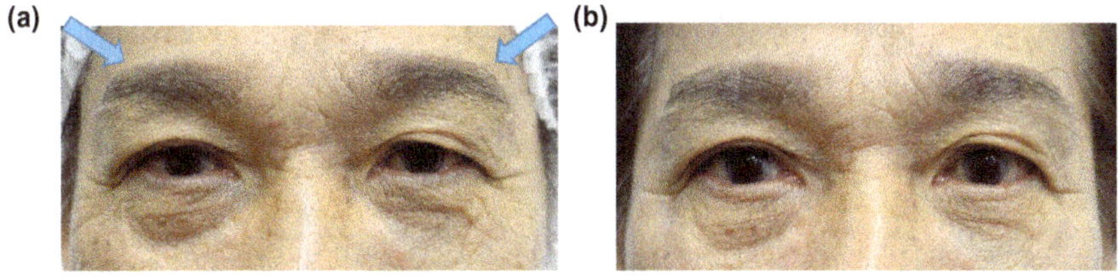

Figure 18.21 (**a**) Before. (**b**) After 1 cc of Juvederm® Volift to both eyebrows. showing modest widening of the palpebral fissures

3) The temporal fossae (the temples)

A marked hollow temple may not be aesthetically pleasing and can disturb the overall contour of the face.

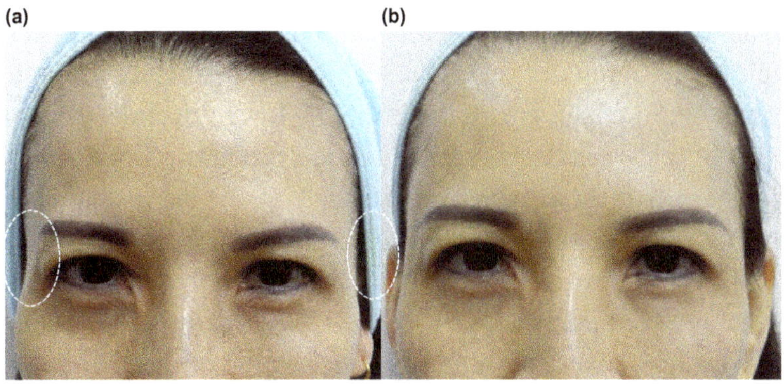

Figure 18.22 (**a**) Before. (**b**) Immediately after 5 cc of Juvederm® Voluma filler to the temporal regions.

4) Cheeks

The cheeks are important areas in facial rejuvenation. Deflated and sunken cheeks exaggerate age, give the appearance of fatigue and emphasizes the infraorbital eye bags.

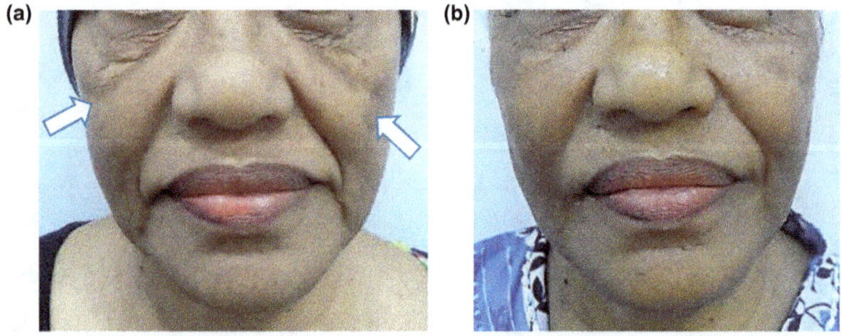

Figure 18.23 (**a**) Before filler. (**b**) Two months after 4 cc filler of Juvederm® Voluma to each cheek to eliminate the eye bags.

5) Tear trough deformity

The tear trough is formed by an osteocutaneous ligament which extends from below the medial canthus downwards and laterally to the mid-pupillary line. This tear trough ligament is a retaining ligament to which are attached the the lower eyelid (palpebral) part of the orbicularis muscle and the orbital part of the orbicularis oculi muscle which is attached to the periosteum of the orbital margin. The overlying tear trough becomes prominent with age where it joins the lateral palpebromalar groove. This creates a continuous groove which demarcates the bulging orbital fat above from the mid-cheek below. Although a normal anatomical feature it becomes a deformity when it creates prominent eye bags which accentuate dark periorbital circles and make the subject look tired.

Treatment is a "positive" blepharoplasty by the insertion of a filler below the trough whereas the traditional removal of fat above the tear trough ligament, a "negative" blepharoplasty may relapse.

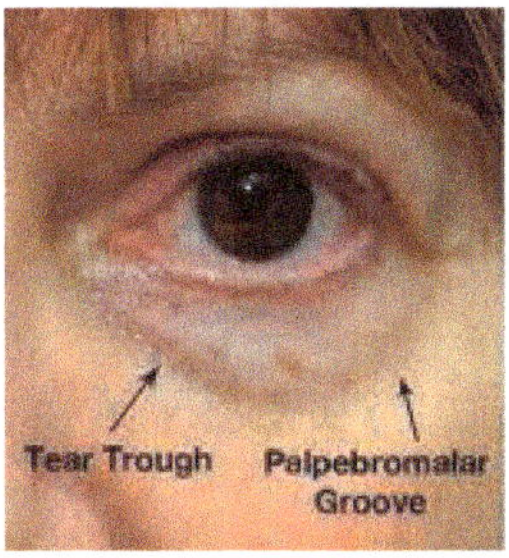

Figure 18.24 (**a**) Shows the fusion of the medial Tear Trough and the lateral Palpebromalar Groove.

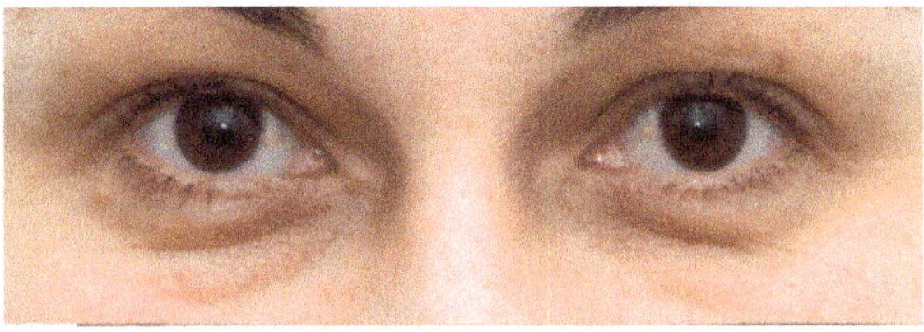

Figure 18.24 (**b**) The marked depression of the tear trough deformity extends downwards and laterally.

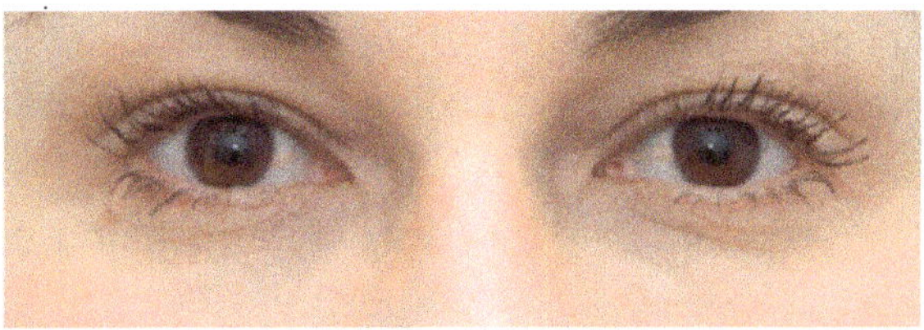

Figure 18.24 (**c**) After elimination by filling with 3 cc Juvederm® Voluma beneath the trough deformity.

Tear trough deformity fillers require experienced assessment and management

The following are important considerations.

1. Skin quality: thick, smooth skin will produce better results than thin wrinkled skin.
2. A defined hollow is more amenable to fillers.
3. Large fat pads and patients with septal fat herniation are difficult to correct with fillers and should be avoided.
4. Low-viscosity hyaluronic acid (HA) can be safely injected but high-viscosity HA and non-biodegradable agents are fraught with complications.
5. Small volumes should be deposited with small syringes and cannullae at the supraperiosteal orbital rim, care being taken to avoid the infraorbital foramen .
6. A post-injection HA filler area should be gently massaged for even distribution.
7. As HA is hydrophilic the absorption of water may cause a swelling .
8. Avoid overcorrection, under correction may be remedied by small repeated administrations
9. Postoperative pain can be avoided by HA fillers with lignocaine, for example, Juvederm® Ultra XC,
10. Erythema, swelling and bruising can be minimised by the application of icepacks pre and postinjection.
11. Anticoagulant aspirin should be discontinued for 7days. Other anticoagulants must be avoided completely.
12. Inadvertent superficial injection scan lead to a bluish discolouration under the skin
13. Iatrogenic blindness due to embolization of filler into the ophthalmic artery is uncommon. It has been reported after

injections of adipose tissue, corticosteroids, paraffin, silicone oil, bovine collagen, polymethylmethacrylate, hyaluronic acid, and calcium hydroxyapatite. Hence the need for expertise and experience.

14. Use a blunt cannula especially when treating the medial aspects of the tear trough deformity. Inject slowly, with minimal pressure and minute quantities of the filler at a time at one site.
15. Local preinjection infections must be avoided
16. Avoid eyelid festoons which are redundant folds of lax skin and orbicularis muscle of the upper or lower eyelids. Using HA which is highly hydrophilic may exacerbate the condition.
17. Follow-up review is essential

6) Naso-labial folds

The naso-labial fold is a common aesthetic concern as a characteristic of the aging face. Factors that contribute to a deep naso-labial fold include gravitational skin laxity, descent of the facial fat pads, anorexia nervosa and maxillary hypoplasia.

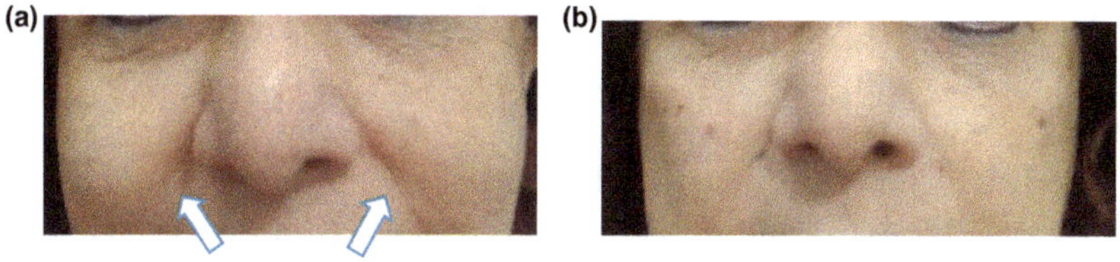

Figure 18.25 (**a**) Before. (**b**) After the injection of 1 cc Juvederm® Ultra Plus to the naso-labial fold depression.

7) Marionette lines

The marionette lines at the corners of the mouth are accentuated by the sagging of the cheeks and get more prominent with age. Fillers are able to soften the lines and improve the overall appearance of the lower face.

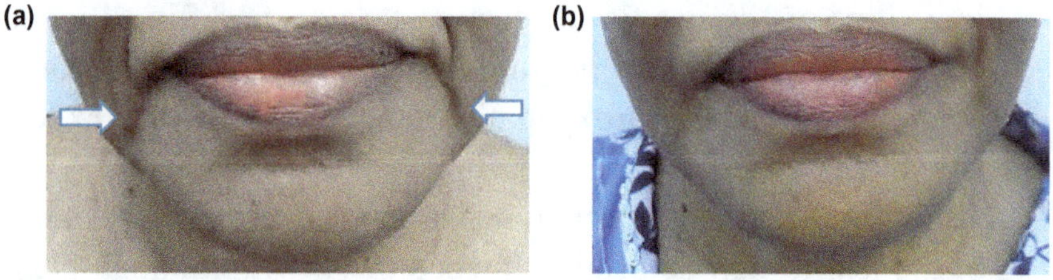

Figure 18.26 (**a**) Before. (**b**) Two months after the injection of 1 cc Juvederm® Voluma beneath bilateral marionette lines.

8) The chin

A pointed chin is often associated with feminine beauty. But a retruded chin has a negative aesthetic effect and in men, can "weaken" the male facial image.

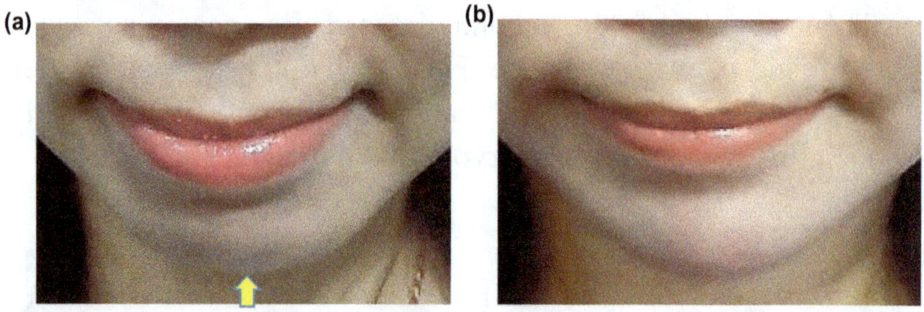

Figure 18.27 (**a**) Before: A retruded small chin (micrognathia). (**b**) Two weeks after the injection of 2 cc Juvederm® Voluma directly to the pogonium of the chin.

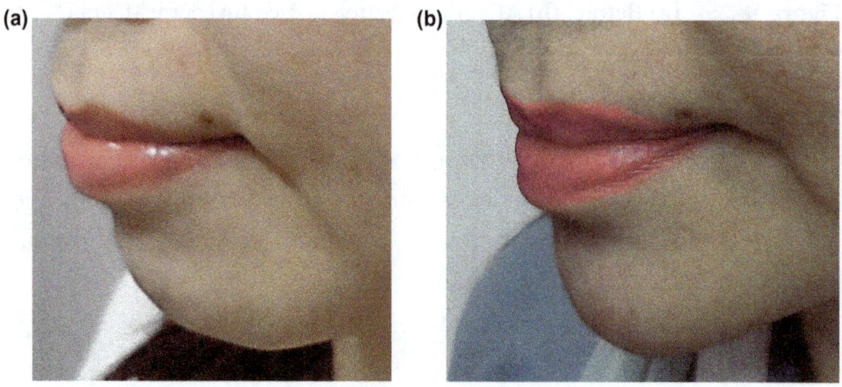

Figure 18.28 Latera views. (**a**) Before. (**b**) After.

9) **Lips**
The lips can be augmented to enhance appearance. Fuller lips are considered to be aesthetically more appealing and youthful.
With age, the lips get thinner and perioral vertical rhytides form barcode wrinkles.
The improvement is especially apparent in the upper lip that was thin prior to filler injection. Besides the improvement in volume, note also the enhanced eversion of the vermillion border.

(a) (b)

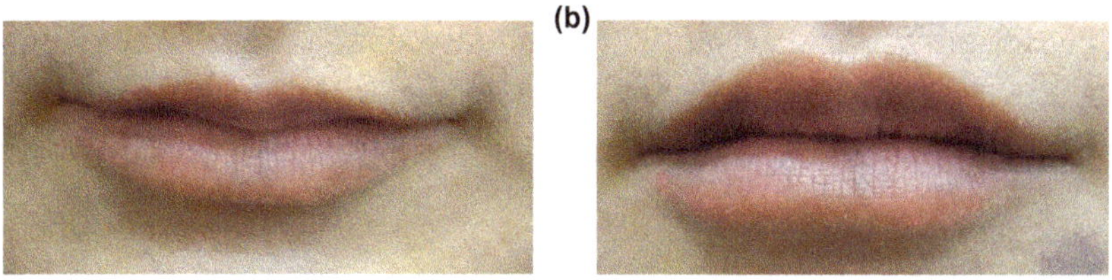

Figure 18.29 (**a**) Before. (**b**) After the administration of 1 cc Juvederm® Volift filler to the upper and lower lips.

Cosmeceuticals

Facial aesthetics includes the maintenance of a healthy-looking youthful skin. It is important to maintain a topical regimen with proven cosmeceuticals to support anti-aging treatments. A widely accepted mechanism of skin aging is the effect of Reactive Oxygen Species (ROS) that cause oxidative damage to the skin cells and collagen, and increase matrix metalloproteinases (MMPs) that potentiate collagen degradation and decrease collagen production. ROS can accumulate over time with advanced age, and are generated when the skin is exposed to ultraviolet radiation. Only those therapeutic agents that are evidence based will be briefly discussed in this section.

Sunscreen

A broad spectrum sunscreen that shields the skin from both UVA and UVB rays must be used with a Sun Protective Factor (SPF) of at least 30 and be applied when exposed to UV rays.

Retinoids

Retinoids such as tretinoin reduce the breakdown of the dermal matrix and increases collagen production.

Its anti-aging effects include:

- improvement in rhytides
- improvement in dyspigmentation
- improvement in texture of the skin

Retinoids must be applied topically over several weeks before its effects are appreciated. Apply just enough cream to cover the affected areas, and rub in gently.

L-Ascorbic Acid

L-Ascorbic acid exerts its anti-aging effects by acting as an antioxidant to reactive oygen species (ROS), helps to stimulate collagen production and inhibits matrix metalloproteinases (MMPs). L-Ascorbic acid requires several weeks of application and effects seen are improvement in wrinkles and skin texture. Skin brightening has also been observed with L-Ascorbic acid due to its inhibitory effects on melanogenesis. It is also commonly used in combination with Vitamin E (tocopherol).

Tocopherol

Tocopherol has antioxidant, moisturizing and photo-protective properties. It is commonly used together with L-ascorbic acid to potentiate the anti-aging effects of these two antioxidants.

Hyaluronic Acid

Hyaluronic acid (HA) is a glycosaminoglycan in the extracellular matrix that has powerful water-binding capabilities that keeps the skin hydrated. Topical HA aims to draw water from the dermis to the epidermis and in so doing, improves the texture of the skin and helps ameliorate the fine wrinkles of the skin.

Peptides

Peptides are used in cosmeceuticals for their anti-aging effects mainly by promoting collagen stimulation. They are found in preparations aimed at treating fine wrinkles and for achieving a youthful skin.

There are three main types of peptides:

1) Carrier peptides
   These peptides serve to deliver anti-aging agents into the skin. An example is GHK-Cu that delivers copper into the skin for anti-inflammatory and collagen stimulating effects.
2) Neurotransmitter peptides
   These peptides are believed to act on the neuromuscular junction to inhibit acetylcholine release thereby improving fine lines and wrinkles.
3) Signal affecting peptides
   Signal peptides serve to downregulate collagenase and stimulate collagen thereby improving texture and fine lines.

   It may take several weeks of application before improvements are seen. Peptides that are well documented include the oligopeptides, pentapeptides and hexapeptides.

Conclusion

Cosmeceuticals are useful in skin health as a non-invasive topical maintenance option. However they have been replaced by radiofrequency and ultrasonic technology for neocollagenesis and the extension of the skin surface.

Chapter 19

Non Surgical Facial Aesthetics — Part 3 Radiofrequency versus Ultrasound Therapy

Malcolm Harris and Rui Ming Ho

Introduction

The dermis is principally collagen types 1 and 3 which diminishes each year after the age of 20. One reason is decreased postmenopausal oestrogen levels which leaves the skin dry, thin, and lax. Many see the facial aging process as wrinkles, laxity, and fragility rather than a loss of collagen, elastin, proteoglycans, and fat from the dermis, and underlying subcutaneous tissues (Figure 19.1). Despite this loss, new collagen and elastin can be promoted in the dermis to lift and tighten the overlying loose skin. Advances in rejuvenation include lasers and LED photomodulation and more recently the introduction of skin tightening by non ablative radiofrequency and ultrasound therapy (Figure 19.2). Both radiofrequency and ultrasound can generate areas of heat within the dermis and SMAS which denature the aging collagen.

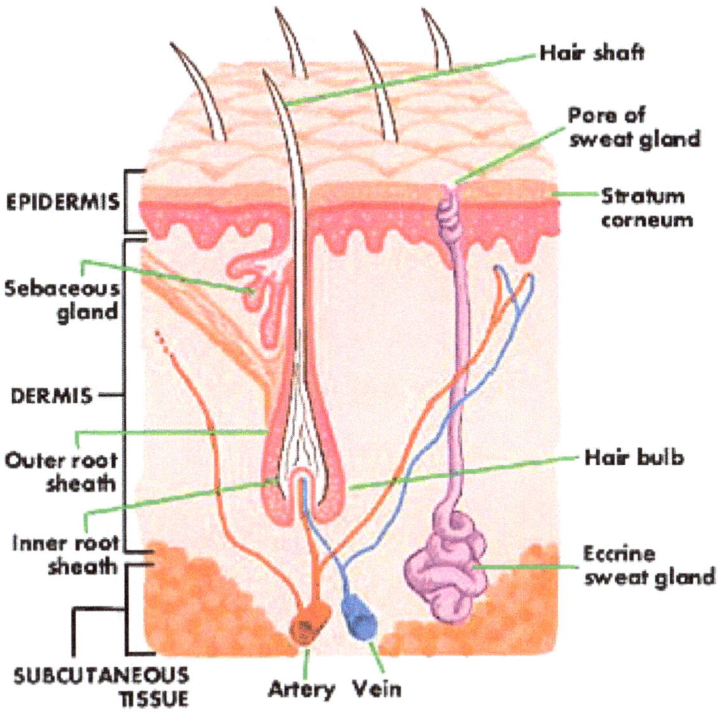

Figure 19.1 The layers and structure of the skin showing the epidermis, dermis and subcutaneous tissue.

This disruption of its molecular structure initiates new collagen and fibrin formation which tightens the skin and creates a "non-surgical face lift" (Figures 19.3a and 19.3b).

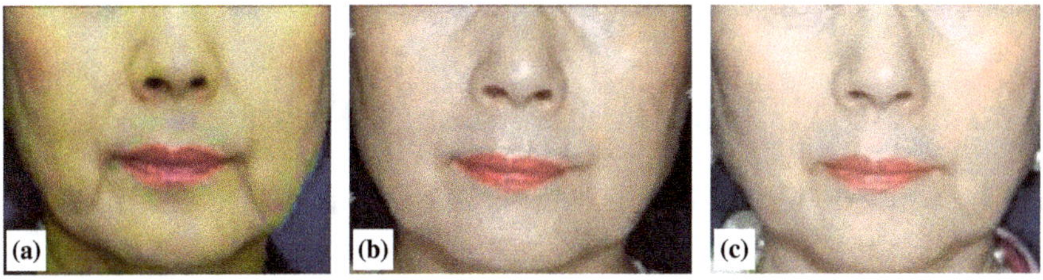

Figure 19.2 **(a)** Before, **(b)** 3 months after and **(c)** 6 months after facial rejuvenation with new collagen and elastin induced by high-intensity focused ultrasound heat.

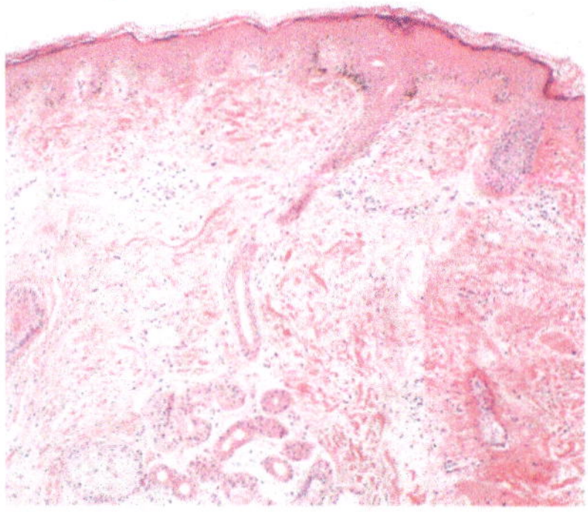

(a)

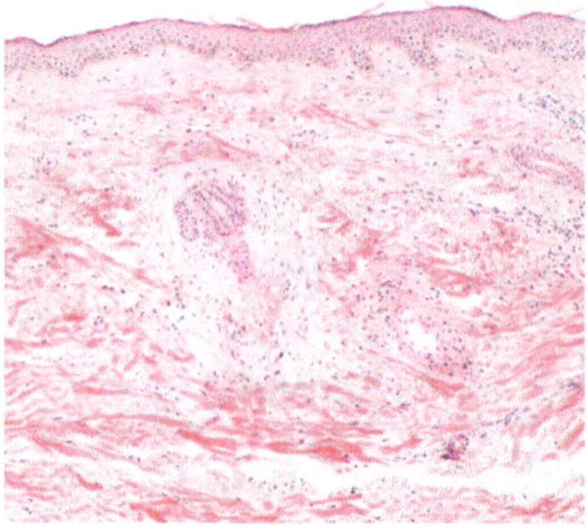

(b)

Figure 19.3 **(a)** A pre-treatment section of the aging facial skin which shows an area of deficient dermis collagen (H&E stain). **(b)** Histology after focused ultrasound treatment which shows a significant accumulation of new horizontal collagen fibres (H&E stain).

Non-ablative High Radiofrequency Treatment (RF)

High radiofrequency (RF) is widely used in medicine and surgery. In 2002 this alternating current therapy was approved by the American Food and Drug Administration (FDA) for cosmetic treatment. Nonablative high radiofrequency (RF) instruments are

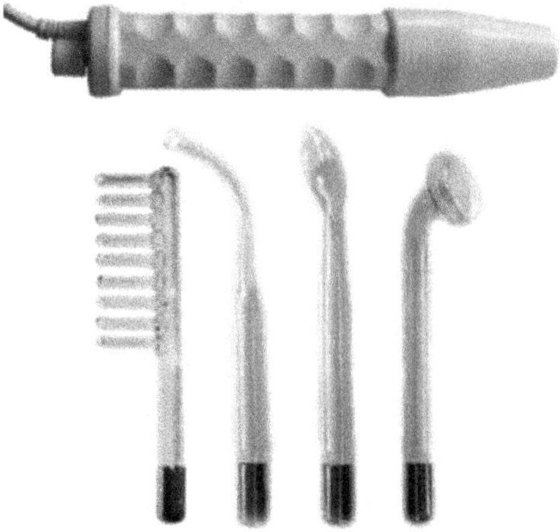

Figure 19.4 This "New Spa" (Skin Care Collection) high frequency portable facial device is equipped with glass electrodes which are refered to as wands which contain argon and are designed to conform with the surface anatomy of the face. The power emission is indicated by an argon violet light.

now a commonly used procedure for the treatment of skin laxity. The devices vary from a hand held "wand" electrode (Figure 19.4) to more complex designs.

The RF is 0.3 to 10 MHz, where 1 MHz is one million cycles per second and can generate heat within the dermis, the superficial musculo-aponeurotic system (SMAS) and the subcutaneous tissues (Figure 19.8).

The heat denatures the sparse aging collagen which then promotes the production of new collagen and elastin as well as inducing lipolysis, and vascularity. This radiofrequency can heat a deep connective tissue stratum from 65°C to75°C, compared to 35°C to 45°C in the overlying epidermis.

The precise mechanism is still uncertain but is attributed to the radiofrequency denatured collagen which releases inflammatory heat shock proteins (HS) such as HSO 70 together with transforming growth factors (TGF). It is TGF β which appears to play a crucial role for the enigmatic promotion of new collagen and elastin.

The Application of Non-ablative Radiofrequency

Currently there are over 10 non-ablative radiofrequency devices which deliver electrical currents to be transformed into thermal energy. These vary from a unipolar system where the current is driven by the voltage difference between the electrode and the patients earthing plate. This unidirectional radiofrequency is comparable to the function of a light bulb. Bipolar, tripolar, and devices that deliver up to 8 power poles of skin tightening electrical current are currently used (Figure 19.5).

Multiple poles have the advantage of delivering lower energy from each pole with less side effects. Another means of reducing side effects is the combination of radiofrequency and photoelectric energy. Furthermore the lower energy means of tissue damage

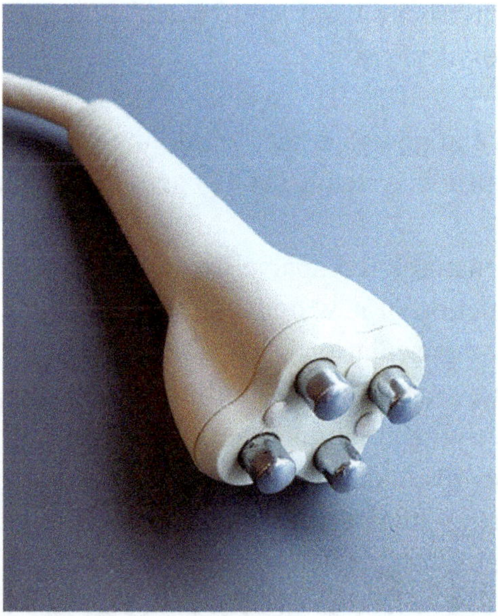

Figure 19.5 A quadruple radiofrequency device.

also conserves epidermal melanocytes and avoids disturbing skin pigmentation.

Such devices can be used for sagging jowls, wrinkle reduction and for volumetric heating of adipose tissue, whereas bipolar RF is suitable for more superficial, non-volumetric heating. The bipolar modality of RF delivery utilizes two electrodes, a positive and negative; and the alternating current flows back and forth between these points. The depth of the tissue heated is determined by the distance of the electrodes from each other.

Fractionated RF is a variant of bipolar RF, where the electrode arrangement is patterned to divide the treatment field into multiple RF thermal zones (RFTZs) with intervening areas of untreated tissue. Again this delivers low energy reduction of tissue damage which also conserves epidermal melanocytes and skin pigmentation.

A basic non ablative monopolar radiofrequency (RF) device is considered to be adequate for skin-tightening and delivers uniform heat to the dermis at a controlled depth with a low wattage of 10 watts with few complications. The glass probe may also be an orange neon design which is believed to be more suitable for aging skin.

A treatment programme can be a total of 8 to12 sessions each of 5–10 minutes, carried out 1 to 3 times a week. After completion of such a course, a maintenance session is recommended every 4–6 weeks and the beneficial results are claimed to last for up to 3 months.

Radiofrequency is recommended for early, and mild to moderate wrinkles or for a recurrence after a surgical face lift. An eyebrow lift of 4 mm can be expected after a single RF application to be compared with 1 cm after minimally invasive surgery.

The current flows through the applicator when in contact with the skin. It requires the application of a topical coupling gel which enables it to sweep over the skin in a circular motion as it generates heat in the dermis. As stated the consequent collagen denaturation provokes a localised inflammatory response and it is the phagocytosis that is capable of stimulating new collagen and elastin. Elastin differs from collagen in that it has a design structured to stretch and recoil whereas collagen has no such capacity. However the elastin fibre response is immediate so that the skin may appear tighter from the first treatment.

Despite the imprecise understanding of the mechanism, high radiofrequency is a safe non-operative procedure for patients with aging facial skin. However at the moment one important feature of RF heat production is that the depth of penetration is less precise than that of ultrasound.

Radiofrequency therapy — Contra indications and complications

Radiofrequency treatment can promote a wide range of side effects and complications although the prevalence is low. They include;

- Transient redness and swelling, common to all energy treatments, which can be managed with topical steroids.
- Operative and postoperative errors due to inadequate training
- Damage due to energy release close to the underlying zygoma, mandible, and frontal bone,
- Insufficient coupling gel to prevent epidermal overheating,
- The need to ensure even energy application to prevent scarring
- Avoidance of any patient predisposed to hypertrophic or keloid scar formation,
- Electrode surface contact with alcohol can be inflammable or with acid based molecules like Retin-A or L-ascorbic acid which can damage the tip and irritate the skin.
- Radiofrequency is to be avoided with vascular diseases, immunosuppression and diabetes,
- High-energy radiofrequency may be painful and require sedation or even a local anaesthetic.

- Radiofrequency therapy requires extensive clinical training.
- **A detailed informed consent form is essential**

Radiofrequency Summary

The high radiofrequency device can eliminate fine lines and wrinkles (rhytids), stimulate the cutaneous circulation and convert oxygen to anti-bacterial ozone. On the neck, deep RF is highly successful for tightening the skin and superficial RF for wrinkled crepe skin (Figure 19.6).

Other applications include elimination of acne by opening skin pores for the penetration of retinol or other creams. High radiofrequency can also be applied to cellulite which forms in the dermis due to the herniation of subcutaneous fat from its fibrous connective tissue compartments. This is seen as skin dimpling especially on the buttocks, lower limbs, and abdomen and has a myriad of names including adiposis oedematosa, dermopanniculosis deformans, status

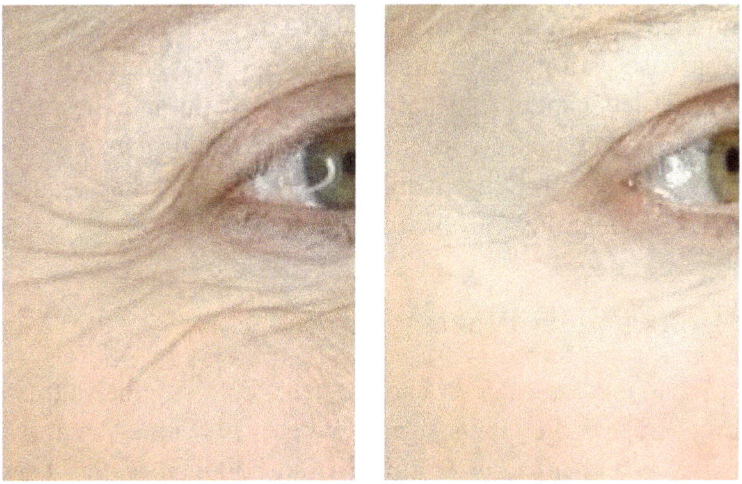

(a) (b)

Figure 19.6 (**a**) Pre-radiofrequency treatment of crows foot rhytids. (**b**) Post radiofrequency treatment of the rhytids protrusus cutis, gynoid lipodystrophy, and orange peel syndrome! Its management requires care as inappropriate radiofrequency application may result in surface irregularities and atrophic scarring due to uneven healing of the fat necrosis.

In summary non ablative radiofrequency (RF) is considered to be a useful skin-tightening device that delivers uniform heat to the dermis at a controlled depth with few complications.

Micro focused Ultrasound Therapy

Introduction

High intensity focal ultrasound therapy (US) uses sound waves above the range of human hearing and its tissue penetration is considered to be superior to radiofrequency for the treatment of the aging face. Despite the fact that ultrasound has a multitude of clinical and non clinical applications its production is a mystery to many clinicians. The simplest explanation is that ultrasonic waves are generated by an electric driven piezoelectric crystal which can convert an electric current to mechanical energy. This energy is transmitted as oscillations by a transducer to an accurately determined site where it denatures old collagen and elastin and the resultant phagocytosis initiates the synthesis of new collagen and elastin. The US Food and Drug Administration (FDA) has issued 18 approved applications for ultrasound therapy.

The Collagenesis Process

The ultrasound transducer shown here delivers the ultrasound energy to bypass the skin's surface where it becomes heat, in the deep skin layers in order to liquefy old collagen of the Thermal Coagulation Zone and new collagen and fibrin will be produced to tighten and lift the overlying skin (Figure 19.7).

Collagen is made up of three polypeptide chains stabilized by cross-linking. One recognisable cause of facial rhytids is that aging

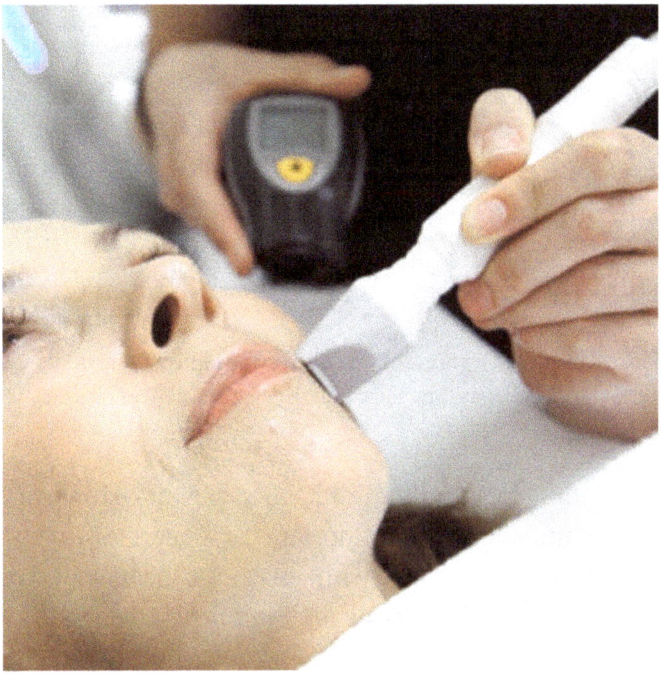

Figure 19.7 This ultrasound transducer delivers ultrasound energy to bypass the skin's surface as heat, into the deep skin layers in order to denature old collagen of the Thermal Coagulation Zone where new collagen and fibrin will be produced to tighten and lift the overlying skin.

reduces the stability of this cross-linking. However despite this process, complete denaturation of the dermis collagen is prevented by heat-stable bonds.

The accuracy of the cosmetic denaturation process is achieved by the delivery of the ultrasound energy to a precise site by "micro-focussed ultrasound with visualization". This unfortunate title "micro focussed ultrasound with visualization (MFU-V)") is a technique that can focus ultrasound waves to precise areas in the dermis and subcutaneous tissues to create thermal coagulation points (TCPs). Heat is generated at these TCPs and produces microcoagulation zones at selected depths which can be 4.5, 3.0, and 1.5 mm from the epidermis surface. Such depths are aimed to target structures such as the superficial musculo-aponeurotic

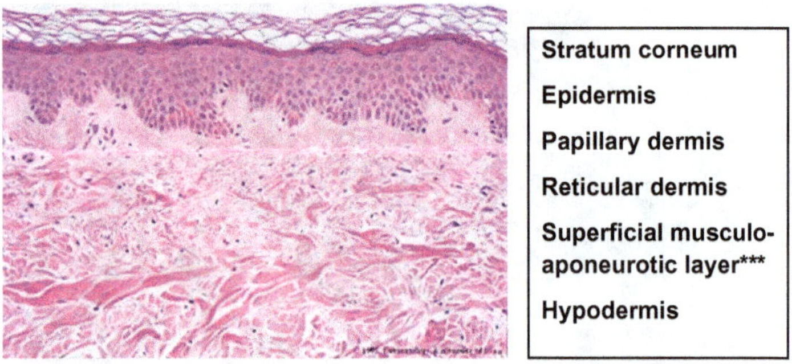

Figure 19.8 This section shows the layers of the skin with restored collagen in the deep reticular dermis and the superficial musculo-aponeurotic layer***.

system, and the deep and mid-dermis planes. However before treatment commences it is important to generate an ultrasound image to confirm the relationship of the transducer on the skin surface to the precise depths of the epidermis, dermis, fascia and the bony interfaces (Figure 19.8). The focused ultrasound is then accurately applied as 50 millisecond bursts to produce the thermal lesion that denatures the aging collagen and stimulates the formation of new collagen and elastin to achieve a non operative face-lift or brow elevation. However this nonsurgical facial rejuvenation process may require additional procedures for optimal results. For instance the combination of 'microfocussed ultrasound with visualisation' is used with 1:1 diluted calcium hydroxyapatite filler (CaHA) which is effective for improving the appearance of a neck with lines and wrinkles and may last 3 months after treatment.

Ultrasound versus nonablative radiofrequency

1. Ultrasound energy with visualisation is ideal for skin tightening as the heat is accurately delivered to the deep subcutaneous layers of the face (Figure 19.8). It can also accurately localise the skin and soft-tissue interfaces before the therapy is activated. This is important to ensure safe delivery of the thermal injury to the appropriate levels of the dermis or superficial

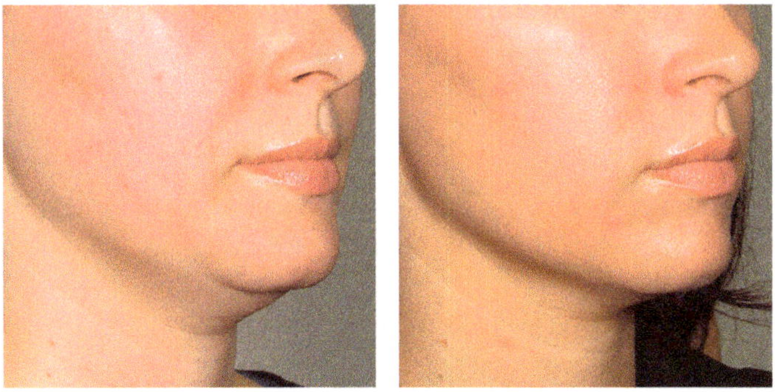

(a) (b)

Figure 19.9 This is a case of sagging jowl treated with ultrasound 18 months previously. Unlike the brow-lift, jowl tightening is not amenable to measurement relative to fixed landmarks: **(a)** before and **(b)** after.

musculo-aponeurotic system with minimal risk to the facial nerve. This precision also avoids heat scatter with its absorption by the basal layer of the epidermis which can produce cutaneous injury and scarring.

2. However both non-ablative radiofrequency and ultrasonic therapy are effective for the cosmetic rejuvenation of aging skin collagen. Radiofrequency treatment time ranges from 5 to 10 minutes per unit area (10 cm^2 quadrants) and the temperature is maintained at 40°C in the dermis. This application of RF is not completely painless and discomfort can be felt due to the temperature rise which may need analgesia or local anaesthetic. The ultrasound power ranges from 50 W to 150 W.
3. Monopolar RF produces new collagen (neocollagenesis) in the papillary, and the upper, mid, and deep reticular dermis. It also produces new elastin (neoelastogenesis) in the papillary dermis, and the upper and mid reticular dermis. However monopolar RF also affects deep tissues diffusely and involves a larger dermal area.
4. This Thermage machine is designed to deliver radiofrequency energy into the skin uniformly heating the dermis while cooling

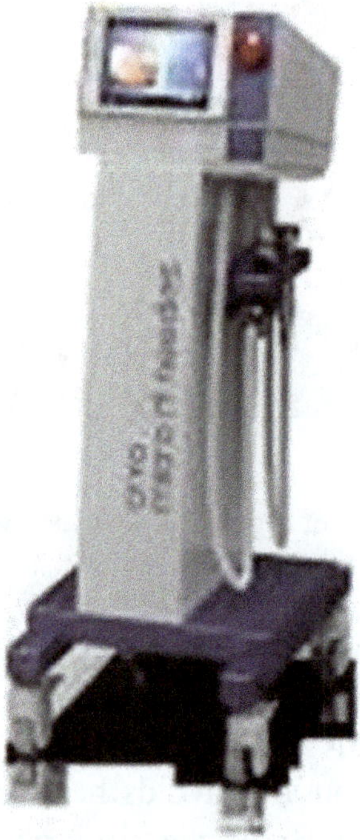

Figure 19.10 Thermage machine designed to deliver radiofrequency energy into the skin uniformly heating the dermis while cooling and protecting the epidermis

and protecting the epidermis. The deep uniform heat in tissue underneath the skin's surface produces immediate thickening and tightening of collagen fibers with further increased production of collagen over time. This smoothes out wrinkles and loose skin. Without surgery and is ideal for treating cellulite involving the legs and abdomen (Figure 19.10).

5. The High Intensive Focal Ultrasound (HIFU — Ultherapy) by comparison;

    i. Utilizes ultrasound technology to visualize and confirm the treatment area
    ii. Tightens the skin and deeper soft tissues.

iii. The benefit of Ultherapy is the accuracy of depth which is not possible with lasers or radiofrequency.
iv. It stimulates new collagen and elastin production in the mid and deep reticular dermis and can focus ultrasonic waves between 4 and 7 mHz at precise coagulation points 3 to 4.5 mm. below the skin surface.

With such accuracy Ultherapy functions 2.5% above and 2.5% below the treatment zone such as the superficial musculo aponeurotic layer, which is the optimum layer for a surgical face lift, and where there is little risk to the epidermis above or the deeper structures below.

It is also safe for all skin types, since with sound waves, there is no risk of hyper or hypo-pigmentation.

The Psychological Aspects of NSFA Treatments

The demand for cosmetic treatments has risen exponentially over recent years. This is influenced by advances in technology the media which publicise its availability and acceptability. The message is that facial appeal is socially advantageous and the unattractive or aging

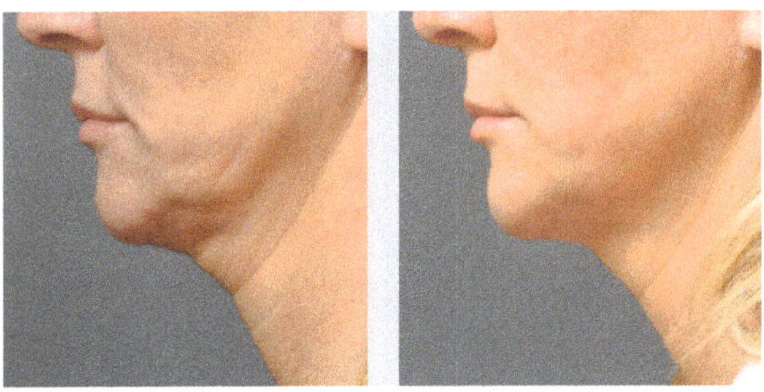

(a) (b)

Figure 19.11 (**a**) A failed surgical face lift. (**b**) Corrected with ultrasound. 3/12 postreatment.

face a disadvantage. The clinician must be aware that all who seek NSFA are psychologically motivated and must judge whether such treatment is desirable and achievable. The importance of psychological assessment is dealt with in Chapter 16.

Clinical Governance in Aesthetic Practice

Clinical governance differs amongst different health care systems but is an essential framework to maintain and improve the quality of service to the patient.

Ideally clinicians who perform facial aesthetic procedures should be certified competent by an appropriate body and have done an adequate number of supervised cases with satisfactory results before they are allowed to perform such procedures independently. As a consequence certain procedures must be performed by specialists whilst others by general practitioners.

Clinicians who fall short of these regulations may be subject to censure and penalties. With such guidelines, patients can be assured that an approved standard of care is in place and will be offered to them.

Chapter 20

Nutrition Support for Osteotomy Patients

Tara Brantley and Sabah Kalamchi

Introduction

Postoperative nutritional care is of critical importance for a patient's psychological well being, immune competence, hard and soft tissue healing and optimum recovery time. However, feeding is hindered by post-osteotomy orofacial pain and paraesthesia, impaired mastication and in some cases jaw immobilizations, all of which are overlooked because the patients are considered to be young and healthy.

The energy and protein needs of the patient are determined by age, weight and activity. This chapter provides an overall feeding regimen however all the surgical team must be involved in nutrition management supported by specialist dietary advice. Paradoxically aggressive overfeeding can have dangerous consequences although this is unlikely in the short term recovery after maxillofacial surgery.

Preoperative assessment: The basic parameters for a nutritionally fit patient include:

i. A normal adult haemoglobin as a simple measure of serum iron and oxygen transport:
   Men: 14.0 to 16.0 g/dL (140 to 160 g/L)
   Women: 12.0 to 15.0 g/dL (120 to 150 g/L)
   Children: 11.0 to 16.0 g/dL (111 to 160 g/L)
ii. Serum albumin as a reliable measure of nutrition with levels between 33 to 55 g/L
iii. The white blood cell count (WBC): 3.5–11.0 × 10^9/L.
iv. Inadequately controlled diabetics are not suitable for orthognathic surgery until completely stable. The blood glucose levels and insulin requirements must be monitored pre, intra, and postoperatively by the anaesthetist and the maxillofacial surgeon until the patient is well enough to resume a normal regimen. Again all must have a confident knowledge of diabetes management.

Hyperglycemia will result in polyuria and electrolyte disturbances, an impaired immune response, infection, and delayed wound healing. Hypoglycemia due to a normal or high insulin dosage and a low blood glucose will lead to a comatose state.

Nutritional Guidelines

These guidelines assume osteotomy patients are not chronically undernourished. Preoperative assessment includes a baseline body weight record. Although the body mass index (BMI) has been criticized, it is a useful baseline with a range of 20 to 23 for females, and 20.5 to 23.5 for males. This can be calculated on a BMI website by entering the patients age, gender, weight and level of activity.

Five to ten percent of total body weight may be lost after surgery and so nutrition should be maintained at 20% protein, 30% fat, and 50% carbohydrates. Protein is needed for tissue repair and to slow muscle catabolism. Young adolescents undergoing secondary cleft repair from 10 to 14 years may weigh 35 to 45 kg and require 2,500 to 3,000 kcal and 45 to 50 g of protein a day.

Adult males from 18 to 22 years who weigh 67 to 75 kg require 2,800 kcal and 1–2 g of protein per kilogram per day. Whereas females aged 18 to 22 years in the region of 58 kg require 2,000 kcals and 1–2 g of protein per kilogram per day. In addition all patients require 30 to 40 mls/kg fluid replacement totalling 2.5 litres per day.

In order to ensure this regimen, patients and families must be given nutritional advice verbally and as a clear information leaflet before surgery. There are also various external aids that can help patients to track their nutritional intake. Many online companies such as Habit or SuperTracker can help patients log their dietary intake, and its nutritional value. Many restaurants and vending machines display nutritional information for food items which include total calories, carbohydrates, protein, and fats.

Immediate Postoperative Nutrition

0–24 Hours Postoperation

Antiemetic medication is given immediately following the operation to prevent nausea and vomiting and to promote pyloric emptying. Metoclopramide 10 mg is more effective given intravenously or as a suppository rather than orally which can exacerbate nausea.

Replacement of blood loss will vary with the complexity and length of the procedure and the skill of the surgeon. A simple consideration is that a 50 kg patient will be deficient of 1000 mls fluid, 8 hours after surgery.

Another means of calculating blood deficit is 2 mL/kg for each hour which can be reduced or avoided by the slow intraoperative intravenous administration of an antifibrinolytic agent such as tranexamic acid or aprotonin. All important is that only a maximum of 500 mls blood loss can be safely replaced by intravenous 5%

dextrose saline or compound sodium lactate (Hartmann's) solution. Greater blood loss with a Hb >6 g/dl will not require transfusion, however if Hb <6 g/dl then consider packed RBCs.

The fluid balance record must record postoperative urinary output, vomit and the anticipated transpiratory loss and ensure a total of 2–3 litres replacement a day.

However a fully compliant patient may be able to drink postoperative clear fluids such as water, tea or fruit juices, gradually within the first postoperative day, in order to reduce the need for intravenous fluids.

After 24 Hours

The patient is encouraged to begin a liquid diet to restore electrolytes and nutrition with an adult feeding cup with a spout (Figure 19.1), or a broad bore straw or a syringe and quill. Intravenous fluids are not needed once an adequate oral feeding rate is achieved. Dietary options at this stage will consist of pureed foods (see details below). Patients who cannot manage to drink and swallow require enteral

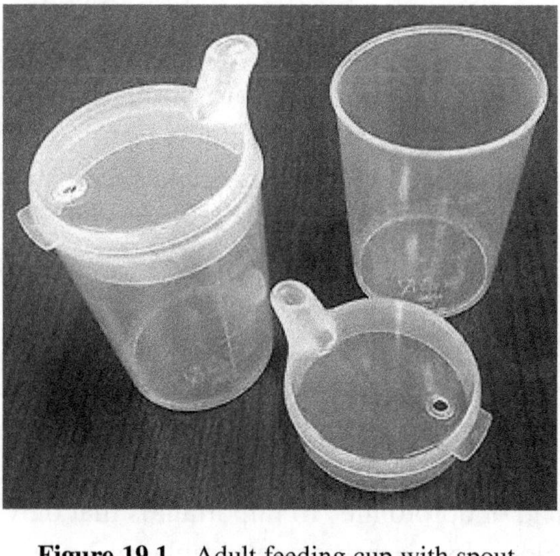

Figure 19.1 Adult feeding cup with spout.

feeding with a fine bore nasogastric tube especially in cases with continued nausea, vomiting, and diarrhea. It is essential that the surgeon is familiar with the insertion and management of the fine bore nasogastric tube.

After 48 Hours

Patients must continue with a fine bore nasogastric feeding tube until an adequate daily oral intake has been achieved to avoid dehydration, electrolyte imbalance and to maintain nutrition. For adequate oral feeding, a full liquidized diet may be augmented by high calorie supplements such as *Ensure*®, which come in a wide variety of contents and palatable flavours. In this way patients may receive half of their calorie intake and maintain essential minerals and protein. Small frequent liquid feeds are more comfortably absorbed and do not suppress appetite.

Philosophical and Religious Dietary Restrictions

Respect for animal rights or religious beliefs should be identified preoperatively and respected postoperatively

i. Vegans can enjoy a well balanced diet but avoid all animal-derived foodstuffs which include meat, eggs, dairy products and honey.
ii. Vegetarians abstain from the consumption of any animal derived food or fish but most ingest eggs and milk products.
iii. Judaism/Kashrut is a complex exclusion of pork and shell fish together with the assurance of religious supervised animal slaughter and meat preparation. Orthodox patients need to be provided with a vegan or a vegetarian diet.
iv. Islam/Halal ordinances exclude pork and animal slaughter requires religious supervision. Muslim patients need to be provided with a vegan or vegetarian diet.

v. Hinduism: Beef is prohibited, as the cow is considered sacred. Many practice a lactovegetarian diet which would make vegan or vegetarian postoperative nutrition acceptable.

vi. Buddhism: A lacto-vegetarian diet which excludes eggs is followed by many Buddhists and so a postoperative vegan or vegetarian diet is appropriate.

In summary vegetarian nutrition is acceptable for many but a vegan diet with B12 supplements is appropriate for all.

Nutrition After Discharge

Patients and their families need clear dietary information on food preparation before leaving the hospital. The patient's weight will be

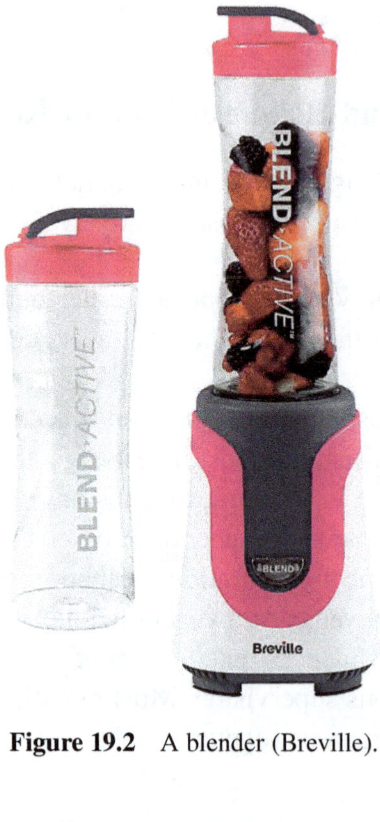

Figure 19.2 A blender (Breville).

monitored at discharge and at each follow up appointment. The largest decrease in nutrient intake occurs during the first week post-operatively. This must be anticipated and prevented with a high calorie, high protein, low volume regimen. Patients must be encouraged to eat small meals frequently as a liquid diet decreases appetite. Without the problem of intermaxillary fixation patients will be able to progress from liquidised to soft pureed foods from the first week, to be continued for the first three months postoperatively to ensure bone healing.

Written Instructions for the Patient and Family

- A hand blender or food processor and a fine sieve are necessary kitchen utensils to prepare a liquidized diet. A measuring jug is invaluable.
- Equal amounts of liquid and solid food should be added into a bowl or food processor for preparation. A very fine texture can be obtained by compressing the blended mixture through a sieve although many soup consistencies do not require this.
- Drinking is facilitated by a feeding cup for adults which has a broad spout.
- Save extra blended food in the refrigerator for later small meals (every 2 to 3 hours).
- Variety will ensure a full range of nutrients and promote an appetite.
- A typical liquidized meal equals three to five 250 ml cupfuls.
- Avoid all foods containing nuts, seeds, skins, peels, or bones. If the food cannot be blended, it is not a dietary choice.
- Most foods are more appetizing if liquidized individually, which preserves their flavours and colours.
- It is important to include Vitamins C and D for wound healing, which are contained in fruit juice, fresh fruit, vegetables and milk products.

Appropriate Diet Guidance

The quoted measure of a cup is 250 mls

The Carnivore (Meat and Fish)

Liquidised tender, well-cooked meat and sausages or fish with no bones, or skin, in addition to any contents of the following regimens.

The Vegetarian

- All whole milk and milk products such as cream cheese, yogourt and ice-cream which can then be flavored with fruit purees, coffee extract, or chocolate.
- Patients with lactose intolerance must use soy or almond milk.
- Liquidized poached or scrambled eggs prepared with milk and butter in addition to the contents of the vegan diet regimen.

The Vegan

High protein and carbohydrate pulses such as well cooked lentils, beans, chick peas (hummus), tehina (sesame seed), and tofu (soya bean curd). All readily liquidize.

- Vegans require soy or almond milk unless allergic. Unsweetened almond milk contains 40 calories per 250 ml cup and soy milk has double the amount. Both are sources of B vitamins and essential minerals.
- Liquidized cooked cereals such as unpolished rice, oatmeal, and couscous.
- Cooked fresh or canned vegetables.
- Fresh fruits without skins or seeds which can be easily blended.

- Smooth nut butters can be blended with cooked vegetables and cereals.
- Miso (fermented soya beans).
- Liquid supplement food beverages such as *Ensure*®.

Most of these can be prepared for hot or cold meals.

Sample Liquidized Meal Menus

Breakfast

- One 250 ml cup oatmeal porridge cooked with dairy milk or vegan soy or almond milk flavoured with salt or sugar or jam or stewed fruit. Other cereals can be prepared with hot or cold milk
- One 250 ml cup of dairy milk, yoghurt or vegan soya or almond milk
- One 250 ml cup of fruit juice
- Tea or coffee with or without milk

Mid-morning — carnivore or vegetarian

- Poached or soft boiled egg
- 1 ripe banana or half a 250 ml cup sieved stewed fruit
- 1 cup whole milk

or vegan

- 1 cup almond milk
- 1/2 a 250 ml cup of soup — lentil, bean or tomato fortified with liquidized peanut butter
- 1 ripe banana or half a 250 ml cup sieved stewed fruit

Lunch

- Half a 250 ml cup cream of chicken soup or vegan miso or lentil soup

- Half a 250 ml cup tender-cooked chicken or vegan hummous and tehina
- Half a 250 ml cup mashed potatoes
- Half a 250 ml cup cooked vegetables
- One 250 ml cup orange-pineapple juice

Afternoon snack

- One 250 ml cup of liquid supplement such as fruit or savoury *Ensure*®.

Dinner

- One 250 ml cup cooked pasta or rice
- One 250 ml cup of pasta sauce
- Half a 250 ml cup of tender cooked minced lamb/beef or vegan bean or chick pea stew

Evening snack

- Half a 250 ml cup dairy ice cream (or vegan soy ice cream)
- 1 cup milk or hot milk beverage or soy or almond milk drink

All diets require a strict oral hygiene routine, with a fine interdental tooth pick or interdental brush and a soft toothbrush and a chlorhexidine mouthwash after meals to reduce plaque accumulation.

Information for Patients Undergoing Orthognathic Surgery

It is essential that all patients are provided with as much information as possible when considering orthognathic surgery which will change their face and their body image. In other words how one sees one self.

As surgery will risk complications there are, several on-line and hardcopy information handouts available. In addition the British Orthodontic Society has produced a 'My jaw surgery' programme which can be accessed at, https://www.bos.org.uk/Public-Patients/Your-Jaw-Surgery1

However the following must be included as minimum information.

****

Orthognathic surgery corrects the relationship of the jaws to give improved jaw function and facial appearance.

Orthodontics

In almost all cases orthodontic treatment is required before the operation for 8–24 months in order to ensure that the teeth can be placed in the ideal relationship afterwards. This dental correction also helps to give the best facial appearance, jaw function and stability following the operation.

Fixed braces are the standard means of orthodontic treatment and they are also invaluable during the operation to correct the relationship of the jaws.

The Operation

This is carried out under a general anaesthetic and carries minimal risk in a fit young adult. In most cases the patient needs to be in hospitalfrom 1–3 days after the operation, although operations on one jaw only are undertaken on a day-stay basis.

The bones are fixed during the procedure by miniature titanium plates and screws which are left in place without any harm or inconvenience. Occasionally a plate or screw may need to be removed if it causes discomfort or gets infected. There are situations where the jaws need to be fixed together with wire or elastics after the operation for up to 4 weeks.

It is essential to bring a small, soft tooth brush into hospital to keep your teeth and orthodontic wires clean. An antiseptic mouth wash, for example chlorhexidine is important after your last meal.

Problems

Postoperative swelling is to be expected, which may give way to bruising over a period of 2 weeks. In most cases, pain is not a problem and can be controlled with painkillers such as ibuprofen.

Most patients need to be away from work for 10 days to 2 weeks depending on their job and how they feel.

Numbness of the lower lip, upper lip and palate is possible depending on the operation. More than half of patients have some degree of short term numbness which in most cases gradually disappears. Small persistent areas tend to diminish in time and are generally not noticeable. There is no disturbance in muscle function.

Oral hygiene and diet

It is important to keep your teeth free of decay throughout the treatment period and a careful choice of a sugar free diet is essential. You must avoid sweet sticky foods, sweet drinks and acid fruit juice.

Hard food will need to be cut up before chewing as it may damage the orthodontic brace. Tooth brushing twice a day with a fluoride tooth paste is essential and patients should spit and not rinse the mouth out after brushing in order to achieve its maximum protective effect against decay.

It is important to have a high protein appetising diet after the operation but this may need to be liquidised for 1–2 weeks. However early movement of the lower jaw is important for the recovery of muscle function. Our dietician will advise you and a diet sheet will be given with this handout.

Postoperative Orthodontics

After the operation there is a short period of orthodontic treatment to fine tune the tooth relationship for about 6–8 months before the braces are removed. This programme ensures that the combination of orthodontics and surgery improves both your appearance and jaw function.

The details will depend on the procedure and must be discussed with the orthodontist and surgeon before treatment so that you know what to expect.

Most cases take around 3 years for completion. During thistime regular appointments with be required to adjust the braces andreview progress.

It is also essential that you have regular dental check-ups to avoiddental decay.

Please contact your treatment team for any advice or help.

Index

www.ingramcontent.com/pod-product-compliance
Lightning Source LLC
LaVergne TN
LVHW020043201125
826049LV00011B/417